D0113823

ANNUAL PROGRESS IN CHILD PSYCHIATRY AND CHILD DEVELOPMENT

ANNUAL PROGRESS IN CHILD PSYCHIATRY AND CHILD DEVELOPMENT 1998

Edited by

MARGARET E. HERTZIG, M.D.

Professor of Psychiatry
Weill Medical College
Cornell University

and

ELLEN A. FARBER, Ph.D.

Clinical Assistant Professor of Psychology in Psychiatry
Weill Medical College
Cornell University

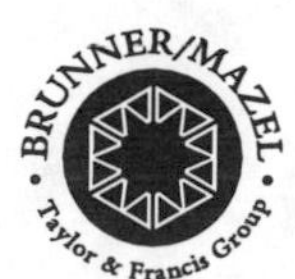

USA	Publishing Office:	BRUNNER/MAZEL *A member of the Taylor & Francis Group* 325 Chestnut Street Philadelphia, PA 19106 Tel: (215) 625-8900 Fax: (215) 625-2940
	Distribution Center:	BRUNNER/MAZEL *A member of the Taylor & Francis Group* 47 Runway Road, Suite G Levittown, PA 19057 Tel: (215) 269-0400 Fax: (215) 269-0363
UK		BRUNNER/MAZEL *A member of the Taylor & Francis Group* 1 Gunpowder Square London EC4A 3DE Tel: +44 171 583 0490 Fax: +44 171 583 0581

ANNUAL PROGRESS IN CHILD PSYCHIATRY AND CHILD DEVELOPMENT 1998

1 2 3 4 5 6 7 8 9 0

Printed by Braun-Brumfield, Ann Arbor, MI, 1999. Cover design by Michelle Fleitz.

A CIP catalog record for this book is available from the British Library.
⊗ The paper in this publication meets the requirements of the ANSI Standard Z39.48-1984 (Permanence of Paper).

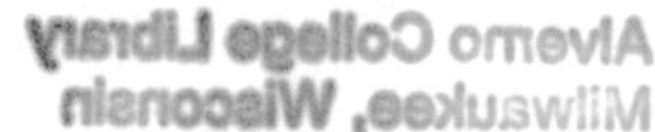

ISBN 0-87630-992-9 (case)

CONTENTS

Part I
DEVELOPMENTAL ISSUES

The research reported in Part I spans the age range from infancy to adolescence. The first paper describes a model for explaining the mechanism of infant facial imitation and its role in later social cognition and social awareness. Facial imitation is parsed out as a separate and unique area because the infant does not have the same feedback mechanisms as with vocal and manual (hand) imitation. Meltzoff and Moore coin three terms for understanding the process by which very young infants imitate facial acts by adults: *organ identification, body babbling*, and *organ relations*. Infants have to relate parts of their own bodies to the corresponding parts of adults', to practice using these organs, and then to match the movement they see adults make with the action they feel themselves making. Imitation is believed to be not reflexive but rather the result of intrauterine body-babbling experience.

Meltzoff and Moore incorporate much of their previous research on infant imitation. They go further in showing how observing another sufficiently to imitate specific movements leads to representations of others. Meltzoff and Moore describe the developmental changes that occur in imitation over the first year and a half of life, and they extend their findings from a specific behavior to describing the purpose of that behavior in later social development. This paper serves as a reminder of the need for more public awareness of the value of face-to-face interaction with very young infants.

The next paper addresses a critical question in attachment research. What is the association of maternal sensitivity and attachment security? De Wolff and van IJzendoorn provide a meta-analysis of approximately 60 studies of maternal behavior and attachment security. They replicated the findings of a previous meta-analysis of 13 studies. In general and not surprisingly, studies that showed the strongest association between parenting and attachment were those that most closely replicated Ainsworth's (1978) original Baltimore study.

De Wolff and van IJzendoorn describe two studies. In the first, they and experts in the attachment field sorted and rated the maternal interactive behaviors measured in each study to create nine "homogenous" sets of studies. That is, they grouped studies that assessed similar aspects of maternal behavior. The constructs were labeled *sensitivity, contiguity of response, physical contact, cooperation, synchrony, mutuality, positive affect, emotional support*, and *stimulation*.

The second study provides a clear description of the meta-analytic procedure, including the selection of studies, the file-drawer problem (unpublished studies are more likely to have zero effect sizes), and the calculation of effect sizes. After sensitivity, effect sizes were highest for two categories of maternal behavior: mutuality and synchrony. However, effect sizes were fairly modest ($rs = .24$ and $.26$, respectively). There is an interesting discussion of the meaning and significance of these numbers. Infants whose mothers responded sensitively to their signals improved their chances of developing a secure relationship from 38% to 62%. De Wolff and van IJzendoorn conclude that although sensitivity is important, it is not the only factor in the development of attachments; other aspects of maternal behavior are also contributory.

Child Development published commentaries on the De Wolff and van IJzendoorn article as well as a rejoinder by the authors. The comments included the fact that the meta-analysis eliminated the influence of developmental change by including mean effect sizes across age in studies with multiple assessment points. Also noted was the primary focus on mother–child dyads to the exclusion of factors and of family units. This is an important paper that will be cited often for its thoughtful reanalysis of attachment and sensitivity.

The third paper in this section is an unusual review that compares children's and adults' ability to distinguish fantasy and reality. Young children are often thought to have difficulty with the reality–fantasy distinction, particularly when they imitate dangerous behavior observed on television. Wooley reviews the evidence on "magical thinking" and concludes that both children and adults are capable of distinguishing fantasy and reality, yet both engage in magical thinking.

The review starts by defining fantastical or magical thinking as ways of reasoning about the physical world that violate known physical principles. Wooley differentiates between fantastical thinking and thinking about fantasy and goes on to describe the ages and stages at which children are able to differentiate real from nonreal, yet believe in fantasy figures and imaginary companions. There have been studies of children's reasoning about wishing and about magic. She then describes the fantastical beliefs that adults engage in, including ESP, astrology, witches, and ghosts. Wooley describes how adults' and children's magical thinking differs. For example, adults have a larger knowledge base and broader social context in which to test the reality of ideas. When children attempt to test the reality of ideas, such as Santa Claus and the tooth fairy, they are encouraged to engage in fantastical thinking by adults rather than discouraged from engaging in it. Wooley suggests that children are more likely to appear credulous because they entertain the possibility of fantasy figures or of magical processes before they are able to generalize from one instance to another.

Child Development also published commentaries on Wooley's paper that further elucidate this research area. For example, Boyer (1997) noted the need to differentiate fantasy events and to treat children's reactions to counterintuitive physical events, such as magic, as different from their beliefs in imaginary figures. Taylor (1997) noted how difficult it can be to test children's understanding of the reality–fantasy distinction because children may continue to play along with imaginary games, not realizing that the adult is now being serious. In sum, this is an interesting topic that draws from numerous areas of child development.

The fourth paper presents a survey study of "compulsive-like" behavior in young children. Although it has long been known that such behaviors are prominent among 2- to 3-year-olds (e.g., Gesell, 1928), there has been little attempt to document the frequency of these behaviors in a nonclinical population. Evans, Leckman, Carter, and colleagues sent a 19-item questionnaire, the Childhood Routines Inventory, to families agreeing to participate in university research. Needless to say, there are limitations to this method when one is studying compulsive behavior. Fifteen percent of those contacted from birth announcements returned the card agreeing to participate in university research and 40% of that 15% were "compulsive" enough to complete and return the questionnaire. The 19 items on the questionnaire were chosen by Evans et al. to reflect childhood versions of *Diagnostic and*

Statistical Manual of Mental Disorders (4th ed.; American Psychiatric Association, 1994) symptoms. The items were best represented by two factors. "Just right" behaviors included preferring things done in a particular way, lining up objects in patterns, and being very aware of how clothes feel. The "repetitive behavior and insistence on sameness" component included preferring a daily routine, acting out the same thing over and over in play, repeating actions, and indicating a strong preference for certain foods. It might have been preferable to parcel out routines that most parents impose, such as a bedtime routine, from routines that children develop, such as turning lights on and off repeatedly.

The children in the Evans et al. study ranged in age from 8 to 72 months. Two-, 3-, and 4-year-olds had more repetitive and just right behaviors than did 1-year-olds or 5- and 6-year-olds. Approximately 60% of those 2–4 years old engaged in some of these behaviors. Repetitive behaviors emerged a few months earlier, on average, than just right behaviors. There were no concurrent or follow-up data to rule out that some of the children did indeed have pathological conditions. However, given prevalence rates for obsessive–compulsive disorder of less than 3% of children and adolescents, in the majority of cases these had to be normally developing children. A community sample drawn from pediatric clinics or day care and Head Start programs might be informative about the frequency of compulsive-like behaviors in the broader population. Evans et al. describe some of the possible mechanisms that compulsive-like behavior serves for preschoolers. This study is an interesting look at a normal behavior that is adaptive but that in some children persists beyond a developmentally appropriate age and becomes maladaptive.

The final paper in this section is about normative development in adolescence. Harter, Bresnick, Bouchey, and Whitesell present a theoretical paper on the development of the self-system. Harter has published many papers on the development of the self, beginning with development in early childhood. Her multidimensional model supplants other investigators' unidimensional models of global self-esteem. She proposes that by middle childhood, children make evaluative distinctions about different domains of their lives. Differentiation increases with age such that the number of dimensions people evaluate themselves on increases.

Harter et al.'s paper deals specifically with adolescent development. In previous research, Harter described the various domains in which people make evaluations about their competence, such as cognitive, athletic, and social. In this paper, Harter and colleagues describe how adolescents present themselves to different people, that is, the various roles that develop with age. Some of the roles considered are self with friends, with parents, in the classroom, and in romantic relationships. Of interest is how people deal with multiple selves and the contradictory attributes accompanying those selves (e.g., being happy with friends and depressed with family). Harter et al. conducted various exploratory studies. One of the interesting findings was that teenagers often described opposing attributes in their relationships with their mothers and their fathers. The difference between self with parent and self with friends was an expected finding. Girls were more likely to describe opposing attributes and role conflicts than boys. The paper also speculates about the presentation of the true and false self and the pathological symptoms that may develop from adopting a false sense of self. Overall, this paper is an interesting discussion of a critical developmental task of adolescence, the construction of multiple selves in different roles and relationships.

REFERENCES

Ainsworth, M., Blehor, M., Waters, E., & Wall, S. (1978). Patterns of attachment: A psychological study of the strange situation. Hillsdale, NJ: Erlbaum.

American Psychiatric Association. (1994). *Diagnostic and Statistical Manual of Mental Disorders* (4th ed.) Washington, DC: Author.

Boyer, P. (1997). Further distinctions between magic, reality, religion, and fiction. *Child Development, 68,* 1012–1014.

Gesell, A. (1928). *Infancy and human growth.* New York: Macmillan.

Taylor, M. (1997). The role of creative control and culture in children's fantasy/reality judgments. *Child Development, 68,* 1015–1017.

PART I: DEVELOPMENTAL ISSUES

1

Explaining Facial Imitation: A Theoretical Model

Andrew N. Meltzoff and M. Keith Moore
University of Washington, Seattle, Washington

A long-standing puzzle in developmental psychology is how infants imitate gestures they cannot see themselves perform (facial gestures). Two critical issues are: (a) the metric infants use to detect cross-modal equivalences in human acts and (b) the process by which they correct their imitative errors. We address these issues in a detailed model of the mechanisms underlying facial imitation. The model can be extended to encompass other types of imitation. The model capitalizes on three new theoretical concepts. First, organ identification *is the means by which infants relate parts of their own bodies to corresponding ones of the adult's. Second,* body babbling *(infants' movement practice gained through self-generated activity) provides experience mapping movements to the resulting body configurations. Third,* organ relations *provide the metric by which infant and adult acts are perceived in commensurate terms. In imitating, infants attempt to match the organ relations they see exhibited by the adults with those they feel themselves make. We show how development restructures the meaning and function of early imitation. We argue that important aspects of later social cognition are rooted in the initial cross-modal equivalence between self and other found in newborns.*

Imitation is a mechanism for the intergenerational transmission of acquired characteristics. Before explicit linguistic instruction, infants learn many of the skills, customs, and behaviour patterns of their culture through imitation. In imitating, infants use another's behaviours as a basis for their own, despite differences in body size, perspective of view, and modality through which self and other can be perceived. As ubiquitous and useful as imitation is, how imitation is accomplished poses one of the deeper puzzles in infancy.

All imitative acts are not of the same kind. There are distinctions among manual, vocal, and facial imitation. In manual imitation the infant sees an adult hand movement and must

Reprinted with permission from *Early Development and Parenting*, 1997, Vol. 6, 179–192.

We thank Pat Kuhl, Scott Johnson, and Alan Slater for insightful suggestions on an earlier draft. We are also grateful to Calle Fisher and Craig Harris for help on the experiments. Funding was provided by a grant from NIH (HD-22514).

generate a matching movement. One possible mechanism would be for the infant to look at his or her own hand and use visual guidance as a way of achieving a match between self and other. Vocal imitation also capitalizes on intramodal comparisons, because infants use auditory guidance to help achieve the match (Kuhl and Meltzoff, 1996). However, for the case of facial imitation, a mechanism based on intramodal guidance would be useless. Infants can see the adult's face but cannot see their own faces. They can feel their own faces move, but have no access to the feelings of movement in the other. By what mechanism can they connect the felt but unseen movements of the self with the seen but unfelt movements of the other?

Classical theories such as Piaget's (1962) answered this question through learning experiences with mirrors and tactile exploration of one's own and others' faces. Mirrors made the unseen visible, rendering one's own body and that of the other in visual terms. Tactile exploration of faces rendered both self and other in tangible terms. In the last 20 years, empirical work from many laboratories has revealed that infants too young to have learned from such experience none the less imitate facial gestures.

This work raises several new questions. What motivates young infants to imitate? What functions does early imitation serve? What psychological mechanisms underlie it? Elsewhere we have discussed the questions of motivation and function (Meltzoff and Moore, 1992, 1994, 1995b). The aim of this paper is to tackle the mechanism question. We will consider not only how infants can imitate in the first place, but also how they correct their imitative efforts to more faithfully match what they perceive.

Until recently there was insufficient empirical evidence to resolve the mechanism question. This has now changed, and we capitalize on the new discoveries to propose a model of the mechanism underlying early facial imitation. The paper contains six sections. (1) A synopsis of our viewpoint is provided. (2) We organize 10 key phenomena from recent research allowing us to characterize early imitation as goal directed, generative, and representationally mediated. (3) New theoretical concepts are introduced to encompass these characteristics. (4) These concepts are used to provide a detailed model of the psychological mechanisms underlying facial imitation, specifying the means by which infants render the acts of self and other in commensurate terms. (5) The explanatory value, parsimony, and coherence of the model are assessed. (6) The implications of the model for developmental theory are considered.

CONCEPTUAL SCHEMATIC OF THE AIM HYPOTHESIS

We think that early facial imitation is based on 'active intermodal mapping' (AIM) (Meltzoff and Moore, 1977, 1983, 1994). Figure 1 provides a conceptual schematic of the AIM hypothesis. The key claim is that imitation is a matching-to-target process. The active nature of the matching process is captured by the proprioceptive feedback loop. The loop allows infants' motor performance to be evaluated against the seen target and serves as a basis for correction. According to this view, the perceived and produced human acts are coded within a common (supramodal) framework which enables infants to detect equivalences between their own acts and ones they see. AIM posits an intermodal mechanism for imitation, in contrast to a reflexive or a conditioned basis for generating the matching response.

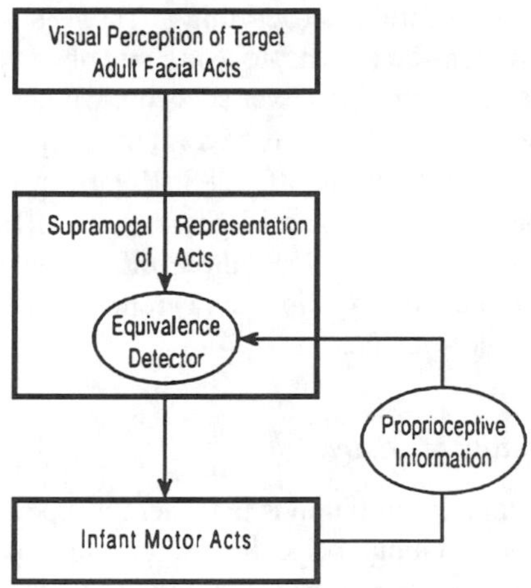

Figure 1. A conceptual schematic of the active intermodal mapping hypothesis (AIM).

ORGANIZING THE EMPIRICAL EVIDENCE

New empirical evidence now allows us to enrich the AIM hypothesis. Ten phenomena bearing on the mechanisms underlying early facial imitation are displayed in Table 1. The entries listed as numbers 1–9 have been demonstrated in infants under 2 months of age. However, there is developmental change in the expression of these competences, as noted in no. 10. For example, neonates can imitate a broad range of facial and manual gestures

TABLE 1
Ten Characteristics of Early Imitation

1. Infants imitate a range of acts[3–5,6,13,14,16,18,20]
2. Imitation is specific (tongue protrusion leads to tongue not lip protrusion)[1,3–6,12,14,16,20]
3. Literal newborns imitate[4,5,7,8,11,13,17,23,25]
4. Infants quickly activate the appropriate body part[13,17,20,22]
5. Infants correct their imitative efforts[13,14,16,17,20]
6. Novel acts can be imitated[6,20]
7. Absent targets can be imitated[6,8,9,12,16,18–20]
8. Static gestures can be imitated[3–5,19]
9. Infants recognize being imitated[15,21,24]
10. There is developmental change in imitation[1–3,6,8,10,13,14,19,21]

Note: Superscripts in the table refer to the following papers: [1]Abravanel and DeYong (1991); [2]Abravanel and Sigafoos (1984); [3]Field et al. (1986); [4]Field et al. (1983); [5]Field et al. (1982); [6]Fontaine (1984); [7]Heimann (1989); [8]Heimann et al. (1989); [9]Heimann and Schaller (1985); [10]Jacobson (1979); [11]Kaitz et al. (1988); [12]Legerstee (1991); [13]Kugiumutzakis (1985); [14]Maratos (1982); [15]Meltzoff (1990); [16]Meltzoff and Moore (1977); [17]Meltzoff and Moore (1983); [18]Meltzoff and Moore (1989); [19]Meltzoff and Moore (1992); [20]Meltzoff and Moore (1994); [21]Meltzoff and Moore (1995a); [22]Meltzoff and Moore (this paper); [23]Reissland (1988); [24]Trevarthen (1980); [25]Vinter (1986).

(no. 1), but young infants do not imitate everything. There is a progression in imitation from pure body actions, to actions on objects, to using one object as a tool for manipulating other objects. Similarly, neonates imitate novel acts (no. 6), but research on older infants reveals a generative imitation of novelty that is beyond the scope of younger infants (Bauer and Mandler, 1992; Barr et al., 1996; Meltzoff, 1988, 1995b). Any adequate theory of early imitation will have to account for at least the 10 phenomena in Table 1.

The phenomena in Table 1 support at least three inferences about the nature of early imitation. We use them to argue that imitation is: (a) representationally mediated, (b) goal directed, and (c) generative and specific.

Imitation is Representationally Mediated

One way of conceiving of early imitation is that there is a perception–production transducer that directly converts visual input to specific motor output. In this view, a seen tongue protrusion yields a tongue protrusion movement by virtue of particular built-in connections between visual and motor centres of the young brain. Two lines of evidence suggest that a more differentiated process than simple transduction is required: (a) the response need not be temporally coupled to the stimulus and (b) imitation is not compulsory; infants need not produce what is given to perception.

In an early study, mouth-opening and tongue-protrusion gestures were shown to 3-week-old infants while they were engaged in the competing motor activity of sucking on a pacifier (Meltzoff and Moore, 1977). The adult terminated the gestural demonstration, assumed a neutral face, and only then removed the pacifier. Three-week-old infants differentially imitated both gestures despite the fact that the adult was no longer showing them. Infants have also been shown to imitate with longer delays. In Meltzoff and Moore (1994) 6-week-old infants saw a person perform a specific gesture on day 1, and then after a 24-hour delay saw the same adult in a neutral pose. Different groups of infants saw different gestures on the first day, and they all saw the same neutral pose on the second day. What differed across the groups was not their current perception but what they had seen the adult do in the past. The results showed that infants differentially imitated the gestures they saw 24 hours earlier. It is difficult to see how direct transduction could account for these data, because the target guiding the infants' action had been absent for 24 hours. Evidently, information gained from vision can be stored and accessed at a later time. One way of achieving this is to represent the adult's act.

There is further evidence that infants' responses are not stimulus bound. Infants sometimes over-ride their current perception. If the situation is arranged correctly, infants will imitate a gesture from the past even when it mismatches what they currently see. A study of 6-week-olds used two people who came and went in front of the infants (Meltzoff and Moore, 1992). One person always demonstrated one gesture and the other a different gesture. After the exchange of people occurred, infants often shut down their ongoing activity stared intently at the new person, and then responded by reproducing the first person's acts. Infants were not imitating what was in current perception; they were overriding what they saw and imitating what the first person did. Imitation of what was in the perceptual field was not compulsory. We have previously noted that this phenomenon has implications for how infants use imitation to individuate people and determine identity across contacts with multiple individuals (Meltzoff and Moore, 1992, 1994, 1995b). For the present purpose, these data show a flexibility between the stimulus and response that is not explained by direct transduction.

Implications. Early imitation is not entirely stimulus bound, directly triggered, or reflexive. There is flexibility inasmuch as infants can imitate the past when shown a neutral face and even override a currently perceived gesture to do something else. We hypothesize that some form of representation stands between perception and production.

Imitation is Goal Directed

Empirical evidence from several independent laboratories shows that the infants' initial imitative responses are often similar to the target but not a complete reproduction. Partial matches along several dimensions are commonly observed (Abravanel and Sigafoos, 1984; Heimann et al., 1989; Jacobson, 1979; Maratos, 1982; Meltzoff and Moore, 1977, 1983). To understand why infants respond with the partial matches, we conducted a study of how 6-week-olds temporally organize their behavior. A microanalysis of the response showed that infants gradually corrected their imitative attempts over time in a sequence of ordered steps (Meltzoff and Moore, 1994). Correction was neither a 'random walk' nor a paring away of irrelevant components from high activity levels, but a generation of novel behaviours not found in baseline activity.

One interpretation that makes sense of this pattern is that the responses are goal directed. The goal organizes these actions by providing a criterion for success and governing the sequence of attempts. The hypothesis that neonatal imitation is organized by a goal is also compatible with other recent findings of primitive goal directedness in newborn motor movements (Butterworth and Hopkins, 1988; van der Meer et al., 1995).

We also discovered something about the nature of the mistakes infants make. When observing an adult sticking his tongue out of the corner of his mouth, 6-week-olds displayed a 'creative error'. Infants poked out their tongues and simultaneously turned their heads to the side, achieving a new kind of 'tongue to the side'. A coder who was blind to the stimulus reviewed the video records and scored every instance in which infants produced a head turn ($>30°$ off midline) simultaneously with a tongue protrusion (HT + TP). The results were that 70% (7 of 10) of the infants shown the tongue protrusion-to-the-side gesture produced the HT + TP response. Only 30% (9 of 30) of control infants shown other facial gestures did so, $p < 0.05$ (see Meltzoff and Moore, 1994, for details of the study).[1] This HT + TP response was not the infants' final effort but occurred early in the test period, as a step towards a more faithful tonge-protrusion-to-the-side response.

The head movement was not in the stimulus, but was an alternative way of getting their bodies to do an act involving both tongue protrusion and an off-midline direction. It is only at the level of goals that head turn is relevant to tongue-protrusion-to-the-side. The adult's

---

[1]The results remained the same when the data were analysed in a different manner. In the alternative analysis, we calculated for each $S(N = 40)$ the number of HT + TP responses as a proportion of the total number of tongue protrusions emitted by each S [HT + TP] ÷ TP). The results showed that these proportional scores were significantly greater for the tongue-protrusion-to-the-side group compared to the controls, Mann–Whitney $U = 92.5$, $p < 0.05$.

movement was a tongue thrust diagonally out of the mouth and the infant's movement was a head rotation to the side. These are different as specific muscle movements, but the tongue protrusion ends up off midline in both cases. Although the literal movements were very different, the final result in terms of the orientation of the tongue was similar, and in this sense it can be seen as an act organized by a goal.

Implications. Both of the foregoing phenomena suggest infants' imitative responses are not motor units akin to reflexes that are simply released by the appropriate input. Rather, early imitation is a goal-directed response whose aim is 'matching the target'. Infants recruit multiple means, some of them not directly given in the stimulus, in attempting to achieve that aim.

Imitation is Generative and Specific

Imitation within the first 2 months of life is not limited to a few privileged gestures. The wide range of gestures that can be imitated suggests a generative process. The list continues to lengthen with successive studies, and to date includes: tongue protrusion, lip protrusion, mouth opening, hand gestures, head movements, eye blinking, cheek and brow motions, and components of emotional expressions (Abravanel and DeYong, 1991; Abravanel and Sigafoos, 1984; Field et al., 1982, 1983, 1986; Fontaine, 1984; Heimann, 1989; Heimann et al., 1989; Heimann and Schaller, 1985; Jacobson, 1979; Kaitz et al., 1988; Legerstee, 1991; Kugiumutzakis, 1985; Maratos, 1982; Meltzoff and Moore, 1977, 1983, 1989, 1992, 1994; Reissland, 1988; Vinter, 1986).

Meltzoff and Moore (1977) selected four gestures to test the specificity of the mapping between the adult's and the infant's bodies: lip protrusion, mouth opening, tongue protrusion, and finger movement. The results showed that infants confused neither organs nor actions. They differentially responded to tongue protrusion with tongue protrusion and not lip protrusion, thus showing that the specific organ could be identified. Infants also differentially imitated two different movements of the same body part, for example, lip opening led to lip opening, not lip protrusion. Such specificity can also be seen in the data from other laboratories (Fontaine, 1984; Maratos, 1982).

Implications. Tongue protrusion is the most studied imitative gesture, and this has sometimes been misinterpreted to mean that it is the only facial gesture that can be imitated. However, as in statistics, the mode does not tell you about the range—and the range of gestures is large. There are limits on what neonates will imitate, but the critical point for theory construction is that early imitation is not limited to a few privileged body parts or salient movement patterns. Moreover, the response is quite specific. There is no global confusion either on the organ side or the movement side. A generative matching-to-target process is indicated.

THEORETICAL CONCEPTS NEEDED TO ACCOUNT FOR FACIAL IMITATION

We are now in a position to flesh out the AIM hypothesis previously presented as a conceptual schematic (Figure 1). An adequate account of the mechanisms underlying early imitation should specify what is present at birth, what is based on early experience, and how cross-modal equivalence can be established. We describe these three aspects next.

Organ Identification

The newborns' first response to seeing a particular facial gesture is activation of the corresponding body part. For example, when they see tongue protrusion, there is often a quieting of the movements of other body parts and an activation of tongue. They do not necessarily protrude the tongue during this initial phase, but may elevate it, wiggle it, or move it slightly in the oral cavity. Likewise, when shown lip protrusion, they produce a marked tension of the lips and even press them together before there is imitation of the movement. It is as if young infants isolate *what* part of their body to move before *how* to move it. We call this 'organ identification'.

Because organ identification occurs in newborns and precedes other imitative efforts, we think that it is the first step in generating an imitative response. We note that an ability to identify corresponding body parts renders self and other in commensurate terms—as movements of tongues, lips, hands, etc. In this view, organs are the cross-modal units of analysis.[2]

We can envision two accounts of how organ identification occurs. The first account is that a delimited set of organs is recognized at birth on the basis of their form ('organs as forms'). It may be that the perceptual context of a face helps identify the whole whose internal parts infants can then parse into facial organs. Some research is compatible with the notion that facial organs may be perceptually identifiable by human newborns, though it is not definitive. Goren et al. (1975), Morton and Johnson (1991), and others report evidence that faces are preferred by newborns over other patterns matched in sensory characteristics. Their claim is that through evolution the structure of a face has become a distinctive perceptual unit responded to at birth.[3] Moreover, neurophysiological data show that visual displays of particular organs, notably parts of the face and hands in monkeys, activate specific brain sites (Desimone, 1991; Gross et al., 1969, 1972; Gross and Sargent, 1992; Perrett et al., 1987, 1992; Rolls, 1992). Gross has also discovered that 'some [face-selective cells] will respond to face components in isolation' (Gross, 1992, p. 5). Thus, specific organs could be neurally represented at birth.

The second account of organ identification is that organs are differentiable because each organ has a unique spatiotemporal pattern of movement ('organs from motion'). Musculature and skeletal structure restrict what body parts can do. Tongues move in and out, but do not flex. Arms are jointed appendages and typically flex. Fingers are a set of three-jointed appendages that can contract on themselves. It may be that infants come to individuate their organs through proprioceptive monitoring of their own actions. The claim is that these unique spatiotemporal movement patterns, which we call 'kinetic signatures', are

---

[2]The reader may wonder what body parts would constitute 'organs'. Preliminary and published studies suggest that the following body parts may be organs that can be identified by young infants: head, brows, jaw, lips, tongue, arms, hands, fingers, trunk, legs, and feet.

[3]There has long been interest in infants' visual preference for faces, and recent progress has been made in understanding this phenomenon (de Boysson-Bardies et al., 1993; Morton and Johnson, 1991; Walton et al., 1992). It is now established that newborns prefer faces over other patterns of about the same size and complexity, scrambled faces, etc. It remains to be determined whether the preference is based on a dedicated 'face detector' or general sensory characteristics such as the visual amplitude spectrum (Kleiner, 1993; Slater, 1993). Regardless of how the preference is mediated, there is a consensus that a face recruits more visual attention than other patterns newborns regularly encounter in the real world.

recognized as cross-modally equivalent when done by self and other. The data are not definitive in showing that infants can map facial organs in this way, but there is compatible evidence. For example, the literature on biological motion using point-light displays shows that the spatiotemporal pattern produced by human movement (such as gait) is a pattern to which infants are acutely attuned (e.g., Bertenthal, 1996).

Both of these accounts serve to differentiate and identify organs. On the first account, organ identification is a perceptual given, preadapted by evolution; on the second account, organ identification emerges from the unique movements each organ can make. Much as we would like to determine which alternative obtains, the available data do not allow a firm decision. The first account perhaps is more compatible with young infants' rapid activation of the correct organ and the findings that they can imitate static facial postures in the absence of kinetic information (Meltzoff and Moore, 1992). The remainder of the essay is written from this perspective, but the account of imitation we are providing is compatible with both alternatives.[4]

Body Babbling: Mapping Movements to End States

An imitative act is not one indissociable unit. It can be differentiated into *organ identification* and *movement* components. This section concerns the movement component. We do not think that infants know *a priori* what muscle movements achieve a particular state of organ relations, such as tongue protrusion, mouth opening, or lip protrusion. This could be learned through experience.

We call this experiential process 'body babbling'. In body babbling, infants move their limbs and facial organs in repetitive body play analogous to vocal babbling. In the more familiar notion of vocal babbling the muscle movements are mapped to the resulting auditory consequence; infants are learning this articulatory–auditory relation (Kuhl and Meltzoff, 1996). Our notion of body babbling works in the same way, a principal difference being that the process can begin *in utero*. What is acquired through body babbling is a mapping between movements and the organ-relation end states that are attained.

By organ-relation end states ('OR end states') we mean a configural relation between organs. For example, three differentiable OR end states differing in extension might be: tongue-to-lips, tongue-between-lips, tongue-beyond-lips. Because both the dynamic patterns of movement and the body end states achieved can be monitored proprioceptively, infants' body babbling builds up a 'directory' mapping movements to OR end states. On this view, the links between specific OR end states and the muscle movements needed to achieve them come from experience rather than being innately given.

Studies of fetal and neonatal behaviour have documented self-generated activity that could serve this hypothesized body babbling function (Hooker, 1952; Humphrey, 1971; Patrick et al., 1982; Prechtl, 1969; Vries et al., 1982, 1985). This is not to say that every possible organ relation is already mapped in the neonatal period. However, the possibility

---

[4]A third possibility is that biologically relevant human acts are redundantly coded, specified both by the configural relations between organs and by kinetic signatures. Such redundancy would allow infants to imitate static gestures as we have reported (Meltzoff and Moore, 1992) and also the dynamic displays discussed by Bower (1982).

of an elementary directory prepared by prenatal experience means that we have identified a developmental process by which newborns could coordinate OR end states with the movements needed to achieve them, without invoking strong nativist claims.[5]

Organ Relations as the Cross-Modal Metric of Equivalence

We now come to the cross-modal metric of equivalence used in imitation. Regarding the visual target, infants parse the adult act they see into the organ relations it exhibits. Regarding infants' own bodies, the consequences of their self-generated movements can be proprioceptively coded in terms of the relations between organs that are attained. Our hypothesis is that *organ relations* provide the common framework in which the acts of self and other are registered. 'Tongue-to-lips', which is an organ relation, would be a description that cuts across modality of perception and could describe both the target and the self. Thus organ relations render commensurate the seen but unfelt act of the adult and the felt but unseen facial act of the infant.

Such mechanisms would allow infants to imitate behaviours practised in body babbling as though looking up the target's OR end state in the 'movement–end state directory' and executing the specified movements. However, results show that infants are not restricted to the imitation of well-practised acts that can be imitated on first try. As we have seen, they are not always satisfied with their initial motor performance. They correct their movements over time. Thus, the infant's criterion for success seems to be achieving 'a match of organ relations', rather than reading out a specific pattern of muscle movements from the directory. Moreover, correction toward a more veridical match implies that representation of the target's organ relations is independent of the infant's motor attempts. In this sense, there is a differentiation between the representation of self and other.

In brief, our hypothesis is that the configural relation between organs serves as the cross-modal equivalence underlying imitation. Infants can perceive organ relations as applying both to adults and themselves. These perceived organ relations are the targets infants attempt to match—an activity observers see as behavioural imitation.

A MODEL OF FACIAL IMITATION

Architecture

Figure 2 provides a detailed model of the mechanism underlying early facial imitation. This model fleshes out the general AIM framework schematized in Figure 1. Figure 2 shows how infants could generate an act that matches a visually perceived facial target. In the model, the equivalence between the infant and adult acts is specified in terms of organ relations. The model depicts the mechanisms underlying facial imitation in the first 2 months of life. Issues of development are addressed in the last section of the paper.

---

[5]Presumably the easiest actions and the most salient proprioceptive outcomes are coordinated first. Simple tongue protrusion may be easily imitated due to prior experience with this movement in the intrauterine environment. It would be a familiar action for neonates, practised in body babbling. Maratos (1982) advanced similar arguments.

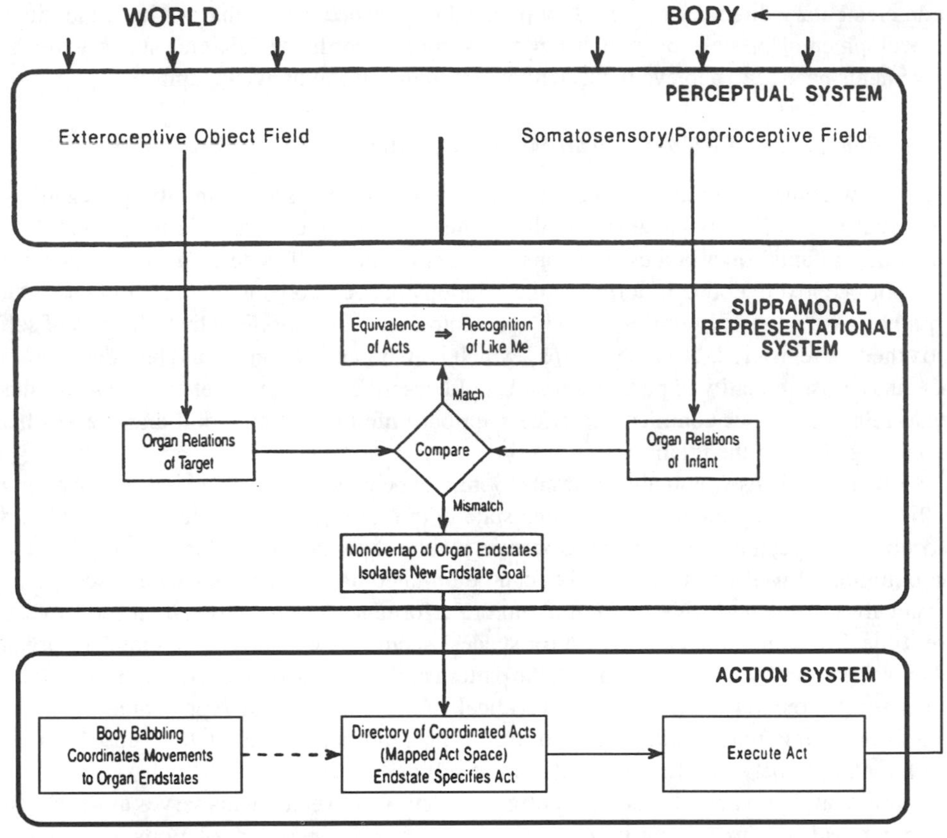

Figure 2. AIM model of the mechanisms underlying early facial imitation. The model depicts the functional relations among the external world, perceptual system, representational system, and action system. Representations of the external target (the adult demonstration) and the infant's body are compared in terms of organ relations (see text). The solid arrows indicate current processing. The dotted arrow indicates prior learning from body babbling experience.

The major components of the model are portrayed by the three bold boxes. The bold box labelled *perceptual system* functions to provide the perception of the infant's own body and the external world. Comparisons between the organ relations of an external target and the current position of the infant's own body are computed in the box labelled *supramodal representational system*. This comparison yields two possible outcomes: a match or mismatch. (1) A mismatch specifies a new configuration of the body, which serves as a goal for the next imitative attempt and is enacted by the box labelled *action system*. The arrow from the action system to the infant's *body* shows that the effect of the act is a change in body configuration. (As already described, the action system box also includes the process of learning to map muscle movements to OR end states through prior body babbling experience.) (2) A match indicates that the motor act seen and the motor act done by the self are equivalent. This recognition of the equivalence of acts is grounds for infants'

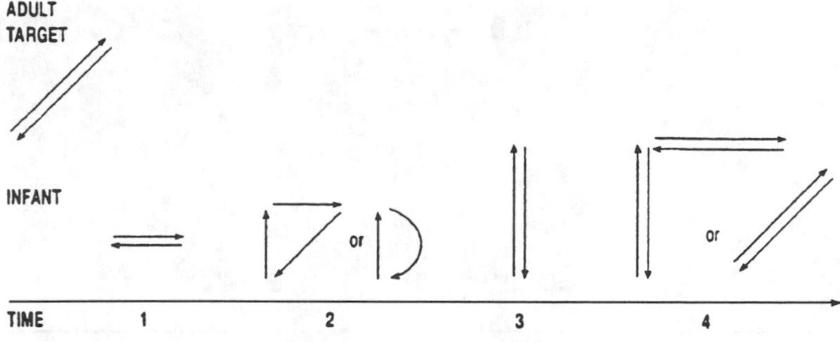

Figure 3. A diagram of infants' correction process. Infants who are shown a novel gesture of tongue-protrusion-to-the-side ('adult target') progress through an ordered series of tongue movements (indicated by '1–4'). The direction and extent of the arrows depict the corresponding dimensions of the infants' tongue protrusion responses. The responses are not randomly ordered, but rather exhibit a systematic convergence toward a more faithful match of the adult target (see text).

apprehension that the other is, in some primitive sense, 'like me' (Meltzoff and Moore, 1995a, 1998).[6]

Operation of the Supramodal Representational System

One challenge for theories of early imitation is the finding that infants correct imitative errors. Consider what happens when a novel gesture such as tongue-protrusion-to the side is presented to 6-week-olds, as was done in Meltzoff and Moore (1994). This target might initially be coded as the familiar organ relation of 'tongue-to-lips'. The movement-end state directory would generate a first response of small tongue movement (assuming this was previously performed in body babbling). In fact, the data from the 1994 study show that 9 of the 10 infants who saw the tongue-protrusion-to-the-side target initially produced a small tongue movement with no lateral component. According to our model, this initial effort is corrected by computing the non-overlap between the organ relations of the visual target and those achieved by these first attempts. This comparison isolates the lateral dimension as a missing component, setting the goal for the next act. Repeated cycles of this process, isolating aspects of the target not captured in the last attempt, give the imitative progression its non-random character.

Meltzoff and Moore's (1994) microanalysis of the correction process revealed four monotonically ordered steps in infants' convergence toward the tongue-protrusion-to-the-side target. As diagrammed in Figure 3, the first step is a lateral movement of the tongue. Step 2 adds a small outward component to the lateral one. Step 3 produces a full tongue protrusion far beyond the lips. Step 4 integrates the lateral component into the full tongue protrusion. This process involves differentiating several dimensions of the target from one another (laterality, forwardness, and extent) and then integrating them into a single act. The process is

[6]Because the adult act is coded in the representational system, and representations persist, the proposed model accommodates the findings of early deferred imitation (e.g., Meltzoff and Moore, 1994). Even after the display has disappeared from view, the representation can be used as a target whenever the infant's attention is drawn to it.

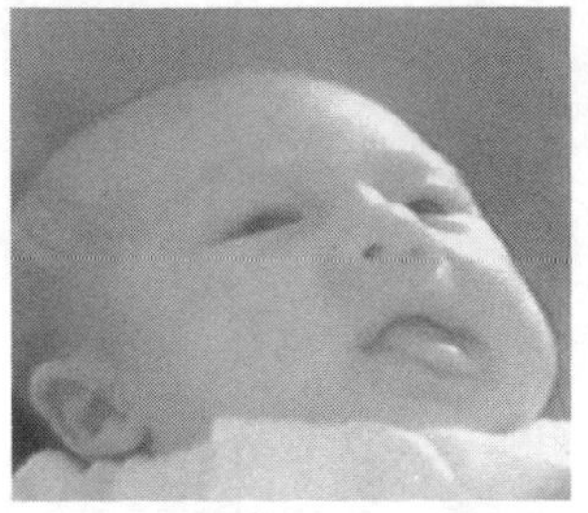
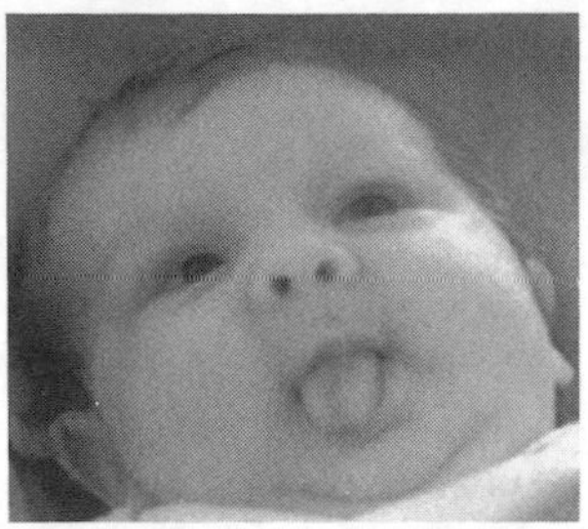
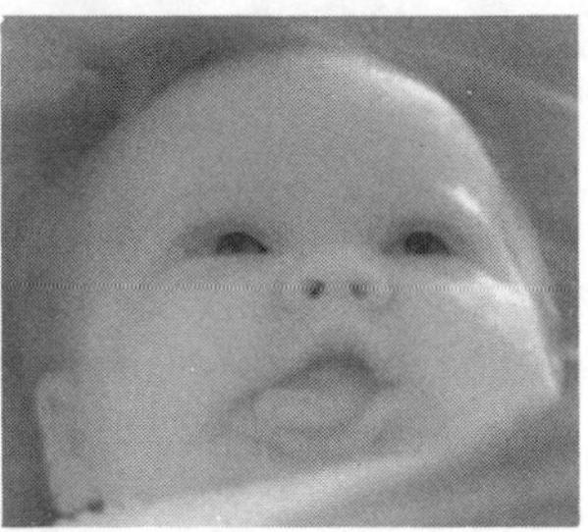

Figure 4. Six-week-old infants imitating the large tongue-protrusion-to-the side gesture demonstrated in the Meltzoff and Moore (1994) study. Such behaviour rarely occurs in baseline activity when infants have not been shown the gesture. Infants produce these imitative matches after correcting earlier approximations. The AIM model of early imitation accounts for such correction by postulating that infants are monitoring their unseen actions through proprioception (see text). The acts shown here correspond to step 4 in Figure 3.

not trial and error or even a simple progression from small to large, but rather an ordered, constructive process.[7] Figure 4 shows the highest-level match to the adult's gesture, which was achieved after the correction process already described.

The correction process results in a novel behaviour that was not initially present. In our terms, it takes infants beyond entries in the directory formed by previous body babbling. Infants do not seem able to generate the novel response *de novo*, on first try, by inferring what movements to make from seeing a new OR end state alone. None the less, imitation is powerful and generative in the sense that a match to novel targets can be achieved without extrinsic reinforcement.

EXPLANATORY VALUE OF THE MODEL

Assessing Parsimony and Coherence

Infant imitation involves an active matching to target in which infants can, at some level, use equivalences between self and other in generating their response. Our initial AIM hypothesis argued that this equivalence is mediated by a supramodal representational system (Meltzoff and Moore, 1977, 1983). Over the past twenty years, we have designed studies investigating the nature of this system. We now think that organ relations are the metric infants use in determining cross-modal equivalence. Organ relations are the *lingua*

[7] The model assumes that infants' comparisons between representations of their own body and the adult target isolate the discrepancies between them (the non-overlap in OR end states), making them salient and recruiting infant attention. Such highlighting, or 'pop out', at the representational level may be similar to infants' increased attention when there is a discrepancy between perception and representation (as in visual dishabituation). In the tongue-protrusion-to-the-side case, the missing lateral component is the first dimension isolated (Figure 3, Time 1). After performing a lateral tongue, what is more discrepant is the missing forward dimension. Having established the relevant directions of the tongue movements (lateral and forward), the *degree* of forward extent beyond the lips next becomes salient. Such a process could underlie the systematic ordering of infants' corrections that was documented in Meltzoff and Moore (1994) and diagrammed in Figure 3.

franca by which acts of self and other can be commonly coded. They are the terms in which a tongue-to-lips by the adult and by the infant can be represented commensurately.

The concept of organ relations unifies three phenomena of early imitation. First, the notion that the adult model is analysed in terms of OR end states would allow infants to imitate static gestures, which has been demonstrated (Meltzoff and Moore, 1992). Second, infants' coding of their own actions in terms of organ relations provides a parsing of their own acts. This creates a directory or 'act space' in which multiple muscle movements are mapped as equivalent paths to the same OR end state (addressing the motor equivalence problem). Such coding of infants' own bodies would allow them to recognize when they are being imitated by another, which has also been reported (Meltzoff, 1990; Meltzoff and Moore, 1995a). Third, given that organ relations represent both self and other in commensurate terms, infants could detect imitative mismatches and correct subsequent imitative attempts (Meltzoff and Moore, 1994).

Assessing Alternatives

Imitation and nativism. Facial imitation is demonstrated by newborns, but it is not completely explained by nativism. We propose important roles for learning and cognition. This may seem counterintuitive: if newborns do it, why invoke learning, no less cognition? The traditional argument seems to be that newborns = built in = reflexive transduction. However, the research findings suggest that this conflates separable terms.

There is no logical necessity that everything newborns do has to be built in, preformed, genetically specified. This ignores any contribution from prenatal experience. In fact, we have argued that intrauterine body babbling experience provides an initial mapping between movements and the OR end states they produce. Similarly, there is no logical necessity that all newborn behaviour—anymore than all 8-month-old behaviour—has to be an automatic, reflexive transduction. This cannot be decided by fiat. It is an empirical issue. For this reason we have carefully investigated newborns. The findings are that early imitation displays both goal-directed correction and temporal flexibility, which are more compatible with interpretive/cognitive processes than direct transduction.

Imitation and amodal perception: The differentiation problem. Imitation requires some cross-modal metric of equivalence. This raises a new problem. If infants can perceive self and other in equivalent terms, can they be told apart? Is there any perceptual distinction between self and other for the young baby? Piaget and Freud wrote elegantly of the initial 'confusion', 'adualism', and lack of distinction between self and other. In more modern terms, if one invokes a thoroughly amodal perceptual system to mediate imitation, this (ironically) recreates a Piagetian lack of differentiation.

A little data goes a long way in sorting this out. As we have seen, imitative acts can be corrected to achieve a more veridical match. Thus information about the infant's acts is available for comparison to a representation of the adult's act. More importantly for the problem at hand, representation of the target derived from the external world is not confused with or modified by the infants' own motor attempts. This suggests a differentiation such that representation of the other's body is separate from representation of the infant's body. Although both representations use the supramodal 'language' of organ relations, self and other are not just one undifferentiated whole.

IMPLICATIONS FOR DEVELOPMENTAL THEORY

Early imitation is not the same as the more mature imitation displayed at 18 months. We believe there are profound developmental restructurings over this period especially in the meaning that imitation has for infants and the functions that it serves. We will discuss how imitation, broadly construed, serves as a 'discovery procedure' for understanding persons. We will also argue that several important aspects of childhood social cognition can be traced back to early imitation and will sketch such development.[8]

Four Developmental Changes in Imitation

According to our model, the newborn initially construes adult behaviours in terms of the organ relations they exhibit. With development, infants come to interpret the behaviour of other people at a higher level, in terms of *human acts*. An elementary human act is not just a movement or an organ relation, but rather a goal-directed organ transformation. Thus the first developmental change is an integration of the OR end state and the movements-to-produce-it into a single unit. Human acts (not simply OR end states in and of themselves) become the new terms of analysis, the meaningful units for parsing the behaviour of self and other. Human acts themselves have characteristics that can be imitated such as speed, duration, and manner. Thus, imitation at the level of acts can yield an increase in fidelity. For example, infants are not confined to imitating mouth opening, but can also imitate the duration of mouth openings. Such imitation has been reported in 6-week-olds (Meltzoff and Moore, 1994). Imitation rapidly shifts in the first weeks of life from being the matching of OR end states to the matching of acts.[9]

A subsequent development is from construing imitation as a matching of specific acts to the more abstract notion of a *matching relationship*. This developmental change is illustrated

---

[8] As in all developmental theories, an interesting case is presented by infants with sensory or motor deficits such as blindness or motor paralysis. Because the present model postulates organ identification and a supramodal framework, the deficits can be compensated for. Development may be slowed, but it would not be blocked. Supramodal representation allows one modality to substitute for another; for example, facial organs may be identified by tactual exploration in the case of blindness. Similarly, as long as the motor deficit does not extend to movements of every organ of the infant's body, some channels for elaborating self–other relations will exist. Even in the Gedanken experiment of a non-comatose infant with complete motor paralysis, the capacity for organ identification would still provide grounds for treating other people as special. As long as the integrity of the central supramodal representational system is not compromised, motor impairments affecting individual body parts can be overcome.

[9] The notion that infants come to construe behaviour in terms of human acts deserves further analysis. Of course even the youngest infants perceive spatiotemporal movements of the face and the OR end states attained. Our point is that newborns do not initially construe the movements and end states as a unitary whole combining them as a single act (the difference between seeing a display as either: tongue movements vs, the configuration of tongue-between-lips vs. the unitary act of tongue protrusion). This developmental change of processing the act as a unitary whole is probably connected to the emergence of an 'act space' from the more primitive movement-to-end state directory. We think that the observation of social others plays an important role in this development. Initially, OR end states are known only in terms of self movement (as a result of producing the movement); observation of others presents OR end states differentiated from the infants' accompanying movements. These differentiated end states help provide the limits and extent (dimensions) of an organ's act space. Given a dimensionalized act space, infants could interpolate new points that lie within the already established space. For example, they could directly and fluidly imitate a novel act which lies within the space, even though they have never practised this particular movement pattern before. Act space thus organizes and represents an organ's transformations (the range of possible end states that can be attained, calibrated with muscle movements).

by infants' reactions to being imitated by adults. Both 1-month-olds and 1-year-olds show marked interest in being copied, but react differently. After a period of being imitated, older infants gleefully 'test' whether they are being copied by abruptly changing acts while staring at the adult to see what he will do (Meltzoff, 1990). Younger infants do not switch to a new behaviour as if testing. They treat the other's particular behaviour as a consequent of their own behaviour—as if their tongue protrusion causes the seen tongue protrusion—and they become upset if the adult starts to do another behaviour. In sum, older infants interpret imitation at a more abstract level than younger infants. The matching relationship transcends particular acts: it is not the notion that (infant) tongue protrusion causes (adult) tongue protrusion—*x* leads to *x*—but rather that the other is doing 'the same as' I do. Interpersonal matching becomes a meaningful unit of analysis, parsing interactions in terms of relationships rather than particular behaviours *per se*.

At about 1 year of age infants show a new interest in imitating the facial actions of others (Uzgiris and Hunt, 1975; Piaget, 1962). We hypothesize that this reinvigoration is due to a new modality-specific understanding of themselves—'my tongue protrusion *looks like* that seen tongue protrusion' (Moore and Meltzoff, 1978). This idea makes sense of the observation that 1-year-olds do more than strictly imitate; they hold out their tongue in exaggerated fashion for an extended period of time. They treat the other as a biological mirror, inducing the adult to hold out his/her tongue for visual inspection. Infants at this age also tactually compare the unseen parts of their bodies with those of adults, feeling the adult's mouth before reaching to their own. This appears to be an active tactual exploration of the similarity between self and the other. In both cases, the developmental change is infants' new interest in the unseen parts of their own bodies. Imitation allows infants to enrich the supramodal perception of themselves with sense-specific information such as what their tongue might *look* like and how their tongue and another's may *feel* the same. This enrichment of the already-established supramodal information with sense-specific information transforms their understanding of themselves and what it means to be like the other.

A further developmental change in imitation involves construing human acts so that the goal of an act can be identified even if it is not seen. This allows *imitation of an inferred act*. The best evidence comes from studies in which 18-month-olds are shown an adult trying, but failing, to perform an act (Meltzoff, 1995a). For example, when an adult's hand slips off a dumbbell he is trying to pull apart, infants infer the adult goal and pull apart the dumbbell themselves. Imitation has developed to the point that infants no longer imitate what they literally see, but what the adult *tried* to do, a step toward understanding the intentions of others.

Imitation as a Discovery Procedure in Human Social Development

The foregoing examples show development in infants' understanding of themselves, others, and interpersonal relationships. This takes us well beyond neonatal imitation as a behaviour, and highlights the significance of imitation in the growth of social cognition.

In our model, the underlying components of newborn imitation are organ identification, body babbling, and supramodal representation. Imitation, in turn, can be deployed as something like a discovery procedure for understanding the actions of people. Through interactions with others and the concomitant growth in self-understanding infants are engaged in an open-ended developmental process.

Such open-ended development continues beyond the changes sketched above and beyond infancy (Gopnik and Meltzoff, 1997). Further developments along this line include taking the perspective of others, role-taking and, eventually, the uniquely human capacity to form moral judgements based on the fundamental equality of persons. Thus development can be characterized as a process of creating equilibrium between self and other at increasing levels of abstraction (Meltzoff and Moore, 1995b). The outcome is a concept of person in which the self is understood as an objective entity in a world of others, and the other is ascribed a subjectivity as rich as one's own. It is our thesis that this developmental pathway is grounded in the initial equivalence of self and other manifest by early imitation.

REFERENCES

Abravanel, E. and DeYong, N. G. (1991). Does object modeling elicit imitative-like gestures from young infants? *Journal of Experimental Child Psychology*, **52**, 22–40.

Abravanel, E. and Sigafoos, A. D. (1984). Exploring the presence of imitation during early infancy. *Child Development*, **55**, 381–392.

Barr, R., Dowden, A. and Hayne, H. (1996). Developmental changes in deferred imitation by 6- to 24-month-old infants. *Infant Behavior and Development*, **19**, 159–170.

Bauer, P. J. and Mandler, J. M. (1992). Putting the horse before the cart: the use of temporal order in recall of events by one-year-old children. *Developmental Psychology*, **28**, 441–452.

Bertenthal, B. I. (1996). Origins and early development of perception, action, and representation. *Annual Review of Psychology*, **47**, 431–459.

Bower, T. G. R. (1982). *Development in Infancy* (2nd ed.). San Francisco: W. H. Freeman.

Butterworth, G. and Hopkins, B. (1988). Hand–mouth coordination in the new-born baby. *British Journal of Developmental Psychology*, **6**, 303–314.

de Boysson-Bardies, B., de Schonen, S., Jusczyk, P., MacNeilage, P. and Morton, J. (1993). *Developmental Neurocognition: Speech and Face Processing in the First Year of Life*. Dordrecht, Netherlands: Kluwer.

Desimone, R. (1991). Face-selective cells in the temporal cortex of monkeys. *Journal of Cognitive Neuroscience*, **3**, 1–8.

Field, T. M., Goldstein, S., Vaga-Lahr, N. and Porter, K. (1986). Changes in imitative behavior during early infancy. *Infant Behavior and Development*, **9**, 415–421.

Field, T. M., Woodson, R., Cohen, D., Greenberg, R., Garcia, R. and Collins, E. (1983). Discrimination and imitation of facial expressions by term and preterm neonates. *Infant Behavior and Development*, **6**, 485–489.

Field, T. M., Woodson, R., Greenberg, R. and Cohen, D. (1982). Discrimination and imitation of facial expressions by neonates. *Science* **218**, 179–181.

Fontaine, R. (1984). Imitative skills between birth and six months. *Infant Behavior and Development*, **7**, 323–333.

Gopnik, A. and Meltzoff, A. N. (1997). *Words, Thoughts, and Theories*. Cambridge, MA: MIT Press.

Goren, C. C., Sarty, M. and Wu, P. Y. K. (1975). Visual following and pattern discrimination of face-like stimuli by newborn infants. *Pediatrics*, **56**, 544–549.

Gross, C. G. (1992). Representation of visual stimuli in inferior temporal cortex. In V. Bruce, A. Cowey and A. W. Ellis (Eds), *Processing the Facial Image*. New York: Oxford University Press, pp. 3–10.

Gross, C. G., Bender, D. B. and Rocha-Miranda, C. E. (1969). Visual receptive fields of neurons in inferotemporal cortex of the monkey. *Science* (Wash.), **166**, 1303–1306.

Gross, C. G., Rocha-Miranda, C. E. and Bender, D. B. (1972). Visual properties of neurons in inferotemporal cortex of the macaque. *Journal of Neurophysiology*, **35**, 96–111.

Gross, C. G. and Sargent, J. (1992). Face recognition. *Current Opinion in Neurobiology*, **2**, 156–161.

Heimann, M. (1989). Neonatal imitation, gaze aversion, and mother–infant interaction. *Infant Behavior and Development*, **12**, 495–505.

Heimann, M., Nelson, K. E. and Schaller, J. (1989). Neonatal imitation of tongue protrusion and mouth opening: methodological aspects and evidence of early individual differences. *Scandinavian Journal of Psychology*, **30**, 90–101.

Heimann, M. and Schaller, J. (1985). Imitative reactions among 14–21 day old infants. *Infant Mental Health Journal*, **6**, 31–39.

Hooker, D. (1952). *The Prenatal Origin of Behavior*. Lawrence, KS: University of Kansas Press.

Humphrey, T. (1971). Development of oral and facial motor mechanisms in human fetuses and their relation to craniofacial growth. *Journal of Dental Research*, **50**, 1428–1441.

Jacobson, S. W. (1979). Matching behavior in the young infant. *Child Development*, **50**, 425–430.

Kaitz, M., Meschulach-Sarfaty, O., Auerbach, J. and Eidelman, A. (1988). A reexamination of newborn's ability to imitate facial expressions. *Developmental Psychology*, **24**, 3–7.

Kleiner, K. A. (1993). Specific vs. non-specific face recognition device. In B. de Boysson-Bardies, S. de Schonen, P. Jusczyk, P. MacNeilage and J. Morton (Eds), *Developmental Neurocognition: Speech and Face Processing in the First Year of Life*. Dordrecht, Netherlands: Kluwer.

Kugiumutzakis, J. (1985). The Origin, Development, and Function of the Early Infant Imitation. Unpublished doctoral dissertation, Uppsala University, Sweden.

Kuhl, P. K. and Meltzoff, A. N. (1996). Infant vocalizations in response to speech: vocal imitation and developmental change. *Journal of the Acoustical Society of America*, **100**, 2425–2438.

Legerstee, M. (1991). The role of person and object in eliciting early imitation. *Journal of Experimental Child Psychology*, **51**, 423–433.

Maratos, O. (1982). Trends in the development of imitation in early infancy. In T. G. Bever (Ed.), *Regressions in Mental Development: Basic Phenomena and Theories*. Hillsdale, NJ: Erlbaum, pp. 81–101.

Meltzoff, A. N. (1990). Foundations for developing a concept of self: the role of imitation in relating self to other and the value of social mirroring, social modeling, and self practice in infancy. In D. Cicchetti and M. Beeghly (Eds), *The Self in Transition: Infancy to Childhood*. Chicago: University of Chicago press, pp. 139–164.

Meltzoff, A. N. (1988). Infant imitation after a 1-week delay: long-term memory for novel acts and multiple stimuli. *Developmental Psychology*, **24**, 470–476.

Meltzoff, A. N. (1995a). Understanding the intentions of others: re-enactment of intended acts by 18-month-old children. *Developmental Psychology*, **31**, 838–850.

Meltzoff, A. N. (1995b). What infant memory tells us about infantile amnesia: long-term recall and deferred imitation. *Journal of Experimental Child Psychology*, **59**, 497–515.

Meltzoff, A. N. and Moore, M. K. (1977). Imitation of facial and manual gestures by human neonates. *Science*, **198**, 75–78.

Meltzoff, A. N. and Moore, M. K. (1983). Newborn infants imitate adult facial gestures. *Child Development*, **54**, 702–809.

Meltzoff, A. N. and Moore, M. K. (1989). Imitation in newborn infants: exploring the range of gestures imitated and the underlying mechanisms. *Developmental Psychology*, **25**, 954–962.

Meltzoff, A. N. and Moore, M. K. (1992). Early imitation within a functional framework: the importance of person identity, movement, and development. *Infant Behavior and Development*, **15**, 479–505.

Meltzoff, A. N. and Moore, M. K. (1994). Imitation, memory, and the representation of persons. *Infant Behavior and Development*, **17**, 83–99.

Meltzoff, A. N. and Moore, M. K. (1995a). A theory of the role of imitation in the emergence of self. In P. Rochat (Ed.), *The Self in Early Infancy: Theory and Research*. New York: North-Holland, pp. 73–93.

Meltzoff, A. N. and Moore, M. K. (1995b). Infants' understanding of people and things: from body imitation to folk psychology. In. J. Bermúdez, A. J. Marcel and N. Eilan (Eds), *The Body and the Self.* Cambridge, MA: MIT Press, pp. 43–69.

Meltzoff, A. N. and Moore, M. K. (1998). Infant intersubjectivity: broadening the dialogue to include intention, identity, and imitation. In S. Bråten (Ed.), *Intersubjective Communication and Emotion in Early Ontogeny: A Sourcebook.* Cambridge, UK: Cambridge University Press.

Moore, M. K. and Meltzoff, A. N. (1978). Object permanence, imitation, and language development in infancy: toward a neo-Piagetian perspective on communicative and cognitive development. In F. D. Minifie and L. L. Lloyd (Eds), *Communicative and Cognitive Abilities: Early Behavioral Assessment.* Baltimore: University Park Press, pp. 151–184.

Morton, J. and Johnson, M. H. (1991). CONSPEC and CONLEARN: a two-process theory of infant face recognition. *Psychological Review*, **98**, 164–181.

Patrick, J., Campbell, K., Carmichael, L., Natale, R. and Richardson, B. (1982). Patterns of gross fetal body movement over 24-hour observation intervals during the last 10 weeks of pregnancy. *American Journal of Obstetrics and Gynecology*, **142**, 363–371.

Perrett, D. I., Hietanen, J. K., Oram, M. W. and Benson, P. J. (1992). Organization and functions of cells responsive to faces in the temporal cortex. In V. Bruce, A. Cowey and A. W. Ellis (Eds), *Processing the Facial Image*. New York: Oxford University Press, pp. 23–30.

Perrett, D. I., Mistlin, A. J. and Chitty, A. J. (1987). Visual neurons responsive to faces. *Trends in Neuroscience*, **10**, 358–364.

Piaget, J. (1962). *Play, Dreams and Imitation in Childhood.* New York: Norton.

Prechtl, H. F. R. (1969). Brain and behavior mechanisms in the human newborn infant. In R. J. Robinson (Ed.), *Brain and Early Behavior*. New York: Free Press, pp. 289–360.

Reissland, N. (1988). Neonatal imitation in the first hour of life: observations in rural Nepal. *Developmental Psychology*, **24**, 464–469.

Rolls, E. T. (1992). Neurophysiological mechanisms underlying face processing within and beyond the temporal cortical visual areas. In V. Bruce, A. Cowey, and A. W. Ellis (Eds), *Processing the Facial Image*. New York Oxford University Press, pp. 11–21.

Slater, A. M. (1993). Visual perceptual abilities at birth: implications for face perception. In B. de Boysson-Bardies, S. de Schonen, P. Jusczyk, P. MacNeilage and J. Morton (Eds), *Developmental Neurocognition: Speech and Face Processing in the First Year of Life*. Dordrecht, Netherlands: Kluwer.

Trevarthen, C. (1980). The foundations of intersubjectivity: development of interpersonal and cooperative understanding in infants. In D. R. Olson (Ed.), *The Social Foundations of Language and Thought: Essays in Honor of Jerome S. Bruner*. New York: Norton, pp. 316–342.

Uzgiris, I. C. and Hunt, J. M. (1975). *Assessment in Infancy: Ordinal Scales of Psychological Development*. Urbana: University of Illinois Press.

van der Meer, A. L. H., van der Weel, F. R. and Lee, D. N. (1995). The functional significance of arm movements in neonates. *Science*, **267**, 693–695.

Vinter, A. (1986). The role of movement in eliciting early imitations. *Child Development*, **57**, 66–71.

Vries, J. I. P. de, Visser, G. H. A. and Prechtl, H. F. R. (1982). The emergence of fetal behaviour. I. Qualitative aspects. *Early Human Development*, **7**, 301–322.

Vries, J. I. P. de, Visser, G. H. A. and Prechtl, H. F. R. (1985). The emergence of fetal behaviour. II. Quantitative aspects. *Early Human Development*, **12**, 99–120.

Walton, G. E., Bower, N. J. A. and Bower, T. G. R. (1992). Recognition of familiar faces by newborns. *Infant Behavior and Development*, **15**, 265–269.

PART I: DEVELOPMENTAL ISSUES

2

Sensitivity and Attachment: A Meta-Analysis on Parental Antecedents of Infant Attachment

Marianne S. De Wolff and Marinus H. van IJzendoorn
Leiden University, Leiden, The Netherlands

This meta-analysis included 66 studies (N = 4,176) on parental antecedents of attachment security. The question addressed was whether maternal sensitivity is associated with infant attachment security, and what the strength of this relation is. It was hypothesized that studies more similar to Ainsworth's Baltimore study (Ainsworth, Blehar, Waters, & Wall, 1978) would show stronger associations than studies diverging from this pioneering study. To create conceptually homogeneous sets of studies, experts divided the studies into 9 groups with similar constructs and measures of parenting. For each domain, a meta-analysis was performed to describe the central tendency, variability, and relevant moderators. After correction for attenuation, the 21 studies (N = 1,099) in which the Strange Situation procedure in nonclinical samples was used, as well as preceding or concurrent observational sensitivity measures, showed a combined effect size of r(1,097) = .24. According to Cohen's (1988) conventional criteria, the association is moderately strong. It is concluded that in normal settings sensitivity is an important but not exclusive condition of attachment security. Several other dimensions of parenting are identified as playing an equally important role. In attachment theory, a move to the contextual level is required to interpret the complex transactions between context and sensitivity in less stable and more stressful settings, and to pay more attention to nonshared environmental influences.

Reprinted with permission from *Child Development*, 1997, Vol. 68(4), 571–591.

Support for this study was provided by a PIONEER award from the Netherlands' Organization for Scientific Research (NWO: PGS 59-256) and by a fellowship from the Netherlands Institute for Advanced Study in the Humanities and Social Sciences (NIAS) to Marinus van IJzendoorn. The authors gratefully acknowledge the thoughtful comments of members of the editorial board and reviewers on an earlier draft of this paper.

INTRODUCTION

In the first volume of his trilogy, *Attachment and Loss*, John Bowlby (1969) signaled an urgent need to determine the antecedent conditions that influence the development of attachment. Bowlby (1969) suggested that one of the conditions contributing to the development of a secure attachment relationship may be the attachment figure's sensitivity in responding to the baby's signals: When infants experience that their social initiatives are successful in establishing a reciprocal interchange with the mother, it is likely that an active and happy interaction between the couple will ensue and that a secure attachment relationship will develop.

After more than 25 years of research on the antecedents of attachment security, we may now be in a position to answer Bowlby's question. Is parental sensitivity indeed an important condition for the development of a secure attachment relationship between infant and parent?

Ainsworth and her colleagues were the first to examine the relation between parental behavior in the home and security of attachment (Ainsworth, Blehar, Waters, & Wall, 1978). They observed 26 middle-class mother-infant dyads from Baltimore throughout the first year of life; more than 70 hr of observation were spent in each home. At the time of the infant's first birthday, mother and infant came to the laboratory for assessment in the Strange Situation. This standardized procedure for assessing the infant-parent attachment relationship was developed in Ainsworth's pioneering study (Ainsworth & Wittig, 1969), and in the past few decades it has been used worldwide (Thompson, in press; van IJzendoorn & Kroonenberg, 1988). Ainsworth and her colleagues assessed a great variety of dimensions of maternal behavior at home. In particular, four rating scales (sensitivity, acceptance, cooperation, and accessibility) were found to be strongly related to attachment security, and the authors concluded that "the most important aspect of maternal behavior commonly associated with the security-anxiety dimension of infant attachment is manifested in different specific ways in different situations, but in each it emerges as sensitive responsiveness to infant signals and communications" (Ainsworth et al., 1978, p. 152).

Two decades after the Baltimore study, however, there is still great controversy over the parental antecedents of the Strange Situation attachment classifications. Gewirtz and Boyd (1977) and Lamb, Thompson, Gardner, and Charnov (1985) sparked this controversy by arguing that in her exploratory study Ainsworth had overgeneralized from the findings of her small sample. Lamb et al. contended that Ainsworth et al.'s (1978) "exciting hypotheses about the specific antecedents of Strange Situation behavior remain unproven except in their most general form" (p. 97). Although many studies had indicated that the infant's prior experiences at home were indeed related to their Strange Situation behavior, according to Lamb et al. it is still unclear which specific maternal behaviors are of formative importance for attachment security. In the first meta-analysis on attachment and sensitivity, Goldsmith and Alansky (1987, pp. 811, 813) also concluded that "many of the studies. . .replicate Ainsworth et al.'s (1978) original findings of the predictive power of maternal sensitivity when replication is evaluated in terms of statistical significance." However, they cautioned that the actual size of the predictive effect of maternal sensitivity is much smaller than once was believed, suggesting only a weak relation between attachment security and parental sensitivity.

Despite all of the skepticism, many authors continue to embrace Bowlby's (1969) original proposition that maternal sensitivity is a crucial antecedent of attachment security (Bretherton, 1985; Main, 1990; Sroufe, 1988). Recently, Isabella (1993) stated that attachment theory and research highlight maternal sensitivity as an all-important characteristic of interaction that has been consistently linked to attachment security. The fact that some studies have yielded much weaker associations than Ainsworth's study can, in this view, be attributed to methodological weaknesses of the replication studies. Some researchers have restricted their observations to a single home visit, whereas others have used brief laboratory assessments of sensitivity instead of extensive home observations (e.g., Frodi, Grolnick, & Bridges, 1985). Some studies included interviews to assess positive parental attitude toward the infant (Benn, 1986), whereas others focused on the frequency of physical contact (Kerns & Barth, 1995). Although these approaches may tap into some dimension of a broad concept of parenting that is pertinent to the development of attachment, they may not capture the original concept of sensitivity. Studies designed according to the basic features and conceptualizations of Ainsworth's Baltimore study (e.g., Belsky, Rovine, & Taylor, 1984; Grossmann, Grossmann, Spangler, Suess, & Unzner, 1985; Isabella, 1993) have yielded results that are closer to the original findings (Pederson et al., 1990). This latter view, which we will refer to as the "orthodox" position, can be summarized as follows: (1) The mother's interactive behavior, in particular, her sensitivity, is considered to be the primary determinant of attachment quality; (2) however, if this association is to be detected, the observations of maternal behavior must be sufficiently intensive and reliable, and the observed dimensions of maternal behavior must be conceptually close to sensitivity.

In this meta-analysis, we integrate the available studies on parenting and attachment in a quantitative manner. In a controversial field like attachment theory, a narrative review may not contribute to resolution of the debate because of its "subjective" and less systematic nature (Bretherton, 1985; Lamb et al., 1985). Meta-analysis offers a way of bringing some degree of order to a large and inconsistent body of findings (Rosenthal, 1991) at the same time that it allows for the testing of specific hypotheses statistically. For example, one might test the idea that studies which show a greater similarity to the Baltimore study show stronger associations between attachment and sensitivity. Almost 10 years after Goldsmith and Alansky's (1987) meta-analysis of 13 studies, it is time to take stock of the growing literature on attachment and sensitivity and to focus on the core issue of variability among the pertinent studies. More than 60 studies have investigated maternal behavior in relation to attachment security. In the current meta-analysis, we address three issues (Mullen, 1989): (1) Central tendency: What is the typical strength of association between maternal behavior and attachment security? (2) Variability: Is the set of study results heterogeneous, in the sense that outcomes are relatively variable across the studies? (3) Prediction: Can the variation between studies be explained by study features that are relevant to the controversy between the skeptical and orthodox positions?

In particular, we test the "orthodox" hypothesis that studies which more closely resemble the original Baltimore study show the strongest associations between parenting and attachment, whereas studies deviating from this intensive, naturalistic longitudinal study yield less impressive results. More specifically, the following hypotheses are tested: (1) Stronger associations between maternal behavior and attachment security are found in studies defining maternal behavior as sensitivity as compared with studies defining maternal behavior differently. (2) Home-based studies show stronger associations between attachment and maternal behavior than do laboratory studies. (3) Long-term home observation studies show stronger relations between maternal behavior and infant attachment than do short-term, home-based studies. (4) Assessments of maternal behavior during the first year of life show stronger associations with attachment security than do assessments after age 1. (5) The longer the time interval between the assessment of maternal behavior and the Strange Situation procedure, the weaker the association between sensitivity and attachment (see Goldsmith & Alansky, 1987). Moreover, we will test whether the association between sensitivity and attachment is dependent on contextual factors such as the socioeconomic or (non-)clinical status of the families involved. The orthodox hypothesis would emphasize a relatively context-free interpretation of this association. It may also be argued, however, that contextual factors partly override the influence of sensitivity on the development of attachment, and that in lower-class or clinical samples the association between sensitivity and attachment would be weaker.

In the first study, we report on the construction of homogeneous sets of concepts related to maternal interactive behavior, through a new method of expert sorting and rating procedures. Meta-analysis has often been criticized for mixing apples and oranges. Careful, systematic *conceptual* analysis is required to establish sets of similar studies that can be included in separate meta-analyses (Cooper & Hedges, 1994). This study paves the way for the second study in which the methods and results of a series of meta-analyses on the association between various aspects of maternal interactive behavior and attachment security are described. In the second study, the crucial issue of homogeneity will be addressed *statistically*.

STUDY 1

Method

Because the grouping of predictor variables may have an important effect on the outcome of a meta-analysis, experts were asked to categorize aspects of maternal interactive behaviors. In sorting the constructs, the experts were blind to the effect sizes associated with the specific constructs. In the total set of pertinent research papers (see Study 2), 55 different constructs were identified, all referring to various aspects of maternal behavior, for example, maternal body contact, maternal involvement, support, stimulation, sensitivity, verbal responsiveness, delight in the interaction, mutuality between mother and child, and frequency of positive responses to child. For each construct, we also identified the formal definition that was presented in the introduction or method sections of the research report, as well as the method of assessing that particular construct. On the basis of these descriptions, the experts were asked to sort the constructs. However, because the task of sorting 55 constructs would have been extremely time consuming, a smaller set was created. The first author identified four groups of constructs that were relatively self-evident. To reduce the total set, 15 constructs were preliminarily assigned to one of the four straightforward categories. These four groups encompassed the following aspects of maternal behavior: (1) Sensitivity, (2) Contiguity of Response, (3) Physical Contact, and (4) Cooperation.

The first group, Sensitivity, included all constructs that conformed to the original definition of Mary Ainsworth and her colleagues (Ainsworth, Bell, & Stayton, 1974): the mother's ability to perceive the infant's signals accurately, and the ability to respond to these signals promptly and appropriately. Constructs that had been assessed with Ainsworth's rating scale (Ainsworth et al., 1974) or a rating scale that was explicitly based on Ainsworth's original rating scale were also assigned to this first group. The second group of constructs was maternal Contiguity of Response, which we defined as promptness or, more generally, frequency of response to the infant's signals. The most important factor distinguishing contiguity of response from sensitivity is the absence of any qualitative assessment of the mother's behavior. Only promptness or frequency of the mother's responses contribute to contiguity of response; appropriateness is irrelevant. In the literature, contiguity of response is often referred to as "responsiveness." Because the term responsiveness is sometimes also used to indicate sensitivity (e.g., "sensitive responsiveness"), the concept "contiguity" was preferred to avoid confusion (see Bornstein, 1989). The third group consisted of all constructs that referred to quality or quantity of Physical Contact. The fourth group, Cooperation, included constructs that bore on the presence or absence of intrusive or interfering maternal behavior. This concept was originally defined and operationalized by Ainsworth (Ainsworth et al., 1974). The second author independently sorted 15 studies in the four categories. The percentage agreement was 93%, which documented the self-evident nature of this preliminary step in the sorting procedure.

Fifteen constructs fitted into one of the four groups; 40 constructs referring to other aspects of maternal interactive behavior remained to be classified. Two methods were used to create conceptually homogeneous groups of concepts: A sorting task in which the experts sorted the concepts into a few subgroups, and a rating task in which the experts rated each concept in terms of its similarity to Ainsworth's sensitivity construct and in terms of its importance for the development of attachment relationships.

Participants. A total of 27 persons who were actively involved in attachment research were asked to participate in the study. Experts were defined as persons who had been actively involved in attachment research for several years and who were at least participating in a graduate program in the behavioral sciences. Complete data were obtained for 19 respondents (12 women). Because the sorting task was rather time consuming, four persons were unable to comply with our request. Four nonrespondents refused for other personal reasons. Almost half of the sample had obtained a doctoral degree ($n = 9$); the remaining participants were graduate students. The respondents had been actively involved in the attachment research for 5 years on average ($SD = 3.89$).

Materials. The Similarity Sorting Task was constructed to investigate how the experts evaluated the conceptual similarities between the concepts. The sorting task consisted of 40 small cards (15 × 10.5 cm), on each of which a particular concept was presented as well as a conceptual definition of that concept and, if necessary, the way in which it was assessed. On the cards, any information about the source of the concept was absent to keep the sorters blind as to the effect sizes related to the concepts. The experts were instructed to sort the cards into maximally 10 groups of relatively similar concepts. The maximum of 10 groups was chosen to facilitate the sorting task and to guarantee the statistical power of the subsequent analyses (Verkes, Van der Kloot, & Van der Meij, 1989). The rating task consisted of the same set of 40 cards with conceptual definitions. We now asked the experts to rate each concept on a 7 point scale in terms of its similarity to Ainsworth's sensitivity construct, which was presented along with the cards. This scale ranged from "not any similarity" (1) to "exact similarity" (7). Besides the similarity to sensitivity, we also asked the experts to rate each concept in terms of its importance for the development of an attachment relationship. Experts could indicate the concept's importance on a 7 point rating scale that ranged from "not at all important" (1) to "very important" (7).

Procedure. The two tasks and a written instruction were sent to the experts. We asked the experts to complete the Sorting Task before starting to accomplish the Rating Task.

Data analysis. The sorting data were analyzed with Homogeneity analysis using alternating least squares (HOMALS; Gifi, 1990). We used the SPSS-PC program HOMALS (SPSS Inc., 1990). HOMALS can be considered as an equivalent to principal components analysis in the case of categorical data. A graphical configuration is constructed in which variables (i.e., the experts who sorted the concepts) and categories (i.e., the groups into which the concepts were sorted) are being represented. In calculating the coordinates of variables and categories, HOMALS uses a distance model: Those concepts that are sorted more frequently into the same group are represented in the configuration relatively close to each other. HOMALS has proved to be a fruitful method for analyzing sorting data of large numbers of stimuli (see Van der Kloot & Van Herk, 1991; Verkes et al., 1989). Following Verkes et al. (1989), we also performed a centroid cluster analysis (Everitt, 1974) on the distances between the 40 concepts in the HOMALS configuration to facilitate the interpretation of its results.

Results

The similarity sorting task. Concepts that were sorted by an expert into the same group received the same numerical code. Concepts that were coded into different groups were given different numerical codes. Those concepts that were not grouped with any other concept were treated as missing data. In this way a 40 (concepts) $\times$ 19 (experts) data matrix was created.

HOMALS yielded a two-dimensional configuration that is shown in Figure 1. The configuration represented the similarities and dissimilarities of the 40 concepts for maternal interactive behavior. The two dimensions had satisfactory eigenvalues of .87 and .81. This means that the 40 concepts are clearly differentiated by the two dimensions of the HOMALS solution. To support the interpretation of the HOMALS configuration, we performed a hierarchical cluster analysis on the distances between all concepts. We used the linkage coefficient to assess the appropriate number of clusters to describe the data optimally (Aldenderfer & Blashfield, 1984). Five clusters were constructed, which are also presented in Figure 1.

Synchrony can be defined as "the extent to which interaction appeared to be reciprocal and mutually rewarding" (Isabella, Belsky, & Von Eye, 1989, p. 13). Asynchronous instances of maternal and infant behavior are "those considered to reflect one-sided, unresponsive, or intrusive behavioral exchanges" (Isabella & Belsky, 1991, p. 376). "Positive mutuality," a concept that was applied by Kiser, Bates, Maslin, and Bayles (1986), exemplifies the cluster *Mutuality*. Positive mutuality is a construct that consists of the following maternal

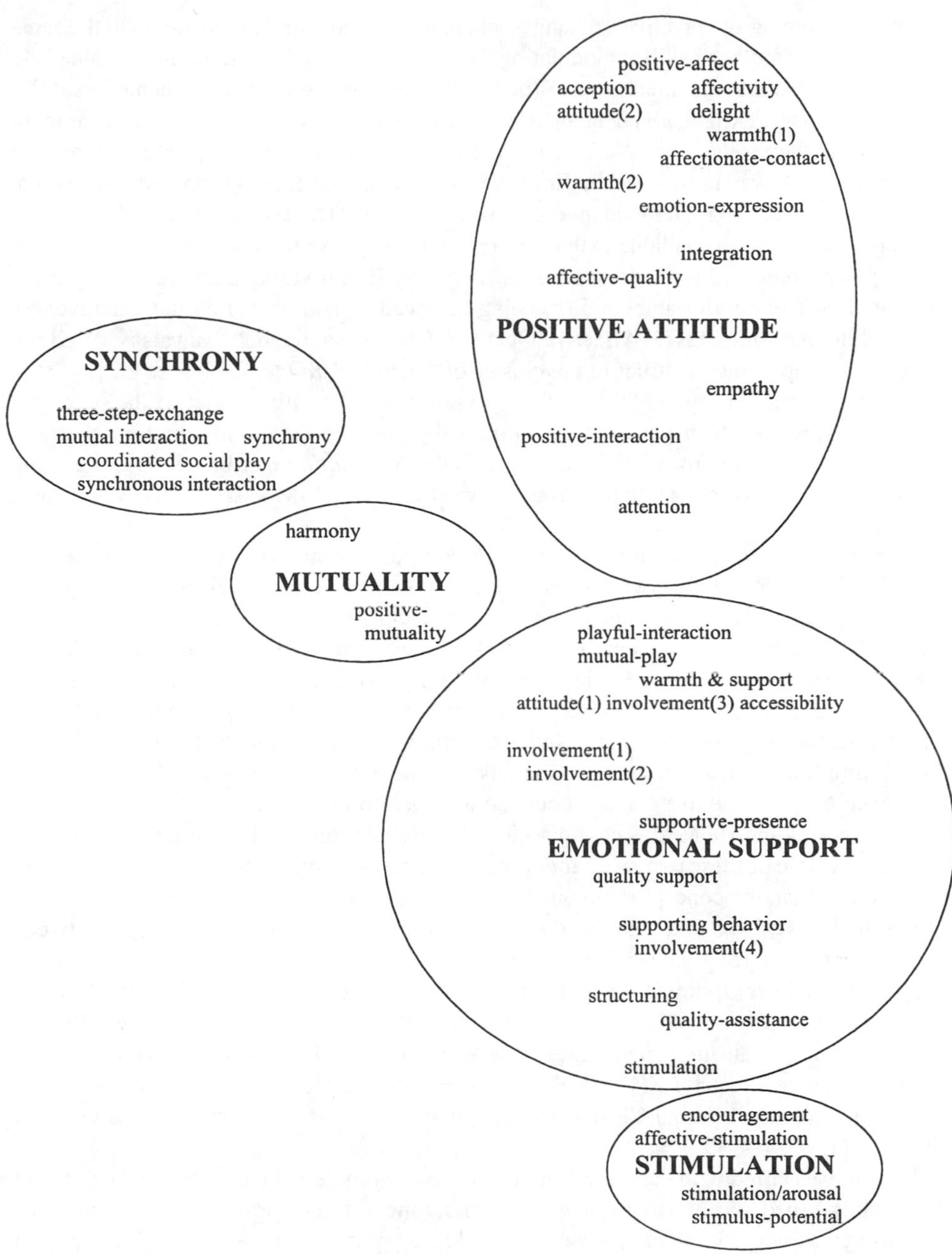

Figure 1. Two-dimensional representation of 40 concepts in the HOMALS solution.

behaviors: Number of "positive exchanges where both mother and infant attend to the same thing," and "the mother's skill at modulating the baby's arousal, her entertainment value, and her responsiveness to the infant's cues" (p. 71); it also includes some infant behaviors: "Expression of positive affect, nonavoidance, active maintenance of the interaction, and amount of gazing at the mother" (p. 71). A central concept in the cluster *Support* is Supportive Presence, which was introduced by Erickson, Sroufe, and Egeland (1985). Matas, Arend, and Sroufe (1978, p. 350) defined this concept as follows: "The extent to which the mothers appeared attentive and available to the children and supportive to their efforts. A high score on supportive presence involved meeting two criteria: (a) Providing a secure base by helping the child feel comfortable, and (b) being involved as manifested by the attentiveness to the child and to the task." Affective Quality (Zaslow, Rabinovich, Suwalsky, & Klein, 1988) is an important construct in the cluster of *Positive Attitude*. Zaslow et al. (1988, p. 290) defined this concept as "the mother's expression of positive affect to the baby, the mother's expression of negative affect to the baby, and the degree to which mother and infant engaged in reciprocal interactions." Finally, *Stimulation* can be described as "any action on the part of the mother directed toward her baby" (Miyake, Chen, & Campos, 1985, p. 292).

The rating task. In a preliminary principal components analysis for categorical data (PRINCALS; Gifi, 1990), it was established that the expert raters were unidimensional in their ratings on the two rating scales (Verkes et al., 1989). The sorting data revealed five distinct clusters of parenting concepts. For each cluster, we computed the mean ratings. The five cluster means were found to differ significantly from each other: On the first rating scale, similarity to Ainsworth's sensitivity concept, the overall $F(4, 35) = 5.52$, $p = .0015$; on the second rating scale, importance for attachment development, the overall $F(4, 35) = 5.03$, $p = .003$. Multiple comparison tests, using the Tukey-HSD procedure, indicated that this overall difference between the five clusters could be ascribed to two clusters that were located at the outer part of the HOMALS configuration: Positive Attitude and Stimulation. Concepts belonging to one of these two broader concepts received significantly lower ratings on both rating scales than the concepts belonging to the other clusters.

On the basis of this outcome, we distinguished in the total set of 40 concepts between a More Optimal Group, consisting of the clusters Synchrony, Mutuality, and Emotional Support, and a Less Optimal Group of concepts, consisting of the clusters Positive Attitude and Stimulation. On the rating scales, the two global clusters were significantly different. On the similarity scale, the group means were $M = 4.10$ and $M = 3.09$ for the More Optimal and Less Optimal clusters, $F(1, 35) = 16.34$, $p = .001$. On the importance scale, the mean rating for the More Optimal Cluster was $M = 4.79$ versus $M = 4.30$ in the Less Optimal Group, $F(1, 35) = 4.89$, $p = .02$.

In sum, we started with the more general construct of maternal interactive behavior, and then distinguished, partly with the help of experts, nine different groups, each referring to a narrower construct. For each group we will conduct a separate meta-analysis. The empirical approach of conceptual analysis through expert ratings enabled us to systematically differentiate between several dimensions of parenting behavior independent of the meta-analytic results. In Study 2, we describe the methods and results of the subsequent meta-analyses.

STUDY 2

Method

Selection of the studies. To identify studies for inclusion in the meta-analysis, we applied three search strategies: Computerized searches, manual search procedures, and consultation of other scientists working in this field.

The following computerized abstracting services were used to locate studies: Psychological Abstracts (from 1974 on), Educational Resources Information Center (from 1983 on), and Social Sciences Citation Index (from 1983 on). Furthermore, we used "World Catalog," a database of the On-Line Contents Library Center (OCLC). The following keywords were used in different combinations: attachment, childrearing practices, infant, mother, mothering, mother-child interactions, mother-child relations, parent-child relations, parenting, responsiveness, and sensitivity.

To supplement these computer searches, we used several manual search procedures. Reference lists from existing reviews were inspected (Goldsmith & Alansky, 1987; Lamb et al., 1985; Lambermon, 1991), as were reference lists of the reviewed articles. In addition, we located unpublished dissertations through a manual search of *Dissertation Abstracts International* (from 1980 on). To locate unpublished research, we also worked through several volumes of conference abstracts (ICIS, SRCD). Finally, we asked two prominent researchers in the attachment field, Drs. M. Main and J. Belsky, to suggest additional studies. They were able to mention three additional studies. One of the reviewers mentioned three additional studies (Fagot & Kavanagh, 1990; Malatesta, Culver, Tesman, & Shepard, 1989; Seifer, Schiller, Sameroff, Resnick, & Riordan, 1996). After submission of the manuscript, we came across two very recent studies (Gunnar, Brodersen, Nachmias, Buss, & Rigatuso, 1996; NICHD Early Child Care Network, 1996).

Each study had to meet three criteria for inclusion in the meta-analysis. The first criterion was that the study contained a measure of the mother's behavior toward her infant, and a measure of the infant's attachment security. The vast majority of maternal behavior measures have been derived from observations of mother-infant interaction. In a few studies, maternal behavior was measured using questionnaires or interviews with the mother. For example, Benn (1986) and Bretherton, Biringen, Ridgeway, Maslin, and Sherman (1989) assessed maternal sensitivity in an interview with mother, whereas Izard, Heynes, Chisholm, and Baak (1991) used a questionnaire to assess the mother's style of emotional expression. In the assessment of attachment security, the Strange Situation procedure was, of course, used in most studies. In some studies, the original procedure was changed because the researchers adapted the procedure to a home situation, or because they wanted to limit the infant's stress (see Capps, Sigman, & Mundy, 1994). In other studies, the Waters and Deane (1985) Attachment Q-Sort for observers was used instead of the Strange Situation (Vaughn & Waters, 1990). We did not include studies using the Mother Attachment Q-Sort, because a recent meta-analysis clearly showed its lack of convergent and discriminant validity (van IJzendoorn, Vereijken, & Riksen-Walraven, in press).

The second criterion for inclusion was that each study should report an association between maternal behavior and infant attachment, so that effect sizes could be calculated. Even if only nonnumerical information was provided (i.e., "no relation" or "significant relation"), we included the study in the meta-analysis and estimated the effect sizes (Mullen, 1989). In some studies in which both maternal behavior and quality of attachment were assessed, however, the researchers did not compute any association between the two assessments, nor did they report on the association (see Easterbrooks & Goldberg, 1985). These studies had to be excluded.

Our third criterion concerned intervention studies. The central hypothesis in our meta-analysis refers to the association between maternal behavior—as it occurs naturally—and infantt attachment. Consequently, if maternal behavior was experimentally influenced through intervention or therapy, we only included data for the nontreated control group. Thus, only those intervention studies that reported separate data for the control group(s) could be included in the meta-analysis (for a meta-analysis of intervention studies, see van IJzendoorn, Juffer, & Duyvesteyn, 1995).

Overall, we adopted a fairly liberal inclusion strategy. No studies were excluded from the meta-analysis on the basis of flawed design. Both Hedges (1986) and Mullen (1989) advise against excluding studies of low quality, because it is very difficult to assess a diffuse dimension like "study quality" directly and appropriately. Instead of using study quality as a criterion for inclusion in the meta-analysis, the meta-analyst is advised to include studies of varying quality. More detailed information on study quality should be included in the coding system, so that the influence of study characteristics on effect size can be examined in the meta-analysis. In the area of attachment research, the quality of the studies remains a hotly disputed issue. The main body of studies on attachment has been published in leading journals such as *Child Development* ($k = 21$), *Developmental Psychology* ($k = 7$), *Infant Behavior and Development* ($k = 6$), the *Monographs of the SRCD* ($k = 3$), and in other refereed journals. A number of studies, however, have been published in less prestigious journals, or remained unpublished. We have addressed the issue of quality of research in three ways. First, the overall quality of the study was estimated in terms of the quality of the publication medium. For journals, the "impact factor," defined as the average number of citations to the papers in a journal, was considered as a proxy of quality (Garfield, 1979). The impact of conference papers and dissertations was set at zero. The overall quality of the studies was then included in the meta-analyses as a moderator variable. Second, we tested the influence of publication status (published versus unpublished) on the size of the combined effects of the associations between attachment and aspects of parenting. Third, we provided combined effect sizes for associations between attachment and sensitivity separately for the total set of pertinent studies, as well as for the subset of studies using the standard assessment of attachment, that is, the Strange Situation procedure, antecedent or concurrent observational assessment of sensitivity, and nonclinical participants. These studies more closely resembled the original Baltimore study in their assessments of predictor and outcome variables.

A total of 66 studies were identified that together involved 4,176 mother-infant pairs. The meta-analytic database included 54 published articles, as well as 12 unpublished conference presentations or dissertations. A common criticism of meta-analysis is that studies with significant findings are overrepresented in the meta-analytic database because studies with significant findings are more likely to be published than studies with nonsignificant findings.

It is assumed that many studies with effect sizes of zero remain unpublished in file drawers. If a meta-analyst relied exclusively on published studies, this could result in an overestimation of population effect sizes. Rosenthal (1979) identified this as the "file drawer" problem. The best solution to the file drawer problem is simply to open the drawers and include as many unpublished studies as possible (Rosenthal, 1991). Unpublished dissertations were located through a manual search of Dissertation Abstracts International (from 1980). We also searched through several conference proceedings (ICIS, SRCD) in which abstracts of presented papers were published.

Another way of dealing with the "file drawer" problem is to estimate the magnitude of the problem by calculating the minimum number of unpublished studies with null results that would be required to turn a significant meta-analytic finding into a nonsignificant one. This number of imaginary unpublished studies is called the "fail safe number" and was introduced by Rosenthal (1979). If this fail safe number is relatively small, a file drawer problem may exist. Calculation of the fail safe number is no definitive solution to the file drawer problem. It only "establishes reasonable boundaries on the file drawer problem and estimates the degree of damage to the research conclusion that could be done by the file drawer problem" (Rosenthal, 1991, p. 104).

Calculation of effect sizes. In the meta-analysis, Pearson's product-moment correlation coefficient (r) was used as the effect size estimate. An effect size indicates the magnitude of the association between two variables, disregarding sample size. If a study reported means and standard deviations, one-directional t values were computed and transformed into r using Schwarzer's (1989) algorithms. If no means and standard deviations were available, the reported test statistics (t, F, or chisquare) or the one-directional p value were transformed into r with Mullen's (1989) computer program.

Because only F tests with 1 degree of freedom in the numerator are appropriate for inclusion in meta-analysis, a contrast F with 1 degree of freedom was computed on the basis of the global F value using the Contrast Analysis procedures (Rosenthal & Rosnow, 1985). Global F tests can be converted to contrast Fs only if group means are available. We applied conservative estimation procedures if a study only reported "no significant effect" ($p = .50$), or "a significant effect" ($p = .05$) in the case of univariate relations (Mullen, 1989).

To compute combined effect sizes, each correlation coefficient was transformed to a Fisher's Z to make the sampling distribution of r more approximate to a Gauss curve. The distribution of r becomes nonlinear at the extreme ends of the scale (Mullen, 1989). Furthermore, in computing the s, individual effect sizes were weighted by sample size, because correlations become more stable as sample size increases and because effect sizes based on large samples deviate less from the population effect size than those based on smaller samples (Mullen, 1989; Rosenthal, 1991). As an indicator of accuracy, we computed the 95% confidence interval around the mean effect size, using Schwarzer's (1989) program.

Combining estimates of effect sizes across studies is reasonable if the studies have a common population effect size. If this is the case, estimates of effect sizes will differ only because of unsystematic sampling error. The crucial question is thus whether the underlying dataset is sufficiently homogeneous. Hedges and Olkin (1985) as well as Rosenthal (1991) advised the use of a test for homogeneity to determine to what extent effect sizes are relatively constant across studies. Regardless of whether this homogeneity test is significant, Johnson, Mullen, and Salas (1995) encouraged the meta-analyst to check for significant moderator variables that may partly account for the variation across studies (see also Rosenthal, 1995). To determine whether a study feature significantly explains a part of the variation in effect sizes, we used Rosenthal's method of focused comparison of combined effect sizes (Mullen, 1989).

Last, blocking was used to reveal moderators in the dataset. Blocking involves grouping study outcomes on the basis of a potential moderator variable. Within each level of the moderator variable, a combined effect size can be computed, and the significance of the differences can be tested (Mullen, 1989).

Multiple outcomes within the primary study. In meta-analysis, the study itself is the unit of analysis. Because the meta-analytic procedures assume independence of units of analysis, we had to deal with the problem of multiple outcomes from single studies. In this meta-analysis, there were three types of multiple outcomes.

First, in several studies the same maternal behavior was assessed at multiple points in time. In these cases we computed a combined effect size over the various measurements; the combined effect size was treated as the outcome of such a study. For example, Isabella (1993) assessed maternal sensitivity at 1, 4, and 9 months of age. The association between maternal sensitivity and the Strange Situation outcome was reported for each age separately. In the meta-analysis, we took the mean outcome across the three times of assessment (see Goldsmith & Alansky, 1987).

Second, several studies examined the relation between a variety of maternal behaviors and attachment security. In the first study, we identified nine categories of predictor variables, each referring to a specific aspect of maternal behavior (see Study 1). After determining the kind(s) of behavior that had been examined in each study, we assigned each behavior to one of our nine categories of maternal behavior. If two maternal behaviors were classified in the same category, we computed the mean effect size. For example, Goldberg, Perotta, Minde, and Corter's (1986) measures of acceptance, delight, perception of the baby, and attitude were all assigned to the category Positive Attitude toward the infant. We therefore computed a mean effect size over these four behaviors.

Third, because many studies assessed different aspects of maternal behavior in their primary analyses, data from a single study were often included in several domains of maternal behavior. For example, the study of Goldberg et al. (1986) provided data for almost every domain of maternal behavior. In case of combining domains into the more and less optimal clusters, we computed means over the study outcomes for the domains so that each study had only one outcome in the meta-analysis.

Fourth, some studies were conducted by the same research team and included the same samples (Isabella & Belsky, 1991, and Isabella et al., 1989; Goossens, 1987, and van IJzendoorn, Kranenburg, Zwart-Woudstra, Van Busschbach, & Lambermon, 1991; Main, Tomasini, & Tolan, 1979, and Londerville & Main, 1981; Miyake et al., 1985, and Nakagawa, Lamb, & Miyake, 1992; Bates, Maslin, & Frankel, 1985, and Kiser et al., 1986, and Frankel & Bates, 1990). In these cases we also computed a mean effect size. In other words, studies involving the same sample were represented by only one effect size in the set of meta-analyses.

Coding the variables. The outcome variable, attachment security, did not need to be coded because it is a sharply defined construct. In the majority of the studies, attachment security was assessed by means of Ainsworth and Wittig's (1969) Strange Situation procedure. In four studies, shortened versions of the Strange Situation procedure were applied (Bohlin, Hagekull, Germer, Andersson, & Lindberg, 1989; Capps et al., 1994; Lewis & Feiring, 1989; Persson-Blennow, Binett, & McNeil, 1988). A total of five studies utilized alternative assessments of attachment, like the Attachment Story Completion Task (Altman, Monk, Jones, & Sosa, 1993; Goodman, Andrews, Jones, Weissman, & Weisman, 1993) and the Attachment Q-Sort (Kerns & Barth, 1995; Pederson et al., 1990; Pederson & Moran, 1996). Recently, van IJzendoorn et al. (in press) showed that the observer Attachment Q-Sort is a reliable and valid measure of attachment security, and they argued that in several respects the Attachment Q-Sort is even preferable to the Strange Situation procedure. In the same meta-analysis, the mother Attachment Q-Sort was shown to be an invalid self-report attachment measure. Studies with the mother version of the Attachment Q-Sort were excluded, therefore, from the current meta-analyses. Furthermore, we focused in the meta-analyses on attachment security (using either the secure-insecure dichotomous variable or security ratings), and we decided not to include the traditional split between insecure attachment classifications because only part of the studies report on the difference between the insecure classifications.

We coded a number of study characteristics. First, some background variables were coded, like publication status (published, unpublished) and year of publication. Second, we coded several characteristics of the sample: sample size, whether the sample was special (i.e., whether the mother or the child suffered from mental or physical handicaps, and whether the family conditions were deviant), socioeconomic status of the sample (middle class, lower class, or heterogeneous), and whether the infants were all firstborn. The most important variables concerned study design. A total of eight design variables were coded: (1) the techniques for measuring maternal behavior (global rating scales, specific behavioral codings based on time or event sampling, or nonobservational techniques like interviews and questionnaires); (2) the exact duration of the observation, in minutes; (3) location where the mother-infant interaction was observed (home or laboratory); (4) the age of the child at the time of the observation; (5) whether the Strange Situation or an alternative measure was used to assess attachment security; (6) the age of the child at the time of assessment of attachment security; (7) time interval in months between the two assessments; and (8) whether the assessments of maternal behavior and infant attachment had been conducted completely independently.

If maternal behavior was assessed at different infant ages, we computed the mean age. For example, in Belsky et al.'s (1984) study, maternal behavior was observed at 1, 3, and 9 months of age. The Strange Situation was assessed at 12.5 months. In this case, we coded the age of the child at the maternal behavior observation (moderator 4) as 4.3 months; the time interval between predictor and outcome assessments (moderator 7) was coded as 8.2 months.

Two persons coded the moderator variables. After a training phase, we performed a reliability check in which each coder independently coded 15 studies. The mean percentage of agreement was 92%. The coding of variables such as publication year, age of the mother, parity, age of the child at predictor, and outcome assessment appeared to be straightforward (for these variables, intercoder agreement was 100%). Most problematic was the coding of the measurement technique used to assess maternal behavior (global versus specific). In this case, intercoder agreement was 67%.

Results

Central tendency and variability. Table 1 presents the mean weighted effect sizes for each domain of maternal behavior, as well as confidence intervals, homogeneity tests, and fail safe numbers. The data pertain to all the studies except the pioneering Baltimore study (Ainsworth et al., 1978) that inspired so many replication studies. Although inclusion of the Baltimore study would not change any of our results drastically, we decided to exclude this study for two reasons. First, it was in the Baltimore study that central measures for sensitivity and attachment were developed and the hypothesis about the association between attachment and sensitivity was generated and specified. Later studies can be considered as replications and extensions. Second, the Baltimore study showed very strong associations between attachment and several aspects of parenting, whereas later studies generally showed less strong relations; in many respects the Baltimore study occupies a somewhat outlying position (see Tables 3 and 4).

As can be derived from Table 1, the combined effect size for the association between maternal sensitivity and attachment was $r(1{,}664) = .22$ ($k = 30, N = 1{,}666$). However, when

TABLE 1
Parenting and Attachment: Meta-Analytic Findings for Each Domain of Parental Behavior

Parental Behavior	Studies (*N*)	Participants (*N*)	Effect Size (*r*)	*p*	95% Confidence Interval	Homogeneity χ^2	Fail Safe (*N*)
Sensitivity	30	1,666	.22	9.12 E-15	.18–.27	43.5[a]	861.8
Ainsworth-scale	16	837	.24	1.55 E-09	.17–.30	18.8	238.9
Contiguity of response	14	825	.10	.01	.03–.17	20.4	38.7[b]
Physical contact	9	637	.09	.04	.01–.17	7.8	14.1[b]
Cooperation	9	493	.13	.007	.03–.21	11.1	17.2[b]
More optimal group	28[c]	1,928	.19	7.77 E-08	.14–.23	63.7[a]	735.6
Synchrony	6	258	.26	.0001	.14–.37	11.9[a]	35.5[b]
Mutuality	3	168	.32	.00003	.18–.46	9.3[a]	17.6[b]
Support	22	1,664	.16	7.41 E-06	.11–.21	37.1	328.2
Less optimal group	24[c]	1,233	.19	7.88 E-10	.14–.26	30.5	377.8
Attitude	21	1,092	.18	3.02 E-08	.14–.25	29.4	273.2
Stimulation	9	422	.18	.0001	.10–.29	7.5	32.0[b]
Total set	123[c]	7,225	.17	8.24 E-24	.15–.19	198[a]	9,923.5
Random set	66	4,176	.19	1.83 E-17	.16–.22	139[a]	3,957.3

[a]Data set is heterogeneous.
[b]File drawer problem is indicated.
[c]Total without overlapping studies.

we adopted a more strict definition of the predictor variable and included only studies that measure sensitivity using Ainsworth's original rating scale, the effect size increased to $r(835) = .24$ ($k = 16$, $N = 837$). The correlation between maternal behavior and infant attachment was highest for the set of studies on Mutuality, $r(166) = .32$. However, this meta-analysis involved only three studies ($N = 168$). Weaker effect sizes were found in the set of studies on Contiguity of response, $r(823) = .10$ (k=14, $N = 825$), and Physical Contact, $r(635) = .09$ ($k = 9$, $N = 637$). The combined effect size for Cooperation was $r(491) = .13$ ($k = 9$, $N = 493$). For Stimulation, a similar combined effect size was found: $r(420) = .18$ ($k = 9$, $N = 422$). For Positive Attitude, the effect size was $r(1{,}090) = .18$ ($k = 21$, $N = 1{,}092$), and for Emotional Support this figure was $r(1{,}662) = .16$ ($k = 22$, $N = 1{,}664$). In the set of studies on attachment and Synchrony, the combinedg effect size appeared to be similar to the outcome in the domain of Sensitivity: $r(256) = .26s$ ($k = 6$, $N = 258$). All effect sizes were significant at the alpha = .05 level.

Besides meta-analyses on each domain, we also performed two meta-analyses on a broader conceptual level. Overall effect sizes, however, did not differ between the more optimal and the less optimal cluster: $r(1{,}926) = .19$ ($k = 28$, $N = 1{,}928$) in the more optimal group, and $r(1{,}231) = .19$ ($k = 24$, $N = 1{,}233$) in the less optimal group. On the most global level, we also computed an overall effect size of the studies, irrespective of their cluster membership: mean $r(7{,}223) = .17$ ($k = 123$, $N = 7{,}225$). This global approach increased, of course, the heterogeneity of the set of studies, and it also led to the inclusion of dependent outcomes of the same studies. Therefore, we randomly selected one effect size per study, in case of multiple outcomes. The resulting overall effect size was $r(4{,}174) = .19$ ($k = 66$, $N = 4{,}176$). In this random set of 66 effect sizes, we tested whether the combined effect size of the sensitivity cluster was significantly different from the other clusters. Because eight comparisons were made, the Bonferroni corrected alpha level was used. The Sensitivity cluster appeared to show a significantly larger effect size than the Contiguity of response cluster ($p = .004$).

The fail safe numbers indicated possible file drawer problems in several domains of maternal behavior: Contiguity of response, Physical Contact, Cooperation, Synchrony, Mutuality, and Stimulation. The combined effect sizes for these domains of parenting need to be considered carefully, as they require further corroboration. In the other domains, fail safe numbers exceeded Rosenthal's (1991) critical value ($5 \times k + 10$). These effect sizes can be considered robust. For example, 862 studies with null results in the file drawers of disappointed researchers would be required to make the effect size for the association between sensitivity and attachment nonsignificant.

Table 1 also presents the test statistic chi-square, which indicates whether the effect sizes within the domain were homogeneous. The combined effect size for heterogeneous clusters constitutes problematic estimates of the population effect size. Therefore, we tried to find homogeneous subsets of studies using disjoint cluster analysis (Mullen, 1989; Schwarzer, 1989). For the Sensitivity domain, we found two significantly disjoint clusters (alpha was set at .05). One small and heterogeneous cluster consisted of the study by Capps et al. (1994) on autistic children, and the study by Benn (1986), who used an interview to assess sensitivity. The remaining studies were homogeneous, $\chi^2(27, N = 1{,}621) = 30.6$, $p = .29$, and the combined effect size was $r(1{,}619) = .21$ ($k = 28$). Including studies similar to the

Ainsworth Baltimore study in terms of (1) the use of the Strange Situation procedure, (2) the application of observational measures of sensitivity, (3) nonclinical participants, and (4) sensitivity assessments preceding or concurrent with the attachment assessment, we found a combined effect size of $r(1{,}097) = .20$ ($k = 21$), and this set of studies was homogeneous, $\chi^2(20, N = 1{,}099) = 25.2$, $p = .19$.

For the Synchrony domain, disjoint cluster analysis showed two different clusters: The study of Isabella et al. (1989) was set apart from the other studies. Isabella et al.'s (1989) study included an equal number of avoidant ($n = 10$), secure ($n = 10$), and ambivalent ($n = 10$) infants, selected from a larger sample of 51 infants. In particular, the secure group contained only the "most secure" B2 and B3 patterns of attachment (Ainsworth et al., 1978). The remaining Synchrony studies constituted a homogeneous set, $\chi^2(4, N = 228) = 3.4$, $p = .39$, and their combined effect size was $r(226) = .19$ ($k = 5$). For the domain of Mutuality studies, the disjoint cluster analysis discriminated the Smith and Pederson (1988) study from the two other studies. This latter set, however, appeared to remain heterogeneous. In the domain of Support, the disjoint cluster analysis set the Matas et al. (1978) study apart from the other studies which constituted a homogeneous set, $\chi^2(20, N = 1{,}616) = 18.4$, $p = .56$. The 21 studies in this set showed a combined effect size of $r(1{,}614) = .14$.

The more optimal group of 28 studies appeared to become homogeneous after exclusion of the Benn (1986), Isabella et al. (1989), and Matas et al. (1978) studies that were identified through the disjoint cluster analysis. The remaining set showed a combined effect size of $r(1{,}818) = .15$ ($k = 25$); $\chi^2(24, N = 1{,}820) = 22.0$, $p = .57$. In five of the domains of maternal behavior (Positive Attitude, Stimulation, Contiguity of response, Cooperation, and Physical Contact), effect sizes appeared relatively constant across studies, even though some of the meta-analyses included a large number of studies. Effect sizes in the "less optimal group" were also found to be homogeneous. We nevertheless performed moderator analyses in these domains because a nonsignificant homogeneity test "does not mean that there is no interesting variability in the research domain" (Mullen, 1989, p. 102).

Prediction. In Table 2, the moderators and their z values are reported for each subset. Again, the Baltimore study (Ainsworth et al., 1978) was not included because of its exploratory nature.

Publication status and impact factor were not significant moderators in any of the nine domains of analysis. In this respect, then, the data do not point to a file drawer or quality problem. Year of publication also was not significant in any domain. The duration of the maternal behavior assessment, the use of the Strange Situation procedure or alternative attachment measures, the independence of parenting and attachment assessments, and whether the sample consisted exclusively of firstborn infants did not emerge as significant moderators as well. In meta-analyses, sample size often is a significant moderator because smaller samples usually tend to show stronger effect sizes than larger samples (see Amato & Keith, 1991). In our case, sample size was a significant moderator in four domains: Sensitivity ($z = 2.02$), Synchrony ($z = 3.39$), Mutuality ($z = 2.36$), and Positive Attitude ($z = 2.06$). Smaller samples indeed showed stronger effect sizes. The remaining moderators will be discussed separately for each domain.

SENSITIVITY. In Table 3, a stem and leaf display of the effect sizes in the most important domain, Sensitivity, is presented. It shows the somewhat outlying position of the Baltimore

TABLE 2

The Effect of Moderators in Different Parenting Domains (z Values)[a]

Moderator	Sensitivity					More Optimal Cluster			Less Optimal Cluster	
	Total ($k = 30$)	Ainsworth Scale ($k = 16$)	Contiguity of Response ($k = 14$)	Physical Contact ($k = 9$)	Cooperation ($k = 9$)	Synchrony ($k = 6$)	Mutuality ($k = 3$)	Support ($k = 22$)	Positive Attitude ($k = 21$)	Stimulation ($k = 9$)
Publication	1.89	.91	.97	.97	—[b]	—[b]	1.49	.21	.61	—[b]
Impact factor	.14	.28	.82	.91	.09	1.34	.46	.26	.27	.61
Year	.97	.92	.14	.31	.52	1.72	.17	1.67	.65	.81
Size	2.02*	.28	1.48	1.76	.81	3.39***	2.36*	1.76	2.06*	.26
SES	2.41*	1.81	.41	1.10	.67	1.86	—[b]	.29	.71	.26
Clinical	.84	.17	.66	.13	2.10*	1.86	1.76	1.10	2.78**	.51
Firstborns	.28	.57	1.36	.79	.76	1.87	—[b]	.19	1.12	.11
Global	.87	—[b]	2.34*	.14	2.59**	—[b]	—[b]	1.12	2.09*	.24
Duration	.27	.99	.30	.19	.78	1.23	1.49	1.42	.46	1.17
Home/lab	.20	.65	1.26	1.65	1.63	1.33	1.49	.93	1.70	2.33*
Age	2.56**	.64	2.58**	1.19	.62	.25	2.19*	1.31	.76	1.89
SSP	1.95	1.32	1.44	1.86	.60	—[b]	—[b]	.05	.98	—[b]
Age-SSP	2.31*	1.35	.95	1.02	.68	.67	1.76	.12	.21	.88
Time interval	2.69**	.79	2.97**	1.28	.33	.40	1.76	.80	1.82	2.20*
Independent	.35	.49	—[b]	—[b]	1.14	—[b]	—[b]	.46	—[b]	—[b]

[a] All computations without the Ainsworth et al. (1978) sample.

[b] No variation in the moderator variable.

$^{*}p < .05$; $^{**}p < .01$; $^{***}p < .001$.

TABLE 3
Stem and Leaf Display of Effect Sizes for the Association between Sensitivity, Contiguity, and Attachment (*r*)

	Leaf	
Stem[a]	Sensitivity[b]	Contiguity
.9		
.8		
.7	8[c]	
.6	5, 8	
.5	1	0
.4	1, 3, 4	8
.3	0, 2, 3, 4	
.2	0, 1, 3, 5, 6, 6, 7	3, 9
.1	2, 4, 4, 5, 6, 7, 8, 9	0, 5
.0	0, 0, 4, 4	0, 0, 1, 5, 6, 7, 8
−.1	2	7

[a]The stem contains the first digit of the correlation coefficient, whereas the leaf contains the second digit.
[b]Underscored figures indicate studies with the Ainsworth et al. (1978) rating scale for sensitivity.
[c]Ainsworth et al. (1978).

study, as well as the Seifer et al. (1996) study with a negative correlation between sensitivity and attachment.

Socioeconomic status appeared to be a significant moderator for the 30 studies assessing sensitivity as defined by Ainsworth et al. (1978) ($z = 2.41$; see Table 2). In the 18 middle-class samples, the effect size was $r(886) = .27$ ($N = 888$), whereas in the eight lower-class samples, this figure was $r(650) = .15$ ($N = 652$). Samples without clearly specified or homogeneous socioeconomic status (e.g., variability from lower to higher class) were excluded from these analyses.

The age of the infants at the time of the sensitivity assessment was also a significant moderator ($z = 2.56$). Contrary to our expectation, samples with older infants (older than 1 year) showed stronger effect sizes, $r(1{,}062) = .27$ ($k = 11$) than samples with younger infants, $r(602) = .20$ ($k = 19$). Also, the age of the infants at the time of the attachment assessment was a significant moderator ($z = 2.31$). Samples with older infants showed stronger effect sizes, $r(847) = .25$ ($k = 16$) than samples with younger infants, $r(817) = .19$ ($k = 14$). A shorter time interval between the sensitivity and attachment assessments led to stronger effect sizes ($z = 2.69$) in the total set of sensitivity studies.

CONTIGUITY OF RESPONSE. In Table 3, a stem and leaf display of the effect sizes for the Contiguity studies is presented. Three moderators were important: Whether contiguity of response was assessed globally ($z = 2.34$), the age of the infant at the contiguity assessment ($z = 2.58$), and the time interval between the contiguity and attachment assessments

($z = 2.97$). More global assessments, $r(363) = .08$ ($k = 8$), showed weaker associations than more specific assessments, $r(458) = .15$ ($k = 8$). Contrary to the moderator results in the domain of sensitivity, a longer time interval, $r(352) = .16$ ($k = 6$), led to a stronger effect size than a shorter interval, $r(469) = .06$ ($k = 9$), and samples with younger infants, $r(501) = .13$ ($k = 7$), yielded somewhat stronger associations than samples with older infants, $r(320) = .06$ ($k = 7$).

COOPERATION. Two moderators were significant ($z = 2.10$ and $z = 2.59$, respectively): Studies with special samples revealed weaker effect sizes, $r(223) = .03$ ($k = 4$), than studies with normal samples, $r(266) = .20$($k = 5$). Global assessments of Coopertion yielded weaker effect sizes, $r(360) = .05$ ($k = 6$), than specific assessments, $r(357) = .32$ ($k = 2$). These results need to be interpreted with caution, however, because only nine studies were included in this dataset. For this small dataset, a stem and leaf display is not presented.

POSITIVE ATTITUDE. Special samples showed significantly ($z = 2.78$) weaker associations between Positive Attitude and attachment, $r(337) = .08$ ($k = 6$), than normal samples, $r(758) = .23$ ($k = 15$). Studies using global attitude assessments, $r(546) = .21$ ($k = 11$), showed significantly stronger effect sizes ($z = 2.09$) than studies with specific assessments, $r(357) = .06$ ($k = 6$).

STIMULATION. Contrary to our expectation, studies on attachment and stimulation at home revealed weaker associations, $r(229) = .07$ ($k = 5$), than studies carried out in the laboratory, $r(169) = .31$ ($k = 3$). Longer intervals again led to smaller effect sizes than shorter intervals ($z = 2.20$). This set of studies was rather small.

The moderator analyses did not uncover significant moderators in the domains of Physical Contact and Emotional Support. In the domain of Synchrony, only sample size appeared to be a relevant moderator. The domain of Mutuality consisted of only three studies; the Smith and Pederson (1988) study showed the strongest effect size, and the characteristics of this study determined the outcome of the moderator analysis.

SYNCHRONY, MUTUALITY, AND EMOTIONAL SUPPORT. The three domains Synchrony, Mutuality, and Emotional Support were considered to be the "more optimal" cluster. In Table 4, the stem and leaf display of the effect sizes in this domain is presented. There were no negative effect sizes, and again, the Ainsworth et al. (1978) study occupied a somewhat outlying position.

We performed a moderator analysis on this cluster because its outcome would be more robust ($k = 28$). Publication status of the study ($z = 2.23$) was a significant moderator. Seven unpublished studies yielded a combined effect size of $r(861) = .11$, whereas the 21 published studies yielded a combined effect size of $r(1{,}063) = .25$.

POSITIVE ATTITUDE AND STIMULATION. The less optimal group was a combination of the domains Positive Attitude and Stimulation ($k = 24$). In Table 4, the stem and leaf display of the effect sizes in this domain is presented. The Ainsworth et al. (1978) study is somewhat of an outlier. Significant moderators were: clinical status ($z = 2.50$), time interval ($z = 2.38$), and global versus specific assessment of maternal behavior assessment ($z = 2.03$). In the 18 normal samples, the combined effect size was $r(896) = .22$, whereas in the six clinical samples it was $r(333) = .10$. Longer time intervals led to somewhat smaller effect sizes than shorter time intervals ($z = 2.38$). Thirteen studies in which maternal behavior was assessed

TABLE 4
Stem and Leaf Display of Effect Sizes for the Association between the Less Optimal Cluster (Positive Attitude, Stimulation), the More Optimal Cluster (Synchrony, Mutuality, Support) and Attachment (r)

	Leaf	
Stem[a]	Less Optimal Cluster	More Optimal Cluster
.9		
.8		
.7	5[b]	7[b]
.6	6	2, 6, 6
.5		
.4	5	7
.3	1, 4, 9	1, 1, 5, 8
.2	2, 3, 3, 4, 6, 6, 7	0, 1, 2, 4, 6, 7
.1	1, 2, 3, 4, 6, 8, 8, 9	0, 2, 4, 5, 6, 7, 9
.0	0, 0, 1, 9	0, 0, 0, 0, 5, 9, 9

[a]The stem contains the first digit of the correlation coefficient, whereas the leaf contains the second digit.
[b]Ainsworth et al. (1978).

globally showed a combined $r(681) = .22$, and the six studies in which maternal behavior was assessed in a specific way yielded a combined $r(342) = .06$.

SPECIAL SAMPLES. In two domains, Cooperation and Positive Attitude, the clinical status of the samples appeared to be a significant moderator: Normal samples revealed stronger associations between attachment and parenting than did special samples. We hypothesized that relatively "mild" factors such as prematurity and adoption have no moderating effect on study outcome, whereas more severe factors like deafness, autism, and maltreatment lead to a weaker association between maternal behavior and attachment. All of the studies using special or clinical groups were combined ($k = 10$). These studies were divided into groups on the basis of whether the sample involved was "mildly" clinical or more severely clinical. However, this distinction did not prove to be a significant moderator variable ($z = .84$, $p = .20$), although the trend was clearly in favor of the hypothesis. The six mildly clinical samples (four premature samples and two adoption samples) yielded a combined effect size of $r(265) = .26$, and four severely clinical samples (maltreatment, cleft palate, deafness, and autism) showed a combined effect size of $r(218) = .16$.

Discussion

Maternal sensitivity, defined as the ability to respond appropriately and promptly to the signals of the infant, indeed appears to be an important condition for the development of attachment security. For the 30 pertinent studies, the combined effect size was $r(1{,}664) = .22$ ($N = 1{,}666$). Including only the 21 studies using the Strange Situation procedure in nonclinical samples, as well as applying observational sensitivity measures preceding or concurrent with the attachment assessment, we found a combined effect size of $r(1{,}097) = .20$ ($N = 1{,}099$). Applying the Hunter and Schmidt (1990) procedures of correcting results for attenuation based on the reliabilities of the measures (mean reliability of the sensitivity measures was .83, and mean reliability of the Strange Situation procedure was .81), we found a "true" population effect size for the association between attachment and sensitivity of $r(1{,}097) = .24$. The 16 studies using the original Ainsworth et al. (1974) sensitivity scale also showed a combined effect size of $r(835) = .24$ ($N = 837$). Cohen (1988, p. 82) has proposed criteria for small, medium, and large effect sizes ($d = .20$, $d = .50$, and $d = .80$, respectively) corresponding to correlations of .10, .24, and .37, respectively. According to these criteria, the size of the association between sensitivity and attachment in the replication studies is medium. After more than 25 years of research, Bowlby's (1969) important question about the role of sensitivity in the development of infant attachment can therefore be answered in the affirmative.

Cohen's (1988) criteria are rather arbitrary, however, even according to the originator (Cohen, 1962). Several authors argue that criteria for the statistical magnitude of effect sizes are not equivalent to criteria for their theoretical or practical importance (Abelson, 1995; Prentice & Miller, 1992; Sechrest & Yeaton, 1982). Rosenthal (1990) criticized simplistic interpretation of the squared correlation coefficient in terms of percentage of explained variation: "From under-graduate days on we have been taught that there is only one proper thing to do when we see a correlation coefficient: We must square it" (Rosenthal, 1990, p. 775). This approach ignores, among other things, the ceiling effect imposed by measurement error. Rosenthal and Rubin's (1982) Binomial Effect Size Display (BESD) is an alternative interpretation of effect sizes. The BESD depicts an effect size (r) in terms of the improvement rate that is attributable to the predictor variable. Applying this approach to the findings of the current meta-analyses, the correlation of $r = .24$ for those studies closely resembling the original Baltimore study represents an improvement in security from 38% to 62%; that is, infants whose mothers respond sensitively to their signals improve their chance of developing a secure relationship from 38% to 62%, whereas infants whose mothers are less sensitive decrease their chance of developing a secure relationship from 62% to 38%. This improvement rate can hardly be considered trivial in a theoretical or practical sense, in particular when we compare this effect size with famous examples from medical research, such as the widely used heart failure reducing drugs Propranolol ($r = .04$) and aspirin ($r = .03$) (Gage, 1996; Rosenthal, 1991).

We therefore cannot agree with Goldsmith and Alansky's (1987) conclusion that there is only a weak association between sensitivity and attachment. In 12 studies, they found an overall effect size of $r = .16$ (without the Ainsworth et al. [1978] study), which is remarkably similar to our overall combined effect size across all study outcomes, $r(7{,}223) = .17$. First, on the basis of the BESD approach, we are inclined to be more impressed with this overall effect size than Goldsmith and Alansky (1987) were. Second, our combined effect size represents somewhat stricter replication studies of the original Baltimore study. Goldsmith and Alansky (1987) derived their combined effect size from 12 studies in which a variety of parenting measures had been examined in relation to attachment security. These disparate measures were combined in a single meta-analysis. For example, behavioral categories such as the frequency of maternal looking or vocalizing were combined with Ainsworth's rating scale for sensitivity. We showed that Contiguity of response is significantly less strongly associated with attachment security than Sensitivity, and that the moderator analysis in the former domain leads to opposite outcomes, in particular with respect to infants' age and time interval between assessments. Hedges (1986) argued that the results of meta-analyses using broad constructs may obscure important differences among narrower constructs subsumed under the broad construct. He recommended including broad constructs in the meta-analysis, but distinguishing narrower constructs in the data and presentation of results.

Third, moderately strong—and even weak—correlations may nevertheless indicate powerful causal mechanisms. The current meta-analyses are based on correlational studies—like the Baltimore study—and it is therefore impossible to derive causal conclusions from its outcome (Cook et al., 1992; Miller & Pollock, 1994; Stroebe & Diehl, 1991). Although most studies on attachment and sensitivity are predictive in the sense that earlier assessments of sensitivity were correlated with subsequent attachment assessments, a requirement of causality is the absence of a third factor explaining the association between sensitivity and attachment. In their meta-analysis of attachment intervention studies, van IJzendoorn et al. (1995) showed that interventions are effective in enhancing maternal sensitivity, and that, in particular, short-term interventions focusing on maternal sensitivity can enhance infants' attachment security. The combined effect size for the effectiveness of the attachment interventions was $d = .48$, which is a medium effect (Cohen, 1988). In fact, the short-term interventions may be considered to be a minimal manipulation of the predictor that still accounts for significant variance in the criterion. Prentice and Miller (1992) argue that this is a plausible reason for interpreting effect sizes as important even when they are small. Combined with the outcome of the current meta-analyses, this attests to the important, but not exclusive, causal role of sensitivity in the development of infant attachment (Ainsworth et al., 1978; Bowlby, 1969).

GENERAL DISCUSSION

Although our results appear to support the "orthodox" position that maternal sensitivity is an important condition of attachment security, the outcome of the Baltimore study itself cannot be considered to be replicated (Goldsmith & Alansky, 1987; Lamb et al., 1985). In the Baltimore study, an effect size of $r(21) = .78$ was found for the association between sensitivity and attachment, which is rather different from the combined effect size of the replication studies, $r(1{,}097) = .24$. Correcting the Baltimore correlation for predictor and criterion unreliability (.89 and .95, respectively) yields a corrected $r(21) = .85$. Logically, a correlation of this impressive magnitude seems to indicate close similarity of the constructs and/or the assessments of attachment and sensitivity rather than an association between independent variables. Furthermore, in a small sample, confidence boundaries around estimated correlations are broad, and outlying observations may be rather influential. Even replication studies with similar longitudinal and intensive designs have failed to replicate the exceptionally strong and striking results of the Baltimore study (e.g., Grossmann et al., 1985; Hubbard & van IJzendoorn, 1991). Paradoxically, the strength of the Baltimore results may have inspired many researchers to document the association between sensitivity and attachment, and at the same time its exploratory design and the size of its results prevented them from strictly replicating the original effect size. Without the Baltimore study, the solid scientific fact of a moderately strong causal association between sensitivity and attachment would not have been established.

The current meta-analyses qualify the original Baltimore results in yet another way. Sensitivity cannot be considered to be the exclusive and most important factor in the development of attachment. Several domains of maternal interactive behavior showed effect sizes that were similar to those for the domain of Sensitivity. For example, Mutuality and Synchrony were quite strongly associated with attachment security, $rs(166, 256) = .32$ and .26, respectively, as were Stimulation, Positive Attitude, and Emotional Support. Contrary to our expectation, the combined effect size of the more optimal cluster of studies on aspects of parenting more closely resembling sensitivity, $r(1{,}926) = .19$, did not differ from the outcome of the less optimal cluster, $r(1{,}231) = .19$. That is, aspects of parenting only indirectly related to the sensitivity concept appear to play a similar role in the development of attachment. The modest correlations between the various aspects of parenting and sensitivity leave room for unique and additional influences on attachment. In six studies, sensitivity was correlated with six other aspects of parenting: mean $r(358) = .34$ ($N = 360$). The original concept of sensitivity may not capture the only mechanism through which the development of attachment is shaped (van IJzendoorn, 1995), and studies combining the promising measures may provide more insight into the additional explanatory value of these alternative approaches over and above sensitivity. Sensitivity has lost its privileged position as the only important causal factor. A multidimensional approach of parenting antecedents should replace the search for the unique contribution of sensitivity. It should be noted that in the current set of attachment studies the concept of parenting is virtually limited to the general domain of parental warmth and acceptance, rather than parental management and control. It is therefore unclear whether these latter aspects of parenting would also contribute to the development of attachment, in particular, after the first year of life.

Contrary to our expectations, the duration of home observations was not related to the magnitude of the association between sensitivity and attachment. It did not appear to matter whether studies were conducted in the laboratory or in the home, except in the case of maternal stimulation. The use of the standard Strange Situation procedure did not lead to different effect sizes compared to the use of alternative attachment measures. The intensive naturalistic design of the Baltimore study does not seem to be essential for the strength of the association between parenting and attachment found in the replication studies. It should be kept in mind, however, that only few replications indeed used an exactly similar design. Furthermore, in samples with younger infants, somewhat weaker associations between sensitivity and attachment tended to be found. Contrary to our hypothesis based on the Baltimore study, we suggest post hoc that these results are theoretically congruent with Bowlby's (1973) view of the development of attachment as contextually labile and flexible in the early years. Because the security of attachment is a characteristic of the dyad more than of the infant in the early years, the development of attachment can easily change direction when family life circumstances, childrearing arrangements or maternal sensitivity change (Thompson, in press; Thompson & Lamb, 1983; Thompson, Lamb, & Estes, 1982). Sensitivity may be an important condition of attachment security only when it remains stable across time, which may occur only in a stable social context (Lamb et al., 1985; Sroufe, 1988).

In this respect, it is important to note that the association between maternal behavior and infant attachment is significantly weaker in studies of lower-class or clinical samples. The measures of maternal behavior and attachment security have been developed and validated in nonclinical, middle-class samples, and they may be less valid in lower-class and clinical samplcs. We also want to suggest that the formation of attachment relationships under complex lower-class or clinical conditions may not be adequately explained in a monocausal and linear way. In their quasi-experimental study of family-based and communal kibbutzim, Sagi and his colleagues (Sagi, van IJzendoorn, Aviezer, Donnell, & Mayseless, 1994) showed that maternal sensitivity may be overridden by an unfavorable childrearing arrangement in which infants have to sleep away from home, and therefore often develop insecure attachments. In a similar vein, it may be expected that the strains and stresses of lower-class life or the problems presented by clinical conditions may overburden potentially sensitive mothers. Davies and Cummings (1994), for example, suggested that unresolved marital conflicts may have a profound negative effect on the children's emotional security even if the bond with the mother is balanced and her interaction style toward the child is sensitive. They proposed to study the development of emotional (in-)security from a family-wide perspective (Cummings & Davies, 1996). The transactions between social context or clinical conditions, on the one hand, and attachment on the other need more careful study to determine the role of sensitivity, and other aspects of parenting and family life in the development of attachment security more precisely (Belsky & Cassidy, 1994; Egeland & Erickson, 1993; Sameroff & Chandler, 1975; Thompson, in press). In attachment theory, a move to the level of context may be necessary, so that the interaction between maternal sensitivity and the accumulation of stresses and risk factors in lower-class or clinical groups can be taken into account.

Even in "normal," nonclinical groups, sensitivity plays an important but not exclusive role in the emergence of attachment security. In cognitive development, genetics may constitute a ceiling effect for the influence of environmental factors, for which less than 50% of the variation in individual differences appears to be left (Plomin, 1994). Attachment security, however, does not seem to be genetically determined in any comparable way. The first, small-scale twin studies on attachment reported only 30%–50% congruence of attachment classifications (Minde, Corter, Goldberg, & Jeffers, 1990; Szajnberg, Skrinjaric, & Moore, 1989; Vandell, Owen, Wilson, & Henderson, 1988). A secondary analysis of the available twin data ($N = 56$) did not support the idea of a genetic basis for individual differences in attachment security (Ricciuti, 1993). Only the variable representing the split between the Strange Situation subclassifications A1-B2 and B3-C2 showed significant genetic influence. This may be due to temperament (e.g., emotional reactivity), which has been shown to be associated with this split (Belsky & Rovine, 1987). Although more research in this area in needed, we suggest that attachment security is especially liable to nongenetic, environmental influences. Nevertheless, behavior genetics may inspire a move toward the contextual level in a specific sense. One of the most intriguing findings of behavior genetics is the crucial role of nonshared environment for child development. Unrelated adoptive siblings appear to develop quite differently, even though they are raised in the same, shared family environment. For example, the correlation between IQ of adoptive siblings is approaching zero when they grow older (Plomin, 1994). In the case of parenting and attachment, the concept of nonshared environmental influences may, for example, lead to more emphasis on the family system and on life events. Although parents may interact equally sensitively with both siblings at the same age, the older sibling also experiences the parents interacting sensitively with the younger sibling—which is a unique and potentially powerful experience that never has been studied thoroughly (Dunn & Plomin, 1990). Life events such as parental loss of attachment figures may affect siblings in different ways, depending on their age. If parents suffered bereavement within 2 years after the birth of a sibling, this sibling—but not the other siblings—may develop dissociative tendencies that may be related to insecure-disorganized attachment (Hesse & van IJzendoorn, 1996; Liotti, 1992). After more than 25 years of research on the important dimension of sensitivity, a move to the level of (nonshared) context should inspire the next wave of studies on the antecedents of attachment security.

REFERENCES[1]

Abelson, R. P. (1995). *Statistics as principled argument.* Hillsdale, NJ: Erlbaum.

Ainsworth, M. D. S., Bell, S. M., & Stayton, D. J. (1974). Infant-mother attachment and social development: "Socialization" as a product of reciprocal responsiveness to signals. In M. P. M. Richards (Ed.), *The integration of a child into a social world* (pp. 99–135). Cambridge: Cambridge University Press.

Ainsworth, M. D. S., Blehar, M. C., Waters, E., & Wall, S. (1978). *Patterns of attachment: A psychological study of the Strange Situation.* Hillsdale, NJ: Erlbaum.

Ainsworth, M. D. S., & Wittig, B. A. (1969). Attachment and exploratory behavior of one-year-olds in a Strange Situation. In B. M. Foss (Ed.), *Determinants of infant behaviour* (Vol. *4*, pp. 11–136). London: Methuen.

Aldenderfer, M. S., & Blashfield, R. K. (1984). *Cluster analysis.* Beverly Hills, CA: Sage.

Altman, S., Monk, C., Jones, P., & Sosa, L. (1993, March). *Children's working models of attachment at 42 months and maternal attitudes and behavior.* Poster presented at the meetings of the Society for Research in Child Development, New Orleans, LA. [7].*

Amato, P. R., & Keith, B. (1991). Parental divorce and the well-being of children: A meta-analysis. *Psychological Bulletin, 110,* 26–46.

Anisfeld, E., Casper, V., Nozyce, M., & Cunningham, N. (1990). Does infant carrying promote attachment? An experimental study of the effects of the increased physical contact on the development of attachment. *Child Development, 61,* 1617–1627. [1, 2].*

Antonucci, T. C., & Levitt, M. J. (1984). Early prediction of attachment security: A multivariate approach. *Infant Behavior and Development, 7,* 1–18. [3, 5].*

Bates, J. E., Maslin, C. A., & Frankel, K. A. (1985). Attachment security, mother-child interaction, and temperament as predictors of behavior-problem ratings at the age of three years. In I. Bretherton & E. Waters (Eds.), Growing points in attachment theory and research (pp. 167–193). *Monographs of the Society for Research in Child Development, 50*(1–2, Serial No. 209). [2, 7, 8].*

[1]References marked with an asterisk indicate studies included in the meta-analyses. We also indicated after these references the numbers of the meta-analytic domains for which the particular study has provided data. The numbers refer to the following meta-analytic domains: (1) Sensitivity, (2) Responsiveness, (3) Physical Contact, (4) Cooperation, (5) Synchrony, (6) Mutuality, (7) Support, (8) Attitude, and (9) Stimulation.

Belsky, J., & Cassidy, J. (1994). Attachment: Theory and evidence. In M. Rutter, D. Hay, & S. Baron-Cohen (Eds.), *Developmental principles and clinical issues in psychology and psychiatry* (pp. 373–402). Oxford: Blackwell.

Belsky, J., & Rovine, M. (1987). Temperament and attachment security in the Strange Situation: An empirical rapprochement. *Child Development, 58*, 787–795.

Belsky, J., & Rovine, M., & Taylor, D. G. (1984). The Pennsylvania Infant and Family Development Project, III: The origins of individual differences in infant-mother attachment: Maternal and infant contributions. *Child Development, 55*, 718–728. [2, 5, 7, 9].*

Benn, R. K. (1986). Factors promoting secure attachment relationships between employed mothers and their sons. *Child Development, 57*, 1224–1231. [1, 8].*

Bohlin, G., Hagekull, B., Germer, M., Andersson, K., & Lindberg, L. (1989). Avoidant and resistant behaviors as predicted by maternal interactive behavior and infant temperament. *Infant Behavior and Development, 12*, 105–117. [1, 2, 3, 4].*

Booth, C. L., Rose-Krasnor, L., & Rubin, K. H. (1991). Relating preschoolers' social competence and their mothers' parenting behaviors to early attachment security and high-risk status. *Journal of Social and Personal Relationships, 8*, 363–382. [7].*

Bornstein, M. H. (Ed.). (1989). Maternal responsiveness: Characteristics and consequences. *New Directions for Child Development*. San Francisco: Jossey-Bass.

Bowlby, J. (1969). *Attachment and loss: Vol. 1. Attachment* (rev. ed.). Harmondsworth: Penguin.

Bowlby, J. (1973). *Attachment and loss: Vol. 2. Separation: Anxiety and anger*. Harmondsworth: Penguin.

Bretherton, I. (1985). Attachment theory: Retrospect and prospect. In I. Bretherton & E. Waters (Eds.), Growing points in attachment theory and research (pp. 3–38). *Monographs of the Society for Research in Child Development, 50*(1–2, Serial No. 209).

Bretherton, I., Biringen, Z., Ridgeway, D., Maslin, C., & Sherman, M. (1989). Attachment: The parental perspective. *Infant Mental Health Journal, 10*, 203–221. [1].*

Burchinal, M. R., Bryant, D. M., Lee, M. W., & Ramey, C. T. (1992). Early day-care, infant-mother attachment, and maternal responsiveness in the infant's first year. *Early Childhood Research Quarterly, 7*, 383–396. [7, 8].*

Butcher, P. R., Kalverboer, A. F., Minderaa, R. B., Van Doormaal, E. F., & Ten Wolde, Y. (1993). Rigidity, sensitivity, and quality of attachment: The role of maternal rigidity in the early socio-emotional development of premature infants. *Acta Psychiatrica Scandinavica, 88*(Suppl. 374), 4–38. [1, 8].*

Caldwell, B. M., & Bradley, R. H. (1984). *Administration manual. Home Observation for Measurement of the Environment*. Little Rock: Department of Psychology, University of Arkansas.

Camfield, E., Brownell, C., Taylor, P., Day, N., Brown, E., & Kratzer. L. (1991, April). *Mediators of relations between maternal behavior at 4 months and infant attachment at 12 months*. Poster presented at the meetings of the Society for Research in Child Development, Seattle. [2, 7].*

Capps, L., Sigman, M., & Mundy, P. (1994). Attachment security in children with autism. *Development and Psychopathology, 6*, 249–261. [1].*

Cohen, J. (1962). The statistical power of abnormal social psychology research: A review. *Journal of Abnormal and Social Psychology, 65*, 145–153.

Cohen, J. (1988). *Statistical power analysis for the behavioral sciences* (rev. ed.). New York: Academic Press.

Cook, T. D., Cooper, H., Cordray, D. F., Hartman, H., Hedges, L. V., Louis, T. A., & Mosteller, F. (1992). *Meta-analysis for explanation: A casebook.* New York: Russell Sage.

Cooper, H., & Hedges, L. V. (Eds.). (1994). *The handbook for research synthesis.* New York: Russell Sage.

Cox, M. J., Owen, M. T., Henderson, V. K., & Margand, N. A. (1992). Prediction of infant-father and infant-mother attachment. *Developmental Psychology, 28,* 474–483. [3, 7, 8].*

Crockenberg, S. B. (1981). Infant irritability, mother responsiveness, and social support influences on the security of infant-mother attachment. *Child Development, 52,* 857–865. [2].*

Cummings, E. M., & Davies, P. T. (1996). Emotional security as a regulatory process in normal development and the development of psychopathology. *Development and Psychopathology, 7,* 123–139.

Davies, P. T., & Cummings, E. M. (1994). Marital conflict and child adjustment: An emotional security hypothesis. *Psychological Bulletin, 116,* 387–411.

Del Carmen, R., Pedersen, F., Huffman, L. C., & Bryan, Y. E. (1993). Dyadic distress management predicts subsequent security of attachment. *Infant Behavior and Development, 16,* 131–147. [2, 8, 9].*

Dunn, J., & Plomin, R. (1990). *Separate lives: Why siblings are so different.* New York: Basic.

Easterbrooks, M. A., & Goldberg, W. A. (1985). Effects of early maternal employment on toddlers, mothers, and fathers. *Developmental Psychology, 21,* 774–783.

Egeland, B., & Erickson, M. F. (1993). Attachment theory and findings: Implications for prevention and intervention. In S. Kramer & H. Parens (Eds.), *Prevention in mental health: Now, tomorrow, ever?* (pp. 21–50). Northvale, NJ: Jason Aronson.

Egeland, B., & Farber, E. A. (1984). Infant-mother attachment: Factors related to its development and changes over time. *Child Development, 55,* 753–771. [1].*

Erickson, M. F., Sroufe, L. A., & Egeland, B. (1985). The relationship between quality of attachment and behavior problems in preschool in a high-risk sample. In I. Bretherton & E. Waters (Eds.), Growing points in attachment theory and research (pp. 147–166). *Monographs of the Society for Research in Child Development, 50*(1–2, Serial No. 209).

Everitt, B. (1974). *Cluster analysis.* London: Heineman Educational Books.

Fagot, B. I., & Kavanagh, K. (1990). The prediction of antisocial behavior from avoidant attachment classifications. *Child Development, 61,* 864–973. [7, 8].*

Fracasso, M. P., Busch-Rossnagel, N. A., & Fisher, C. B. (1994). The relationship of maternal behavior and acculturation to the quality of attachment in Hispanic infants living in New York city. *Hispanic Journal of Behavioral Sciences, 16,* 143–154. [1].*

Frankel, A., & Bates, J. E. (1990). Mother-toddler problem solving: Antecedents in attachment, home behavior, and temperament. *Child Development, 61,* 810–819. [7].*

Frodi, A., Grolnick, W., & Bridges, L. (1985). Maternal correlates of stability and change in infant-mother attachment. *Infant Mental Health Journal, 6,* 60–67. [1].*

Gage, N. L. (1996). Confronting counsels of despair for the behavioral sciences. *Educational Researcher, 25,* 5–15

Garfield, E. (1979). *Citation indexing: Its theory and application in science, technology, and humanities.* New York: Wiley.

Gewirtz, J. L., & Boyd, E. F. (1977). Does maternal responding imply reduced infant crying? A critique of the 1972 Bell and Ainsworth report. *Child Development, 48,* 1200–1207.

Gifi, A. (1990). *Non-linear multivariate analysis*. New York: Wiley.

Goldberg, S., Perotta, M., Minde, K., & Corter, C. (1986). Maternal behavior and attachment in low-birth-weight twins and singletons. *Child Development*, *57*, 34–46. [1, 2, 3, 4, 7, 8, 9].*

Goldsmith, H. H., & Alansky, J. A. (1987). Maternal and infant predictors of attachment: A meta-analytic review. *Journal of Consulting and Clinical Psychology*, *55*, 805–816.

Goodman, G., Andrews, T., Jones, S., Weissman, J., & Weissman, A. (1993). *Maternal play behavior and children's representations as mediators of developmental outcomes among high-risk dyads*. Manuscript in preparation. [1].*

Goossens, F. A. (1987). Kwaliteit van de hechtingsrelatie van jonge kinderen aan hun moeder, vader en crècheleidster. [Quality of infants' attachment to father, mother, and caregiver in daycare]. *Nederlands Tijdschrift voor de Psychologie*, *42*, 308–320. [1].*

Grossmann, K., Grossmann, K. E., Spangler, G., Suess, G., & Unzner, L. (1985). Maternal sensitivity and newborns' orientation responses as related to quality of attachment in northern Germany. In I. Bretherton & E. Waters (Eds.), Growing points in attachment theory and research (pp. 233–268). *Monographs of the Society for Research in Child Development, 50*(1–2, Serial No. 209). [1].*

Gunnar, M. R., Brodersen, L., Nachmias, M., Buss, K., & Rigatuso, J. (1996). Stress reactivity and attachment security. *Developmental Psychobiology*, *29*, 191–204. [1].*

Hedges, L. V. (1986). Issues in meta-analysis. *Review of Research in Education*, *13*, 353–399.

Hedges, L. V., & Olkin, I. (1985). *Statistical methods for meta-analysis*. Orlando, FL: Academic Press.

Hesse, E., & van IJzendoorn, M. H. (1996). *Parental loss of close family members within two years preceding or following participants' birth is related to absorption*. Unpublished manuscript, Center for Child and Family Studies, Leiden University.

Hoeksma, J. B., & Koomen, M. M. Y. (1991). *Development of early mother-child interactions and attachment*. Unpublished doctoral dissertation, Free University of Amsterdam, The Netherlands. [1, 6].*

Hubbard, F. O. A., & van IJzendoorn, M. H. (1991). Maternal unresponsiveness and infant crying across the first nine months: A naturalistic longitudinal study. *Infant Behavior and Development*, *14*, 299–312.

Hunter, J. E., & Schmidt, F. L. (1990). *Methods of meta-analysis: Correcting error and bias in research findings*. Beverly Hills, CA: Sage.

Isabella, R. A. (1993). Origins of attachment: Maternal interactive behavior across the first year. *Child Development*, *64*, 605–621. [1, 8, 9].*

Isabella, R. A., & Belsky, J. (1991). Interactional synchrony and the origins of infant-mother attachment: A replication study. *Child Development*, *62*, 373–384. [5].*

Isabella, R. A., Belsky, J., & Von Eye, A. (1989). Origins of infant-mother attachment: an examination of interactional synchrony during the infant's first year. *Developmental Psychology*, *25*, 12–21. [5]*

Izard, C. E., Heynes, O. M., Chisholm, G., & Baak, K. (1991). Emotional determinants of infant-mother attachment. *Child Development*, *62*, 906–917. [8].*

Johnson, B. T., Mullen, B., & Salas, E. (1995). Comparison of three meta-analytic approaches. *Journal of Applied Psychology*, *80*, 94–106.

Juffer, F. (1993). *Verbonden door adoptie: Een experimenteel onderzoek bij gezinnen met een adoptiebaby*. [Attached through adoption: An experimental study on attachment and competence in families with an adopted baby]. Amersfoort, The Netherlands: Academische Uitgeverij. [1, 4].*

Kerns, K. A., & Barth, J. M. (1995). Attachment and play: Convergence across components of parent-child relationships and their relations to peer competence. *Journal of Social and Personal Relationships, 12*, 243–260. [3].*

Kiser, L. J., Bates, J. E., Maslin, C. A., & Bayles, K. (1986). Mother-infant play at six months as a predictor of attachment security of thirteen months. *Journal of the American Academy of Child Psychiatry, 25*, 68–75. [6].*

Krentz, M. S. (1982). *Qualitative differences between mother-child and caregiver-child attachment of infant in family day care*. Unpublished doctoral dissertation, California School of Professional Psychology. [2, 7].*

Kveton, E. M. (1989). The quality of infant-parent attachment at 17 months as related to the quality of parent-infant interaction and prenatal parenting attitudes (Doctoral dissertation, Virginia Consortium for Professional Psychology, 1989). *Dissertation Abstracts International,s 50*, 5884B. [1].*

Lamb, M. E., Hopps, K., & Elster, A. B. (1987). Strange Situation behavior of infants with adolescent mothers. *Infant Behavior and Development, 10*, 39–48. [2, 5, 8, 9].*

Lamb, M. E., Thompson, R. A., Gardner, W., & Charnov, E. L. (1985). *Infant-mother attachment: The origins and developmental significance of individual differences in Strange Situation behavior*. Hillsdale, NJ: Erlbaum.

Lambermon, M. W. E. (1991). *Video of folder? Korte-en langetermijn effecten van voorlichting over vroegkinderlijke opvoeding*. [Video or booklet? Short-term and long-term effects of information about early childhood education]. Unpublished doctoral dissertation, University of Leiden, The Netherlands. [1, 7].*

Lederberg, A. R., & Mobley, C. E. (1990). The effect of hearing impairment on the quality of attachment and mother-toddler interaction. *Child Development, 61*, 1596–1604. [4, 7, 8, 9].*

Lewis, M., & Feiring, C. (1989). Infant, mother, and mother-infant interaction behavior and subsequent attachment. *Child Development, 60*, 831–837. [2, 3].*

Lieberman, A. F., Weston, D. R., & Pawl, J. H. (1991). Preventive intervention and outcome with anxiously attached dyads. *Child Development, 62*, 199–209. [7, 9].*

Liotti, G. (1992). Disorganized/disoriented attachment in the etiology of the dissociative disorders. *Dissociation, 5*, 196–204.

Londerville, S., & Main, M. (1981). Security of attachment, compliance, and maternal training methods in the second year of life. *Developmental Psychology, 17*, 289–299. [4].*

Lyons-Ruth, K., Connell, D. B., Zoll, D., & Stahl, J. (1987). Infants at social risk: Relations among infant maltreatment, maternal behavior, and infant attachment behavior. *Developmental Psychology, 23*, 223–232. [1, 3, 4, 8].*

Main, M. (1990). Cross-cultural studies of attachment organization: Recent studies, changing methodologies, and the concept of conditional strategies. *Human Development, 33*, 48–61.

Main, M., Tomasini, L., & Tolan, W. (1979). Differences among mothers of infants judged to differ in security. *Developmental Psychology, 15*, 472–473. [1, 3, 8].*

Malatesta, C. Z., Culver, C., Tesman, C., & Shepard, B. (1989). The development of emotion expression during the first two years of life. *Monographs for the Society for Research in Child Development, 54*(1–2, Serial No. 219). [8].*

Mangelsdorf, S., Gunnar, M., Kestenbaum, R., Lang, S., & Andreas, D. (1990). Infant proneness to distress temperament, maternal personality, and mother-infant attachment: Associations and goodness of fit. *Child Development, 61*, 820–831. [7].*

Matas, L., Arend, R. A., & Sroufe, L. A. (1978). The relationship between quality of attachment and later competence. *Child Development, 49*, 547–556. [7].*

Meij, J. (1991). *Sociale ondersteuning, gehechtheidskwaliteit en vroegkinderlijke competentie-ontwikkeling*. [Social support, quality of attachment, and early development of competence in infants]. Unpublished doctoral dissertation, University of Nijmegen, The Netherlands. [1].*

Miller, N., & Pollock, V. E. (1994). Meta-analytic synthesis for theory development. In H. Cooper & L. V. Hedges (Eds.), *The handbook of research synthesis* (pp. 457–483). New York: Russell Sage.

Minde, K., Corter, C., Goldberg, S., & Jeffers, D. (1990). Maternal preference between premature twins up to age four. *Journal of the American Academy of Child and Adolescent Psychiatry, 29*, 367–374.

Miyake, K., Chen, S. J., & Campos, J. J. (1985). Infant temperament, mother's mode of interaction, and attachment in Japan: An interim report. In I. Bretherton & E. Waters (Eds.), Growing points in attachment theory and research (pp. 276–297). *Monographs of the Society for Research in Child Development, 50*(1–2, Serial No. 209). [2, 4, 7, 9].*

Mullen, B. (1989). *Advanced BASIC meta-analysis*. Hillsdale, NJ: Erlbaum.

Nakagawa, M., Lamb, M. E., & Miyake, K. (1992). Antecedents and correlates of the Strange Situation behavior of Japanese infants. *Journal of Cross-Cultural Psychology, 23*, 300–310. [1, 4, 7, 8].*

NICHD Early Child Care Network. (1996, April). *Infant child care and attachment security: Results of the NICHD study of early child care*. Symposium presented at the International Conference on Infant Studies, Providence, RI. [7].*

Pederson, D. R., & Moran, G. (1996). Expressions of the attachment relationship outside of the Strange Situation. *Child Development, 67*, 915–967. [1].*

Pederson, D. R., Moran, G., Sitko, C., Campbell, K., Ghesquire, K., & Acton, H. (1990). Maternal sensitivity and the security of infant-mother attachment: A Q-sort study. *Child Development, 61*, 1974–1983. [1].*

Persson-Blennow, I., Binett, B., & McNeil, T. F. (1988). Offspring of women with nonorganic psychosis: Antecedents of anxious attachment to the mother at one year of age. *Acta Psychiatrica Scandinavica, 78*, 66–71. [2, 3, 8].*

Plomin, R. (1994). The Emanuel Miller Memorial Lecture 1993: Genetic research and identification of environmental influences. *Journal of Child Psychology and Psychiatry, 35*, 817–834.

Prentice, D. A., & Miller, D. A. (1992). When small effects are impressive. *Psychological Bulletin, 112*, 160–164.

Ricciuti, A. E. (1993). Child-mother attachment: A twin study. *Dissertation Abstracts International, 54*, 3364.

Roggman, L. A., Langlois, J. H., & Hubbs-Tait, L. (1987). Mothers, infant, and toys: Social play correlates of attachment. *Infant Behavior and Development, 10*, 233–237. [5, 9].*

Rosenboom, L. G. (1994). *Gemengde gezinnen, gemengde gevoelens? Hechting en competentie van adoptiebaby's in gezinnen met biologisch eigen kinderen*. [Mixed families, mixed feelings? Attachment and competence of adopted babies in families with biological children]. Unpublished doctoral dissertation, University of Utrecht, The Netherlands. [1, 7].*

Rosenthal, R. (1979). The "file drawer problem" and tolerance for null results. *Psychological Bulletin, 86*, 638–641.

Rosenthal, R. (1990). How are we doing in soft psychology? *American Psychologist, 45*, 775–777.

Rosenthal, R. (1991). *Meta-analytic procedures for social research*. Newbury Park, CA: Sage

Rosenthal, R. (1995). Writing meta-analytic reviews. *Psychological Bulletin, 118*, 183–192.

Rosenthal, R., & Rosnow, R. L. (1985). *Contrast analysis: Focused comparisons in the analysis of variance*. New York: Cambridge University Press.

Rosenthal, R., & Rubin, D. B. (1982). Comparing effect sizes of independent studies. *Psychological Bulletin, 92*, 500–504.

Sagi, A., van IJzendoorn, M. H., Aviezer, O., Donnell, F., & Mayseless, O. (1994). Sleeping out of the home in a kibbutz communal arrangement: It makes a difference for infant-mother attachment. *Child Development, 65*, 992–1004.

Sameroff, A. J., & Chandler, M. J. (1975). Reproductive risk and the continuum of caretaking casualty. In F. D. Horowitz (Ed.), *Review of child development research* (Vol. *4*, pp. 187–244). Chicago: University of Chicago Press.

Schneider Rosen, K., & Rothbaum, F. (1993). Quality of parental caregiving and security of attachment. *Developmental Psychology, 29*, 358–367. [7, 8].*

Schwarzer, R. (1989). *Meta-analysis programs*. Unpublished manual, University of Berlin, Department of Psychology.

Sechrest, L., & Yeaton, W. H. (1982). Magnitudes of experimental effects in social science research. *Evaluation Review, 6*, 579–600.

Seifer, R., Schiller, M., Sameroff, A. J., Resnick, S., & Riordan, K. (1996). Attachment, maternal sensitivity, and infant temperament during the first year of life. *Developmental Psychology, 32*, 12–25. [1].*

Shaw, D. S., & Vondra, J. I. (1995). Infant security and maternal predictors of early behavior problems: A longitudinal study of low-income families. *Journal of Abnormal Child Psychology, 23*, 335–357. [2].*

Smith, P. B., & Pederson, D. R. (1988). Maternal sensitivity and patterns of infant-mother attachment. *Child Development, 59*, 1097–1101. [4, 6].*

SPSS, Inc. (1990). *SPSS categories*. Chicago: SPSS, Inc.

Sroufe, L. A. (1988). The role of infant-caregiver attachment in development. In J. Belsky & T. Nezworski (Eds.), *Clinical implications of attachment* (pp. 18–40). Hillsdale, NJ: Erlbaum.

Stifter, C. A., Couleham, C. M., & Fish, M. (1993). Linking employment to attachment: The mediating effects of maternal separation anxiety and interactive behavior. *Child Development, 64*, 1451–1560. [1, 4].*

Stroebe, W., & Diehl, M. (1991). You can't beat good experiments with correlational evidence: Mullen, Johnson, and Salas' meta-analytic misinterpretations. *Basic and Applied Social Psychology, 12*, 25–32.

Szajnberg, N. M., Skrinjaric, J., & Moore, A. (1989). Affect attunement, attachment, temperament, and zygosity: A twin study. *Journal of the American Academy of Child and Adolescent Psychiatry, 28*, 249–253.

Teti, D. M., Nakagawa, M., Das, R., & Wirth, O. (1991). Security of attachment between preschoolers and their mothers: Relations among social interaction, parenting stress, and mothers' sorts of attachment Q-set. *Developmental Psychology, 27*, 440–447. [7].*

Thompson, R. A. (in press). Early socio-personality development. In W. Damon (Ed.), *Handbook of child psychology: Vol. 3. Social, emotional, and personality development*. New York: Wiley.

Thompson, R. A., & Lamb, M. E. (1983). Security of attachment and stranger sociability in infancy. *Developmental Psychology, 19*, 184–191.

Thompson, R. A., Lamb, M. E., & Estes, D. (1982). Stability of infant-mother attachment and its relation to changing life circumstances in an unselected middle-class sample. *Child Development*, *53*, 144–148.

Ungerer, J. A., Dolby, R., Waters, B., Barnett, B., Kelk, N., Lewin, V., & Blaszczynski, A. (1990). The early development of empathy: Self-regulation and individual differences in the first year. *Motivation and Emotion*, *14*, 93–106. [8].*

Vandell, D. L., Owen, M. T., Wilson, K. S., & Henderson, V. K. (1988). Social development in infant twins: Peer and mother-child relationships. *Child Development*, *59*, 168–177.

van den Boom, D. C. (1988). *Neonatal irritability and the development of attachment: Observation and intervention*. Unpublished doctoral dissertation, University of Leiden, The Netherlands. [1].*

Van der Kloot, W. A., & Van Herk, H. (1991). Multidimensional scaling of sorting data: A comparison of three procedures. *Multivariate Behavioral Research*, *26*, 563–581.

van IJzendoorn, M. H. (1990). Attachment in Surinam-Dutch families: A contribution to the cross-cultural study of attachment. *International Journal of Behavioral Development*, *13*, 333–344. [1].*

van IJzendoorn, M. H. (1995). Adult attachment representations, parental responsiveness, and infant attachment: A meta-analysis on the predictive validity of the Adult Attachment Interview. *Psychological Bulletin*, *117*, 387–403.

van IJzendoorn, M. H., Juffer, F., & Duyvesteyn, M. G. C. (1995). Breaking the intergenerational cycle of insecure attachment: A review of the effects of attachment-based interventions on maternal sensitivity and infant security. *Journal of Child Psychology and Psychiatry*, *36*, 225–248.

van IJzendoorn, M. H., Kranenburg, M. J., Zwart-Woudstra, H. A., Van Busschbach, A. M., & Lambermon, M. W. E. (1991). Parental attachment and children's socio-emotional development: Some findings on the validity of the Adult Attachment Interview in the Netherlands. *International Journal of Behavioral Development*, *14*, 375–394. [1].*

van IJzendoorn, M. H., & Kroonenberg, P. M. (1988). Cross-cultural patterns of attachment. A meta-analysis of the Strange Situation. *Child Development*, *59*, 147–156.

van IJzendoorn, M. H., Vereijken, C. M. J. L., & Riksen-Walraven, J. M. A. (in press). Is the Attachment Q-sort a valid measure of attachment security in young children? In B. E. Vaughn & E. Waters (Eds.), *Patterns of secure base behavior: Q-sort perspectives on attachment and caregiving*. Hillsdale, NJ: Erlbaum.

Vaughn, B. E., & Waters, E. (1990). Attachment behavior at home and in the laboratory: Q-sort observations and Strange Situation classifications of one-year-olds. *Child Development*, *61*, 1965–1973.

Verkes, R. J., Van der Kloot, W. A., & Van der Meij, J. (1989). The perceived structure of 176 pain descriptive words. *Pain*, *38*, 219–229.

Waters, E., & Deane, K. E. (1985). Defining and assessing individual differences in attachment relationships: Q-methodology and the organization of behavior in infancy and early childhood. In I. Bretherton & E. Waters (Eds.), Growing points in attachment theory and research (pp. 39–40). *Monographs of the Society for Research in Child Development*, *50*(1–2, Serial No. 209).

Wille, D. E. (1991). Relation of preterm birth with quality of infant-mother attachment at one year. *Infant Behavior and Development*, *14*, 227–240. [6, 7, 8].*

Zaslow, M. J., Rabinovich, B. A., Suwalsky, J. T. D., & Klein, R. P. (1988). The role of social context in the prediction of secure and insecure/avoidant infant-mother attachment. *Journal of Applied Developmental Psychology*, *9*, 287–299. [3, 7, 8].*

3

Thinking About Fantasy: Are Children Fundamentally Different Thinkers and Believers From Adults?

Jacqueline D. Woolley
University of Texas, Austin, Texas

Young children are often viewed as being unable to differentiate fantasy from reality. This article reviews research on both children's and adults' beliefs about fantasy as well as their tendency to engage in what is thought of as "magical thinking." It is suggested that children are not fundamentally different from adults in their ability to distinguish fantasy from reality: Both children and adults entertain fantastical beliefs and also engage in magical thinking. Suggestions are offered as to how children and adults may differ in this domain, and an agenda for future research is offered.

INTRODUCTION

Children are often thought to live in a world in which fantasy and reality are undifferentiated—a world in which horses can talk, fish can fly, and wishes come true. This is usually a harmless assumption; in fact, many adults often feel somewhat envious of a life so free of the constraints of everyday reality. However, in recent years, a series of traumatic events involving young children and television has served to focus attention on children's ability to make the fantasy-reality distinction and the potential negative consequences of not doing so. In one of the most highly publicized cases, a child, purportedly after watching a comedy show in which the characters talked about how fun it was to set things on fire, set fire to the trailer in which he lived, resulting in serious injury. Many have suggested that this act resulted from the child being unable to distinguish the fantasy world of television from the

---

Reprinted with permission from *Child Development*, 1997, Vol. 68 (6), 991–1011.

Preparation of this manuscript was supported in part by NIH grant R29 HD30300-01. Many thanks are due to Marc Bruell, Angeline Lillard, Karl Rosengren, and Eugene Subbotsky, who provided very valuable feedback on earlier drafts of the manuscript. I would also like to thank Alison Gopnik and two anonymous reviewers for numerous extremely insightful and constructive suggestions. Finally, many thanks are also due to all the graduate students in my fantasy-reality seminar, whose stimulating discussions helped to inspire many of the thoughts expressed herein.

real world. The more general claim underlying this argument is that young children differ in important ways from older children and adults in their ability to distinguish fantasy from reality.

The purpose of this article is to evaluate this claim. To do so, I present findings from a variety of literatures dealing with children, including their understanding of mind, their beliefs about magic, and their understanding of fantasy characters. I also review research from the adult literature, including magical thinking and superstition. Because I have included these diverse literatures, the reader must keep track of a large number of terms (e.g., fantastical, magical, superstitious). To aid the reader in this task, a few words about the interrelations among these various terms, as they are used in this article, are in order. What these terms have in common is that they represent belief in an entity or process that is unsupported by what we generally consider to be the principles of nature. Broad (1953, p. 9) describes these sorts of phenomena as violating certain "basic limiting principles," which he defines as principles that are "...commonly accepted either as self-evident or as established by overwhelming and uniformly favorable empirical evidence." Thus one might think of these phenomena as violating, or at least being inconsistent with, our naive theories of the world. It is these phenomena to which I refer when I use the term "fantasy."

One can consider where these different phenomena fit on a continuum of ontological commitment to what we think the world is really like. At one end of the continuum lie those entities and processes that are in line with our theories of the world, and are supported by empirical evidence. These are things we mark with the term "real." At the opposite end of the continuum we might find those sorts of processes to which we make no ontological commitment, like the sheer fantasy in which we participate when reading a novel or going to the movies, or that a young child engages in when pretending. Between these two end points lie a number of different kinds of beliefs. Toward the "real" end are beliefs that are consistent (or at least not inconsistent) with our theories of the world, yet for which we lack adequate empirical evidence to call them "real." An example of this for myself might be the possibility that UFOs containing aliens from other planets have visited the Earth. It is something that I consider possible, yet I do not have satisfactory evidence to claim with any confidence that the phenomenon exists. Toward the "unreal" end of the continuum lie a number of beliefs that may violate my theories, but to which I may still be willing to make some sort of commitment. Magical, superstitious, and possibly even religious[1] beliefs may fit here. For example, a young child who understands that the mind cannot directly cause events in the world may still believe in wishing. Similarly, an adult who understands basic principles of cause and effect may still avoid walking under ladders. Individual difference factors may affect where these beliefs will be placed on the continuum. The UFO believer and I, for example, may have different requirements for what counts as good evidence, which will affect how far toward the "real" end we place UFOs. The young child and I may have different theories about magic, and hence have different commitments to a process such as wishing. Regardless of where these many phenomena lie on an individual's continuum, what they all share is their utility for the individual in explaining the world. I will attempt

---

[1]See the section "Adults' Beliefs about Fantastical Entities" for a brief discussion of relations between magic and religion.

to examine research with both children and adults to address the claim that children use principles from the domain of fantasy to explain their world, and that they differ from adults in doing so. I will also attempt to explore the individual and situational factors that affect people's thoughts and beliefs.

In examining the empirical evidence concerning fantasy and reality, I begin by distinguishing two dimensions of this distinction: (1) "fantastical thinking" and (2) "thinking about fantasy." This distinction parallels that made by Chandler and Lalonde (1994, p. 84): We must "... be clear about whether we intend to characterize children as prone to magical thinking, or prone to think about the possibility of magic." "Fantastical thinking" (which will be taken in this article to be synonymous with magical thinking) refers to ways of reasoning about the physical world that violate known physical principles, whereas "thinking about fantasy" is considered to refer to knowledge of the real and fantastical status of a variety of fantastical entities. This is essentially a process/content distinction: We can "think fantastically" (process), and we can think about fantasy (content). Next, I move to consider possible developmental relations between children and adults, addressing both the possibility that they do not differ on either of these dimensions, and that they differ qualitatively and importantly on both. I conclude with a number of suggestions for how children and adults differ in their ability to distinguish the realms of fantasy and reality.

THE VIEW OF CHILDREN AS "FANTASY PRONE"

Recent years have witnessed a growing body of literature demonstrating children's impressive proficiency in making a variety of reality-nonreality distinctions. By the age of 3, children can distinguish a mental entity, such as a thought or an image, from the real physical object it represents (Estes, Wellman, & Woolley, 1989; Wellman & Estes, 1986). At about this same age, children, in their everyday talk, discuss the contrasts between reality and pretense, reality and toys, and reality and pictures (Woolley & Wellman, 1990). By the age of 4, children also have a fairly solid understanding of the distinction between reality and deceptive appearances (Flavell, Green, & Flavell, 1986). Despite these impressive achievements, the view of children as "fantasy bound" still persists, not only in the popular media, but in the scientific literature as well. Astington (1993, p. 63), for example, in her recent book on children's understanding of mind, acknowledges children's good performance on tasks assessing the issues just discussed, yet still maintains that "the boundary between reality and fantasy may still not be clearly drawn" and "reality and imagination are not always kept strictly apart in the child's world."

Research on a variety of aspects of children's everyday behavior lends support to the suggestion that children live in a world in which fantasy and reality are more intertwined than they are for adults. Perhaps the most documented evidence of the pervasive role of fantasy in children's lives is the amount of time they spend engaged in pretend play. Most children begin pretending toward the end of their second year of life. The amount of time children spend in pretend play peaks during the preschool years and, according to most accounts, decreases in frequency between the ages of 5 and 8. A somewhat less well-documented phenomenon is that of children's imaginary companions. Recent estimates of the frequency of children having imaginary companions range between 25% and 65% (Singer & Singer,

1990; Taylor, Cartwright, & Carlson, 1993). Here too, the highest incidence is between 3 and 8 years of age, with most children abandoning their imaginary companions by the age of 10. Additionally, there is a growing literature on children's beliefs in fantasy figures such as Santa Claus and supernatural beings such as monsters and witches (Clark, 1995; Harris, Brown, Marriot, Whittall, & Harmer, 1991; Rosengren & Hickling, 1994). These sorts of beliefs also appear to be strongest between the ages of 3 and 8. Finally, recent studies have demonstrated that children hold a variety of beliefs in magical events and processes (Johnson & Harris, 1994; Phelps & Woolley, 1994; Rosengren & Hickling, 1994; Subbotsky, 1994). These observations and findings taken together appear to suggest that children may be very different from adults when it comes to distinguishing fantasy from reality.

But how different are they? And if they are different, in what specific sense(s) do they differ? As noted earlier, it is important to make a distinction between "thinking about fantasy" and "fantastical thinking." This distinction is important because children and adults could potentially differ on one or the other, or both (or neither), of these. When discussing thinking about fantasy, I will be concerned with beliefs about the real versus fantastical nature of various entities. One way children might differ from adults is that they may not make the fantasy-reality distinction at all, and so may believe everything that adults know to be fantastical to be real. In defining fantastical thinking, I will consider reliance on a set of principles that violate accepted views of reality. These are principles such as nonpermanence, permeability, transmogrification, and animism (see e.g., Johnson & Harris, 1994; Piaget, 1929; Subbotsky, 1993).[2] Children may differ from adults in that they might explain their world using these principles, whereas adults presumably explain their world in terms of the laws of physics (permanence, impermeability, and so on).

I will now consider the possible ways that children might differ from adults. The first possibility is simply that children and adults do not differ. But clearly they do; as noted earlier, children engage in pretend play, children believe in Santa Claus, children wish for things, children are afraid of monsters. The traditional view of how children differ from adults is that there are qualitative differences between them. As stated earlier, there could be qualitative differences between children and adults in terms of "fantastical thinking" (process), and children and adults could also differ qualitatively in terms of "thinking about fantasy" (content). Finally, children and adults could differ on both; children may not make the fantasy-reality distinction, and they may also marshal what we consider to be irrational explanations for events in their world. In the sections below, I will first review the relevant evidence for each of these possibilities, and then within each of these sections, whenever possible, I will discuss three additional issues: (1) task concerns, (2) possible sources of concepts, and (3) individual differences.

---

[2]In a sense, this is also "thinking about fantasy," as use of these principles presumably often implies some conscious beliefs about their real-world relevance. It is important to state here that, in reality, "thinking about fantasy" and "fantastical thinking" are certainly very intertwined. My distinguishing them in this article is not meant to imply that they are orthogonal, but to identify a difference that has tended to be overlooked and that has led to various inconsistencies and contradictions in the literature.

DO CHILDREN AND ADULTS DIFFER QUALITATIVELY IN TERMS OF FANTASTICAL THINKING?

In this article, fantastical thinking is considered to be synonymous with magical thinking. There are numerous definitions of magical thinking in the literature. Alcock (1995, p. 15) defines it as "the interpreting of two closely occurring events as though one caused the other, without any concern for the causal link." Keinan (1994, p. 48) defines magical thinking as "any explanation of a behavior or experience that contradicts the laws of nature. . .usually refers to powers, principles, or entities that lack empirical evidence or scientific foundation." Zusne and Jones (1989, p. 13) define it as "a belief that (a) transfer of energy or information between physical systems may take place solely because of their similarity or contiguity in time and space, or (b) that one's thoughts, words, or actions can achieve specific physical effects in a manner not governed by the principles of ordinary transmission of energy or information." All of these have in common that magical thinking involves reasoning without knowledge of, or on the basis of some sort of misconception about, causality, or about natural laws more generally. In this next section I review research that can be considered evidence for the claim that children think fantastically, both about mind-reality relations and about the behavior and interactions of physical objects.

Children's Beliefs About Mind-Reality Relations

According to Piaget (1929), young children's confusion between thoughts and things results in a variety of mistaken beliefs about the relations between the mind and the physical world. These include beliefs that reality can be modified by a thought ("magic by participation between thoughts and things"); believing that an action or mental operation, such as counting to 10, can exert an influence on a desired event ("magic by participation between actions and things"); and beliefs that an object can be used to influence another object ("magic by participation between objects"). Piaget's interviews with children suggested to him that such beliefs are present through the concrete operations period, that is, until age 11 or 12. More recently, Rothbaum and Weisz (1988, p. 20) described a "magical stage" from 2 to 6 years of age in which "the fate of external objects and events is determined by various thoughts (e.g., wishes) and actions (e.g., not stepping on cracks in the sidewalk) that, in reality, have no influence over the outcome."

Most adults have clear beliefs about basic causal relations between the mind and the world. Although adults know that thought can indirectly cause events to happen (e.g., I want something, and eventually I may work to obtain it), most eschew beliefs in direct mental-physical causality. That is, our commonsense psychology does not assume that simply thinking about something can make it happen. Recent research indicates that by age 3 children understand that imagined and dreamed-of entities have different properties than physical things (Estes et al., 1989; Harris et al., 1991; Wellman & Estes, 1986). However, it appears that they may not be sure about whether simply imagining something can cause it to come into existence. Woolley and Wellman (1993) report that many young 3-year-olds tend to believe that imagination reflects or creates reality; these young children make what Woolley and Wellman call the true fiction error. After imagining an object inside an empty box, these children claimed that the object would then appear inside. Harris, Brown, Marriot, Whittall, and Harmer (1991) report similar claims from slightly older children. They found that 4- to 6-year-olds, when asked to pretend that a monster or a bunny was inside a box, would act as if they believed the creatures to be inside the boxes. When left alone in the room with the boxes, children often peaked inside the "bunny" box and acted afraid of the "monster" box. Thus it appears that children between the ages of 3 and 6 do exhibit fantastical thinking concerning imagination-reality relations.

However, in contrast with these findings, Golomb and Galasso (1995), in an attempt to replicate Harris et al., found that very few children ever acted this way. They presented children with a similar situation to that used by Harris et al., with the addition of what they considered a more clear message to children that the pretend "game" was over before observing their behavior and asking questions. They submit that, when it is made clear to children that the pretense mode has come to an end, they do not behave as if they believe imagination creates reality. However, Golomb and Galasso's procedure differed from that of Harris et al. in another important way that they neglected to address. Whereas in Harris et al.'s studies children were left alone in the room with the boxes, children in Golomb and Galasso's studies were never left alone. Research by Subbotsky (1993) indicates that the presence or absence of an adult can have a substantial effect on children's behavior, with the presence of an adult often inhibiting magical thinking.

Results from two studies by Woolley and Phelps (1994) also call into question the extent to which children really believe their imagination creates reality. In these studies, in addition to obtaining verbal judgments as to the existence of imagined objects (e.g., "Will the pencil be in the box, or will the box be empty?"), researchers used a behavioral measure that they argued assessed "practical reasoning." After children had imagined an object inside a box, the experiment was interrupted by an unfamiliar person. This person requested the object that the child had imagined in the box, and couched her request in terms of a real-world need (e.g., after the child had imagined a pencil in the box, the unfamiliar experimenter knocked on the door and said, "Excuse me. I'm sorry to bother you, but I'm working at my desk, and I can't find my pencil. Do you have a pencil that I could borrow?"). Woolley and Phelps found that, although numbers of children comparable to those in the Woolley and Wellman study verbally claimed that the imagined pencil was in the box, very few ever chose to hand the experimenter the box in which they had imagined the object. They interpret these findings as indicating that although children may often entertain fantastical beliefs when there is little cost of doing so (e.g., as in one-on-one informal questioning situations), they are fully able to reason rationally in a situation that appears to have practical consequences.

Clearly there are also many instances in children's everyday lives in which they do not act as if they believe imagination creates reality. If a child wants a cookie, it seems much more likely that she will ask for one than that she will try to get one through imagining! What sorts of factors govern when children think fantastically about imagination and when they do not? First, the type of entity children imagine, whether it is an everyday item versus a supernatural entity, may affect children's claims about whether they believe the object can be created through their imagination. Children may be more likely to believe they can create a fairy with their imagination than that they can create a cookie. However, there are mixed results regarding this factor. Harris et al. (1991) report that the type of entity makes no difference; children equally deny that imagined everyday and supernatural entities are real. In contrast, Phelps and Woolley (1995) found that 3-year-olds are more likely to claim that imagined, positively charged fantastical entities are more likely to exist than imagined, negatively charged ordinary objects. Effects of emotional valence were also found by Samuels and Taylor (1994). They found that when pictured events had a negative emotional valence, children were more likely to make incorrect judgments about their reality status. It is possible that children's judgments about imagined entities may reflect whether or not they *want* the entity to appear, as well as their beliefs.

A third factor that may affect children's claims that imagination creates reality may be whether or not the imagined entity is projected outside the head. Wellman and colleagues (Estes et al., 1989; Wellman & Estes, 1986) have primarily asked children to imagine in their heads, whereas the studies that find claims that imagination can create reality ask children to imagine things in boxes. When the outcome of their imaginative efforts is uncertain (e.g., when visual confirmation is lacking), children may respond in terms of possibility; even the faintest possibility of the object's existence might inspire an affirmative response. However, imaginary companions may be the clearest case of something that is projected outside the head. According to Taylor et al. (1993), children are not confused about the fantasy status of their imaginary companions; they know that these companions are different from real friends.

As stated earlier, one reason young children might claim that imagined objects really exist is that they are wishing or hoping for the object. Certainly most young children are thought to believe in wishing to some degree. There have been very few experimental studies of children's beliefs about wishing. Vikan and Clausen (1993) conducted a study in which children were shown drawings of children and scenes, and told that the child in the drawing was making a wish in an attempt to influence the person depicted in the scene. Children were then asked to indicate the effectiveness of the wish. Results indicated that 4- and 6-year-olds believe they can influence others by thinking (wishing); 94% of the 4- to 6-year-old children tested professed a belief in what Vikan and Clausen term "control by thinking" at at least one point in the testing session. They interpret their results as indicating that "despite all modern evidence that suggests children are precocious rationalists, it would appear that the 'childish' young child is still with us" (p. 310). Vikan and Clausen also gathered information on children's knowledge of realistic influence methods, and conclude that children are aware both of realistic and magical influence methods; thus they do not see children's thinking as dominated only by magical thinking.

Woolley, Phelps, and Davis (1995) report the results of an interview given to 3- to 6-year-old children. Their results reveal significant beliefs in wishing; they also reveal, however, that beliefs in the efficacy of wishing decrease during these years. With regard to whether children's beliefs about wishing involve faulty beliefs about mental-physical causality, their data indicate that children do believe wishing to involve thinking about something and then getting it. In a second study, Woolley et al. addressed whether children believe thinking to be the sole cause of obtaining an object through wishing or simply a component (i.e., is thinking sufficient or just necessary?). A combination of interview questions and story tasks assessed the extent to which children see wishing as a process that also requires magic.

Their data indicate that children see wishing as both mental and magical, and as something that requires a certain degree of skill or know-how. Thus, in line with Vikan and Clausen's conclusions, children do not think of wishing as an ordinary way to get something; rather, they think of it as a magical process, and one that requires some degree of skill to execute.

Subbotsky (1993, 1994) directly investigated children's beliefs in the second type of process discussed by Piaget—"magic by participation between actions and things." He first assessed children's beliefs about whether saying magic words could transform a drawing of something into the object it depicted. He then told children a story about a girl with a magic box that would transform drawings of objects into the things they depicted. A few days later, he invited children back to the experimental room, showed them a box that purportedly was the same box as that in the story, and gave them a number of drawings of objects. The experimenter then left the room and observed the children's behavior. He found that, whereas almost all children denied the possibility of magic in the initial interview, 90% of the children tested attempted some form of magical transformation when left alone with the box. Many selected an item (usually a positive one), made various gestures, said magic words, and then expressed clear disappointment when they opened the box and found only a drawing inside. Subbotsky interprets these results as revealing that magical causality is a viable principle in young children's thinking.

There are also numerous task issues that must be considered in evaluating conclusions about children's beliefs in mental-physical causality. One of these issues is whether experimenters request verbal judgments or observe a child's behavior. In Harris et al. (1991), children's initial verbal judgments revealed a clear distinction between reality and imagination, yet in subsequent behavior these same children appeared to be confused about the boundary between the two. Then in their final judgments the children also appeared confused or, as Harris et al. term them, credulous. Hence, Harris et al. argue that the nature of children's response, verbal or behavioral, is not a critical factor. However, Subbotsky argues that different levels of knowledge are revealed in verbalizations and behavior. According to Subbotsky (1993), children's understanding of the nature of reality is first revealed in verbal judgments and only later in behavior. Thus, according to his argument, these different measures could lead to different estimates of the age at which children make certain important distinctions. A related issue is whether researchers are obtaining conceptual knowledge or simply emotional responses. Behavioral measures may tap emotional responses more than conceptual understanding. The simple observation that an adult cries during an emotionally charged movie certainly does not indicate that the person believes that the depicted events are real.

An additional task issue is the situation in which children are asked to make this differentiation. Woolley and Wellman (1993) suggest that whether or not children make the true fiction error depends on the situation. However, they do not speculate on the conditions that would or would not lead to the error. Woolley and Phelps (1994) argue that, in situations where it is clear to them that their actions have real-world consequences, children will not make the true fiction error. They contrast this with situations in which magical or fantastical thinking is encouraged. One way in which a child might perceive magical thinking to be encouraged is if another person first professes some magical belief. Work by Subbotsky (1993, 1994) suggests that this is in fact the case. When children are asked to judge whether a particular event that violates physical principles is possible, they are much more likely to claim the event is possible after hearing a story in which another child experienced this type of event. Thus, children do appear to be more likely to engage in magical thinking if they are in a situation in which magical beliefs are first professed by someone else. Consideration of these factors together suggests that it is less fruitful to ask simply whether children make the imagination-reality distinction, and more interesting and important to ask what types of situations inspire which ways of thinking, and what types of entities appear to confuse children, as well as exploring relations between verbal responses and actual behavior.

The issue of individual differences is one that has been grossly overlooked by investigators in this area. This is troublesome, as a close look at the research reveals that individual differences are pervasive. Woolley and Wellman (1993) found that, of 19 3-year-olds, eight consistently made the true-fiction error, whereas nine did not. In Woolley and Phelps (1994), although few children indicated behaviorally that they believed imagination could create reality, between 23% and 38% indicated so verbally, whereas the remainder did not (Study 1). In Harris et al. (1991, Study 4), when left alone with the "monster" box, 10 (of 20) 4-year-olds and 10 (of 24) 6-year-olds touched or opened the box. Finally, Johnson and Harris (1994) categorized children in their studies as either "credulous" or "skeptical." Credulous children were those who wondered whether the entity they imagined might really be in the box, and skeptical children were those who claimed that the box was empty. They found that, of 3-year-olds, 15 were considered credulous, whereas nine were considered skeptical; among 5-year-olds, 15 were credulous and seven skeptical, and among 7-year-olds, nine were credulous and 11 skeptical. What factors are responsible for these individual differences? Woolley and Wellman (1993) neglect to address the issue of what might underlie individual differences. Harris et al. (1991) acknowledge them as interesting, but also do not attempt to investigate them, nor do Johnson and Harris (1994). Golomb and Galasso (1995) state, regarding their findings, that "the individual differences that emerged, however, are as yet an uncharted domain that must be more closely examined." With regard to imaginary companions, Taylor et al. (1993) investigate whether children who have an imaginary companion are better at making the imagination-reality distinction, but find that there is no difference between them and children without imaginary companions. However, they do find that children who have imaginary companions engage in more fantasy play, and that their fantasy play is more sophisticated than the fantasy play of children who do not have imaginary companions. The nature of individual differences in beliefs about mental-physical causality is clearly an area worthy of further investigation.

Children's Beliefs About the Behavior and Interactions of Physical Objects

Children are often believed to think fantastically about the behavior of and interactions between physical objects. According to Johnson and Harris (1994), 3- to 5-year-old children make a distinction between the types of processes that happen in the real world versus the types of processes that "could only happen with magic." Given hypothetical events, such as a toy car moving across the table by itself, children reason that events that would violate familiar physical principles such as inertia, constancy, and permanence must be magic. Rosengren, Kalish, Hickling, and Gelman (1994) similarly found that young children make a clear distinction between possible and impossible events, yet leave open the door to magic. Their data show that children understand, for example, that animals generally cannot be made smaller or undergo changes in shape, yet they accept the idea that these sorts of changes could happen with the aid of a magician.

These studies were concerned with children's hypothetical reasoning about the possibility of magical events. Two later studies addressed whether children also evoke magical explanations when they attempt to explain events they actually observe. Phelps and Woolley (1994) presented 4- to 8-year-old children with a series of physical events, some for which they expected children to have adequate physical explanations and some that they reasoned children would find perplexing. They were interested in whether children would explain the perplexing events in terms of magic. They found that, when faced with events that violated their expectations (e.g., a glass bottle with a thin spiral top in which, when held in one's hand, the blue liquid inside rose to the top instead of staying at the bottom), children of all ages tested tended to offer magical explanations. Interestingly, Phelps and Woolley argue that age is not the critical factor in children's tendency to use magic to explain events; instead, it is children's physical knowledge about the event that is critical in predicting whether magic will be afforded an explanatory role. However, children's concept of what magic is does appear to change with age. In a study similar to that of Phelps and Woolley, Rosengren and Hickling (1994) presented children with "extraordinary" events, such as heat causing paint on a toy car to change color, and solicited explanations. They found that, whereas many 4-year-olds explained the events as magic, many 5-year-olds claimed the events were tricks. Follow-up interviews revealed that whereas 4-year-olds view magic as involving special powers, most 5-year-olds view it as consisting of tricks that can be learned by anyone.

Task issues with regard to these studies again center on whether the studies assess verbal claims of magic versus behavior. As noted earlier, in his studies of magical thinking, Subbotsky (1993) measures both verbal responses and behavior, and argues that the difference is critical. Phelps and Woolley (1994) and Rosengren and Hickling (1994) assess only verbal responses. An important question that is raised by this issue is how often in their daily lives children evoke magic as a force (versus in an experimental setting). Could children in experimental settings evoke magic simply because they are asked for an explanation and feel compelled to say something? Relatedly, might they be more likely to evoke magic in situations where it appears to be valued? In studies by Subbotsky, conducive contexts were created in three ways: (1) Children were told a story in which a magical event takes place, (2) children were given adult instruction about magic, and (3) children were shown a "magic box." Under these conditions, children claimed that various physical principles could be violated and appeared to espouse magic.

As with children's beliefs about mental-physical causality, there is little information on individual differences. Rosengren and Hickling (1994) failed to find a relation between parental perceptions or encouragement of fantasy and children's performance on magic tasks. Thus, they suggest, "the relation between parents' perceptions and encouragement of social magical beliefs (i.e., beliefs in fantasy figures) and children's magical beliefs and explanations of causal events may be both subtle and complex" (p. 1622). This is undoubtedly the case. One individual difference factor that Phelps and Woolley (1994) argue is critical in children's explanations of causal events is children's level of knowledge of physical mechanisms. Children with more physical knowledge should be less likely to evoke magic. Level of knowledge should also be related to magical explanations in other domains, such as biology and psychology. For example, if given the sorts of events used by Rosengren et al. (1994), children with less biological knowledge should be more prone to offer magical explanations if and when they encounter anomalous transformations. Likewise, children's level of understanding of mind should be related in the same way to their use of magical explanations for anomalous psychological events. Future studies should investigate the relations between knowledge and magic in these other domains. Researchers should also assess the ways in which general fantasy proneness might interact with such knowledge in children's magical explanations.

Summarizing, young children often do appeal to magical forces to explain and predict events in the real world; in other words, they do engage in "fantastical thinking." But with the exception of some children younger than age 4, this tendency does not appear to result from a confusion between fantasy and reality. If a general confusion about the fantasy-reality distinction was at the root of children's magical thinking, it would be unlikely that we would observe the selective uses of magical thinking found in these studies. That is, it appears that children's tendency to explain events using magical forces is related to their knowledge of particular mental and physical phenomena, not to a general fantasy-reality confusion. Also important is the finding that children are aware of the magical nature of such beliefs. As Woolley et al. (1995) demonstrate, children believe wishing to be a magical process; they understand that simply thinking about something cannot cause it to happen, but claim that magic can make it possible. An awareness of the extraordinary must be predicated on knowledge about what is ordinary.

Evidence of Fantastical Thinking in Adults

The simple fact that children do resort to magical explanations and do believe in wishing still appears to set them apart in important ways from adults. However, it is also clear that children do not always think fantastically, which is the implication of claiming that they are unable to distinguish fantasy from reality. It seems more accurate to say that children think fantastically about certain things and in certain situations. But still they might differ from adults in that adults may not think this way at all. So to endorse the claim that children and adults are categorically different, we would need to show that, in contrast to children, who think fantastically even a little bit, adults do not think in such ways at all.[3]

[3]One way to approach this issue is to consider the frequency of adults' involvement in the realm of fiction. According to Singer and Singer (1990, p. 32), regarding make-believe play, "the urge to play in this way may persist into adolescence, and indeed, where social circumstances permit, even surface in adult life." Singer and Singer cite a variety of examples that illustrate how pantomime, dressing up, and playacting have been a feature of adult society through the centuries. Adults' engagement in daydreaming, reading, film, and theatergoing can also be viewed as involvement in fantasy. From a philosophical perspective, Walton (1990) argues that adults' interest in art, including visual, musical, and theater arts, is essentially the equivalent of the child's fascination with make-believe. Currie (1990, p. 19) echoes this sentiment in suggesting that "our daydreams and fantasies, as well as our encounters with fiction, involve us in 'making-believe' that such and such is the case." Although these arguments are convincing from a theoretical and philosophical standpoint, the bulk of the review that follows deals with empirical evidence that adults engage in behaviors that are more universally considered fantastical.

Unfortunately for such a claim there is ample evidence that adults also engage in fantastical thinking about certain things and in certain situations. A number of different situations have been hypothesized to lead to, or have been shown to lead to, "magical thinking" in adults. According to both Freud (1919/1955) and Werner (1948), there is a stage in children's development in which magical thinking is dominant. As such, when adults are faced with a threat that arouses anxiety, they will regress to this mode of thinking (see also, e.g., Keinan, 1994). According to Piaget (1929), magical thinking in adults represents a momentary loss of the distinction between thoughts and reality. He hypothesized that situations in which magical thinking may occur in adults include the following: (1) involuntary imitation (e.g., when someone on television has a husky voice and one finds oneself clearing one's own throat),[4] (2) anxiety (e.g., nervousness about giving a talk may result in superstitious behavior), and (3) desire or fear, or situations in which one really wants or does not want something to happen (e.g., the belief that if one brings one's umbrella to work it will guarantee a sunny day).

There is considerable empirical research on the types of situations that lead to magical thinking in adults, although space considerations prohibit a detailed review of this literature here. Most notably, adults have been shown to have a tendency toward magical thinking in situations where perception of control is lacking (Langer, 1975). People who engage in such magical thinking tend to believe that their thoughts or actions alone can change their situation. These sorts of situations include games of chance (Weisz, 1981), illness (Taylor, 1983; Taylor, Lichtman, & Wood, 1984), stress (Keinan, 1994), death (Persinger & Makarec, 1990), and, in general, when faced with threat or anxiety. For example, Taylor (1983) describes how a substantial number of women with breast cancer maintain illusions that, for example, if they simply have a positive attitude, they can control their cancer and keep it from coming back. This process also appears to operate on a societal level. By looking at the number of articles, books, television shows, and other forms of media on superstition and related issues during a given period, it is possible to gauge the level of interest in these sorts of phenomena at different periods in our culture. Studies using these techniques have found that level of economic threat in a society is related to the amount of or level of interest in magical thinking (Zusne & Jones, 1989). Inasmuch as economic threat leads to increases in an individual's uncertainty about his or her well-being, these trends reflect the same sorts of factors as discussed above.

A number of the characteristics that are considered to lead to magical thinking in adults are exactly those that are often thought to characterize children's thinking more generally: lack of information, conditions of uncertainty, and inability to explain phenomena. This might appear to indicate a strong continuity between children and some adults. However, in adults, the relation between these conditions and magical thinking is mediated by a feeling of lack of control. To argue for continuity between children and adults, the relation between

---

[4]Another perhaps more commonly observed example of involuntary imitation, also given by Piaget, is the case when someone is bowling and has thrown the ball slightly off course. One will often see individuals leaning their body in the direction in which they want the ball to go. In both examples, we engage in an action "which consists in trying to affect the external world by some action on one's own body." However, as Piaget claims, whereas in minds that are "less conscious of the self" (e.g., infants) these would continue unchecked, in adults they are "instantly checked by our habits of thinking" (1929, p. 163).

these should be mediated similarly in children. Although adults may often perceive children in this way, there is scant evidence that children perceive themselves as often being in such a state or position. It is, of course, also theoretically possible that these sorts of situations result directly in magical thinking in children. At this point, the exact nature of possible continuities between adult magical thinking and that seen in children is unclear and worthy of further investigation.

There is also considerable evidence that adults often use fantastical processes and forces to explain and predict their world. This is seen most clearly in superstitious behavior. Superstition is defined by Adorno, Frenkel-Brunswik, Levinson, and Sanford (1950, p. 236) as "the belief in mystical or fantastical external determinants of the individual's fate." A more thorough definition is provided by Zusne and Jones (1989, p. 242): "(a) specific, circumscribed belief or act that (b) involves magical thinking, either actually or as a remnant, held or engaged in because (c) it is culturally transmitted or learned through fortuitous reinforcement and (d) it is resorted to under conditions of uncertainty." According to Keinan (1994), superstitions are likely to be rooted in magical thinking (see also Jahoda, 1969; Zusne & Jones, 1989). In an investigation of adults' superstitious beliefs, Blum and Blum (1974) report that the percentage of people who held partial or strong beliefs about walking under a ladder was 47%, for knocking on wood was 41%, and for breaking a mirror was 41%. In a follow-up study, Blum (1976) reports the following strong or partial beliefs: walking under a ladder, 46%; knocking on wood, 46%; crossing fingers, 35%; breaking a mirror, 35%. Gallup and Newport (as cited in Stanovich, 1994) report that 46% of the respondents they surveyed believed in faith healing, 49% believed in demonic possession, and 14% believed in fortune telling. Finally, there is widespread evidence that many people believe in astrology, perhaps the most notable in recent years being Nancy Reagan. In addition to Mrs. Reagan, Frazier (as cited in Stanovich, 1994) reports that 58% of adults believe in astrology. Regarding younger adults, a Gallup poll of teenagers aged 13 to 18, conducted in June 1984, reports that 55% believe that astrology works. Results of various other studies that have investigated superstitious behavior can be seen in Table 1.

Many adults also hold beliefs that appear to contradict everyday commonsense knowledge about the mind. One example of this is reported by Cottrell, Winer, and Smith (1996). They find that many adults claim to believe that they can feel the unseen stares of another person, that is, they are aware when someone else is looking at them, even if their back is turned. Although not considered superstitious beliefs in the same sense as those reported above, these beliefs seem related to superstition in the sense that many superstitions concern emissions from the eye, for example, the concept of the evil eye, bewitching, and the like. These beliefs also appear to violate knowledge about mental-physical causal relations, in that with these beliefs often comes a feeling that persistent gazing at the back of another person can make that person turn around. Interestingly, Cottrell et al. find the highest incidence of these arguably irrational beliefs in their oldest participants. They endorse a position similar to Subbotsky's (1993), but which they attribute to Werner (1948, 1957, cited in Cottrell et al., 1996), in which "intuitive" or "primitive" modes of thought coexist with more rational ones, and vary as a function of situation and individual differences.

All of the above results were obtained using surveys or questionnaires. As with children's magical beliefs, it is also important to demonstrate that these sorts of beliefs are present in

TABLE 1

Percentage of Survey Informants Endorsing Selected Magical Beliefs

Survey	Sample	ESP[a]	Ghosts	Communication with Dead	Astrology	Witchcraft	Lucky Charms	Have Personal Psychic Power	Had Psychic Experience
Warner & Clark, 1938	352 APA members	8							2
Warner, 1952	349 APA members	17							8
Jahoda, 1968	280 West African students					76			
Salter & Routledge, 1971	98 students	12			4	4			
Evans, 1973	1,416 *New Scientist readers*	67							51
Current Opinion, 1974, 2, 36	±1,000 adults	45	11	12	22	10	16		
Greeley, 1975									58
Polzella, Popp, & Hinsman, 1975	Students	58							44
McConnell, 1977	Parapsychological Association members								71
Jones, Russell, & Nickel, 1977	475 students	58% endorsed 50% or more of 22 items							
Bainbridge, 1978a	226 students	64							
Gallup, 1978	1,553 adults	51	11		29	10			
Gallup Youth Survey, 1978	1,174 teens	67	20			25			
Wagner & Monnet, 1979	1,188 college professors	65							11
Bainbridge & Stark, 1980	1,056 students	22							54

Leland, Patterson, & Clark (Marks & Kammann, 1980)	619 students	26					50	
Marks & Kammann, 1980	304 students	80				38	31	
McConnell & Clark, 1980	203 members of Parapsychological Association	93						
Profiles, 1981	80 members of Parapsychological Association	88						
Alcock, 1981	272 students	80						
McClenon, 1982	353 elite AAAS members	29						
Schouten, 1983	126 students	87						22
Gallup Youth Survey, 1984	506 teens	59			55			
Not-so-skeptical inquirers, 1984	±600 *Psychology Today* readers	83	50+		39			
Gallup Youth Survey, 1986	504 teens	46	15		52	19		
Harrold & Eve, 1986	409 students	59	35	38	8	34		
R. Eve & D. Dunn, Univ. of Texas at Arlington, 1988	±400 high school biology teachers	34		27				

Source: From Zusne and Jones (1989, pp. 233–234). Copyright 1989 by Lawrence Erlbaum Associates, Inc.
[a]Includes endorsements of telepathy, clairvoyance, precognition, and PK, singly.

actual behavior. Studies by Rozin and colleagues (Rozin, Markwith, & Ross, 1990; Rozin, Millman, & Nemeroff, 1986; Rozin & Nemeroff, 1990) indicate that they are. In one study, adults showed a reluctance to drink sugar water from a container labeled "cyanide," even though the label was arbitrarily placed on the sugar container by the participants themselves (Rozin et al., 1986). Rozin et al. interpret these findings as indicating a level of belief in the laws of sympathetic magic, that is, that an image or label of an object contains certain properties of the object itself. In other studies (Rozin, Nemeroff, Wane, & Sherrod, 1989), Rozin and colleagues probed adults' beliefs in a related magical law, that of contagion. Here the belief is that when two objects come into contact with one another, there is a permanent exchange of properties between them. They found that adults were, for example, unwilling to use a hairbrush that had been previously used by someone they disliked, even though the brush had been thoroughly sterilized. They were also unwilling to drink juice that had been contacted by a cockroach, even though the roach was dead and sterilized. They conclude that the magical law of contagion has a significant influence on the way adults react to objects they encounter in their everyday lives.

Subbotsky (1993) has also conducted experiments with adults, patterned after those discussed earlier. In one, he presented adults with a box that appeared to transform a postage stamp in various ways, including through the "psychic efforts" of the experimenter. He found that a majority of the adult participants acknowledged the possibility that mental effort was involved in transforming the postage stamp. He notes that this is dependent on certain conditions, including, first, that participants have to observe an event that they are unable to explain, and, second, that some action of the experimenter must render such an explanation legitimate. These conditions are similar to those necessary to evoke magical explanations in children, as discussed earlier. In another study (Grivtsov, 1988, cited in Subbotsky, 1993), adults were given a task that was insoluble, although it was presented to them as a test of intelligence and creativity. Many of them, after working on the task for a substantial amount of time, eventually admitted, in response to the experimenter's suggestion, that telekinesis might be the way to solve the task. Subbotsky (1993) suggests that the participants' frustration with the task caused them to turn to this sort of means that, in most cases, they had rejected at the outset. Subbotsky concludes from his work that magical thinking is an important component of consciousness in both children and adults.

A number of individual differences in adults have been hypothesized or shown to be related to magical thinking. A "fantasy-proneness" construct or personality dimension was defined by Wilson and Barber (1983). Persons who are fantasy-prone report vivid imagery, are susceptible to hypnosis, and often report telepathic and psychic experiences. They are reported to differ from non-fantasy-prone individuals on measures of imagination, creativity, suggestibility, and also in childhood experiences (Lynn & Rhue, 1988). Regarding people who believe in UFOs (discussed in a later section), Spanos, Cross, Dickson, and DeBreuil (1993) find that, with such people, the intensity of their UFO experiences correlates significantly with inventories that assess fantasy-proneness. According to Keinan (1994) and others, people with lower tolerance for ambiguity may be more likely to engage in magical thinking, particularly in stressful situations. Zusne and Jones (1989) propose that a number of personality factors are related to magical thinking, including feelings of uncertainty, the belief that one's fate is controlled externally, and social marginality. They suggest that these feelings might be facilitated by factors such as authoritarianism, externalization, life change, and emotional instability. Finally, addressing developmental antecedents, Persinger and Makarec (1990) report that people who reported that they had their first religious experience before adolescence were more likely as adults to hold superstitious beliefs (and to hold religious beliefs) than people who did not. It is interesting to note that various studies that have looked at the potential effects of years of education on superstitious beliefs have found no relation between the two (see e.g., Persinger & Makarec, 1990). Relatedly, studies by Emme (1940, and others, cited in Zusne & Jones, 1989) have found that whereas specific instruction aimed at reducing superstition has an effect, general instruction in science does not.

In summary, results on children's and adults' fantastical thinking indicate that, in certain situations, certain children and certain adults will engage in magical thinking. In no study do all children engage in such behavior, and in no study do all adults surveyed profess superstitious beliefs. How different is the child's wish for a baby sister from the adult's avoidance of walking under a ladder? Or the child's tendency to explain magically an event for which she lacks knowledge of a physical mechanism from our ancestors' explanation of the sunrise as an act of God? Magical thinking is something in which many of us engage, to different degrees, and with more or less conviction, as individuals and as cultures, throughout the life span and throughout history.

DO CHILDREN AND ADULTS DIFFER QUALITATIVELY IN TERMS OF HOW THEY THINK ABOUT FANTASY?

Children's Beliefs About Fantastical Entities

Anecdotal and empirical evidence alike tells us that children commonly believe in the reality of fantasy figures. However, there is considerable inconsistency in the findings in this literature as a whole; some studies argue that children are quite adept at differentiating fantastical entities and events from real ones, and others argue that children are confused by this task. One of the earliest studies of this issue was conducted by Taylor and Howell (1973). They presented children with fantastical pictures of animals who had human characteristics, along with pictures presenting animals and humans in their normal activities, and asked children to state whether the scenes depicted in the pictures could really happen. They report that 3-year-olds had considerable difficulty differentiating real events from fantastical events, and that ability improved with age.

More recently, Samuels and Taylor (1994) used a similar method, with some methodological improvements, to assess the effects of emotional content on such differentiation. They found that younger preschool age children had difficulty distinguishing fantastical pictures from pictures of events that were possible in the real world; 40% of their younger children (M age = 3,10) claimed four out of five times that emotionally charged fantasy pictures could happen in real life. This ability improved with age, with only 13% of the older children (M age = 5,0) making this claim. They also found that children were most confused when events were perceived as frightening, with children often claiming that real negative events could not take place in the real world.

Morison and Gardner (1978) also assessed children's understanding of the reality status of a variety of entities. Children were presented with pictures of generic supernatural creatures such as witches and dragons, specific fantasy figures from popular culture such as Big Bird and Smoky the Bear, and real entities such as birds and frogs. Children received both free sorting tasks, in which they were asked which pictures went together, and a task in which they were asked to categorize each item as being "real" or "pretend." On the categorization tasks, even kindergartners were able to properly place these entities into piles of "real" and "pretend," with this ability continuing to develop through the grade-school years. However, the authors report that, up until grade 6, children rarely spontaneously used fantasy status as a dimension with which to categorize entities into distinct types. Morison and Gardner conclude that it is misleading to claim that children cannot distinguish reality and fantasy. Rather, they suggest that in young children the distinction is less well articulated and less firmly established. Although I am in full agreement with this conclusion, it leaves open the issue of what it means for this distinction to be "less well articulated" and "less well established." Suggestions to this end are offered toward the end of the present article.

Evidence can also be found regarding children's understanding of the fantasy status of specific event-related fantasy figures, most notably, Santa Claus, the Easter bunny, and the tooth fairy (Clark, 1995; Prentice, Manosevitz, & Hubbs, 1978). Belief in these figures and behaviors associated with them (e.g., putting teeth under the pillow, leaving a cookie by the chimney for Santa) conceivably plays a very important role in the fantasy lives of young children. Early studies of this question attempted to relate children's degree of belief in these figures to their cognitive developmental stage, as determined through Piagetian measures. Blair, McKee, and Jernigan (1980), for example, found that age, but not cognitive developmental stage, was a significant determinant of the degree of children's beliefs in these figures. Parents also report that their young children believe that event-related figures such as Santa, the tooth fairy, and the Easter bunny are real (e.g., exist in the real world), and report a lesser degree of belief in non-event-related figures such as dragons, witches, ghosts, monsters, and fairies (Rosengren & Hickling, 1994).

These sorts of fantasy figures are often strongly tied to religious beliefs, and, as such, it is possible that non-Christian children lack many of the associated experiences. Prentice and Gordon (1986) interviewed Jewish children 3 to 10 years of age about their beliefs in Santa Claus and the tooth fairy, and also administered a questionnaire to parents about their encouragement of these figures. Interestingly, parental encouragement of belief in these fantasy figures was not found to be related to children's beliefs. Prentice and Gordon's primary hypothesis was that Jewish children's belief in the tooth fairy would be greater than their belief in Santa Claus. They found, as in other studies, that belief in these figures decreased with age. However, they also found equal degrees of belief in Santa and the tooth fairy, with the degree of disbelief in both myths much higher than in Christian children. They suggest an interesting developmental hypothesis with respect to Jewish children's disbelief in the tooth fairy: A child's first experience with fantasy figures may color attitudes toward subsequent ones. Children learn about Santa Claus first, and to Jewish children he is presented as unreal. When they later hear about the tooth fairy, they may also assume that she is unreal.

One explanation for the inconsistency in the claims made in this literature rests upon task issues. Investigators attempting to address these issues have really asked children three different questions. Blair et al. (1980), Morison and Gardner (1978, Pt. II), Prentice and Gordon (1986), and Samuels and Taylor (1994) asked children to categorize various entities as real or fantastical. This sort of procedure requires children to identify as fantastical a variety of specific entities, many of which are presented to the child through his or her immediate and broad culture as being real (e.g., Santa Claus). Because children are finding out about the reality status of these figures on a case-by-case basis, results of studies like these will show a large variation, depending upon the particular fantasy figures and populations that are probed. This sort of variation is even found within studies, as evidenced by Morison and Gardner's finding that children were more likely to give fantastical explanations when characters came from fairy tales than when they came from popular culture.

Studies that show early abilities in this domain tend to be those in which children are required to identify attributes of an entity that has already been characterized by an adult. For example, in the studies by Estes et al. (1989) reviewed earlier, the experimenter identified a mental entity or a real entity as such and then asked the child to say, for example, whether it can be seen, touched, and so on. Because the entities are already categorized for the child, retrieval of proper attributes is facilitated, revealing sophisticated fantasy-reality knowledge. Finally, other studies have assessed the extent to which young children spontaneously use the fantasy-reality distinction as a dimension with which to categorize stimuli (e.g., Morison & Gardner, 1978, Pt. I; Taylor & Howell, 1973). Clearly this type of study goes beyond assessing children's basic ability to differentiate and delves into their beliefs about the relevance of this dimension in different situations. As such, children have not been shown to perform well until much later than on other sorts of tasks. Finally, all the studies discussed use verbal responses to assess children's beliefs; none uses the sort of behavioral measure used by Subbotsky (1993) in his studies. This literature might benefit from the use of behavioral measures in tandem with verbal ones.

As with research on children's fantastical thinking, there appear to be considerable individual differences in children's beliefs about fantasy figures and events. These differences are rarely even acknowledged, let alone probed. Of the 15 younger participants in Samuels and Taylor (1994), six consistently made fantasy-reality confusions throughout the experiment, whereas seven rarely or never made them. Prentice and Gordon (1986) report that 23% of their sample believed in Santa Claus, and 25% believed in the tooth fairy. Because most studies only report mean scores on their items, it is difficult to determine the extent of individual differences, but it is clear that they do exist.

To what degree are children's beliefs in these entities a direct product of the culture in which they are immersed? This is a critical question, as it is conceivable that children's beliefs are as much a product of being immersed in this culture as they are reflective of some cognitive limitations. As we know from anecdotal evidence, children in our culture are "invited" by parents and other authority figures to participate in a variety of cultural rituals, for example, putting their tooth under the pillow, hanging Christmas stockings, and making wishes. Additionally, children hear stories from parents and others, see films, and hear tales from other children about monsters and ghosts. What is the role of parents specifically in instantiating and maintaining (and eventually debunking) beliefs in fantasy figures?

According to Rosengren and Hickling (1994), parents report low levels of encouragement of belief in supernatural beings. Only between 5% and 10% reported encouraging belief in dragons, witches, ghosts, and monsters, and only slightly more reported encouraging belief in fairies and magicians (28%). However, they also report fairly high levels of encouragement regarding event-related figures, with 63%–72% reporting encouraging beliefs in the tooth fairy, the Easter bunny, and Santa. Importantly, Rosengren and Hickling found that the number of fantasy characters in which parents reported that they encouraged belief, as well as the number of fantasy characters parents themselves reported believing in as a child, were related to the number of characters they reported that their children believed were real. Recall, however, that in the Prentice and Gordon (1986) study discussed earlier, children's beliefs did not appear to be related to parental encouragement. Clearly, children's conceptions are a product of a number of influences, and the relation between parent and child beliefs is likely to be more subtle and complex than can be revealed through the sorts of questionnaire measures that have been used.

Adults' Beliefs About Fantastical Entities

Are children unique in holding such beliefs about fantastical entities? Here I review evidence that the beliefs many adults hold about fantastical entities differ only in content, and not in kind, from children's beliefs. At first glance, it might seem ridiculous to even ask the question of whether adults believe in monsters, witches, or ghosts. We would all most likely aver that we have outgrown such "childish" beliefs. However, the numbers of young and older adults who claim to believe in such creatures are not all that different from the percentages we just reviewed for children. Reporting the results of the Gallup Youth Survey in 1988, Frazier (1989) discusses trends in the beliefs of teenagers aged 13 through 17. He reports that 22% of the teenagers surveyed by Gallup believe in Big Foot, 22% believe in ghosts, and 16% believe in the Loch Ness monster. Gallup and Newport (1991) report the following percentages from a telephone survey of 1,236 adults: 29% believe that houses can be haunted, 25% believe in ghosts, 55% believe in the devil, and 10% claim to have spoken with or been spoken to by the devil.

Even if we do not accept these data, it is still difficult to argue that adults are that different from children. It may be that a child's fairy or ghost is an adult's UFO, for example.[5] In fact, some have made this claim. Shaeffer (1981), for example, considers UFO believers to be very much like children believing in monsters, goblins, witches, and other mythical creatures. Regarding adults' belief in UFOs, a Gallup pole (reported in Zimmer, 1985) reports that 57% of those surveyed claim that UFO sightings are real, and Zimmer (1985) reports 38% claiming that UFOs are alien spaceships. In addition, Gallup and Newport (1991, cited in Stanovich) find that 47% even claim that extraterrestrials have visited the earth at some point in time.

---

[5] It is undoubtedly a fact that there are objects in the sky and that sometimes these objects cannot be identified. It is also highly possible that there is life in other solar systems. As Zusne and Jones (1989, p. 3) suggest, "The UFOs acquire psychological interest when misperception of objects under difficult viewing conditions is involved or when beliefs and expectations affect that which is perceived."

Beliefs in UFOs arguably comprise the closest parallel to children's beliefs in fantasy figures, in large part due to the degree with which they have permeated contemporary popular culture. Zimmer (1985) discusses three different models of what UFO beliefs in adults represent. One model is that UFO believers are "simply those caught up in the excitement and awe of science fiction and perhaps also in the aura of the occult" (p. 407). Menzel and Taves (1977) similarly assert that UFO believers are also likely to believe in astrology, witches, occultism, and parapsychology. According to this explanation, adults believe because they want to and are caught up in the excitement of believing, perhaps not unlike children. A second model proposes that adults who believe in UFOs are those who feel alienated from society; adopting unconventional beliefs helps such "outsiders" affirm their status as different. This model receives little empirical support and does not appear to suggest any continuities between children and adults. Finally, a third explanation of UFO beliefs is that their holders are mentally disturbed in some way (see also Spanos ct al., 1993). In this vein, Shaeffer (1981) considers UFO believers as engaging in prescientific thinking and as being irrational and emotional. To the degree that one characterizes children's thinking as prescientific, irrational, and emotionally driven, this model may hold some parallels with childhood. However, this is a view of childhood that does not receive much popularity nowadays. There is also little empirical evidence to support this view of adult UFO believers. In Zimmer's (1985) research, support is marshaled only for the first of these, leading to the conclusion that adult UFO believers are those who are fascinated with the mental excitement generated by the possibility of alternative realities.

Most of the beliefs discussed above, however, are often considered marginal or at least not mainstream. A more appropriate parallel may be seen in the thinking of children and adults if we focus our attention on *faith*. Faith is most commonly defined as the acceptance of the existence of a supernatural being without clear empirical support for that being's existence. Inherent in this definition is that such empirical support is irrelevant to maintenance of the belief. Detailing the similarities and differences between magical and religious beliefs is a task that has captivated religious scholars, historians, and anthropologists alike (see, e.g., Neusner, Frerichs, & Flesher, 1989). As Neusner et al. state, "A convention of the history of religion in the west . . . is that one group's holy man is another group's magician: 'What I do is a miracle, but what you do is magic'" (pp. 4–5). In other words, magic and religion have historically served similar functions, and much of correct attribution has to do with who is performing the deed. Neusner et al. also state that "In any given system, persons know the difference between acts of religion (that is, miracles) and those of superstition (namely magic) by reference to the source and standing of the one who does a deed deemed out of the ordinary" (p. 61). Magical and religious beliefs may serve similar functions ontogenetically as well as historically. It is conceivable that children's early beliefs in cultural fantasy figures such as Santa Claus may form the foundation for later beliefs in God. For children who believe in Santa, he is the one who rewards their good behavior and punishes their misdeeds; he is the one who watches over them all year long; he is the one who "knows if you've been bad or good." God serves many of these same functions for many adults. Some have even proposed that God appears first to children as but one of many superhuman beings or fantasy characters, from which he is later individuated (Rizzuto, 1979). If religious beliefs are conceptualized in this way, a considerable degree of consistency can be seen between the nature of children's early beliefs in supernatural beings and adults' beliefs in deities and related supernatural figures.

Summarizing, the literature reviewed in this section should cause us to reject the hypothesis that children and adults differ qualitatively both in terms of fantastical thinking and in terms of thinking about fantasy. Yet we have also rejected the claim that children and adults do not differ at all. This leaves us with the task of proposing exactly how children and adults do differ. In this next section I offer some suggestions and speculations.

HOW DO CHILDREN AND ADULTS DIFFER?

Children might differ from adults regarding fantasy-reality differentiation in a number of ways. Some of the suggestions made following are specific to the fantasy-reality distinction and some are suggestions about general developmental changes. They are not necessarily mutually exclusive or orthogonal; it is possible that all or none are involved. It is hoped that these suggestions will inspire further research and theorizing in this area.

1. *Differences between children and adults are due to cultural context.* It may be that children and adults are equipped with the same cognitive apparatus for distinguishing fantasy and reality, and that perceived differences in their thinking and behavior are entirely due to the subculture in which children are immersed. Adults encourage fantastical thinking in children. Children view adults as authority figures. Children's beliefs in fantasy figures arguably can be viewed as rational acceptance of beliefs presented to them by their culture. What if adults were encouraged by an authority figure to believe in something like Santa Claus? A case in point might be the infamous "War of the Worlds" radio broadcast, which caused many adults to flee from their homes when they misperceived a fantasy tale as a news broadcast. A parallel could also be drawn with the perpetuation of fantasy by religious cult figures to their members. To many adults, the media, as well as our political and religious leaders, represent authority, perhaps not unlike the way parents are thought of by young children. One could imagine a professor at a university introducing her students to a fantastical concept. How would a student evaluate such information? One process would certainly involve encounters with others outside the classroom; such interactions would presumably serve to engender disbelief. The effectiveness of this mechanism is presumably why cult leaders often seek to limit contact of members with people outside the cult. Arguably, young children are in a somewhat similar situation. Fantasy beliefs encouraged in the home are likely to be encouraged outside the home as well, at day-care, at school, at the homes of friends, and in public venues. Additionally, adults have the advantage of being able to evaluate such information by comparing it to their much larger knowledge base. This inspires the next suggestion.

2. *Differences between children and adults are in domain-specific knowledge.* The research reviewed in this article indicates that by the age of 3 children have the basic ability to distinguish fantasy and reality. Taking the perspective of the "child as scientist," children have to accrue evidence, test their theories, and make decisions about the reality status of a variety of entities. With regard to learning the fantastical nature of various supernatural and event-related figures, children most likely acquire knowledge on a case-by-case basis. In arguing against traditional claims that young children do not distinguish real from

unreal, Shweder and Levine (1975, p. 225) state, regarding children's early understanding of dreams, that "...they distinguish by some criteria the real and unreal but have no good reasons to view dream-events as anything but real." My argument here is in line with this view and suggests that it can be applied even more widely. Children accept many fantastical entities as real at first, but rather than reflecting an inability to differentiate reality from fantasy, this sort of judgment represents an incorrect assignment of an object or entity to a category. Thus, development in thinking about fantasy can be viewed as acquisition of domain-specific knowledge. Whether or not such knowledge acquisition inspires more global theory change regarding fantasy is a question that could be explored in future research.

This view of course begs the question of why it is that children make the incorrect assignment in the first place. Why is it that children might first view dream events as real, or first believe Santa Claus to be real? One suggestion may be that viewing events this way is consistent with children's existing beliefs. It may be that having a larger set of beliefs in fantastical entities and processes affects evaluation of new information. Because young children tend to believe in the existence of more of these sorts of things, when introduced to a new fantastical entity or process, a child may be more likely to accept it, perhaps because its existence is consistent with more of his or her beliefs. This view would explain not just children's easy acceptance of fantastical entities and processes, but also the ease with which certain adults often endorse magical beliefs. According to Zusne and Jones (1989), adults' beliefs in magical phenomena such as ESP, astrology, witches, and ghosts tend to be highly intercorrelated, indicating that acceptance of one sort of fantastical belief often engenders endorsement of others. An important task for the future is to try to understand how knowledge and theories about the physical (and mental and biological) world coexist with such cohesive interconnected fantastical beliefs.

Results from some of the studies reviewed in this article indicate that the more knowledge children do have about particular physical phenomena, the less likely they are to resort to magical explanations of such events. Regarding beliefs in mental-physical causality specifically, development may involve increased understanding of the relation between mental states and reality (e.g., a decrease in beliefs that there is a strict correspondence between the two). Woolley et al. (1995), however, suggest that ways of thinking about mental-physical causality may not actually change, that beliefs in direct mental-physical causality persist throughout the life span, but are applied to different domains. For example, whereas some very young children believe in imagination-reality causation, many slightly older children believe in wishing, and many adults believe in prayer.

3. *Differences between children and adults may reflect a gradual shift in certainty.* Rather than viewing children's and adults' categorization of fantasy figures and magical processes as dichotomous, with children considering them real and adults understanding them to be not real, it may make more sense to situate children's and adults' beliefs on a continuum of certainty or possibility. Because much research has relied on dichotomous scoring systems (e.g., asking children whether this or that entity is real or not real, ascertaining whether children say an event is magic or not magic), children and adults often appear to be categorically different in their responses. Yet children may appear to be credulous regarding fantasy figures and magical processes not because they are *certain* of the existence of fantasy

creatures, but because they are more likely than adults to consider the *possibility* that they might exist. Their initial response in a particular situation, rather than being "yes, there really is a monster in the box," may be "maybe, let's see," allowing the possibility that, for example, a monster *might* be in a box. Although most adults do not even entertain this initial suggestion, it is very different from claiming that children are misclassifying the entity.

The development of such a model is clearly linked to domain-specific knowledge acquisition. Children may decide, on a case-by-case basis, that this or that monster, that particular ghost, and so on are not real. This, of course, still leaves open the possibility that the next monster or ghost *is* real. At some point, when the child has encountered and correctly classified enough instances, generalizations may develop and enable a stronger feeling of certainty that monsters and ghosts in general are not real. This may even, at some point, take the form of a definition or logical necessity. Although speculative, it may be that it is important to children at a certain age to be very clear that monsters are, by definition, not real. At this point, though, although a given child understands that monsters and ghosts generally speaking or by definition are not real, she may still believe in Santa Claus or other fantasy figures. Supportive of this, Morison and Gardner (1978) found that individual participants' use of a fantasy explanation for one item did not predict its subsequent use on other similar items.

To assess whether this sort of continuous progression is operating, researchers need to develop more sensitive measures beyond the yes/no, real/not real response options used in most studies. Children could be allowed to say "sometimes" and "maybe," for example. More easily quantifiable estimates could also be generated by having children indicate how many times something would happen. For example, regarding children's beliefs in wishing, rather than simply asking whether wishes come true, a child could be asked, "If we made five wishes right now, how many would come true?" Intermediate numbers might yield evidence of different levels of certainty or possibility.

4. *Children and adults differ in belief-consistency detection.* This suggestion focuses on the type of information processing that may be involved in making a correct judgment about the status of a particular fantastical entity or process. As discussed earlier, in determining whether a fantastical being or process can exist or operate in the real world, children need to evaluate its consistency with the beliefs or world knowledge that they already hold. For example, beliefs that would be relevant to determining whether Santa Claus exists might include knowledge that most animals cannot fly, that no one could realistically travel to all the houses on the earth in one night, that fat people cannot fit through small places, and so on. So belief-inconsistency detection is clearly dependent on domain-specific knowledge. However, it may also involve various information-processing abilities, such as working memory, long-term memory retrieval speed and accuracy, and comparison and matching procedures. Deficiencies in any or all of these could affect belief consistency detection. But belief consistency detection also has a motivational component. Children must first be motivated in some way to detect inconsistency and then to resolve it once detected. It seems clearly possible that children might be perfectly good at detecting inconsistency but simply be bothered less by it than adults. Alternatively, it is also possible that the motivational component may work, not to detect inconsistency, but to avoid it. Laboratory studies of ESP

believers (versus disbelievers) presented with apparent demonstrations of ESP failures have shown that ESP believers often distort actual outcomes to fit with their beliefs. That is, they perceive failed ESP attempts to be successful (Zusne & Jones, 1989). This would suggest an attempt to maintain consistency perhaps not unlike that which operates in resistance to scientific theory change (see also Chinn & Brewer, 1993, regarding theory change in response to anomalous data).

5. *Children and adults differ in terms of discounting ability.* Regardless of the empirical data presented here, few would dispute that many young children often sincerely fear the "monsters" under their beds. One explanation for children's fears of supernatural and imaginary creatures may be the following: When children think about monsters, a certain amount of negative emotion is generated, simply by entertaining the very faint possibility that they might exist. Children may understand that these entities generally are not real, but may be less good at saying "it's not real" to themselves and comforting themselves with this knowledge. That is, they may be less able to discount the possibility of the monsters' existence. Harris et al. (1991) have suggested that increased discounting ability may also produce decreased susceptibility to availability effects, which he posits are responsible for children's magical thinking. As children get older, they get better at recruiting knowledge to offset shifts in subjective likelihood. Children might, for example, get better at reminding themselves that monsters do not exist. The development of discounting ability is most likely linked to developments in basic information-processing ability as well as increased domain-specific knowledge. One might consider that availability effects are also operating in adults' judgments about children's fantasyproneness; the one event in which a child gets her pretend monster mixed up with the real world may be much more available to a parent than the countless other times she is able to keep these two worlds separate and distinct.

6. *Differences between children and adults are due (in part) to the acquisition of foundational concepts.* Carey (1985) proposes (and rejects) the idea that children and adults are fundamentally different thinkers due to the acquisition, at some point in development, of certain foundational concepts. One of these is the appearance-reality distinction. Despite Carey's conclusions, it seems very plausible that a relevant acquisition in children's understanding of fantasy is their understanding of the appearance-reality distinction and, relatedly, their understanding of misrepresentation. That is, many not-real things may seem real in certain ways, and so may be taken as such at face value. For example, Big Bird and other characters on television have many of the same characteristics as real people; they talk, walk, eat, and so on. Regarding children's beliefs about magic, certainly the magician *appears* to pull a rabbit out of his hat. But does he really? It seems plausible that a large component of the shift in children's belief in magic as a real force to viewing it as tricks could be an understanding of deceptive appearances and misrepresentations. Regarding children's fears of imaginary creatures, the fear children experience when they think about a monster is very real to them, and hence so must seem the monster. A developing understanding that the world is not always as it seems, that appearances and other representations can misrepresent reality, may help children to conceptualize the existence of a not-real world.

Directions for Future Research

One goal of this article was to suggest an agenda for future research in this area. I have tried to offer specific suggestions throughout; however, in this last section I also indicate several general areas in which more research is needed.

1. *What do the very early stages look like?* Little research has addressed fantasy-reality issues in toddlers. By around 18 months of age, most children are beginning to engage in pretend play and to be introduced to some fantasy figures. From the research reviewed in this article, children by the age of 3 have considerable knowledge about fantasy and reality. It may be that much of the boundary confusion between real and fantasy worlds that pervades lay conceptions about children actually occurs between the ages of 18 months and 3 years, when children are first encountering the world of fantasy.

2. *What happens between the ages of 8 and adulthood?* Very little research has concentrated on older school-age children and adolescents. Is this a latent period? Because by this age most children have outgrown beliefs in Santa Claus, the tooth fairy, imaginary companions, wishing, and more, most researchers have neglected to address what sort of thinking about the unseen world might be going on during this period. One possibility is that superstitious beliefs and/or beliefs in religion are filling the void left by earlier beliefs in fantasy. Suggestive of this, Clark (1995, p. 58) reports a conversation with an 8-year-old boy who is beginning to question the existence of Santa Claus. He says, "Some people think it's not real. . .Santa Claus. . . . When the presents are there on Christmas, I don't know where he is. . . . Probably it's God doing all this stuff, and it's Santa Claus who's not real." Clark proposes that the imaginal experience involved in believing in Santa Claus and other fantasy figures actually increases children's capacity for later faith in other forms. Probing the interrelatedness of magic and religion in the child's world is a question that has received almost no attention in the developmental literature.

Yet as Singer and Singer (1990) argue, fantastical thinking does not really stop at this age, it simply may be less overt and hence harder to observe. They suggest a number of ways that children of this age engage in fantasy, including group games such as pirates and rescue missions, board games, and video and computer games. Most of these games, as they state, "contain a fanciful element of fairy tale or myth" (p. 239). School plays, books, and television also provide forums for engaging in fantasy. Television can occupy much of children's attention at this age; this is also one area in which fantasy-reality differentiation has received considerable attention by researchers (for an excellent example of this research see Wright, Huston, Reitz, & Piemyat, 1994). Clearly, this is not a latent period, but one that is ripe for empirical investigation of children's thinking about fantasy.

3. *How do children make fantasy-reality decisions?* Verifying the nonexistence of things that do not exist is a tricky problem. As Morison and Gardner (1978, p. 647) state, ". . . the child is expected to sort experience in the absence of obvious perceptible cues; in fact, the final cue to fantasy status is often the lack of confirmation in the world of the entity in question." How this process might differ from the more mundane task of verifying the existence of things that exist is an intriguing question. For example, in Samuels and Taylor (1994), children were shown a picture of a moose cooking and asked whether it could happen in the real world. Clearly children have never seen a moose cooking, but how are they to

know that it is fantastical to think of such an event? Presumably there are many other things that moose actually do that children also have never seen. Even more problematic is the fact that children's books are rife with examples of animals doing all sorts of human-like things.

Relatedly, research on children's beliefs about magic indicates that between the ages of 3 and 6 children change from thinking of magic as real to thinking of it as a trick. How does this transformation occur? What, if any, beliefs in real magic remain? How would children arrive at the belief that magical forces are unlikely to exist? Longitudinal and perhaps also microgenetic studies of children's beliefs most likely hold the answers to these questions.

4. *What role does emotion play in distinguishing fantasy and reality?* There are many important unanswered questions here. Does emotion disrupt the ability to distinguish reality and fantasy? Are children more prone to its effects than adults, perhaps because adults are better at discounting? Alternatively, might emotion facilitate making this distinction in some situations? One possibility is that heightened arousal may serve to cause one to pay greater attention to certain aspects of a situation—fantasy-reality status being one. Morison and Gardner (1978) predicted that children will master the fantasy-reality status of scary events earlier than nonscary events. This might be an example of emotion acting to facilitate such judgments, and it seems a sensible prediction from an evolutionary standpoint. However, research has not supported this prediction (e.g., Prawat, Anderson, & Hapkiewicz, 1985; Samuels & Taylor, 1994).

In fact, most research with both children and adults suggests that emotion may disrupt these boundaries. A standard tenet in clinical psychology, for example, is that in instances of insecurity, emotional reactions are strong, and individuals may interpret reality according to the emotions they are experiencing. Although more research needs to be done to come to any definite conclusions about the effects of emotion on children's fantasy-reality differentiation, various prominent researchers in the field (e.g., Bretherton & Beeghly, 1982; Harris et al., 1991; Lillard, 1994) have suggested that children are facile at determining the boundary between fantasy and reality, except when the situation is emotionally charged. In fact, Samuels and Taylor (1994) found that children deemed all scary events to be unreal. However, as Lillard (1994) notes, such judgments do not necessarily reflect confusion about the fantasy-reality boundary. Rather it is very possible that, while keeping the boundary in place, in the aim of coping with difficult emotions, children simply move these events across the boundary into the realm of pretend. It would be worth looking at whether children would be more or less willing to evoke magical explanations when an unexplainable event is scary. With regard to beliefs in mental-physical causality, research could also address whether children are more likely to believe in the efficacy of positive wishes than of negative wishes, for example.

However, there are other studies that suggest that emotional content does not affect children's ability to distinguish between reality and fantasy. Prawat et al. (1985) found no effect of the emotional content (scary versus not scary) of various pictures of monsters on children's judgments of their fantasy-reality status. Harris et al. (1991) found that making mental images scary did not affect children's ability to make the fantasy-reality distinction in the case of imagined or pretended entities. Golomb and Galasso (1995) also found no effect of emotion on children's ability to distinguish imagination from reality in a pretend context. A particularly illustrative case is that of children's imaginary companions. Imaginary companions are highly positively charged, yet Taylor et al. (1993) report that children are not confused about their reality status. Researchers need to address when emotion does and does not affect fantasy-reality differentiation, as well as how it "works its magic."

5. *What sorts of individual differences exist and what is their nature and course?* The majority of studies in this domain reveal considerable and significant individual differences, yet researchers rarely acknowledge them and even more rarely try to explain them. Researchers need to address the nature and possible origins of these individual differences, as well as their developmental trajectories. Substantial individual differences in parental encouragement of fantasy figures were reported by Rosengren and Hickling (1994). What might be the effects of this on children's beliefs? What effects are there of environmental factors? Are there individual differences in information-processing abilities that might affect these sorts of beliefs? Are some children simply born credulous and others skeptical? There is also the issue of continuity. One question to be asked here is whether children who early in life are more fantasy prone grow up to be adults who believe in UFOs, for example. One study cited earlier (Persinger & Makarec, 1990) found that adults who reported having a religious experience before adolescence were more likely both to believe in religious tenets and to have superstitious beliefs than those who had not had such an experience. Others have hypothesized a "fantasy-proneness" personality dimension. What were people who have been classified this way like as children?

6. *What sort of variability is evident in children's developing conceptions?* Recently, Siegler (1996) has proposed that children's thinking is much more variable than the developmental psychology literature suggests. He proposes that documenting the variability in children's knowledge can lead to important clues about mechanisms of change. His work inspires new questions regarding children's development in a variety of domains. He focuses on three issues: variability, choice, and change. Some of these questions can and should be applied to children's beliefs in fantasy. For example, regarding variability, research on children's magical thinking has found that in some tasks children appear to be credulous and in others skeptical. Questions to be answered include: Under what situations do children appear to espouse magical beliefs? Woolley and Phelps (1994) suggest that the child's perception of the practical nature of the situation is important. Some clues may also be available from studies of children's humor. McGhee and Johnson (1975) note that if available cues suggest to the child that the situation is a serious one, she will not perceive a violation of her physical knowledge as funny, and will go about trying to solve the problem (or, as Woolley and Phelps argue, not resort to a magical explanation). On the other hand, children are able to respond to cues that signal that a situation should be perceived as non-serious or funny, and they respond appropriately. Further, why and when do children persist with one way of thinking when their behavior in other situations suggests that they are aware of others? Regarding Siegler's second issue, choice, what are the respective roles of domain-specific knowledge and temperament or other personality styles? When faced with a new fact or a new entity, how do children evaluate its fantasy status? Which plays a larger role—their existing beliefs about fantastical entities, or something like a "fantasy-prone" disposition? Regarding the third issue, change, what is the experience of discovery like? This question was identified earlier, in number 3. How is the discovery that Santa Claus is not real constrained by domain-specific knowledge? How might this discovery (and others)

be generalized to related issues? Acknowledging the variability in children's conceptions can open the doors to numerous important questions in this domain.

CONCLUSIONS

In conclusion, in this article I have reviewed evidence on the issue of magical thinking and thoughts in children and adults. I conclude that differences between children and adults reflect continuous rather than discontinuous development. Although I have proposed a number of possible forms such development might take, which of these best characterizes development is unknown. Future studies should aim to reveal the various contributions of some or all of these processes to our changing views of reality across individuals and across the lifespan. It is very likely that explanations of the world in terms of magic, science, and religion coexist, as they have throughout history, in the minds of children and adults alike throughout the lifespan.

REFERENCES

Adorno, T. W., Frenkel-Brunswik, E., Levinson, D. J., & Sanford, R. N. (1950). *The authoritarian personality.* New York: Harper.

Alcock, J. E. (1995). The belief engine. *Skeptical Inquirer, May/June, 19,* 14–18.

Astington, J. W. (1993). *The child's discovery of the mind.* Cambridge, MA: Harvard University Press.

Blair, J. R., McKee, J. S., & Jernigan, L. F. (1980). Children's belief in Santa Claus, Easter Bunny, and Tooth Fairy. *Psychological Reports, 46,* 691–694.

Blum, S. H. (1976). Some aspects of belief in prevailing superstitions. *Psychological Reports, 38,* 579–582.

Blum, S. H., & Blum, L. H. (1974). Do's and don'ts: An informal study of some prevailing superstitions. *Psychological Reports, 35,* 567–571.

Bretherton, I., & Beeghly, M. (1982). Talking about internal states: The acquisition of an explicit theory of mind. *Developmental Psychology, 18,* 906–921.

Broad, C. D. (1953). *Religion, philosophy, and psychical research.* New York: Harcourt, Brace.

Carey, S. (1985). Are children fundamentally different kinds of thinkers than adults? In S. Chipman, J. W. Segal, & R. Glaser (Eds.), *Thinking and learning skills* (Vol. 2). Hillsdale, NJ: Erlbaum.

Chandler, M. J., & Lalonde, C. E. (1994). Surprising, miraculous, and magical turns of events. *British Journal of Developmental Psychology, 12,* 83–95.

Chinn, C. A., & Brewer, W. F. (1993). The role of anomalous data in knowledge acquisition: A theoretical framework and implications for science instruction. *Review of Educational Research, 63*(1), 1–49.

Clark, C. D. (1995). *Flights of fancy, leaps of faith: Children's myths in contemporary America.* Chicago: University of Chicago Press.

Cottrell, J. E., Winer, G. A., & Smith, M. C. (1996). Beliefs of children and adults about feeling stares of unseen others. *Developmental Psychology, 32,* 50–61.

Estes, D., Wellman, H. M., & Woolley, J. (1989). Children's understanding of mental phenomena. In H. Reese (Eds.), *Advances in child development and behavior* (pp. 41–86). New York: Academic Press.

Flavell, J. H., Green, F. L., & Flavell, E. R. (1986). Development of knowledge about the appearance-reality distinction. *Monographs of the Society for Research in Child Development, 51* (1, Serial No. 212).

Frazier, K. (1989). Gallup poll of beliefs: Astrology up, ESP down. *Skeptical Inquirer, 13,* 244–245.

Freud, S. (1955). *The "uncanny."* London: Hogarth Press/Institute of Psychoanalysis. (Original work published 1919).

Gallup, G. H., & Newport, F. (1991). Belief in paranormal phenomena among adult Americans. *Skeptical Inquirer, 15,* 137–146.

Golomb, C., & Galasso, L. (1995). Make believe and reality: Explorations of the imaginary realm. *Developmental Psychology, 31,* 800–810.

Harris, P. L., Brown, E., Marriot, C., Whittall, S., & Harmer, S. (1991). Monsters, ghosts, and witches: Testing the limits of the fantasy-reality distinction in young children. *British Journal of Developmental Psychology, 9,* 105–123.

Jahoda, G. (1969). *The psychology of superstition.* New York: Penguin.

Johnson, C., & Harris, P. L. (1994). Magic: Special but not excluded. *British Journal of Developmental Psychology, 12,* 35–51.

Keinan, G. (1994). Effects of stress and tolerance of ambiguity on magical thinking. *Journal of Personality and Social Psychology, 67,* 48–55.

Langer, E. J. (1975). The illusion of control. *Journal of Personality and Social Psychology, 32,* 311–328.

Lillard, A. (1994). Making sense of pretense. In C. Lewis & P. Mitchell (Eds.), *Children's early understanding of mind: Origins and development.* Hove, UK: Earlbaum.

Lynn, S. J., & Rhue, J. W. (1988). Fantasy proneness: Hypnosis, developmental antecedents, and psychopathology. *American Psychologist, 43,* 35–44.

McGhee, P. E., & Johnson, S. F. (1975). The role of fantasy and reality cues in children's appreciation of incongruity humor. *Merrill-Palmer Quarterly, 21,* 19–30.

Menzel, D. H., & Taves, E. (1977). *The UFO enigma: The definitive explanation of the UFO phenomenon.* New York: Doubleday.

Morison, P., & Gardner, H. (1978). Dragons and dinosaurs: The child's capacity to differentiate fantasy from reality. *Child Development, 49,* 642–648.

Neusner, J., Frerichs, E. S., & Flesher, P. V. M. (Eds.). (1989). *Religion, science, and magic: In concert and in conflict.* Oxford: Oxford University Press.

Persinger, M. A., & Makarec, K. (1990). Exotic beliefs may be substitutes for religious beliefs. *Perceptual and Motor Skills, 71,* 16–18.

Phelps, K. E., & Woolley, J. D. (1994). The form and function of young children's magical beliefs. *Developmental Psychology, 30,* 385–394.

Phelps, K. E., & Woolley, J. D. (1995). *Effects of animacy and emotionality on children's beliefs about imagination.* Unpublished manuscript, University of Texas.

Piaget, J. P. (1929). *The child's conception of the world.* London: Routledge & Kegan Paul.

Prawat, R. S., Anderson, A. H., & Hapkiewicz, W. (1985). Is the scariest monster also the least real? An examination of children's reality justifications. *Journal of Genetic Psychology, 146,* 7–12.

Prentice, N. M., & Gordon, D. (1986). Santa Claus and the Tooth Fairy for the Jewish child and parent. *Journal of Genetic Psychology, 148*(2), 139–151.

Prentice, N. M., Manosevitz, M., & Hubbs, L. (1978). Imaginary figures of early childhood: Santa Claus, Easter bunny, and the tooth fairy. *American Journal of Orthopsychiatry, 48,* 618–628.

Rizzuto, A.-M. (1979). *The birth of the living God: A psychoanalytic study.* Chicago: University of Chicago Press.

Rosengren, K. S., & Hickling, A. K. (1994). Seeing is believing: Children's explorations of commonplace, magical, and extraordinary transformations. *Child Development, 65,* 1605–1626.

Rosengren, K. S., Kalish, C. W., Hickling, A. K., & Gelman, S. A. (1994). Exploring the relation between preschool children's magical beliefs and causal thinking. *British Journal of Developmental Psychology, 12*(1), 69–82.

Rothbaum, F., & Weisz, J. R. (1988). *Child psychopathology and the quest for control.* New York: Sage.

Rozin, P., Markwith, M., & Ross, B. (1990). The sympathetic magical law of similarity, nominal realism, and neglect of negatives in response to negative labels. *Psychological Science, 1*(6), 383–384.

Rozin, P., Millman, L., & Nemeroff, C. (1986). Operation of the laws of sympathetic magic in disgust and other domains. *Journal of Personality and Social Psychology, 50*(4), 703–712.

Rozin, P., & Nemeroff, C. (1990). The laws of sympathetic magic: A psychological analysis of similarity and contagion. In J. W. Stigler, R. A. Shweder, & G. Herdt (Eds.), *Cultural psychology: Essay on comparative human development* (pp. 205–232). Cambridge, MA: Cambridge University Press.

Rozin, P., Nemeroff, C., Wane, M., & Sherrod, A. (1989). Operation of the sympathetic magical law of contagion in interpersonal attitudes among Americans. *Bulletin of the Psychonomic Society, 27,* 367–370.

Samuels, A., & Taylor, M. (1994). Children's ability to distinguish fantasy events from real-life events. *British Journal of Developmental Psychology, 12,* 417–427.

Shaeffer, R. (1981). *The UFO verdict: Examining the evidence.* New York: Prometheus.

Shweder, R. A., & Levine, R. A. (1975). Dream concepts of Hausa children. *Ethos, 3,* 209–230.

Siegler, R. S. (1996). *Emerging minds: The process of change in children's thinking.* New York: Oxford University Press.

Singer, D. G., & Singer, J. L. (1990). *The house of make-believe: Children's play and the developing imagination.* Cambridge, MA: Harvard University Press.

Spanos, N. P. Cross, P. A., Dickson, K., & DeBreuil, S. C. (1993). Close encounters: An examination of UFO experiences. *Journal of Abnormal Psychology, 102,* 624–632.

Stanovich, K. E. (1994). Reconceptualizing intelligence: Dysrationalia as an intuition pump. *Educational Researcher, 22,* 5–21.

Subbotsky, E. V. (1993). *Foundations of the mind: Children's understanding of reality.* Cambridge, MA: Harvard University Press.

Subbotsky, E. V. (1994). Early rationality and magical thinking in preschoolers: Space and time. *British Journal of Developmental Psychology, 12,* 97–108.

Taylor, B. J., & Howell, R. J. (1973). The ability of three-, four-, and five-year-old children to distinguish fantasy from reality. *Journal of Genetic Psychology, 122,* 315–318.

Taylor, M., Cartwright, B. S., & Carlson, S. M. (1993). A developmental investigation of children's imaginary companions. *Developmental Psychology, 29,* 276–285.

Taylor, S. E. (1983). Adjustment to threatening events. *American Psychologist, 38,* 1161–1173.

Taylor, S. E., Lichtman, R. R., & Wood, J. V. (1984). Attributions, beliefs about control, and adjustment to breast cancer. *Journal of Personality and Social Psychology, 46,* 489–502.

Vikan, A., & Clausen, S. E. (1993). Freud, Piaget, or neither? Beliefs in controlling others by wishful thinking and magical behavior in young children. *Journal of Genetic Psychology, 154*(3), 297–314.

Walton, K. L. (1990). *Mimesis as make-believe.* Cambridge, MA: Harvard University Press.

Weisz, J. R. (1981). Illusory contigency in children at the State Fair. *Developmental Psychology, 17,* 481–489.

Wellman, H. M., & Estes, D. (1986). Early understanding of mental entities: A reexamination of childhood realism. *Child Development, 57,* 910–923.

Werner, H. (1948). *Comparative psychology of mental development.* New York: International Universities Press.

Wilson, S. C., & Barber, T. X. (1983). The fantasy-prone personality: Implications for understanding imagery, hypnosis, and parapsychological phenomena. In A. A. Sheikh (Ed.), *Imagery: Current theory, research, and application* (pp. 340–390). New York: Wiley.

Woolley, J. D., & Phelps, K. E. (1994). Young children's practical reasoning about imagination. *British Journal of Developmental Psychology, 12,* 53–67.

Woolley, J. D., Phelps, K. E., & Davis, D. L. (1995). *Children's beliefs about wishing as a mental and magical process.* Unpublished manuscript, University of Texas.

Woolley, J. D., & Wellman, H. M. (1990). Young children's understanding of realities, nonrealities, and appearances. *Child Development, 61,* 946–961.

Woolley, J. D., & Wellman, H. M. (1993). Origin and truth: Young children's understanding of imaginary mental representations. *Child Development, 64,* 1–17.

Wright, J. C., Huston, A. C., Reitz, A. L., & Piemyat, S. (1994). Young children's perceptions of television reality: Determinants and developmental differences. *Developmental Psychology, 30,* 229–239.

Zimmer, T. A. (1985). Belief in UFOs as alternative reality, cultural rejection, or disturbed psyche. *Deviant Behavior, 6,* 405–419.

Zusne, L., & Jones, W. H. (1989). *Anomalistic psychology: A study of magical thinking.* Hillsdale, NJ: Erlbaum.

4

Ritual, Habit, and Perfectionism: The Prevalence and Development of Compulsive-Like Behavior in Normal Young Children

David W. Evans
University of New Orleans, New Orleans, Louisiana
James F. Leckman, Alice Carter, J. Steven Reznick, Desiree Henshaw, Robert A. King, and David Pauls
Yale University, New Haven, Connecticut

Young children engage in a significant amount of ritualistic, repetitive, and compulsive-like activity that appears to be part of their normal behavioral repertoire. Empirically, little is known about the onset, prevalence, and developmental trajectory of these phenomena. A parent-report questionnaire, the Childhood Routines Inventory (CRI), was developed to assess compulsive-like behavior in young children, and was administered to 1,492 parents with children between the ages of 8 and 72 months. The CRI has strong overall internal consistency and a distinct two-factor structure. The frequency of compulsive-like behaviors changes with age: Two-, 3-, and 4-year-olds engaged in more compulsive behavior than children younger than 1 year of age and older than 4 years of age. Results are discussed from a developmental psychopathology framework and for their implications for future research in this area.

INTRODUCTION

In his pioneering work documenting the emergence of various motor, cognitive, and social abilities in children, Arnold Gesell (Ames, Ilg, & Frances, 1976; Gesell, 1928; Gesell, Ames, & Ilg, 1974) noted that normal $2\frac{1}{2}$- to 3-year-old children exhibit marked compulsive behavior. Strong preferences for sameness in the environment; repetitive, ritualized

Reprinted with permission from *Child Development*, 1997, Vol. 68(1), 58–68. Copyright © 1997 by the Society for Research in Child Development, Inc.

Portions of this manuscript were presented at the biennial meetings of the Society for Research in Child Development, Indianapolis, IN, March 30–April 2, 1995. For copies of the CRI please contact the first author at the address below. The authors thank William Kessen, Elisabeth Dykens, Robert M. Hodapp, and Lawrence Scahill for their comments. Special thanks go to Harry W. Evans for his editorial expertise and insightful comments.

behavior; rigidity in terms of likes and dislikes; and the sometimes acute sensory perceptual awareness of minute details or imperfections in toys or clothes are all examples of normative behavior in the young child that Gesell termed the "rituals of the ritualist" (Gesell et al., 1974).

In the context of psychopathology, compulsions refer to repetitive behaviors, such as checking or washing, that are performed to reduce anxiety (APA, 1994). Other obsessive-compulsive behaviors include arranging objects or performing certain tasks until they satisfy some subjective, sensory-perceptual criteria as being "Just Right" (Leckman, Walker, Goodman, Pauls, & Cohen, 1994). Some research with adolescents and adults has studied the continuities and discontinuities between pathological and nonpathological (i.e., that which is thought to represent certain personality styles) obsessive-compulsive behavior (Flament, Whitaker, Rapoport, Davies, et al., 1988; Niler & Beck, 1989; Rachman & de Silva, 1978; Salkovskis & Harrison, 1984). Whereas the compulsions of OCD are maladaptive responses to uncontrollable intrusive thoughts, nonclinical compulsive behavior is believed to be more adaptive, with greater control over intrusive thoughts.

Aside from these studies comparing OCD and subclinical OC behavior in adults, little research has studied compulsivity as a normative phenomenon during childhood—a time when such behavior is thought to be quite prevalent (Leonard, Goldberger, Rapoport, Cheslow, & Swedo, 1990; Marks, 1987).

Compulsivity in Childhood

Ritualistic and compulsive-like behavior can readily be observed in children's games (King & Noshpitz, 1991; Leonard et al., 1990; Marks, 1987; Rachman & de Silva, 1978). Playing tag or hopscotch, or reciting rhymes like "step on a crack, break your mother's back," are common activities that resemble the ritualism and magical thinking that occur in OCD (Bolton, 1996; King & Noshpitz, 1991). In these childhood rituals, as in OCD, certain behaviors are enacted for the purpose of warding off harm to self or others, especially parents (King & Noshpitz, 1991; Marks, 1987). Even before middle childhood, however, children exhibit repetitive, compulsive-like behavior. Ritualization may be particularly prevalent in children at times of transition (bedtime, mealtime, bath), or when transitions are accompanied by normative fears or anxieties (e.g., fears of the dark; Garber, Garber, & Spizman, 1993). Regardless of the function that rituals may serve, consider the compulsive nature of the following example of a bedtime ritual: "Saying goodnight to the people downstairs will have to be done in just a certain way, and these goodnights will have to be said in a certain order. A certain number of kisses. The exact same words to be said by everyone" (Ilg, Ames, & Baker, 1981, p. 90).

Requests to hear the same story, or to watch the same video over and over, are common examples of the "insistence on sameness" and repetition that characterize the behavior of many, if not all, young children. Other compulsive-like behaviors in childhood seem to mirror sensory-perceptual and "Just Right" phenomena of OCD (Leckman, Goodman, et al., 1994). Whereas the parents may insist that the child eat his vegetables at dinner, the child may insist that the potatoes be placed only in a certain part of the plate and must not touch any other food; should the potatoes land outside of this area, the child may seem to experience a sense of near-contamination, setting off a tirade of fussiness for which many 2- and 3-year-olds are notorious.

Preference for balance, symmetry, and wholeness is common in OCD; this, too, is shared by many young children: "The two year old, with his rigid sense of just how he wants everything to be, may insist, as when he has a cookie, on having one for each hand. He may also be much upset, as again when he has a cookie, if a bite is taken out or a piece broken off, insisting that everything be whole and round and unbroken" (Ilg et al., 1981).

The child may exhibit "Just Right" phenomena by imposing relatively strict and circumscribed ways of arranging his or her favorite objects (see also Garrison & Earls, 1982; Passman, 1976, 1977, 1987; Winnecott, 1953). Other examples of "Just Right" behaviors include attention to detail: a heightened awareness of the way certain clothes feel (e.g., being bothered by the feel of tags on the neck of a shirt, or other minute imperfections), the ordering of objects in symmetrical patterns, and the general structuring of the world around him or her. The child may insist that the bedroom door be left open just a certain amount of space, or that the window shades be drawn to a particular level.

Some researchers (Leonard et al., 1990; Rachman & de Silva, 1978) have compared retrospective accounts of childhood rituals and superstitions reported by adolescents with OCD and those reported by normal controls. This research indicates that adolescents with OCD engaged in the "normal" rituals of early childhood (e.g., eating food in a certain order, timeconsuming hobbies) and were comparable to a control group when OCD symptoms per se (e.g., hand washing) were accounted for.

Markt and Johnson (1993) found that even college students (roughly 20%) may engage in certain presleep rituals, possibly in an effort to ward off fears or anxieties that accompany bedtime. The exact nature and developmental course of compulsive behavior as a phenomenon of normal childhood has not attracted research, however (Leonard et al., 1989). Thus we know very little about the age limits, origin, or possible relation between early compulsivity and later obsessive-compulsive problems (Marks, 1987, p. 118). This study attempted to address some of these aspects of the normative course of compulsive-like behaviors in early childhood.

The first goal of the study was to construct a measure to assess compulsive behaviors in young children and to explore the psychometric properties of this instrument. The second goal was to estimate the prevalence of compulsive-like behaviors in young children. Comparisons of the mean scores and subscores on this measure afford a view of the developmental course of compulsive-like behaviors.

METHOD

Participants

Parents with children between the ages of 8 months and 72 months were identified from town records and published birth announcements in the New Haven, CT, area. Parents were initially contacted by mail following the birth of their infant and asked whether they were interested in participating in research on child development. The names and addresses of those who responded affirmatively (approximately 15% of the population) were entered into a database ($N = 3{,}712$). Questionnaires were sent out in two waves. The first wave included those parents with children aged 8 months to 31 months; the second wave was sent 14 weeks later to parents of children aged 32 to 72 months. Complete data are available on 1,488 (40%) respondents. Participants were divided into six age groups for analyses based on traditional age cut points. The gender distribution within each age group is as follows: <12 months (85 males, 77 females); 12–23 months (203 males, 211 females); 24–35 months (158 males, 145 females); 36–47 months (110 males, 145 females); 48–59 months (89 males, 109 females); 60–72 months (74 males, 71 females). Participants in these age groups did not differ significantly on birth order, maternal education (mean = 15.35 years), or paternal education (15.13 years). Although all two-parent families with children who were in the target age range and who had been born in New Haven County were initially invited to participate, those responding to our mailing represent a bias toward well-educated, white, middle-class families (see Table 1 for demographic information).

Measures

The Childhood Routines Inventory (CRI) is a 19-item parent-report questionnaire that was designed to assess children's compulsive-like behaviors. The CRI affords three indices of the presence of compulsive-like behavior in young children: How much/how often the child has engaged in ritualistic behavior (frequency/intensity), when the behavior began (onset), and whether the child currently engages in compulsive-like behavior (current). Parents also indicate whether a given behavior ever caused them concern (a component of the CRI that will be addressed at a later point). The CRI items were originally chosen

TABLE 1
Demographics: Education Levels and Ethnic Backgrounds of New Haven Sample Compared with 1990 U.S. Census Data (%)

	New Haven		
	Mothers	Fathers	U.S. Census
Education:			
<12 years	.7	2.0	23.2
H.S. diploma	16.1	22.3	42.0
Some college	22.6	18.8	16.9
College degree	61.2	56.9	17.9
	New Haven		U.S. Census
Ethnicity:			
White	95.4		80.3
Black	2.0		12.1
Asian	1.0		2.9
Hispanic	1.0		9.0[a]
Other	.6		3.9

[a]According to U.S. Census, persons of Hispanic origin may be of any race; therefore, percentages may total more than 100%.

by the authors as reflecting DSM IV symptoms for compulsivity, placed in the context of childhood, and phrased so as to avoid casting the items in a pathological framework.

Procedure

The CRI was mailed to parents along with a letter of introduction and a description of our study. Parents also received questionnaires relevant to other aspects of child development research. A self-addressed, stamped envelope was included in the mailing, and parents were encouraged to return the completed questionnaires within 2 weeks. As compensation/incentive for participation, parents received coupons for discounts from local merchants.

RESULTS

The first goal of the study was to explore the internal consistency of the CRI using the 1 to 5 metric representing the frequency/intensity with which the children engaged in compulsive-like behavior at any point in the past. An average frequency/intensity score was created by adding the scores from each item and dividing by the number of items on the CRI. These scores were normally distributed. The CRI demonstrated good overall internal consistency (Cronbach's alpha = .89), suggesting the usefulness of the single construct of "compulsive-like behavior."

Age × Gender Comparisons of Frequency/Intensity of Compulsive-like Behaviors

The mean frequency/intensity scores of the CRI were compared across the six age groups (<12 months, 12–23, 24–35, 36–47, 48–59, 60–72) and revealed an effect of age, $F(5, 1421) = 38.16$, $p < .01$. Post hoc analyses indicated that 2-, 3-, and 4-year-olds had frequency/intensity scores that were significantly higher than those of younger (<12 months, 12–23 months) and older (60–72 months) children. No main or interaction effects with sex emerged.

Factor Structure of the CRI

We next explored subconstructs of the CRI. Given the relatively large sample size, we were able to use a two-step process to explore the factor structure. Exploratory factor analysis (principal components) with Varimax rotation was performed on one-half of the sample chosen at random. The intial criterion for retaining a principal component was an eigenvalue >1.00. A scree test (Cattell, 1966) indicated that two principal components be retained. An item from the CRI was considered part of a factor if its factor loading was ≥.5 and did not load on another factor.

The principal components revealed two constructs that are central to the phenomenology of obsessive-compulsive disorder. The first principal component comprises items on the CRI that can be characterized as "Just Right" features. "Just Right" phenomena refer to carrying out certain behaviors (e.g., arranging objects) until they satisfy some sensory-perceptual criteria for being "just so" (Leckman, Goodman, et al., 1994; Leckman, Walker, et al.,

1994). The "Just Right" factor on the CRI includes: (1) "prefers to have things done in a particular order or in a certain way"; (2) "arranges objects or performs certain behaviors until they seem 'Just Right' "; (3) "lines up objects in straight lines or symmetrical patterns"; (4) "insists on having certain belongings around the house 'in their place' "; (5) "seems very aware of how certain clothes feel." This component accounts for 33% of the variance.

The second principal component included items that relate to repetitive behavior and insistence on sameness: (1) "Prefers the same household schedule or routine every day"; (2) "Acts out the same thing over and over in pretend play"; (3) "Repeats certain actions over and over"; (4) "Has strong preferences for certain foods." This second component accounted for 8% of the variance.

The validity of these two factors was corroborated by expert agreement. Two child psychologists and one child psychiatrist were asked to categorize each item of the CRI as to whether it belongs in a "Just Right" category, a "repetitive behaviors" category, both, or neither category. Perfect interrater agreement was achieved for all of the "Just Right" items from the principal components analyses such that all those items that loaded on the "Just Right" factor were rated as being "Just Right" items by these experts. All raters agreed that an additional item—"seems very concerned with dirt, cleanliness, or neatness"—belonged in the "Just Right" factor as well, which was then included in this factor. Raters all agreed that "prefers same household routine every day," "acts out same thing over and over in pretend play", and "repeats certain actions over and over" all belong in the "repetitive behaviors" factor, but did not include "strong preferences for wearing (or not wearing) certain articles of clothing" in this factor. Indeed, two of the three raters indicated that this item was a "Just Right" variable. Moreover, all three raters agreed that "prepares for bedtime by engaging in a special activity or routine or by doing or saying things in a certain order or certain way" belonged in the "Just Right" factor. "Has strong food preferences" and "bedtime routines" were included, then, in the repetitive behaviors factor in subsequent analyses.

In order to determine how well this two-factor model fit the data at each age group, two sets of analyses were performed. First, confirmatory factor analyses tested the two-factor model (above) at each of six age groups, and also tested whether two alternate models (a one-factor and a three-factor solution) better fit the data. The three-factor model included a factor that emerged from the initial principal components analyses. This factor (attached to one favorite object; collects/stores objects; is concerned with dirt, cleanliness, or neatness) had an eigenvalue greater than 1.00, but did not appear to account for significant additional variance beyond the two principal components. The two-factor model yielded relatively good fit indices across all six age groups. The chisquare/degrees of freedom ratio was <2.00 for children in the age groups <12 months, 24–35 months, 48–60 months, and 70–72 months, indicating an excellent fit. Although children in age groups 12–23 months and 36–47 had chi/*df* ratios greater than 2.00, other indices indicated that the two-factor model was a relatively good fit to the data for these age groups. Moreover, the one- and three-factor models yielded chi/*df* ratios well above 2.00 in most cases, and greater than 3.00 in some instances. For children less than 12 months, however, the one- and two-factor models were similar (one-factor chi/*df* = 1.82). The three-factor model chi/*df* ratio was 1.83 for the oldest age group, which is greater than the 1.58 that emerged in the two-factor model for this age group. Thus, as a whole, the two-factor model provides the best fit to the data with this replication sample (see Table 2).

TABLE 2
Goodness-of-Fit Indices[a] for Confirmatory Factor Analysis of the Two-Factor Model

Age Group (Months)	Chi-square	Chi/*df*	GFI	RMSR
>12	99.71	1.88	.87	.08
12–23	121.96	2.30	.95	.04
24–35	105.33	1.98	.94	.05
36–47	128.40	2.42	.91	.058
48–59	95.84	1.81	.92	.057
60–72	83.52	1.58	.90	.06

[a]Goodness-of-Fit Index (GFI) $\geq$ .90, chi-square/degrees of freedom ratio (Chi/*df*) $\leq$ 2.00, and Root Mean Square Residuals (RMSR) $\leq$ .05 are considered excellent fit. Degrees of freedom = 53.

Similar "goodness-of-fit" analyses were performed to compare the matrices across age groups, using Green's Test (Green, 1992). In general, the pattern of correlations among the CRI items was somewhat different for the youngest children (<12 months) compared to all other age groups. Comparison of the older age groups to each other (3- with 4-year-olds, 3-with 5-year-olds, 4-with 5-year-olds, and so on) indicated that the patterns of correlation among CRI items were similar across these ages (see Table 3).

Age × Gender Effects for "Just Right" and "Repetitive Behaviors" Factors

Findings similar to those of the total CRI frequency/intensity score emerged for the "Just Right" and Repetitive Behaviors factors: Age group had a significant main effect: $F(5, 1420) = 43.22$, $p < .01$; $F(5, 1420) = 10.62$, $p < .01$, for the "Just Right" and Repetitive Behaviors factors, respectively. Again 2-, 3-, and 4-year-olds were reported to engage in compulsive-like behaviors with greater frequency/intensity than younger or older children. A significant quadratic age effect for both factors emerged as well, reflecting an increase in these phenomena with age, followed by a decrease at the oldest age groups. A factor × age group interaction revealed that the "Just Right" factor is marked by a more dramatic ascent in the early ages, $F(1, 5) = 16.78$, $p < .01$. No significant age × gender interaction or gender main effects emerged.

Comparisons of CRI Means: Child's Current Status

Next, age-related differences in children's *current* status on each of the three CRI indices described above (overall score, "Just Right," and "Repetitive Behaviors" factors) were examined across the six age groups. These indices are based on the cumulative number of dichotomous items that parents endorsed ("Child currently engages in this behavior; 'Yes' or 'No' "). Age differences emerged on all three indices: total score, $F(5, 1416) = 23.45$, $p < .0001$; "Just Right," $F(5, 1397) = 39.04$, $p < .0001$; and Repetitive Behaviors, $F(5, 1402) = 10.75$, $p < .0001$ (see Tables 4, 5, and 6 for means and standard deviations and Duncan groupings). The age group × sex interaction and main effect for sex were

TABLE 3
Goodness-of-Fit Comparisons of CRI Correlation Matrices by Each Age Group[a]

Age Group	Chi-square	p	GFI	RMSR
1 vs. 2[b]	115.72	.0001	.99	.035
1 vs. 3	141.79	.0001	.98	.048
1 vs. 4	163.66	.0001	.96	.067
1 vs. 5	123.05	.0001	.96	.070
1 vs. 6	130.90	.0001	.94	.090
2 vs. 3	93.30	.001	.98	.033
2 vs. 4	93.90	.001	.96	.052
2 vs. 5	86.10	.005	.95	.059
2 vs. 6	55.90	.471	.95	.066
3 vs. 4	62.42	.229	.97	.033
3 vs. 5	62.90	.217	.97	.040
3 vs. 6	57.18	.394	.96	.065
4 vs. 5	67.29	.124	.98	.041
4 vs. 6	57.88	.369	.96	.045
5 vs. 6	48.44	.722	.97	.047

[a]Probability of chi-square $> .001$, Goodness-of-Fit Index (GFI) $\geq .90$, and Root Mean Square Residuals (RMSR) $\leq .05$ are considered excellent fits.
[b]1 = <12 months, 2 = 12–23, 3 = 24–35, 4 = 36–47, 5 = 48–59, 6 = 60–72.

not significant. On all three indices, the means for children in age groups 3, 4, and 5 (2-, 3-, and 4-year-olds) were higher than for children at the older (5- and 6-year-olds) and younger (<2 years) ages. For the total score, 2-, 3-, and 4-year-olds were reported to currently engage in significantly more compulsive-like behaviors than children in other age groups. Children from the youngest age groups (less than 12 months) engaged in less compulsive-like behavior than did the 5- and 6-year-olds, who did not differ from each other. Similarly, on the "Just Right" factor, 2-, 3-, and 4-year-olds engaged in significantly more "Just Right" behaviors than did children in all other age groups, quadratic $F(1, 5) = 115.47$, $p < .01$. One-year-olds engaged in similar levels of "Just Right" behaviors as did 6-year-olds, and both 1- and 6-year-olds engaged in more "Just Right" behaviors when compared with children less than 1 year of age (see Table 4 for means, standard deviations, and Duncan groupings).

Consistent with the findings from the "Just Right" factor, 2-, 3-, and 4-year-olds engaged in a similar number of Repetitive Behaviors, whereas children from the youngest and oldest age groups engaged in the fewest, quadratic $F(1,5) = 32.20$, $p < .01$. These quadratic analyses revealed that the "Just Right" factor begins a more dramatic (steeper) ascent, whereas the "Repetitive Behaviors" factor, though following a similar quadratic pattern, has a more gradual ascent by virtue of higher scores on this factor for the youngest age group.

TABLE 4
Means, Standard Deviations, Sample Sizes, and Duncan Groupings for Total CRI Score, "Just Right," and Repetitive Behaviors Factors

	Age Group (Months)					
	<12	12–23	24–35	36–47	48–59	60–72
Total CRI score:						
M	4.57	7.54	9.53	9.04	8.37	6.98
SD	3.63	4.72	4.93	4.85	4.99	4.61
n	118	418	304	231	198	153
Duncan grouping[a]	E	C,D	A	A,B	B,C	D
"Just Right":						
M	1.93	2.14	3.06	2.81	2.56	1.98
SD	1.17	1.78	1.83	1.82	1.87	1.77
n	117	411	300	230	192	153
Duncan grouping[a]	D	C	A	A,B	B	C
Repetitive:						
M	1.85	2.45	2.71	2.45	2.31	1.82
SD	1.66	1.77	1.85	1.77	1.80	1.61
n	117	413	300	228	198	152
Duncan grouping[a]	D	A,B	A	A,B	B,C	D

[a]Groups with the same letter are not significantly different.

TABLE 5
Raw Scores and Percentiles for Total, "Just Right," and Repetitive Behaviors by Age Group and for Total Sample

	Age Group (Months)						
	<12	12–23	24–35	36–47	48–59	60–72	Total
Total scale:							
95%	10	16	18	18	17	15	17
75%	8	11	13	13	12	10	12
50%	4	7	10	9	8	6	8
25%	2	4	5	6	5	3	4
5%	0	0	1	1	0	0	0
"Just Right":							
95%	3	6	6	6	6	6	6
75%	2	3	5	4	4	3	4
50%	1	2	3	3	2	2	2
25%	0	1	2	1	1	1	1
5%	0	0	0	0	0	0	0
Repetitive:							
95%	5	6	6	6	6	5	6
75%	3	4	4	4	4	3	4
50%	1	2	2	2	2	1.5	2
25%	1	1	1	1	1	0	1
5%	0	0	0	0	0	0	0

TABLE 6
Mean Age of Onset (Months) for Each Item on the CRI

	CRI Item	Mean Age of Onset (*SD*)
Q2	Been very attached to one favorite object?	13.85 (9.11)
Q7	Preferred the same household schedule or routine every day?	15.43 (11.06)
Q5	Had Persistent habits?	15.80 (11.44)
Q11	Had strong preferences for certain foods?	17.14 (10.78)
Q19	Prepared for bedtime by engaging in a special activity or routine, or by doing or saying things in a certain order or certain way?	17.43 (11.17)
Q10	Repeated certain actions over and over?	18.09 (10.46)
Q12	Liked to eat food in a particular way?	18.68 (10.84)
Q16	Seemed very aware of certain details at home (such as flecks of dirt on the floor, imperfections in toys and clothes)?	19.58 (11.28)
Q1	Preferred to have things done in a particular order or in a certain way (i.e., is he/she a "perfectionist"?)	21.10 (10.92)
Q3	Seemed very concerned with dirt, cleanliness, or neatness?	21.75 (10.44)
Q4	Arranged objects or performed certain behaviors until they seem "just right" to him/her?	22.45 (10.45)
Q17	Strongly preferred to stick to one game or activity rather than change to a new one?	22.96 (12.18)
Q6	Lined up objects in straight lines or in symmetrical patterns?	23.65 (10.03)
Q9	Insisted on having certain belongings around the house "in their place"?	23.92 (10.89)
Q8	Acted out the same thing over and over in pretend play?	24.14 (10.79)
Q15	Collected or stored objects?	25.26 (12.03)
Q13	Seemed very aware of, or sensitive to, how certain clothes feel?	25.29 (12.65)
Q14	Had a strong preference for wearing (or not wearing) certain articles of clothing?	25.92 (12.32)
Q18	Made requests or excuses that would enable him/her to postpone going to bed?	26.19 (11.68)

Note: Items are arranged in order from earliest to latest onset.

Frequency of Endorsement Across the Age Groups

In addition to exploring whether children at certain ages engage in more compulsive-like behavior than do children at other ages, we were interested in the frequency of endorsement of each item by age. Whereas the above analyses addressed differences in the intensity and number of items endorsed, we next explored data akin to prevalence rates of each compulsive-like behavior across the ages. Across the 19 items that comprise the CRI, more parents with children in the 24–35 month age range endorsed items (on average, 62%) indicating that their children currently engage in such behaviors (*range* = 38%–83%). This figure is considerably lower for children less than 1 year of age ($M = 27\%$, *range* = 4%–60%) and 12- to 23-month-olds ($M = 47\%$, *range* = 27%–81%). Three- and 4-year-olds

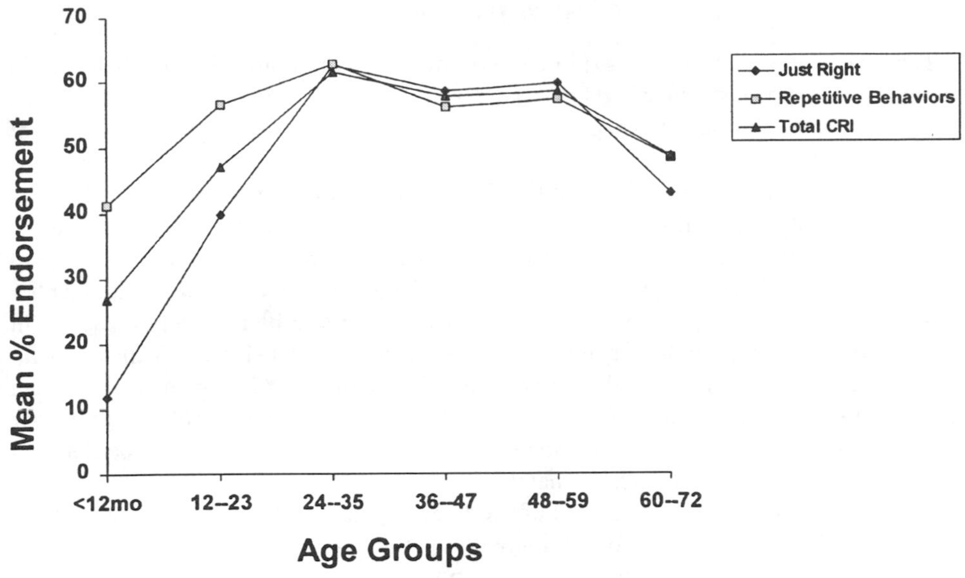

Figure 1. Percentage of participants engaging in compulsive-like behaviors across age groups.

were comparable to 2-year-olds, with an average of 58% and 59% of parents (respectively) reporting that their children currently engage in such behaviors (*ranges* = 34%–82% and 36%–86%). Forty-nine percent of the oldest group (ages 60–72 months) on average were reported to engage in these compulsive-like behaviors (*range* = 17%–84%). Results presented in Figure 1 are expressed as the mean percentages of parents at each age group who report that their child engages in compulsive-like behavior (a dichotomous variable). These average mean percentages were calculated for each of the two factors and for the total CRI scale.

Percentiles in Relation to Raw Scores

Next, analyses were conducted to determine percentile scores of the three "current" factors for particular levels of raw scores. For the sample as a whole, endorsement of 17 of the 19 CRI items places an individual in the ninety-fifth percentile; 12, 8, and 4 items endorsed place an individual in the seventy-fifth, fiftieth, and twenty-fifth percentiles, respectively. For the six items from each of the two factors, 6, 4, 2, and 1 items mark the ninety-fifth, seventy-fifth, fiftieth, and twenty-fifth percentiles. These percentiles are age dependent such that endorsement of a greater number of items for each index is required to achieve these percentiles for the middle age groups than for the younger and older age groups (see Table 5).

Finally, parents reported the age at which their children began to engage in particular behaviors. On average, parents reported that their children began engaging in these behaviors at 20.98 months of age (*range* = 13.85–26.19). The Repetitive Behaviors factor had a significantly earlier age of onset (18.28 months) compared to the "Just Right" factor (21.85), $F(1, 1028) = 144.16$, $p < .01$ (see Table 6 for mean ages of onset for each item).

DISCUSSION

The goal of this study was to explore the phenomenon of compulsive-like behavior in young children. Because few efforts have attempted to quantify these phenomena (Marks, 1987), little is known about the prevalence, age of onset, or developmental course of compulsive-like behavior.

A measure intended to assess compulsive-like behavior in young children (the CRI) was developed and its age-related parameters explored. The main findings indicated that (1) the CRI demonstrated good internal consistency, and two factors emerged—"Just Right" and "Repetitive Behaviors." These factors correspond to constructs that underlie the phenomenology of OCD; (2) compulsive-like behavior appears to be relatively prevalent in early childhood; (3) 2- to 4-year-old children engage in compulsive-like behavior with greater frequency/intensity than do younger and older children; (4) a greater percentage of 2- to 4-year-olds engage in compulsive-like behavior compared with older and younger children; and (5) repetitive-oriented compulsive-like behaviors tend to emerge earlier than the sensory-perceptual "Just Right" behaviors.

The results speak not only to an area of child development that has received little attention, but also have implications for the study of repetitive, sensory-perceptual compulsive behaviors in the context of disorder. The CRI promises to be useful in identifying age-inappropriate levels of compulsive-like behavior. Thus the CRI would allow for the early identification of overly rigid or repetitive behavior characteristic of certain disorders of childhood onset (e.g., Pervasive Developmental Disorder, OCD).

The CRI was found to be internally consistent, indicating that the construct of "compulsive-like behavior" has some reliability during this developmental epoch. The factor structure of the CRI suggests that two constructs found in the OCD literature—repetition and sensory perceptual phenomena—are relevant to normative development. Some researchers and theorists (Carter, Pauls, & Leckman, 1995; King & Noshpitz, 1991; Leonard et al., 1990) have debated the relation between compulsive behaviors of "normally" functioning individuals and those more extreme, pathological variants of OC behavior. These early compulsive behaviors bear a strong similarity to pathological expressions of OC behavior, though their etiological similarities require further study. Compulsive-like behavior in early childhood could possibly provide researchers with a model for the study of OCD and its possible adaptive origins.

The two-factor structure was found to be relatively stable across the age groups, although a single factor might better describe the structure of the CRI for younger, preverbal children, with the two factors emerging as differentiated constructs with age. Thus, compulsive-like behavior seems to follow the orthogenetic trend of other developmental phenomena (Werner, 1948, 1957).

Subsequent analyses of this study explored age-related trends for compulsive-like behavior. The results for the total CRI score and the "Just Right" factor indicate that compulsive-like behavior is significantly more prevalent in children aged 24 to 47 months than for younger and older children. For the "Repetitive Behavior" factor, 12- to 23-month-old children engaged in similar amounts of such behavior as did the 24- to 47-month-olds, which was significantly more than children <12 months, or greater than 60 months.

Compulsive-like behavior shows age-related trends such that fewer children at the youngest and oldest age groups engage in compulsive-like behaviors compared to those in the middle ages (24–47). Indeed, for many items, over 75% of children in the 24–35 and 36–47 month age groups were reported to engage in compulsive-like behaviors (e.g., "perfectionistic"; "bedtime routines"; "strong preferences for certain foods"; "strong preferences for certain clothes"). Despite an eventual decrease in compulsive-like behavior with age, this phenomenon remains relatively common through age 5. Because the frequency/intensity questions assess whether a child had "ever" engaged in a given behavior, it is likely that the decreases observed at the oldest age groups are due to retrospective reporting bias. The CRI questions assessing the child's current status may, then, be a more valid index of compulsive-like behavior than the portion assessing whether the behavior "ever" occurred.

These findings support Gesell's early work finding that repetitive, ritualistic behaviors are more prevalent in 2- to 3-year-old children than in children at other ages. Whether compulsive-like behavior in young children is a mechanism for organizing, accommodating to, and eventually mastering the environment, as Gesell theorized, is not clear from the results of this study. Given the high rates of compulsive-like behavior in 2- to 4-year-olds, it is likely, however, that such compulsivity is serving some adaptive function. Piaget (1952) recognized that repetition in infancy develops from reflexive to more purposeful, intentional activities that lie at the root of adaptation to a changing environment. To others, repetitive, ritualistic behaviors and other "transitional phenomena" serve a child's social and emotional need to gain a sense of self-control and regulate emotional states (Kopp, 1982, 1989). Or, in the case of bedtime rituals and requests, such behaviors may simply allow the child to spend more time with his or her parents (Albert, Amgott, Krakow, & Howard, 1979).

Alternatively, some of the compulsive-like behavior reported may not be a too-distant relative of certain repetitive, fixed-action patterns with possible biological or biochemical origins found in other species, and relating to affiliation (in humans, attachment or maternal behaviors) (Insel, 1992; Insel & Shapiro, 1992; Leckman, Mayes, & Insel, 1996; Leckman et al., 1994a) or fear responses (anxiety) (Marks, 1987). All are possible explanations that require further study.

Sociologists and anthropologists (e.g., Albert et al., 1979) argue that certain childhood rituals parallel "rites of safe passage" that are used in many cultures to mark change while preserving continuity and sameness. Perhaps these various examples of repetitive behaviors share common underlying features, or at least their similarities may serve as a heuristic for future research in this area. Cross-cultural studies are a necessary step toward understanding the biological, social, or cultural significance of compulsive-like behavior in young children.

Parents estimated that, on average, the behaviors of the CRI first appear around the age of 18 to 21 months. These estimates vary across the two factors, with repetitive behavior reportedly having earlier onset than "Just Right" behaviors. As mentioned above, the repetitive behaviors may reflect the very early biologic rhythmicity and repetition seen in infants (see also Berkson, 1983). "Just Right" behaviors, on the other hand, require slightly more sophisticated and intentional motor, sensory, and perceptual abilities; this would account for their later onset.

The results of this study have implications for the study of OCD and other disorders characterized by repetitive compulsive-like behavior. The few studies examining the prevalence rates of OCD during childhood and adolescence have yielded estimates ranging from less than 1% (Rutter, Tizard, & Whitmore, 1970) to 2% or 3% (e.g., Flament et al., 1988). The majority of individuals with OCD report first symptoms as occurring in childhood (Beech, 1974; Black, 1974), and many researchers report a general trend toward the realization that OCD is much more common in childhood than previously thought (Carter et al., 1995). Indeed, accurate prevalence rates in childhood OCD may be obscured by the lack of sensitive measures and by problems in distinguishing clinically relevant behavior from normal childhood activity. Among the many possible directions for future research noted above, it will be necessary to establish representative community and clinic-referred norms for the CRI in order to fulfill its use as a screener for vulnerability to later psychopathology.

Future work might also look to other periods in normal development where OC-like behavior becomes particularly salient. The preoccupations with self and others and grooming behaviors associated with adolescence (Elkind, 1967, 1978), and the preoccupations and compulsive-like behaviors that are thought to accompany the pre, peri-, and postpartum experience, are both likely candidates for developmentally related normative variants of obsessive-compulsive behavior (Leckman et al., 1994a, 1996). Studying the developmental correlates of these normative phenomena may similarly yield insights into the phenomenology and pathogenesis of OCD (Leckman, Walker, et al., 1994).

Behavioral observations are needed to validate further the construct of compulsive-like behavior, as parental reports present a risk of attenuated reliability. Given, however, that some aspects of compulsive-like behavior are manifested in private contexts (e.g., mealtime, bedtime), the potential loss of reliability inherent in parental reports brings with it an increase in ecological validity. Nonetheless, these data call for further research in the way of behavioral validation. We are currently working to establish measures to complement parental reports of compulsive-like behavior.

Although a primary goal of this study was to explore the developmental course of compulsive-like behavior, the cross-sectional design employed here has obvious limitations in our ability to speak to development per se; this can be ameliorated only by longitudinal studies and by using established indices of development in addition to chronological age.

In conclusion, this study represents a first step in the assessment and analysis of compulsive-like behavior in young children. This aspect of behavior is relatively common in early childhood, and appears to be part of a normal sequence of early development. Beyond a certain point, however, compulsive and ritualistic behavior becomes somewhat less prevalent, and may be indicative of an overly rigid style at a time when greater flexibility is required to master the more complex tasks of later childhood.

This brief parent-report inventory may prove useful to parents, clinicians, pediatricians, and day-care providers as a context for addressing questions about their children's compulsive behavior, such as, "Is this behavior of a typical magnitude?" or "Is the behavior(s) following a normal developmental course?" The data presented in this study can address these questions only within the limitations of the sociodemographic strata represented in this sample. More research is needed to explore the utility of this measure with clinic populations, and also to understand its possible adaptive function in a normative context.

REFERENCES

Albert, S., Amgott, T., Krakow, M., & Howard, M. (1979). Children's bedtime rituals as a prototype rite of safe passage. *Journal of Psychological Anthropology, 2,* 85–105.

American Psychiatric Association. (1994). *Diagnostic and statistical manual of mental disorders* (4th ed.). Washington, DC: APA.

Ames, L. B., Ilg, F. L., & Frances, L. (1976). *Your two-year-old.* New York: Dell.

Beech, H. R. (1974). Approaches to understanding obsessional illness. In H. R. Beech (Ed.), *Obsessional states* (pp. 3–17). London: Methuen.

Berkson, G. (1983). Repetitive stereotyped behaviors. *American Journal of Mental retardation, 88,* 239–246.

Black, A. (1974). The natural history of obsessional neuroses. In H. R. Beech (Ed.), *Obsessional states* (pp. 19–54). London: Methuen.

Bolton, D. (1996). Annotation: Developmental issues in obsessive-compulsive disorder. *Journal of Child Psychology and Psychiatry and Allied Disciplines, 37,* 131–137.

Carter, A., Pauls, D., & Leckman, J. F. (1995). The development of obsessionality: Continuities and discontinuities. In D. Cicchetti & D. Cohen (Eds.), *Handbook of developmental psychopathology* (Vol. 2, pp. 609–632). New York: Wiley.

Cattell, R. (1966). The scree test for number of factors. *Multivariate Behavioral Research, 1,* 245–276.

Elkind, D. (1967). Egocentrism in adolescence. *Child Development, 38,* 1025–1034.

Elkind, D. (1978). Understanding the young adolescent. *Adolescence, 13,* 127–134.

Flament, M., Whitaker, A., Rapoport, J. L., Davies, M., & Zaremba Berg, C. (1988). Obsessive-compulsive disorder in adolescence: An epidemiological study. *Journal of the American Academy of Child and Adolescent Psychiatry, 27(6),* 764–771.

Garber, S. W., Garber, M. D., & Spizman, R. F. (1993). *Monsters under the bed and other childhood fears.* New York: Villard.

Garrison, W., & Earls, F. (1982). Attachment to a special object at age three years: Behavior and temperament characteristics. *Child Psychiatry and Human Development, 12,* 131–141.

Gesell, A. (1928). *Infancy and human growth.* New York: Macmillan.

Gesell, A., Ames, L. B., & Ilg, F. L. (1974). *Infant and the child in the culture today.* New York: Harper & Row.

Green, J. A. (1992). Testing whether correlation matrices are different from each other. *Developmental Psychology, 28,* 215–224.

Ilg, F. L., Ames, L. B., & Baker, S. M. (1981). *Child behavior.* New York: Harper Collins.

Insel, T. R. (1992a). A neuropeptide for affiliation: Evidence from behavioral, receptor, autoradiographic, and comparative studies. *Psychoneuroendocrinology, 17,* 3–35.

Insel, T. R., & Shapiro, L. E. (1992). Oxytocin receptor distribution reflects social organization in monogamous and polygamous voles. *Proceedings of the National Academy of Sciences USA, 89,* 5981–5985.

King, R., & Noshpitz, J. D. (1991). *Pathways of growth: Essentials of child psychiatry.* New York: Wiley.

Kopp, C. (1982). Antecedents of self-regulation: A developmental perspective. *Developmental Psychology, 18,* 199–214.

Kopp, C. (1989). Regulation of distress and negative emotions: A developmental view. *Developmental Psychology, 21,* 343–354.

Leckman, J. F., Goodman, W. K., North, W. G., Chappell, P. B., Price, L. H., Pauls, D., Anderson, G. M., Riddle, M., McSwiggan-Hardin, M., McDougle, C. J., Barr, L. C., & Cohen, D. J. (1994a). The role of central oxytocin in obsessive-compulsive disorder and related normal behavior. *Psychoneuroendocrinology, 19,* 723–749.

Leckman, J. F., Mayes, L., & Insel, T. R. (1996). *Preoccupations and behaviors associated with early phases of romantic love and early parental love: Evolutionary, neurobiological, and psychopathologic perspectives.* Manuscript submitted for publication.

Leckman, J. F., Walker, D., Goodman, W., Pauls, D., & Cohen, D. J. (1994). "Just Right" perceptions associated with compulsive behavior in Tourette's syndrome. *American Journal of Psychiatry, 151,* 675–680.

Leonard, H., Goldberger, E. L., Rapoport, J. L., Cheslow, B. S., & Swedo, S. (1990). Childhood rituals: Normal development or obsessive-compulsive symptoms? *Journal of the American Academy of Child and Adolescent Psychiatry, 29,* 17–23.

Marks, I. (1987). *Fears, phobias and rituals.* Oxford: Oxford University Press.

Markt, C., & Johnson, M. (1993). Transitional objects, presleep rituals and psychopathology. *Child Psychiatry and Human Development, 23,* 161–173.

Niler, E. R., & Beck, S. J. (1989). The relationship among guilt, dysphoria, anxiety and obsessions in a normal population. *Behavior Research and Therapy, 27,* 213–220.

Passman, R. H. (1976). Arousal-reducing properties of attachment objects: Testing the function limits of the security blanket relative to the mother. *Developmental Psychology, 12,* 421–436.

Passman, R. H. (1977). Providing attachment objects to facilitate learning and reduce distress: Effects of mother and security blanket. *Developmental Psychology, 13,* 25–28.

Passman, R. H. (1987). Attachment objects: Are children who have security blankets insecure? *Journal of Consulting and Clinical Psychology, 55,* 825–830.

Piaget, J. (1952). *The origins of intelligence in the child.* New York: Basic.

Rachman, S. J., & de Silva, P. (1978). Abnormal and normal obsessions. *Behavior Research and Therapy, 16,* 233–248.

Rutter, M., Tizard, J., & Whitmore, K. (1970). *Education, health and behavior.* London: Longmans.

Salkovskis, P. M., & Harrison, J. (1984). Abnormal and normal obsessions—a replication. *Behavior Research and Therapy, 22,* 549–552.

Sperling, M. (1963). Fetishism in children. *Psychoanalytic Quarterly, 32,* 374–392.

Werner, H. (1948). *The comparative psychology of mental development.* New York: International Universities Press.

Werner, H. (1957). The concept of development from a comparative and organismic point of view. In D. B. Harris (Ed.), *The concept of development* (pp. 125–148). Minneapolis: University of Minnesota Press.

Winnecott, D. W. (1953). Transitional objects and transitional phenomena: A study of the first not-me possession. *International Journal of Psychoanalysis, 34,* 89–97.

PART I: DEVELOPMENTAL ISSUES

5

The Development of Multiple Role-Related Selves During Adolescence

Susan Harter, Shelley Bresnick, Heather A. Bouchey, and Nancy R. Whitesell
University of Denver, Denver, Colorado

The organization of the adolescent self-portrait is discussed within a framework that focuses on the construction of multiple self-representations across different relational contexts. Contradictions between self-attributes in different contexts create conflict, beginning in midadolescence when cognitive-developmental structures allow one to detect but not resolve opposing attributes. Conflict is greater across roles than within roles. Moreover, for certain roles (e.g., self with mother vs. self with father) conflict is higher. Females, particularly those with a feminine gender orientation, report greater conflict involving attributes in more public contexts. Opposing self-attributes also raise concerns for adolescents about which attributes reflect true versus false self-behaviors. Conflict is more frequent for opposing attributes that pit true against false self-characteristics. False self-behavior is associated with liabilities including devaluation of false self-attributes, low self-esteem, and depressive reactions. Perceived support across relational contexts is highly predictive of favorable evaluations of attributes, high self-esteem, and true self-behavior within corresponding contexts. Strategies for resolving potential contradictions in self-attributes would appear to emerge as one moves into late adolescence and adulthood, when multiple self-representations are perceived as both appropriate and desirable, and the individual can achieve some degree of integration through higher level abstractions and the narrative construction of his or her life story.

INTRODUCTION

The study of the self-system has witnessed a number of shifts within the last two decades (see Harter, in press-a). Of particular relevance to this article is the shift from a focus on more global representations of the self to a multidimensional framework. Earlier theorists (e.g.,

---

The research reported in this article was supported by an NIH grant awarded to the first author.

Coopersmith, 1967; Rosenberg, 1979) emphasized constructs such as global self-esteem, namely the individual's overall sense of worth as a person. However, such an approach has been challenged on the grounds that it masks important evaluative distinctions that individuals, beginning in middle childhood, make about their adequacy in different domains of their lives. The prevailing zeitgeist, supported by extensive data, underscores the fact that multidimensional models of self far more adequately describe the phenomenology of self-evaluations than do unidimensional models (see Bracken, 1996; Damon & Hart, 1988; Harter, 1982, 1990, 1993; Hattie, 1992; Marsh, 1987, 1989; Mullener & Laird, 1971; Oosterwegel & Oppenheimer, 1993; Shavelson & Marsh, 1986). Moreover, differentiation increases with age, such that the number of domains that can be evaluated increases across the periods of childhood, adolescence, and adulthood.

From a developmental perspective, multiple self-representations can also be observed in the proliferation of role-related selves during adolescence. Thus, adolescents come to describe themselves quite differently across different interpersonal contexts, for example, with parents, teachers, classmates, close friends, and those in whom they are romantically interested. Historically, William James (1890) set the stage for the consideration of the multiple selves that may be manifest in different interpersonal roles or relationships. James (1890) concluded that "A man has as many social selves as there are individuals who recognize him and carry an image of him in their mind" (p. 190). Moreover, James noted that these multiple selves may not all speak with the same voice. For example, he observed that "Many a youth who is demure enough before his parents and teachers, swears and swaggers like a pirate among his tough young friends" (p. 169). James noted that multiplicity could be harmonious, as when an individual is tender to his children but also stern with the soldiers under his command. Alternatively, there may be a "discordant splitting" if one's different selves are experienced as contradictory. James conceptualized such incompatibility as the "conflict of the different Me's."

Despite historical precedent for considering the multiplicity of the self, theoreticians in the first half of the century did not embrace James' contentions. As Gergen (1968) has observed, there was historical resistance to such a stance in the form of a "consistency ethic." Thus, many scholars placed major emphasis on the integrated, unified self (Allport, 1961; Horney, 1950; Jung, 1928; Kelly, 1955; Lecky, 1945; Maslow, 1961; Rogers, 1951). For Allport, the self includes all aspects of personality that make for a sense of inward unity. Lecky (1945) fashioned an entire theory around the theme of self-consistency, emphasizing how behavior expresses the effort to maintain the integrity and unity of the self. Epstein (1973, 1981) has more recently argued that an important criterion that an individual's self-theory must meet is *internal consistency*. Thus, one's self-theory will be threatened by evidence that is inconsistent with the portrait one has constructed of the self, or by postulates within the theory that appear to be contradictory. Epstein (1981) has formalized these observations under the rubric of the "unity principle," emphasizing that one of the most basic needs of the individual is to maintain the coherence of the conceptual system that defines the self.

More recently, the pendulum would appear to have swung back to an emphasis on multiplicity, with increasing zeal for models depicting how the self varies across situations. In contrast to the emphasis on unity, several social psychologists (Gergen, 1968; Mischel,

1973; Vallacher, 1980) have argued that the most fruitful theory of self must take into account the multiple roles that people adopt. Thus, Gergen contended that the "popular notion of the self-concept as a unified, consistent, or perceptually whole psychological structure is possibly ill-conceived" (1968, p. 306). Although consistency *within* a relationship was deemed desirable, consistency *across* relationships was viewed as difficult, if not impossible, and in all likelihood damaging. That is, people are compelled to adjust their behavior in accord with the specific nature of the interpersonal relationship and its situational context. In the extreme, high self-monitors (Snyder, 1987) frequently and flexibly alter their self-presentation in the service of creating a positive impression, enacting behaviors that they feel are socially appropriate, and that will preserve critical relationships. For Gergen, such multiplicity is not only a response to the demand characteristics of differnt interpersonal contexts, but also rests heavily on social comparison. As Gergen (1977) observes, "In the presence of the devout, we may discover that we are ideologically shallow; in the midst of dedicated hedonists, we may gain awareness of our ideological depths" (1977, p. 154).

Gergen (1991) has more recently elevated his argument to new heights in his sociocultural treatise on the "saturated" or "populated" self. Gergen observes that in our current era of postmodernism, individuals have been forced to contend with a swirling sea of multiple social relationships, which in turn requires the construction of numerous, disparate selves. In the face of this multiphrenia, individuals are forced to suspend any demands for personal coherence. Lifton (1993) develops a similar theme in his analysis of the emergence of the postmodern "protean self," named after Proteus, the Greek sea god who possessed many forms. For Lifton, the protean self emerges out of "confusion, from the widespread feeling that we are losing our psychological moorings" (p. 1). He attributes this confusion to unmanageable historical forces, rapid societal and economic changes, and social uncertainties. Lifton is a bit more sanguine than Gergen, however, emphasizing the flexibility and resilience of the protean self, whereas Gergen focuses more on the erosion of the belief in one's essential self.

Other social psychologists have also turned their attention to the investigation of multiple self-representations in adults (e.g., Ashmore & Ogilvie, 1992; Higgins, Van Hook, & Dorfman, 1988; Kihlstrom, 1993; Markus & Cross, 1990; Rosenberg, 1988). Each of these investigators agree that the self is multifaceted, rather than a monolithic, unitary cognitive structure. However, there is less unanimity on the nature of the structure of such selves and on the extent to which multiple representations are integrated. For some, the notion of a hierarchy is preserved (e.g., Kihlstrom). For others (e.g., Ashmore and Ogilvie), multiple selves form a somewhat loose "confederation." Still others believe that certain (but not all) subsets of self-attributes are interconnected (Higgins et al., 1988). In the extreme, theorists such as Kagan (1991) assert that the multiple representations of self are not integrated into an abstract, unitary self.

DIFFERENTIATION OF MULTIPLE SELVES DURING ADOLESCENCE

From a developmental perspective, there is considerable evidence that the self becomes increasingly differentiated. As stated previously, in addition to domain-specific self-evaluations, findings reveal that during adolescence there is a proliferation of selves that vary as a function of social context. These include self with father, mother, close friend, romantic partner, peers, as well as the self in the role of student, on the job, and as athlete (Bresnick, 1986, 1995; Gecas, 1972; Griffin, Chassin, & Young, 1981; Hart, 1988; Harter & Monsour, 1992; Smollar & Youniss, 1985). For example, the adolescent may be depressed and sarcastic with parents, caring and rowdy with friends, curious and attentive as a student, and flirtatious but also self-conscious with someone in whom one is romantically interested. A critical developmental task of adolescence, therefore, is the construction of multiple selves in different roles and relationships.

Developmentalists highlight both cognitive and social processes that contribute to this proliferation of selves. Cognitive-developmental advances allow the adolescent to make greater differentiations among role-related attributes (see Fischer, 1980; Fischer & Canfield, 1986; Harter, 1990; Harter & Monsour, 1992; Keating, 1990). Moreover, these advances conspire with socialization pressures, leading to the emergence of different selves in different relational contexts (see Erikson, 1959, 1968; Grotevant & Cooper, 1983, 1986; Hill & Holmbeck, 1986; Rosenberg, 1986). For example, bids for autonomy from parents make it important to define oneself differently with peers in contrast to parents (see also Steinberg & Silverberg, 1986; White, Speisman, & Costos, 1983). Rosenberg (1986) points to another component of the differentiation process in observing that as one moves through adolescence, one is more likely to be treated differently by those in different relational contexts. Such differentiation should produce less overlap in those role-related attributes that are identified as salient self-descriptors, which is precisely what our research reveals. In two studies from our own laboratory (Harter & Monsour, 1992; Bresnick, 1986) we have found that the percentage of overlap in self-attributes generated for different social contexts decreases during adolescence, from 25% to 30% for young adolescents to a low of approximately 10% among older teenagers.

Contradictions and Conflict Between Attributes

The fact that adolescents perceive themselves differently in different relational contexts sets the stage for attributes to be considered contradictory. Indeed, James' "conflict of the different Me's" would appear to be particularly salient during adolescence. A certain level of intrapsychic conflict over opposing attributes in the adolescent self-portrait would appear to be normative. However, excessive conflict experienced by particular individuals may put one at psychological risk (as will become more evident later in this article).

There has been little in the way of systematic, empirical efforts that explore the extent to which opposing role-related attributes provoke conflict in the developing adolescent. Thus, we have embarked upon a program of research to address these issues. In an initial study from our laboratory (Harter & Monsour, 1992) we focused on the phenomenological conflict provoked by the identification of opposing or contradictory role-related attributes (e.g., cheerful vs. depressed, rowdy vs. calm, studious vs. lazy, at ease vs. self-conscious) within the adolescent self-portrait. Adolescents at three grade levels (7th, 9th, and 11th) first generated lists of self-descriptors for four roles: self with friends, with parents, in romantic relationships, and in the classroom. They then transferred each attribute to a large circle, which allowed for a spatial representation of their self-portrait. They were asked to arrange their attributes in one of three concentric circles (center, intermediate, and outer) corresponding to importance of each attribute. They were then asked to identify pairs of attributes that represented *opposing* characteristics, as well as which of these opposites they experienced as conflicting or clashing.

Across five converging indices (mean number of opposites, mean number of conflicts, percent of opposites in conflict, percent of subjects reporting that at least one opposite caused conflict, and percent of subjects reporting that opposites made them feel confused), the same pattern emerged. Attributes identified as contradictory and experienced as conflicting did not appear with great frequency among young adolescents. However, they peaked for those in midadolescence, and then showed a slight decline for older adolescents. Examples of conflicting attributes included being serious at school but fun-loving with friends, being happy with friends but depressed with family, being caring with family but inconsiderate with peers, being talkative as well as shy in romantic relationships, and being both attentive and lazy at school.

From a cognitive-developmental perspective, how might an increase in contradictions and conflict within the adolescents' self-portraits be explained? Why do their self-theories not meet the criterion of *internal consistency* (Epstein, 1973)? Those of a Piagetian persuasion would argue that with the advent of formal operations in early adolescence, one should have the cognitive tools necessary to construct an integrated theory in which the postulates are internally consistent, and therefore not troublesome. However, our findings critically challenge such an expectation, and therefore demand an explanation that moves beyond classic Piagetian theory.

Thus, in interpreting the developmental data, we initially turned to Fischer's neo-Piagetian cognitive-developmental theory (Fischer, 1980; Fischer & Lamborn, 1989). Unlike classic Piagetian theory which posits the single stage of formal operations for the period of adolescence and beyond, Fischer identifies four stages through which development proceeds, beginning in early adolescence. Moreover, there are liabilities associated with the stage observed in midadolescence. According to this formulation, early adolescent thought is characterized by "single abstractions" in which one can construct rudimentary, abstract self-descriptors, for example, self-conscious, at-ease, awesome, dorky, cheerful, depressed, etc. However, young adolescents do not yet have the cognitive ability to simultaneously compare these abstractions to one another, and therefore they tend not to detect, or be concerned over, self-attributes that are potential opposites (e.g., self-conscious vs. at ease). As one young adolescent put it, when confronted with the fact that he had indicated that he was both "nice" and "mean," "Well, you are nice to your friends and then mean to people who don't treat you nicely; there's no problem. I guess I just think about one thing about myself at a time and don't think about the other until the next day." When another young adolescent was asked why opposing attributes did not bother her, she succinctly exclaimed: "That's a stupid question, I don't fight with myself!"

During midadolescence, the cognitive skills (namely, "abstract mappings") necessary to compare single abstractions begin to emerge. This particular substage should usher in the need to integrate multiple attributes into a theory of one's personality that is coherent and unified. However, the ability to "map" constructs about the self onto one another for the purposes of comparison also represents a liability since the adolescent does not yet possess the ability to integrate seemingly opposing postulates (e.g., depressed and cheerful). As a result, they are experienced as contradictions with the self-system that may also provoke intrapsychic conflict. As one 14-year-old put it, "I really think I am a happy person and I want to be that way with everyone but I get depressed with my family and it really bugs me because that's not what I want to be like." Another 15-year-old, in describing a conflict within her romantic relationships, exclaimed, "I hate the fact that I get so nervous! I wish I wasn't so inhibited. The real me is talkative, I just want to be natural but I can't." Another 15-year-old girl explained that, "I really think of myself as friendly and open to people, but the way the other girls act, they force me to become an introvert, even though I know I'm not." In exasperation, one ninth grader observed of the self-portrait she had constructed, "Its not right, it should all fit together into one piece!"

According to Fischer's theory, consolidation and coordination should be more likely in later adolescence, with the emergence of "abstract systems," since they allow one to integrate or resolve seeming contradictions within the self-theory. For example, the tendency to be both cheerful and depressed can be coordinated under higher order abstractions such as "moody" or "temperamental." As one older adolescent explained, "Sometimes I'm really happy and sometimes I get depressed, I'm just a moody person." Older adolescents also can and do (Harter & Monsour, 1992) normalize or find value in seeming inconsistency, suggesting that it would be unnatural if not weird to act similarly with everyone. Rather, they report that it is desirable to be different across relational contexts. One teenager indicated that, "You can be shy on a date, and then outgoing with friends because you are just different with different people; you can't always be the same person and probably shouldn't be." As another older adolescent put it, "There's a time you should listen and a time you should talk. You can do both."

The major developmental differences, therefore, reflect an increase in the detection of opposing attributes and the associated phenomenological experience of conflict associated with multiple role-related selves. particularly as individuals move from early- to midadolescence. Such a developmental shift can be interpreted within neo-Piagetian models that identify cognitive advances and liabilities that reflect substages during the period of adolecence. For those older adolescents who can normalize seeming contradictions or integrate them at more abstract levels of thought, there may be some reduction in the conflict experienced, although these processes can be expected to continue well into adulthood.

Are there more contradictions across or within roles? We have also extended our analysis to parameters of the conflict experienced between opposing attributes that go beyond cognitive-developmental explanations. Thus, we were curious about whether there are more opposing attributes and associated conflict within particular roles (e.g., rowdy vs. quiet with friends) or across different roles (e.g., tense with a romantic other but relaxed with friends). This issue has been briefly addressed in the adult (although not the adolescent) literature. Among those social psychologists who have focused on the adult self, it has been argued that consistency within a particular relationship is critical; therefore, perceived violations of this consistency ethic, where one displays opposing attributes within the same role, should be particularly discomforting to the individual (Gergen, 1968; Vallacher, 1980). According to these theorists, the adoption of different behaviors in different roles should be less problematic or conflictual for adults, since they represent an appropriate adaptation to different relational contexts rather than inconsistency.

From a developmental perspective, we did not expect these particular processes to be in place during adolescence. Adolescents are actively concerned with creating, defining, and differentiating role-related selves. As reported earlier, this preoccupation results in relatively little overlap in the self-attributes associated with different roles, particularly as one moves through adolescence. As our cognitive-developmental analysis indicated, perceived opposition between differing attributes across relational contexts should become more marked or salient, beginning in midadolescence when teenagers develop the cognitive ability to detect seeming contradictions. Thus, the salience of these differences should cause adolescents to identify more opposing attributes across roles than within roles. Perceived conflict caused by opposing attributes should also be greater across roles, particularly with the onset of midadolescence, when teenagers can begin to compare characteristics across such roles but cannot integrate these salient and seemingly contradictory self-attributes.

Findings from two different studies conducted in our laboratory (Bresnick, 1986, 1995) confirmed these expectations in that there were significantly more opposing attributes and a greater percentage of opposing attributes in conflict identified across, compared to within, roles. In the first study, which included six different roles (self with mother, father, friends, in the classroom, in romantic relationships, and on the job), across-role opposing attributes were more frequent ($M = 3.68$) than were within-role opposites ($M = 1.56$). This pattern was confirmed in a second study which included five roles, all of which represented interpersonal relationships (self with mother, father, best friend, a group of friends, and a romantic interest) as opposed to more general contexts such as the classroom or on the job. In this second study, opposing attributes across roles attributes ($M = 2.72$) were significantly more frequent than were within-role contradictions ($M = .50$). Those opposing attributes experienced as in conflict followed the same pattern.

Figure 1 presents the data for opposing attributes both across- and within-roles as a function of developmental level. Consistent with our earlier work (Harter & Monsour, 1992), young adolescents reported fewer opposing attributes than either those in mid- or late adolescence. However, the slight decline in opposing attributes and conflicts found for older adolescents in the earlier study was only obtained for the within-role characteristics. As can be seen in Figure 1, for those across-role attributes, there was a systematic developmental increase in opposing attributes, particularly noteworthy between early- and midadolescence. The fact that six roles were included in the first Bresnick study (compared to only four in the original Harter and Monsour study) may have been partly responsible for the increase into late adolescence, since the inclusion of additional roles increased the probability that opposing attributes might be detected. That is, there were 15 possible role pairs that might contain contradictions compared to only 6 role pairs in the original study. (However, as will become apparent, this increase is primarily because of the reports of female adolescents.)

Rosenberg (1986) points to a feature of the socialization process during adolescence that may contribute to the greater number of contradictory attribute pairs, coupled with conflict, that were reported across roles. He observes that as the individual moves through the adolescent years, he/she is more likely to be responded to differently by those in different

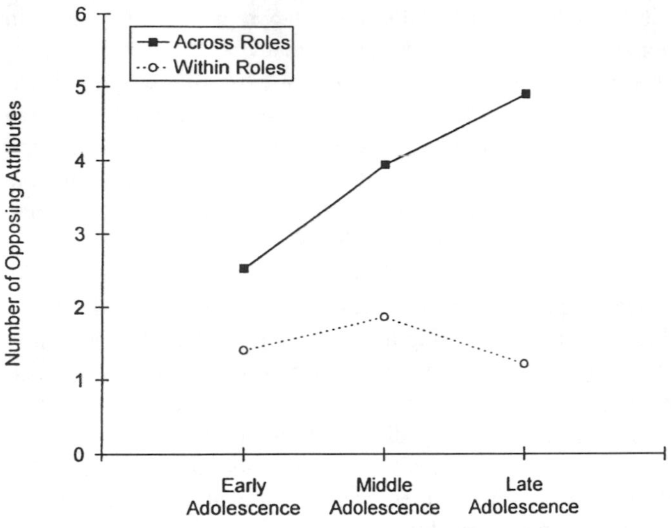

Figure 1. Mean number of opposing attributes across and within roles at three periods of adolescence.

relational contexts. Thus, significant others across varying relationships increasingly pull for the display of different personal attributes, leading to what Rosenberg labels the "barometric self" of the adolescent. This volatility, in turn, should contribute to the perception that one's differing characteristics are in conflict. Thus, it would appear that a combination of cognitive and social factors lead to developmental increases in the number of opposing and conflicting attributes identified across role-related, multiple self-representations.

Are more opposites and conflicts reported across some roles compared to others? The demonstration that opposing attributes, accompanied by conflict, may be more frequent across *particular* role pairs would suggest the need to move beyond mere cognitive-developmental explanations. Since the original study (Harter & Monsour, 1992), we have broadened the range of roles and focused on whether some role combinations are more problematic than others. In increasing the number of roles, we separated reports of self-attributes with mother and with father (whereas initially we merely enquired about self with "parents"). The separation of attributes with each parent thus enhances the likelihood that characteristics with each may contradict attributes in roles with peers; it also creates the potential for attributes with mother versus with father to be in opposition to each other. Along with increasing the number of roles, we have modified our procedure somewhat to facilitate adolescents' understanding of the task and their ability to manage more roles. A sample protocol from an older female adolescent is presented in Figure 2. Adolescents are first asked to generate six attributes for each role, writing them on the lines associated witheach interpersonal context. They then, as in the previous procedure, identify any pairs of attributes that are perceived to reflect opposites by connecting them with lines. Next they indicate whether any of these opposites are experienced as clashing or in conflict with each other, by putting arrow-heads on the lines connecting those pairs of opposites.

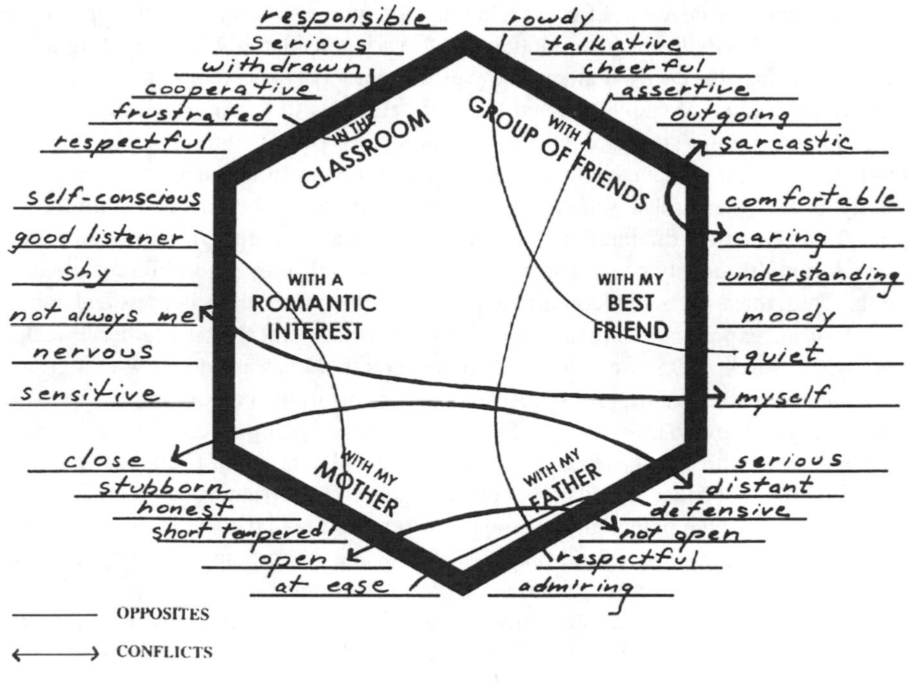

Figure 2. Sample protocol of an older adolescent female.

Across three different studies (Bresnick, 1986, 1995; Carson, 1985) we have consistently found that opposing attributes were most frequent for the combination of self with mother versus self with father. Examples have included being close with mother but distant with father, stubborn with mother versus respectful with father, open with mother but not open with father, at ease with mother but defensive with father, hostile with mother but cheerful with father. Opposing attributes with mother versus father greatly contributed to the developmental differences in across-role opposites depicted in Figure 1, as well as to gender differences that will be discussed.

Also contributing to increases in opposing attributes and conflicts with age was the tendency for opposites between attributes involving self with a given parent to conflict with attributes in peer relationships. Examples included being short-tempered with mother versus a good listener in romantic relationships, respectful with father but assertive with friends, distant from my father but attentive with a romantic interest. Adolescent bids for autonomy from parents (Cooper, Grotevant, & Condon, 1983), coupled with the increasing importance of the peer group (Brown, 1990; Savin–Williams & Berndt, 1990), would lead to the expectation that attributes expressed with mother and father might well differ from those displayed with peers (namely, friends and romantic partners), leading to a greater potential for contradictions.

However, why should adolescents report increasingly different characteristics with mother and father? Here, we can only speculate. Family therapists observe that children and adolescents typically develop different relationships with each parent, which in turn may cause the salient attributes in each relationship to vary considerably. Contributing to these dynamics is the fact that each parent may have a different set of expectations about those child characteristics that he or she values and therefore attempts to foster. Thus, the adolescent may become caught in a struggle between two parents who are encouraging and reinforcing different facets of his/her personality, provoking opposing attributes and resulting conflict. Secondly, both of these roles, self with mother and self with father, occur within the same general context, namely the family; however, behaviors across other multiple roles are not as likely to simultaneously occur, since they are typically displayed in different situational contexts. Thus, these particular conditions may exacerbate the contradictions and conflicts that adolescents experience in their respective roles with mother versus father. Finally, in one study (Bresnick, 1995) we included two contexts that contrasted self with a group of friends and self with one's best friend. Attributes in opposition and conflict were relatively frequent across these two roles as well. Examples included being sarcastic with a group of friends but caring with a best friend, and being rowdy with a group of friends but quiet with a best friend. If a best friend is also part of one's larger circle of friends, behaving differently toward each in the same potentially overlapping contexts may be particularly distressing.

In this study we also asked participants to rate the importance of being consistent across each of the role pair combinations ("how important is it to you to act the *same* with ______ and ______?"). Adolescents reported that it was significantly more important to be consistent with mother and with father ($M = 3.0$), as well as with a best friend and a group of friends ($M = 3.0$), than in all other role pairs ($M = 2.3$, combined). Thus, more opposites and associated conflict may be experienced because adolescents feel they are violating their goal of acting consistently across these contexts.

Are there gender differences in opposites and conflicts? Although no gender differences were initially anticipated, we have documented the fact that females report significantly more opposites and conflicts than do males, a finding obtained in every study we have conducted (Bresnick, 1986, 1995; Carson, 1985; Harter & Monsour, 1992). In addition to highly significant main effects for gender, the pattern reveals that gender differences increase during mid- and late adolescence. In our more recent studies in which we have separated the roles of mother versus father, we find that the developmental increases in the opposites and conflicts reported for this particular role pair were significantly greater for females compared to males. Moreover, we have recently documented (Bresnick, 1995) that females become more upset over conflicting attributes across early, mid-, and late adolescence, whereas males systematically become less upset.

To date, we have offered only a general interpretation of these gender differences, drawing upon those frameworks that emphasize the greater importance of relationships for females than males (Chodorow, 1989; Eichenbaum & Orbach, 1983; Gilligan, 1982; Jordan, 1991; Miller, 1986; Rubin, 1985). These theorists posit that the socialization of girls involves far more embeddedness within the family, as well as more concern with connectedness to others. Boys, in contrast, forge a path of independence and autonomy in which the logic of moral and social decisions takes precedence over affective responses to significant others. In extrapolating from these observations, we have suggested that in an effort to maintain the multiple relationships that girls are developing during adolescence, and to create harmony among these necessarily differentiated roles, opposing attributes within the self become particularly salient as well as problematic. Boys, in contrast, can move more facilely among their different roles and multiple selves to the extent that such roles are logically viewed as more independent of one another. However, these general observations require further refinement, including an empirical examination of precisely which facets of the relational worlds of adolescent females and males are specifically relevant to gender differences in opposing attributes displayed across different contexts.

Closer examination of gender effects reveals that it is a subset of female adolescents who report more opposites and greater conflict, compared to males (Bresnick, 1995). In another recent dissertation (Johnson, 1995), we have determined that adolescent females who endorse a feminine gender orientation may be particularly vulnerable to the experience of opposing attributes and associated conflict. Feminine adolescent females, compared to females who endorse an androgynous orientation, report more conflict, particularly in roles that involve teachers, classmates, and male friends (as compared to parents and female friends). Several hypotheses are worth pursuing in this regard. Is it that feminine girls report more contradictions in contexts where they feel they may be acting inappropriately by violating feminine stereotypes of behavior? Given that femininity on sex-role inventories is largely defined by caring, sensitivity, and attentiveness to the needs and feelings of others, might female adolescents who adopt this orientation (and eschew masculine attributes) be more preoccupied with relationships, making opposing attributes and accompanying conflict more salient? Moreover, might it be more important for feminine girls to be consistent across relationships, a stance that may be difficult to sustain? These are new directions in which this work needs to proceed.

TRUE VERSUS FALSE SELF-BEHAVIOR

The construction of multiple selves in which different attributes are perceived as contradictory should understandably provoke some concern over which of the opposing attributes in a given pair reflects one's "true self." Our own work has revealed that this proliferation of selves does engender problematic questions for adolescents about which is "the real me," particularly when attributes in different roles appear contradictory (e.g., cheerful with friends but depressed with parents). During our multiple-selves procedure, a number of adolescents spontaneously agonized over which of the attributes represented their "true self." The salience of this issue has been further documented by our subsequent findings demonstrating that adolescents can readily distinguish true and false self-behaviors.

When asked to define true self-behavior, adolescents' descriptions include the "real me inside," "saying what you really think," "expressing your opinion." In contrast, false self-behavior is defined as "being phony," "not stating your true opinion," "saying what you think others want to hear" (Harter, Marold, Whitesell, & Cobbs, 1996). These observations converge with what Gilligan and colleagues (Gilligan, 1982; Gilligan, 1993; Gilligan, Lyons, & Hanmer, 1989) have referred to as "loss of voice," namely the suppression of one's thoughts and opinions. In developing questionnaires that specifically address the extent to which adolescents engage in false self-behavior, we have found that many sixth graders do not embrace this concept. They will enquire into what it means, or state that it doesn't make sense because they are always their true selves. The distinction between true and false self behavior is, however, well understood by seventh graders, and becomes increasingly salient among those in midadolescence and beyond.

Our contextual approach to adolescent self-processes has prompted us to enquire, in recent studies of the multiple selves that adolescents construct, whether they display more false self-attributes in some contexts compared to others. Across these studies, each of which has addressed slightly different roles, there is a general pattern. The highest levels of false self-behavior (30% to 40% of attributes) are displayed with one's father and (for female adolescents from an all-girls school environment) with boys in social situations (Johnson, 1995). (We have not yet asked male adolescents to report on females in social situations.) Lower levels of false self-behavior (20–25%) are reported with classmates, teachers, and one's mother. The least false self-behavior is reported in relationships with close friends (10–15%). Thus, true self-behavior (the reciprocal of false self-behavior) increases across these three types of relational contexts. A similar pattern is obtained in our studies of the extent to which adolescents are able to voice their opinions (Harter et al., in press).

Does the perceived authenticity of attributes predict conflict? In two recent studies of multiple self-representations across roles, we have asked adolescents to indicate whether each attribute they generate represents true or false self-behavior. With these evaluations, we have been able to address the authenticity of attributes in pairs judged to be conflictual. We were curious about whether conflicts were more frequent between pairs of attributes in which one was judged true and the other false, between two true self-attributes, or between two false self-attributes. In both studies (Bresnick, 1995; Johnson, 1995) the pattern was the same. Conflict is significantly more likely to occur among attribute pairs in which one characteristic of the self was judged to be true self-behavior, whereas the other was deemed false self-behavior (58% and 60% of all conflicts, respectively, across the two studies). Less common were conflicts between two attributes both judged to reflect true self-behavior (29% and 34%). Conflicts between two false self-attributes were negligible (13% and 6%). Thus, it is those opposing attribute pairs representing one false and one true self-behavior that are particularly problematic in provoking conflict within the adolescent's self-theory.

We have also, in some studies, enquired into the *reasons* that adolescents report for why opposing attributes cause conflict, and these reasons parallel the findings cited above. In two such studies (Bresnick, 1986; Harter & Monsour, 1992) the largest reason category included explanations in which a behavior violated the adolescent's perception of who he/she was or wanted to be (53% and 44% of all reasons, respectively). As one adolescent put it, "I really think of myself as a happy person and I want to be that way with everyone because I think that's my true self, but I get depressed with my family and it bugs me because that's not what I want to be like or who I am." Another subject explained that "I hate the fact that I get so nervous on a date, so inhibited. The real me is talkative, I just want to be natural." Another observed: "I am a patient person, particularly with friends, and want to be, but then I get impatient with my mom." In these reasons it would appear that the conflicts represent a behavior experienced as "false," which clashes with an attribute that is perceived to reflect more true self-behavior.

A second category of reasons offered for conflict seems to reflect opposing attributes where each member of the pair represents true self behaviors; the frequency across the same two studies was 36% and 29%, respectively. As one adolescent explained, "I'm close with my family and fun-loving with my friends, and that's how I want to be, but sometimes these work against each other." Another observed, "I'm glad I can be emotional with my mother but I'm more naturally reserved with my father."

A third category of reasons offered for why opposing attributes conflict is that the significant others in each relational context expect or elicit different behaviors (11% and 20%, respectively). For example, one adolescent noted that "My teachers expect me to be serious but my friends want me to be rowdy." Another explained how "On a date I get withdrawn and self-conscious and just the opposite with my friends where I can get very sarcastic, but I don't like being either way, that's not me." Although adolescents providing such reasons do not always explicitly indicate that each opposing attribute represents a form of false self-behavior, the implication in their explanations is that they are behaving in ways that others call for, rather than how they feel they really are, or would prefer to act.

In a recent study (Bresnick, 1995), in which adolescents were asked to rate each attribute with regard to whether it reflected true versus false self-behavior, we also included a checklist of reasons for why attributes conflicted. One reason specified that "How I act isn't how I really am, it isn't my true self." We found that adolescents checked this reason for 69% of the conflicts that involved one true and one false self-behavior, suggesting their awareness of why these attributes clashed. A second reason in the checklist was that "One part of me wants to be one way and another part wants me to be a different way." This reason was endorsed for 77% of the conflicts that involved two true self-attributes, suggesting at least their preference that these be manifestations of their true self. Finally, a third reason specified that "Certain people expect me to be one way and other people expect me to be different." This reason was checked for 65% of the conflicts involving two false self-attributes, suggesting that attributes elicited by the demands of others are more likely to be experienced as false. Thus, the findings for the reasons offered for conflict provide converging evidence that dimensions involving the authenticity of one's behavior are quite salient.

HOW MUCH DO ADOLESCENTS LIKE THE ATTRIBUTES THEY DISPLAY ACROSS ROLES?

We have recently extended our contextual approach to multiple self-representations by enquiring into whether adolescents *like* their attributes more in some relationships compared to others. Thus, in two studies (Bresnick, 1995; Johnson, 1995) we asked participants to rate how much they liked each attribute, on a 4-point scale (where a score of 4 reflected the most positive evaluation and a score of 1 represented the most negative evaluation). The roles varied somewhat across the two studies. In the first (Bresnick, 1995), self-attributes with father were rated most negatively ($M = 2.78$), self with mother as well as with a group of friends was given slightly higher ratings ($M = 2.90$), whereas self-attributes with close friend were rated the most desirable ($M = 3.27$). In the Johnson dissertation, where female subjects from an all-girls high school were polled, the attributes they liked least ($M = 2.64$) were displayed with boys in social situations. Attributes with classmates, parents (no distinction between mother and father), and teachers were rated more positively

($M = 3.10$, combined), and attributes with close friends were evaluated the most positively ($M = 3.55$). This pattern directly parallels that obtained for the percentage of true and false self-attributes reported in that the greater the percentage of true self-attributes displayed, the more positively the attributes were evaluated. More direct confirmation for this link is documented by the correlations between the percentage of true self-behavior and the liking ratings. In the Bresnick study, these correlations ranged from .47 to .58 across relational contexts; in the Johnson study, the range was from .53 to .60. Thus, adolescents find their true self-attributes to be more desirable, while they devalue those judged to reflect false self-behavior.

Relational Self-Esteem

The fact that adolescents evaluate their attributes more positively in some relational contexts than others converges with other evidence (Harter, Waters, & Whitesell, in press) that adolescents report differing levels of *self-esteem* across different relationships. In this study, we examined high school students' perceptions of their worth as a person across four contexts, with parents, teachers, male classmates, and female classmates. We obtained a clear, four-factor solution with negligible cross-loadings, reflecting the fact that older adolescents make distinctions among their feelings of self-esteem in these relationships. Across the sample, the average discrepancy between adolescents' highest and lowest self-esteem scores was 1 (where the maximum could be 3). In the extreme, some adolescents did report the maximum. For example, one subject reported the lowest possible self-esteem (1.0) with her parents in contrast to the highest possible value (4.0) with female classmates. More recently, we have examined our relational self-esteem construct in a middle school population, where the contexts included mother, father, siblings, peers, and close friends. Once again, a very clear factor structure emerged, revealing that younger adolescents also make distinctions in their perceptions of worth as a person, across relational contexts.

Why should adolescents evaluate their attributes differently across contexts? With regard to factors that might be responsible for why individuals evaluate both their specific attributes as well as overall self-esteem differently across contexts, we have adopted Cooley's (1902) looking-glass self-perspective as one framework for explaining these differences. According to this model, the opinions of significant others, who serve as social mirrors into which one gazes, become incorporated into evaluations of self. Considerable evidence now reveals that perceived approval or validation from significant others, notably parents and peers for adolescents, is a powerful predictor of global self-esteem (Harter, 1990, in press-a; Rosenberg, 1979). We reasoned that context-specific support should be even more predictive of adolescents' perceptions of worth, as well as the evaluation of specific attributes, in the corresponding context compared to other contexts. The findings clearly confirm this expectation (Harter et al., in press). The correlations between validation support and relational self-esteem in the corresponding contexts range from .49 to .64 ($M = .54$). In contrast, the correlations between validation support in given contexts and the relational self-esteem in different contexts range from .22 to .41 ($M = .33$).

Similar links between support and self-evaluations have been demonstrated when we ask adolescents to rate how much they like their specific attributes across multiple roles. In one such study (Johnson, 1995) participants were also asked to rate the level of support that they received from others in each context. Across six different contexts, the pattern was the same. Those reporting low support liked their attributes least well ($M = 2.64$ across contexts, combined). Those acknowledging moderate support evaluated their attributes more positively ($M = 3.01$), and those reporting high levels of support found their attributes to be the most favorable ($M = 3.27$). As would be expected, given the correlation between the positivity of evaluations and the percentage of true self-attributes, higher levels of support are associated with more true self-behavior. A similar pattern has been obtained in other studies of true self-behavior (see Harter et al., 1996) as well as in our examination of the ability to voice one's opinions where higher levels of "voice" are associated with higher levels of support (Harter, Waters, & Whitesell, 1997). However, these studies do not speak directly to the directionality of these effects. Is it that displays of true self-behavior and voice garner more approval, or is it that if one receives support, one is more likely to display true self-behaviors, including the expression of one's opinion? It is likely that both processes are operative and reinforce each other within a given context, perpetuating differences in the level of true self-behavior as well as the evaluation of attributes and self-esteem across contexts.

SELF-ORGANIZATION DURING ADOLESCENCE: NORMATIVE AND PATHOLOGICAL IMPLICATIONS

Given normative cognitive-developmental advances as well as socialization pressures during adolescence, it is inevitable that multiple context-dependent selves will become differentiated during adolescence. As our findings have revealed, there is decreasing overlap among those attributes that adolescents identify as most salient across relational contexts. Differences in the attributes associated with different contexts, in turn, introduce the potential for some to be viewed as contradictory, leading to perceived conflict between attributes in the adolescent self-portrait. Such conflict will be exacerbated as one moves into midadolescence, where the emerging cognitive-developmental structures allow one to detect but not resolve such contradictions.

Thus, a certain level of conflict will be normative, particularly during midadolescence. That is, teenagers at this level of development do not yet possess the skills necessary to integrate those opposing attributes that come to define the loose confederation of multiple selves that have proliferated. However, certain individuals, as well as subgroups, may be more vulnerable to conflict. For example, we have identified a subset of girls, namely those with a feminine gender orientation, that are more prone to conflict, particularly among attributes that are displayed in public arenas such as in the classroom, as well as with boys in social situations.

The challenges posed by the need to create different selves are also exacerbated for ethnic minority youth in this country who must bridge "multiple worlds," as Cooper and her colleagues point out (Cooper, in press; Cooper, Jackson, Azmitia, Lopez, & Dunbar, 1995). Minority youth must move between multiple contexts, some of which may be with members of their own ethnic group, including family and friends, and some of which may be populated by the majority culture, including teachers, classmates, and other peers who may not share the values of their family of origin. Rather than assume that all ethnic minority youth will react similarly to the need to cope with such multiple worlds, Cooper and colleagues have highlighted several different patterns of adjustment. Some youth are able to move facilely across the borders of their multiple worlds, in large part because the values of the family, teachers, and peers are relatively similar. Others, for whom there is less congruence in values across contexts, adopt a bicultural stance, adapting to the world of family, as well as to that of the larger community. Others find the transition across these psychological borders more difficult, and some find it totally unmanageable. Particularly interesting is the role that certain parents play in helping adolescents navigate these contextual waters, leading to more successful adaptations for some than others.

The differentiation of multiple selves will be of particular concern to developmental psychopathologists to the extent that it is associated with a number of negative correlates and outcomes. These include excessive conflict between attributes in multiple roles, high levels of false self-behavior, and the devaluation of those characteristics that define one's role-related behavior. Moreover, each of these variables is, in turn, associated with lower levels of social support as well as low relational self-esteem in the corresponding context. In addition, we know from previous studies (see Harter, in press-a; Harter et al., 1996) that low self-esteem and high levels of false self-behavior are predictive of depressive reactions including depressed affect, low energy level, and hopelessness. The perception that certain self-attributes are false would seem to be very central to this constellation of liabilities.

A basic claim of theorists concerned with false self-behavior is that lack of authenticity has negative outcomes or correlates. Gilligan and colleagues (Gilligan et al., 1989; Gilligan, 1993), as well as others (see Jordan, 1991; Jordan, Kaplan, Miller, Stiver, & Surrey, 1991; Lerner, 1993; Miller, 1986, 1991) observe that suppression of the self leads to lack of zest which, in the extreme form, will be manifest as depressive symptoms and associated liabilities such as low self-esteem. In our own studies of self-reported level of false self-behavior (e.g., Harter et al., 1996), we have demonstrated that adolescents highest in false self-behavior reported the lowest level of global self-esteem and were the most likely to report depressive affect. Moreover, they acknowledged that they were much less likely to be in touch with their true self-attributes. With adults, we have demonstrated that those reporting lack of authenticity with a spouse or partner also report lower self-esteem and more depressed affect than those who were able to be their true selves (Harter, Waters, Pettitt, Whitesell, Kofkin, & Jordan, 1997). Thus, the pattern reveals that those who experience greater levels of false self-behavior are at risk for negative outcomes than can be quite debilitating, from a mental health perspective.

Origins of False Self-Behavior

In a previous section it was observed that the very proliferation of multiple selves during adolescence, including the detection of contradictory attributes in different roles, raises concerns for the adolescent about which attributes are the "real me." Gergen (1991) echoes this theme in noting that the need to craft different selves to conform to the particular relationship at hand leads to doubt about one's true identity. That is, the sense of an obdurate, core self is compromised in playing out one's role as "social chameleon." These processes would appear to reflect normative developmental change, against a sociocultural structure that contributes to the concern over behaviors that may lack authenticity. Thus, normative processes highlight the salience of false self-behaviors. However, individual differences in the level of perceived false self-behavior are of particular concern to developmental psychopathologists since the higher this level, the greater the potential for conflict between multiple selves. As we have demonstrated, the majority of perceived conflicts involve clashes between true and false self-behaviors.

It becomes critical, therefore, to enquire into the causes of individual differences in the *level* of false self-behavior that is displayed. There is considerable evidence that the origins of inauthenticity involve socialization practices that begin in childhood (see Harter, in press-b, in press-c). For example, attachment theorists (see Bowlby, 1980; Bretherton, 1991; Crittenden, 1994) and those who study the early construction of autobiographical memory in the form of narratives (see Eisenberg, 1983; Hudson, 1990; Nelson, 1993; Snow, 1990) identify certain early seeds of false self-behavior. They observe that the narratives that are initially constructed by young children are highly scaffolded by parents who dictate which aspects of the child's experience the parents feel are important to codify in the construction of his/her autobiographical memory. Children may receive subtle signals that certain episodes should not be retold or are best "forgotten" (Dunn, Brown, & Beardsall, 1991). Such distortions may well contribute to the formation of false self-behavior, if a child accepts the altered version of his/her experience.

False self-behavior will also emerge to the extent that caregivers make their support primarily contingent upon the child's living up to their particular standards, since the child must adopt a socially implanted self (Deci & Ryan, 1995; Harter et al., 1996). Our own findings reveal that the causes of high levels of false self-behavior not only involve low levels of parent and peer support but "support" that is perceived as conditional upon meeting the demanding and often unattainable expectations of others. Moreover, parenting practices that constitute lack of attunement to the child's needs, empathic failure, lack of validation, threats of harm, coercion, and enforced compliance all cause the true self to go underground (Bleiberg, 1984; Stern, 1985; Winnicott, 1965). In Sullivan's (1953) terminology, they lead to "not me" experiences.

Severe and chronic sexual and/or physical abusive treatment by caregivers also places the child at serious risk for suppressing his/her true self and displaying various forms of false self-behavior (Harter, in press-b). Moreover, such early trauma leads to extremely negative self-evaluations, and serves to exacerbate the fragmentation of multiple selves, rendering them unpredictably inaccessible to consciousness, thereby preventing their integration. For example, secrecy pacts around sexually abusive interactions lead the abused child to defensively exclude such episodic memories from awareness. Moreover, the sexual and physical abusive acts themselves at the hands of family members cause the child to split off experiences, relegating them to either a private or inaccessible part of the self. The very disavowal, repression, or dissociation of one's experiences, coupled with psychogenic amnesia and numbing, as defensive reactions to abuse, therefore set the stage for the loss of one's true self. Herman (1992) describes a more conscious pathway in that the abused child comes to see the true self as corroded with inner badness and therefore it is to be concealed at all costs. Persistent attempts to be good, in order to please the parents, lead the child to develop a socially acceptable self experienced as false or inauthentic.

The persistence in abuse victims of their sense of inner badness, namely that they are fundamentally bad or "rotten to the core," has been documented by numerous other abuse experts (e.g., Briere, 1992; Terr, 1990; van der Kolk, 1987; Westen, 1995). Fischer and his colleagues (Calverley, Fischer, & Ayoub, 1994; Fischer & Ayoub, 1994) have explored the implications of such abuse for the subsequent organization of self-constructs in documenting the sense of profound negativity that female adolescent sexual abuse victims experience with regard to their core self. Their sexual abuse victims had diagnoses of posttraumatic stress disorder. These investigators built upon our multiple selves procedure (Harter & Monsour, 1992) in which adolescents arranged spontaneously generated self-attributes into a self-portrait by identifying attributes that were the most important or central, less important, and least important. Adolescents in our normative sample displayed a positivity bias, placing the majority of favorable attributes at the core of the self, relegating negative attributes to the periphery of their self-portrait in judging them to be their least important characteristics. Fischer and colleagues found that their sexually abused adolescent girls not only reported considerably more negative self-attributes compared to our normative sample but identified their unfavorable characteristics as far more central to their self-concepts, namely, the defining features of the core self.

Moreover, the abuse literature reveals that such core negative attributes are not well integrated with those positive attributes deemed less central, and therefore the more favorable evaluations cannot offset core evaluations of badness. The very dissociative symptomatology mobilized by abuse victims seriously interferes with the integration of self-attributes (see Briere, 1992; Harter, in press-b; Putnam, 1993; Westen, 1995). Splitting, fragmentation, and compartmentalization, the staples in the abuse victim's dissociative armamentarium, all, by definition, preclude a sense of the coherence of the self. These tendencies are further exacerbated among multiple personality disorder victims of severe and chronic sexual abuse. Multiple identities are created to compartmentalize traumatic memories and affects, and these dissociated alters or personality states function as separate entities capable of independent volitional activities. By necessity, they will lead to a fragmented and incoherent self-portrait. The hallmark of such fragmentation among those with multiple personality disorders is that there is little or no awareness or coconsciousness on the part of some personalities for other personalities. In contrast, what we have referred to as the normative differentiation of multiple selves in the adolescent repertoire represents consciously experienced contradictions, typically between one's behaviors and conflicting ideals or intentions. In the concluding section to follow, we return to the more normative processes of differentiation and the possibilities for integration.

Is it possible and/or desirable to integrate the multiple selves that are inevitably constructed? Our cognitive-developmental analysis has suggested that normative limitations during the period of midadolescence will preclude the integration of those attributes that define the multiple selves that are constructed across different contexts. Contradictory attributes are particularly problematic. Advances that begin to emerge in late adolescence and are further developed in adulthood may allow for one type of integration. As observed in an earlier section, older adolescents begin to normalize seemingly opposing attributes, viewing them as appropriate if not desirable.

For example, older adolescents asserted that "it wouldn't be normal to act the same way with everyone, you act one way with your friends and a different way with your parents, that's the way it should be"; "It's good to be able to be different with different people in your life; you'd be pretty strange and also pretty boring if you weren't." Such normalization of different attributes in different roles increased with age suggesting that, developmentally, adolescents come to adopt the stance observed in the adult literature (Gergen, 1968; Vallacher, 1980), namely that consistency across roles may not be appropriate.

With increasing age, adolescents were also more likely to avert conflict by constructing higher order abstractions that serve to integrate seemingly contradictory attributes (e.g., happy and sad don't conflict because they are both part of being moody). The older adolescent can also resolve potentially contradictory attributes by asserting that he/she is flexible or adaptive, thereby subsuming apparent inconsistencies under more generalized abstractions about the self. As a result of these cognitive strategies, seemingly contradictory attributes may persist in the self-portrait; however, they no longer cause conflict.

Another solution for creating some sense of a unified self can be found in the efforts of those theorists who have emphasized the role of autobiographical narratives in the construction of the adult self (Freeman, 1992; Gergen & Gergen, 1988; McAdams, in press; Oyserman & Markus, 1993). In developing a self-narrative, the individual creates a sense of continuity over time as well as coherent connections among self-relevant life events. In constructing such a life story, experiences are temporally sequenced into an integrated self-narrative that provides meaning and future direction. Moreover, narrative construction is a continuous process since we not only craft but revise the story of our lives, creating new blueprints that facilitate further architectural development of the self. This type of narrative integration does not require that one display similar attributes across different relational contexts; thus, seeming inconsistencies can not only be tolerated but may be retained as desirable facets of the self-system.

Multiplicity, as exemplified by the displays of different attributes in different contexts, may well be very adaptive to the extent that characteristics are experienced as more positive in some roles than in others. As was demonstrated, adolescents value their attributes in some contexts over those in others. Thus, an individual may well opt to spend more time in those life niches where favorable self-appraisals are more common. The same point applies to the concept of relational self-esteem. Multiplicity, in the form of the ability to construct different perceptions of one's worth as a person in different relationships, may have similar protective benefits. Our evidence reveals that for the majority of adolescents, there are particular contexts in which individuals experience higher self-esteem, contexts in which they also receive greater support. Thus, an adaptive strategy is to inhabit such domains, either in action or in thought, with greater frequency than contexts in which there is less support and therefore a more negative appraisal of personal worth.

Moreover, one can come to value those more positive contexts, allowing one's sense of worth in those domains to generalize to perceptions of global self-esteem. It is important to appreciate the fact that the concept of global self-esteem is not to be laid to rest in the contemporary shift to contextual and multidimensional frameworks. Such an internment is unlikely given that global self-esteem remains a phenomenological reality in the lives of individuals. Moreover, there is a voluminous literature on its numerous and meaningful correlates. Of interest in our own data (Harter et al., 1996) is the finding that for the vast majority of individuals, self-esteem in one particular relational context is much more predictive of global self-esteem than are relational self-esteem scores in all other contexts. The specific domain occupying this position varies from adolescent to adolescent. Moreover, the relational self-esteem score in that particular context is higher than in other domains. Thus, psychological occupancy in that particular context would appear to be very adaptive in that it should promote more positive feelings of global self-esteem. From this perspective, global self-esteem does not subsume more context-specific evaluations of one's worth as a person; that is, it is not at the apex of an integrated hierarchy of self-constructs. Rather, the more adaptive strategy is to discount contexts where self-evaluations are less favorable.

In summary, the period of adolescence represents normative challenges to the harmonious organization and integration of self-constructs. However, with increasing development, further skills emerge which equip the individual with strategies that normalize the construction of multiple selves, that allow one to selectively occupy those contexts in which self-evaluations are more favorable, and that provide for a phenomenological sense of unity through the construction of a meaningful narrative of one's life story.

REFERENCES

Allport, G. W. (1961). *Patterns and growth in personality*. New York: Holt, Rinehart, & Winston.

Ashmore, R. D., & Ogilvie, D. M. (1992). He's such a nice boy . . . when he's with Grandma: Gender and evaluation in self-with-other representations. In T. M. Brinthaupt & R. P. Lipka (Eds.), *The self: Definitional and methodological issues* (pp. 236–290). Albany, NY: State University of New York Press.

Bleiberg, E. (1984). Narcissistic disorders in children. *Bulletin of the Menninger Clinic, 48,* 501–517.

Bowlby, J. (1980). *Attachment and loss: Vol. 3. Loss, sadness, and depression*. New York: Basic Books.

Bracken, B. (1996). Clinical applications of a context-dependent multi-dimensional model of self-concept. In B. Bracken (Ed.), *Handbook of self-concept* (pp. 463–505).

Bresnick, S. (1986). *Conflict in the adolescent self-theory*. Unpublished honors thesis, University of Denver, Denver, CO.

Bresnick, S. (1995). *Developmental and gender differences in role-related opposing attributes within the adolescent self-portrait*. Unpublished doctoral dissertation, University of Denver, Denver, CO.

Bretherton, I. (1991). Pouring new wine into old bottles: The social self as internal working model. In M. R. Gunnar & L. A. Sroufe (Eds.), *The Minnesota Symposium on Child Development: Vol. 26. Self-processes and development* (pp. 1–42). Hillsdale, NJ: Erlbaum.

Briere, J. (1992). *Child abuse trauma: Theory and treatment of the lasting effects*. Newbury Park, London: Sage Publications.

Brown, B. B. (1990). Peer groups and peer cultures. In S. S. Feldman & G. Elliot (Eds.), *At the threshold: The developing adolescent* (pp. 171–196). Cambridge, MA: Harvard University Press.

Calverley, R. M., Fischer, K. W., & Ayoub, C. (1994). Complex splitting of self-representations in sexually abused adolescent girls. *Development and Psychopathology, 6,* 195–213.

Carson, J. (1985). *Adolescent development: Conflict within the self.* Unpublished manuscript, University of Denver, Denver, CO.

Chodorow, N. J. (1989). *Feminism and psychoanalytic theory.* New Haven: Harper.

Cooley, C. H. (1902). *Human nature and the social order.* New York: Charles Schribner's Sons.

Cooper, C. (in press). *The weaving of maturity: Cultural perspectives on adolescent development.* New York: Oxford University Press.

Cooper, C. R., Grotevant, H. D., & Condon, S. M. (1983). Individuality and connectedness both foster adolescent identity formation and role taking skills. In H. D. Grotevant & C. R. Cooper (Eds.), *Adolescent development in the family: New directions for child development* (pp. 43–59). San Francisco: Jossey–Bass.

Cooper, C. R., Jackson, J. F., Azmitia, M., Lopez, E., & Dunbar, N. (1995). Bridging students' multiple worlds: African American and Latino youth in academic outreach programs. In R. F. Macias & R. G. Garcia–Ramos (Eds.), *Changing schools for changing students: An anthology of research on language minorities* (pp. 211–234). Santa Barbara, CA: University of California Linguistic Minority Research Institute.

Coopersmith, S. (1967). *The antecedents of self-esteem.* San Francisco: W. H. Freeman.

Crittenden, P. M. (1994). Peering into the black box: An exploratory treatise on the development of self in young children. In D. Cicchetti & S. L Toth (Eds.), *Rochester Symposium on Developmental Psycholpathology: Vol. 5. Disorders and dysfunctions of the Self* (pp. 79–148). Rochester, NY: University of Rochester Press.

Damon, W., & Hart, D. (1988). *Self-understanding in childhood and adolescence.* New York: Cambridge University Press.

Deci, E. L., & Ryan, R. M. (1995). Human autonomy: The basis for true self-esteem. In M. H. Kernis (Ed.), *Efficacy, agency, and self-esteem, 2* (pp. 31–46). New York: Plenum Press.

Dunn, J., Brown, J., & Beardsall, L. (1991). Family talk about feeling states and children's later understanding of others' emotions. *Developmental Psychology, 27,* 445–448.

Eichenbaum, L., & Orbach, S. (1983). *Understanding women: A feminist psychoanalytic approach.* New York: Basic Books.

Eisenberg, N. (1983). *Early descriptions of past experiences: Scripts as structure.* Princeton, NJ: Educational Testing Service.

Epstein, S. (1973). The self-concept revisited. *American Psychologist, 28,* 405–416.

Epstein, S. (1981). The unity principle versus the reality and pleasure principles, or the tale of the scorpion and the frog. In M. D. Lynch, A. A. Norem–Hebeisen, & K. Gergen (Eds.), *Self-concept: Advances in theory and research* (pp. 82–110). Cambridge, MA: Ballinger.

Erikson, E. (1959). Identity and the life cycle. *Psychological Issues, 1,* 18–164.

Erikson, E. (1968). *Identity, youth and crisis.* New York: Norton.

Fischer, K. F. (1980). A theory of cognitive development: The control and construction of hierarchies of skills. *Psychological Review, 87,* 477–531.

Fischer, K. W., & Aboub, C. (1993). Affective splitting and dissociation in normal and maltreated children: Developmental pathways for self in relationships. In D. Cicchetti & S. Toth (Eds.), *Rochester Symposium on Developmental Psychopathology: Vol. 5. The self and its disorders* (pp. 149–222). Rochester, NY: University of Rochester Press.

Fischer, K. W., & Canfield, R. (1986). The ambiguity of stage and structure in behavior: Person and environment in the development of psychological structure. In I. Levin (Ed.), *Stage and structure: Reopening the debate* (pp. 246–267). New York: Plenum.

Fischer, K. W., & Lamborn, S. (1989). Mechanisms of variation in developmental levels: Cognitive and emotional transitions during adolescence. In A. de Ribaupierre (Ed.), *Transition mechanisms in child development: The longitudinal perspective* (pp. 37–61). Cambridge, England: Cambridge University Press.

Freeman, M. (1992). Self as narrative: The place of life history in studying the life span. In T. M. Brinthaupt & R. P. Lipka (Eds.), *The self: Definitional and methodological issues* (pp. 15–43). Albany, NY: State University of New York Press.

Gecas, V. (1972). Parental behavior and contextual variations in adolescent self-esteem. *Sociometry, 35,* 332–345.

Gergen, K. J. (1968). Personal consistency and the presentation of self. In C. Gordon & K. J. Gergen (Eds.), *The self in social interaction* (pp. 30–326). New York: Wiley.

Gergen, K. J. (1977). The social construction of self-knowledge. In T. Mischel (Ed.), *The self: Psychological and philosophical issues* (pp. 139–169). Totowa, NJ: Rowman and Littlefield.

Gergen, K. J. (1991). *The saturated self.* New York: Basic Books.

Gergen, K. J., & Gergen, M. M. (1988). Narrative and the self as relationship. In L. Berkowitz (Ed.), *Advances in experimental social psychology* (Vol. 21, pp. 17–56). New York: Academic Press.

Gilligan, C. (1982). *In a different voice.* Cambridge, MA: Harvard University Press.

Gilligan, C. (1993). Joining the resistence: Psychology, politics, girls, and women. In L. Weis & M. Fine (Eds.), *Beyond silenced voices* (pp. 143–168). Albany, NY: State University of New York Press.

Gilligan, C., Lyons, N., & Hanmer, T. J. (1989). *Making connections.* Cambridge, MA: Harvard University Press.

Griffin, N., Chassin, L., & Young, R. D. (1981). Measurement of global self-concept versus multiple role-specific self-concepts in adolescents. *Adolescence, 16,* 49–56.

Grotevant, H. D., & Cooper, C. R. (1983). *Adolescent development in the family: New directions for child development.* San Francisco, CA: Jossey–Bass.

Grotevant, H. D., & Cooper, C. R. (1986). Individuation in family relationships. *Human Development, 29,* 83–100.

Hart, D. (1988). The adolescent self-concept in social context. In D. K. Lapsley & F. C. Power (Eds.), *Self, ego, and identity* (pp. 71–90). New York: Springer–Verlag.

Harter, S. (1982). The perceived competence scale for children. *Child Development, 53,* 87–97.

Harter, S. (1990). Causes, correlates and the functional role of global self-worth: A life-span perspective. In J. Kolligian & R. Sternberg (Eds.), *Perceptions of competence and incompetence across the life-span* (pp. 67–98). New Haven, CT: Yale University Press.

Harter, S. (1993). Causes and consequences of low self-esteem in children and adolescents. In R. F. Baumeister (Ed.), *Self-esteem: The puzzle of low self-regard* (pp. 87–117). New York: Plenum.

Harter, S. (in press-a). The development of self-representations. In W. Damon (Series Ed.) & N. Eisenberg (Vol. Ed.), *Handbook of child psychology: Vol. 3. Social, emotional, and personality development* (5th ed.). New York: Wiley.

Harter, S. (in press-b). The effects of child abuse on the self-system. In B. B. Rossman & M. S. Rosenberg (Eds.), *Multiple victimization of children: Conceptual, developmental, research, and treatment issues.* New York: Haworth Press.

Harter, S. (in press-c). *The personal self in social context: Barriers to authenticity.* In R. D. Ashmore & L. Jussim (Eds.), *Self and identity: Fundamental issues.* New York: Oxford University Press.

Harter, S., & Monsour, A. (1992). Developmental analysis of conflict caused by opposing attributes in the adolescent self-portrait. *Developmental Psychology, 28(2),* 251–260.

Harter, S., Marold, D., Whitesell, N. R., & Cobbs, G. (1996). A model of the effects of parent and peer support on adolescent false self behavior. *Child Development, 67,* 360–374.

Harter, S., Waters, P., & Whitesell, N. R. (in press). Relational self-esteem: Differences in perceived worth as a person across interpersonal contexts. *Child Development.*

Harter, S., Waters, P., & Whitesell, N. R. (1997). Lack of voice as a manifestation of false self behavior: The school setting as a stage upon which the drama of authenticity is enacted. *Educational Psychologist, 32,* 153–173.

Harter, S., Waters, P. L., Pettitt, L. M., Whitesell, N., Kofkin, J., & Jordan, J. (1997). Autonomy and connectedness as dimensions of relationship styles in men and women. *Journal of Social and Personality Relationships, 14,* 147–164.

Hattie, J. (1992). *Self-concept.* Hillsdale, NJ: Erlbaum.

Herman, J. (1992). *Trauma and recovery.* New York: Basic Books.

Higgins, E. T., Van Hook, E., & Dorfman, D. (1988). Do self-attributes form a cognitive structure? *Social Cognition, 6,* 177–207.

Hill, J. P., & Holmbeck, G. N. (1986). Attachment and autonomy during adolescence. In G. J. Whitehurst (Ed.), *Annals of child development* (Vol. 3, pp. 145–189). Greenwich, CT: JAI Press.

Horney, K. (1950). *Neurosis and human growth.* New York: Norton.

Hudson, J. A. (1990). The emergence of autobiographical memory in mother–child conversation. In R. Fivush & J. A. Hudson (Eds.), *Knowing and remembering in young children* (pp. 166–196). New York: Cambridge University Press.

Johnson, E. (1995). *The role of social support and gender orientation in adolescent female development.* Unpublished doctoral dissertation, University of Denver, Denver, CO.

Jordan, J. V. (1991). The relational self: A new perspective for understanding women's development. In J. Strauss & G. Goethals (Eds.), *The self: Interdisciplinary approaches* (pp. 136–149). New York: Springer–Verlag.

Jordan, J. V., Kaplan, A. G., Miller, J. B., Stiver, J. L., & Surrey, L. P. (Eds.). (1991). *Women's growth in connection.* New York: Guilford Press.

Jung, C. G. (1928). *Two essays on analytical psychology.* New York: Dodd, Mead.

Kagan, J. (1991). The theoretical utility of constructs for self. *Developmental Review, 11,* 244–250.

Keating, D. P. (1990). Cognitive processes in adolescence. In S. Feldman & G. Elliot (Eds.), *At the threshold: The developing adolescent* (pp. 54–89). Cambridge, MA: Harvard University Press.

Kelly, G. A. (1955). *The psychology of personal constructs.* New York: Norton.

Kihlstrom, J. F. (1993). What does the self look life? In T. K. Srull & R. S. Wyer, Jr. (Eds.), *The mental representation of trait and autobiographical knowledge about the self: Advances in social cognition* (Vol. 5, pp. 79–90). Hillsdale, NJ: Erlbaum.

Lecky, P. (1945). *Self-consistency: A theory of personality.* New York: Island Press.

Lerner, H. G. (1993). *The dance of deception.* New York: Harper Collins.

Lifton, R. J. (1993). *The protean self.* New York: Basic Books.

Markus, H., & Cross, S. (1990). The interpersonal self. In L. A. Pervin (Ed.), *Handbook of personality: Theory and research* (pp. 576–608). New York: Guilford Press.

Marsh, H. W. (1986). Global self-esteem: Its relation to specific facets of self-concept and their importance. *Journal of Personality and Social Psychology, 51,* 1224–1236.

Marsh, H. W. (1987). The hierarchical structure of self-concept and the application of hierarchical confirmatory factor analysis. *Journal of Educational Measurement, 24,* 17–19.

Marsh, H. W. (1989). Age and sex effects in multiple dimensions of self-concept: Preadolescence to early adulthood. *Journal of Educational Psychology, 81,* 417–430.

Maslow, A. (1961). Peak-experience as acute identity-experiences. *American Journal of Psychoanalysis, 21,* 547–556.

McAdams, D. (in press). The unity of identity. In R. D. Ashmore & L. Jussim (Eds.), *Self and identity: Fundamental issues.* New York: Oxford University Press.

Miller, J. B. (1986). *Toward a new psychology of women* (2nd ed.). Boston: Beacon Press.

Miller, J. B. (1991). The development of women's sense of self. In J. V. Jordan, et al. (Eds.), *Women's growth and connection: Writings from the Stone Center* (pp. 11–26). New York: Guilford Press.

Mischel, W. (1973). Toward a cognitive social learning reconceptualization of personality. *Psychological Review, 80,* 252–283.

Mullener, N., & Laird, J. D. (1971). Some development changes in the organization of self-evaluations. *Developmental Psychology, 5,* 233–236.

Oosterwegel, A., & Oppenheimer, L. (1993). *The self-system: Developmental changes between and within self-concepts.* Hillsdale, NJ: Erlbaum.

Oyserman, D., & Markus, H. R. (1993). The sociocultural self. In J. Suls (Ed.), *Psychological perspectives on the self* (Vol. 7, pp. 187–220). Hillsdale, NJ: Erlbaum.

Putnam, F. W. (1993). Dissociation and disturbances of self. In D. Cicchetti & S. Toth (Eds.), *Rochester Symposium on Developmental Psychopathology: Vol. 5. Disorders and dysfunctions of the self.* Rochester, NY: University of Rochester Press.

Rogers, C. R. (1951). *Client-centered therapy.* Boston: Houghton Mifflin.

Rosenberg, M. (1979). *Conceiving the self.* New York: Basic Books.

Rosenberg, M. (1986). Self-concept from middle childhood through adolescence. In J. Suls & A. G. Greenwald (Eds.), *Psychological perspective on the self, 3* (pp. 182–205). Hillsdale, NJ: Erlbaum.

Rosenberg, S. (1988). Self and others: Studies in Social Personality and Autobiography. In L. Berkowitz (Ed.), *Advances in experimental social psychology* (Vol. 21, pp. 56–96). New York: Academic Press.

Rubin, L. (1985). *Just friends: The role of friendship in our lives.* New York: Harper.

Savin–Williams, R. C., & Berndt, T. J. (1990). Friend and peer relations. In S. S. Feldman & G. Elliot (Eds.), *At the threshold: The developing adolescent* (pp. 277–307). Cambridge, MA: Harvard University Press.

Shavelson, R. J., & Marsh, H. W. (1986). On the structure of the self-concept. In R. Schwarzer (Ed.), *Anxiety and cognition* (pp. 283–310). Hillsdale, NJ: Erlbaum.

Smollar, J., & Youniss, J. (1985). Adolescent self-concept development. In R. L. Leahy (Ed.), *The development of self* (pp. 247–266). New York: Academic Press.

Snow, K. (1990). Building memories: The ontogeny of autobiography. In D. Cicchetti & M. Beeghly (Eds.), *The self in transition: Infancy to childhood* (pp. 213–242). Chicago: University of Chicago Press.

Snyder, M. (1987). *Public appearances, private realities: The psychology of self-monitoring.* New York: Freeman.

Steinberg, L., & Silverberg, S. B. (1986). The vicissitudes of autonomy in early adolescence. *Child Development, 57,* 841–851.

Stern, D. (1985). *The interpersonal world of the infant.* New York: Basic Books.

Sullivan, H. (1953). *The interpersonal theory of psychiatry.* New York: Norton.

Terr, L. (1990). *Too scared to cry.* New York: Basic Books.

Vallacher, R. R. (1980). An introduction to self theory. In D. M. Wegner & R. R. Vallacher (Eds.), *The self in social psychology* (pp. 3–30). New York: Oxford University Press.

van der Kolk, B. A. (1987). *Psychological trauma.* Washington, DC: American Psychiatric Press.

Westen, D. (1995). The impact of sexual abuse on self structure. In D. Cicchetti & S. Toth (Eds.), *Rochester Symposium on Developmental Psychopathology: Vol. 5. Disorders and dysfunctions of the self.* Rochester, NY: University of Rochester Press.

White, K., Speisman, J., & Costos, D. (1983). Young adults and their parents: Individuation to mutuality. In H. D. Grotevant & C. R. Cooper (Eds.), *Adolescent development in the family: New directions for child development* (pp. 61–76). San Francisco: Jossey–Bass.

Winnicott, D. W. (1965). *The maturational processes and the facilitating environment.* New York: International Universities Press.

Part II
CLINICAL ISSUES

The five papers in Part II address a wide array of clinically relevant issues. In the first paper, Graber, Lewinsohn, Seeley, and Brooks-Gunn use data derived from the Oregon Adolescent Depression Project, a large epidemiological study of psychopathology in high school students, to examine associations between the timing of pubertal development and concurrent and prior psychopathology during adolescence. The timing of the pubertal transition has long been held to be of major importance in determining whether pubertal development is associated with psychopathology, with early-maturing girls and late-maturing boys hypothesized as being at greatest risk for the emergence of psychopathology.

The adolescent students of Graber et al.'s paper, who ranged in age from 14 through 18 years old, were drawn from nine senior high schools in urban and rural western Oregon. Sampling within schools was proportional to size of school, size of grade within school, and proportion of boys and girls within grade to obtain a final sample of 1,709 adolescents that was representative of the larger population of students. Adolescents were interviewed using the Schedule for Affective Disorders and Schizophrenia for School-Age Children as adapted for use in epidemiological studies. Adolescents also completed a questionnaire battery covering a range of psychosocial variables as well as an adapted version of the Pubertal Development Scale. Adolescents were specifically asked whether their physical growth and development was early, on time, or late in comparison with that of most teenagers their age. Stability of response to this item over a 1-year period was 83% agreement ($\kappa = .61$) for girls and 77% agreement ($\kappa = .48$) for boys.

Analyses tested whether pubertal timing (early, on time, or late) was associated with present and lifetime history of mental disorders, psychological symptoms, and psychosocial functioning. As hypothesized, adolescents whose pubertal development was "off time" showed more evidence of psychopathology than other same-gender adolescents. Specifically, as compared with on-time girls, those who matured early had significantly elevated lifetime rates of major depression, substance abuse or dependence, disruptive behavior disorders, and eating disorders. Early-maturing girls also reported lower self-esteem, poorer coping skills, and less support from family and friends. They missed more days at school, rated their health as poorer, had higher rates of ever having used tobacco, and had a higher rate of suicide attempts. When compared with on-time girls, those who matured late also had a significantly elevated lifetime rate of major depression. The impact of pubertal timing was less striking in boys. The only significant diagnostic contrast was that late-maturing boys had significantly lower rates of substance abuse or dependence than did on-time boys. Nonetheless, when compared with on-time boys, early-maturing boys tended to report more major life events, a higher level of depressive symptoms, more emotional reliance on others, more physical illness, an elevated hypomanic personality style, and a higher rate of tobacco use. Late-maturing boys reported more daily hassles, higher level of depression, more internalizing behavior problems, more negative cognitions, more self-consciousness, more emotional reliance on others, poorer coping skills, more conflict with parents, and elevated hypomanic personality.

It has been suggested that early-maturing girls, who begin puberty when no other children are yet experiencing these events, may be at greater risk for psychopathology because they are less well prepared for the physical, psychological, and social challenges posed by puberty and entry into adolescence. Conversely, late-maturing boys, who begin and complete puberty after all other adolescents have already passed through this developmental stage, may well experience psychosocial problems or feelings of inferiority as a consequence of their less mature physical appearance and more limited athletic ability. Mechanisms aside, however, the number of adolescents who perceive their pubertal development to be off time is not trivial. In this epidemiological sample, almost 20% of girls reported early-onset puberty and 15% of boys described late-onset puberty. The findings of this study emphasize the importance of including information about pubertal timing in clinical assessments with adolescents. Moreover, age of onset of puberty may serve as a useful screen for the early detection of psychopathology.

In the second paper in this section, Whitaker and colleagues examine the relation of neonatal cranial ultrasound abnormalities to psychiatric disorder at age 6 in a regional birth cohort of low-birthweight children. The introduction of ultrasonography, a noninvasive brain-imaging technique suitable for use with low-birthweight newborns, has greatly expanded researchers' ability to study the sequelae of perinatal brain injury. Although the motor and cognitive sequelae of neonatal cranial ultrasound abnormalities in low-birthweight infants have been extensively studied, the relationship of abnormalities noted during the perinatal period to childhood psychopathology has been a relatively neglected area.

This knowledge gap is addressed in this study of participants in the Neonatal Brain Hemorrhage study birth cohort. That study prospectively enrolled 1,105 consecutive infants with birthweights between 501 and 2,000 grams between September 1, 1984, and June 30, 1997. The cohort was screened with cranial ultrasound scans obtained at 4 hr, 24 hr, and 7 days of life. Of the cohort, 98% were scanned at least once and 47% were also scanned between the 3rd and 5th hospital week, predischarge, or both. Abnormalities were classified as follows: (a) No abnormality; (b) isolated germinal matrix hemorrhage, isolated ventricular enlargement, or both; and (c) parenchymal lesions, ventricular enlargement with or without isolated germinal matrix hemorrhage or isolated ventricular enlargement, or both.

At age 6, 685 children were followed up. Behavioral measures included the Diagnostic Interview Schedule for Children—Parent version and the Riley Motor Problems Inventory, which were administered by a pediatric nurse practitioner who also obtained information on family functioning and parental mental health. Predictor variables included neonatal ultrasound status; prenatal factors including maternal social disadvantage and maternal alcohol and tobacco use; perinatal factors including sex, Apgar scores, gestational age, and fetal growth ratio; neonatal complications of prematurity; and neonatal chronic illness.

Twenty-two percent of the cohort had at least one psychiatric disorder, the most common being attention deficit–hyperactivity disorder (ADHD; 16%). In the sample as a whole, parenchymal lesions and/or ventricular enlargement increased risk relative to no abnormality, independent of other biological and social predictors, and to any disorder (odds ratio

4.4, $p < .001$), ADHD (odds ratio 3.4, $p < .05$), and tic disorders (odds ratio 8.7, $p < .05$). In children of normal intelligence, parenchymal lesions and ventricular enlargement independently increased risk for any disorder (odds ratio 4.8, $p < .01$) and separation anxiety disorder (odds ratio 5.3, $p < .05$). These effects were not affected by female gender or social advantage, and isolated germinal matrix and intraventricular hemorrhage were not related to psychiatric disorder at age 6.

The findings are of particular interest in providing evidence of a direct link between demonstrated and specific damage to the central nervous system (parenchymal lesions and ventricular enlargement) and psychiatric disorder at age 6, most particularly ADHD, tic disorders, and separation anxiety disorders. Moreover, smoking, sex, and social disadvantage were independent predictors of disorder. Conversely, relative social advantage did not function as a protective factor. These findings are not consistent with the more commonly espoused interactional model of biological and social risk. As articulated by Sameroff and Chandler (1975), among children who are not severely disabled, higher rates of psychiatric disorder would be expected with greater social disadvantage, and perinatal brain injury *per se* would have an effect only among socially disadvantaged children. Among advantaged children, inherent "self-righting tendencies" would counteract any adverse effects of perinatal risk factors. The relation of parenchymal lesions and ventricular enlargement to psychiatric disorder at age 6 years is more consistent with a main-effects model than with the more widely accepted interactional model.

In the third paper in this section, "Cognitive Deficits in Parents From Multiple-Incidence Autism Families," Piven and Palmer direct attention toward the problem of defining the boundaries of the phenotype in autism. Results from family and twin studies have established that the etiology of autism—a severe neuropsychiatric disorder defined by the presence of social deficits, communication abnormalities, stereotyped repetitive behaviors, and a characteristic course—is mainly genetic. However, the definition of the phenotype for use in genetic studies has continued to be the subject of debate. Findings of studies directed toward familial aggregation of cognitive deficits and academic- and language-related disorders in families of autistic persons have been difficult to interpret because of variation in the criteria for the selection of probands (autism vs. pervosine developmental disorder) and in the methods used for the assessment of relatives (direct examination vs. family history).

Piven and Palmer address these issues by directly examining cognitive abilities in parents of two or more reliably diagnosed (by means of the Autism Diagnosis Interview and the Autism Diagnostic Observation Schedule) autistic children. The selection of such a sample is advantageous because probands in families with multiple incidences of autism are less likely than probands in families with a single incidence to have autism as a result of nongenetic causes and are therefore likely to represent a more etiologically homogenous sample than those ascertained through a single autistic or pervosinely developmentally disordered (PDD) proband. In addition, relatives ascertained through multiple-incidence autism probands may have a higher genetic liability for autism and the genetically related broader autism phenotype than relatives ascertained through single-incidence autism or PDD probands. Parents ascertained through a child with Down syndrome served as a comparison group, selected to control for the effect of caring for a handicapped child on the emotional and social functioning of parents. In addition, relatives of a Down syndrome child would not be expected to have an increased genetic liability over the general population for social or communication deficits or for stereotyped behaviors characteristic of autism.

In all, 25 mothers and 23 fathers from 25 multiple-incidence autism families and 30 mothers and 30 fathers from 30 Down syndrome families participated. The two groups of parents did not differ significantly with respect to age, level of education, or father's occupation. Measures included the Wechsler Adult Intelligence Scale—Revised, the Woodcock Johnson Tests of Achievement, the Rapid Automatized Naming Test, and the Tower of Hanoi. Parents of autistic children were found to perform significantly more poorly on performance IQ, a test of executive function (the Tower of Hanoi), and passage comprehension and rapid automatized naming. Moreover, scores on the different measures were more likely to be independent of each other in the parents of children with autism and more highly correlated in the parents of children with Down syndrome.

The results are consistent with the premise that cognitive deficits may be an expression of the underlying genetic liability for autism. Moreover, the relationship of the findings to the pattern of cognitive deficits observed to occur in autism *per se*, as well their overlap with those identified in nonverbal learning disability syndrome (Klin, Volkmar, Sparrow, Cicchetti, & Rourke, 1996), are interpreted as lending further support to the emerging descriptions of a broader autism phenotype. Families with multiple incidences of autism were used by Piven and Palmer to examine aspects of social functioning in relatives of autistic probands. The method is potentially very powerful. Examination of the components of the broader autism phenotype in relatives may permit genetically meaningful but distinct aspects of the autistic phenotype to be disentangled. Future studies using this approach are awaited with interest.

In the next paper in this section, Leonard and colleagues provide clinicians with a valuable summary of the pharmacology of the selective serotonin reuptake inhibitors (SSRIs) by detailing what is known about their metabolism in children and adolescents and the practical clinical implications for their use in this age group. More than 300 articles retrieved through *Index Medicus* searches for articles published during the past 10 years were reviewed. The SSRIs represent a new class of antidepressants with distinct advantages in their side effect profile and their broad therapeutic index over that seen with the tricyclic antidepressants. *SSRIs* derive their name from their effect on selective inhibition of serotonin reuptake into the presynaptic terminal, the resultant increase in serotonin concentration at the synaptic cleft, and their limited effect on other monoamines. However, these acute effects probably do not explain the therapeutic effects seen several weeks later, which are hypothesized to involve neuroadaptive changes of a specific receptor subtype, perhaps the delayed desensitization of serotonin autoreceptors.

The SSRIs with the most potent serotonergic reuptake inhibition are (in order of decreasing potency) paroxetine, fluvoxamine, sertraline, clomipramine, and fluoxetine. However, more potency has not been shown to correlate directly with clinical antidepressant and antiobsessional efficacy. At higher dosages, all of the SSRIs will inhibit the reuptake of norepinephrine and, to a lesser degree, dopamine. The selectivity profile between the SSRIs has not been found to be related to clinical efficacy but may affect potential side effects and drug interactions.

Much less is known about the pharmacokinetics of psychotropic medications in children than in adults, and in fact much of the information summarized in the Leonard et al. review derives from the downward extrapolation of the relevant adult literature. All of the SSRIs are metabolized primarily in the liver by the cytochrome P450 system. They are also potent inhibitors of several different isoenzymes. With increased knowledge about the potential for drug–drug interactions, and with limited information about the unique vulnerabilities of children, caution must be exercised in prescribing concomitant medication. Moreover, each SSRI has its own individual pattern of metabolism and inhibition. It is incumbent on the prescribing physician to inquire about all prescription drugs, over-the-counter medications, and illicit drugs that the patient may be taking to avoid potentially toxic combinations.

The SSRI side effect profile of fewer anticholinergic effects, less sedation, less weight gain, and limited cardiovascular and other systemic toxicities affords particular benefit in the pediatric population. Nevertheless, SSRIs do have a distinct pattern of adverse reactions characterized by gastrointestinal (nausea, diarrhea, vomiting) and central nervous system (agitation, disinhibition, jitteriness, headache, insomnia) effects. Rates of side effects appear to differ among the individual SSRIs, although large, direct comparison trials have not been done. In addition, differences between the rates of specific side effects experienced by adults, in comparison with those experienced by children and adolescents, have not been determined.

Although further study of the pharmacokinetics, pharmacodynamics, efficacy, and safety of the SSRIs in the pediatric age group is clearly required, this review provides the current day practitioner with a concise guide to the use of this important class of psychotropic medication in children and adolescents.

In the final paper in this section, Mammen and colleagues describe four cases of ego-dystonic anger attacks in the mothers of young children. Ego-dystonic anger attacks are an underrecognized psychiatric symptom that may occur in association with depression, in association with other psychiatric disorders, and in the absence of comorbid disorders. They are characterized by overwhelming anger and autonomic arousal occurring upon provocation viewed as trivial by the affected individual. The anger experienced during the attack is described as uncharacteristic and accompanying aggressive acts are followed by guilt and regret.

The four case vignettes illustrate how high levels of parental anger may have a negative impact on young children by causing arousal and disregulation of emotions and behavior and by modeling angry responses and aggressive acts for the child. Although there is no evidence that occasional episodes of anger are harmful to children, mothers with anger attacks are likely to respond to provocations with frequent and intense anger outbursts, which may escalate the child's provocative and oppositional behavior. Moreover, mothers experiencing anger attacks report avoiding their children to reduce the likelihood of becoming angry or abusing them. Diagnosing anger attacks is of particular clinical importance because they tend to respond well to treatment with SSRIs, and this may make a dramatic difference in mother–child interactions.

Mammen et al. note that anger has been a generally neglected topic in psychiatric research and practice and suggest that underrecognition of anger attacks may be a particular problem among mothers because women are socialized to deny anger. Anger attacks may be a more common problem than is generally recognized as mothers may not volunteer that they have trouble controlling their anger and may only acknowledge having anger attacks when directly questioned. Although research on the prevalence, correlates, and etiology of parental anger attacks and their relationship to child psychopathology is required, exploration of the possibility of ego-dystonic anger attacks in mothers of young children who present with oppositional and aggressive behavior patterns is clearly indicated.

REFERENCES

Klin, A., Volkmar, F. R., Sparrow, D. V., Cicchetti, D. V., & Rourke, B. P. (1996). Validity and neuropsychological characterization of Asperger syndrome: Convergence with nonverbal learning disabilities syndrome. In M. D. Hertzig & E. Farber (Eds.), *Annual progress in child psychiatry and child development* (pp. 241–259). New York: Brunner/Mazel.

Piven, J., Palmer, P., Jacobi, D., Childress, D., & Arndt, S. (1997). The broader autism phenotype: Evidence from a family history study of multiple-incidence autism families. *American Journal of Psychiatry, 154,* 185–190.

Sameroff, A. J., & Chandler, M. J. (1975). Reproductive risk and the continuum of caretaking casuality. In F. D. Horowitz (Ed.), *Review of child development research* (pp. 187–244). Chicago: University of Chicago Press.

6

Is Psychopathology Associated With the Timing of Pubertal Development?

Julia A. Graber
Columbia University, New York, New York
Peter M. Lewinsohn and John R. Seeley
Oregon Research Institute, Eugene, Oregon
Jeanne Brooks-Gunn
Columbia University, New York, New York

Objective: *This investigation tested whether the timing of pubertal development was associated with concurrent and prior experiences of psychopathology (symptoms and disorders) in adolescent boys and girls.* **Method:** *A large (N = 1,709) community sample of high school students were interviewed using the Schedule for Affective Disorders and Schizophrenia for School-Age Children as adapted for use in epidemiological studies. Adolescents also completed a questionnaire battery covering a range of psychosocial variables.* **Results:** *Analyses tested whether pubertal timing was associated with present and lifetime history of mental disorders, psychological symptoms, and psychosocial functioning. As hypothesized, early-maturing girls and late-maturing boys showed more evidence of psychopathology than other same-gender adolescents.* **Conclusions:** *Early-maturing girls had the poorest current and lifetime history of adjustment problems, indicating that this pattern of pubertal development merits attention by mental health providers and researchers.*

Recent epidemiological studies have begun to document the extent to which psychopathology occurs during adolescence (Bird et al., 1988; Lewinsohn et al., 1993; McGee et al., 1990). Embedded in developmental studies of psychopathology has been the hypothesis that the experience of pubertal development shapes and interacts with other transitions in ways that impact adolescent mental health (Brooks-Gunn et al., 1994). The timing of the pubertal

---

Reprinted with permission from the *Journal of the American Academy of Child and Adolescent Psychiatry*, 1997, Vol. 36(12), 1768–1776.
The OADP was supported by grants from the NIMH (MH40501, MH50522) to Dr. Lewinsohn. The authors also acknowledge the support of the W.T. Grant Foundation Consortium on Adolescent Depression and the NICHD Research Network on Child Well-Being for their influence on this project.

transition (compared with one's peers) has been considered most salient for determining whether or not pubertal development is associated with psychopathology. The earliest-maturing girls begin puberty when no other children are experiencing these events; hence, these girls have been hypothesized to be at risk for psychopathology or lesser problems perhaps because they are less well-prepared for the physical, psychological, and social challenges posed by puberty and the entry into adolescence (Brooks-Gunn et al., 1985). Conversely, late-maturing boys begin (and complete) puberty after all other adolescents have already passed these events and may experience psychosocial problems or feelings of inferiority due to less mature appearance and poorer athletic ability in comparison with peers (Jones, 1965).

Research consistent with the "off-time" hypothesis has shown that girls who are early maturers are more likely than other girls to exhibit depressive, eating, and delinquent symptoms as well as general behavior problems (Attie and Brooks-Gunn, 1989; Caspi and Moffitt, 1991; Graber et al., 1994; Hayward et al., 1997; Petersen et al., 1991; Simmons and Blyth, 1987), with late-maturing girls showing no consistent pattern of adjustment problems in comparison with on-time maturers across these same studies. For boys, Andersson and Magnusson (1990) report that both early- and late-maturing boys began to drink alcohol earlier than their peers and that late-maturing boys may be more likely to develop an alcohol abuse problem in young adulthood ($p < .12$). No studies to date have examined pubertal timing and disorders in both boys and girls.

In this article, we examine whether self-reported pubertal timing is associated with concurrent and prior episodes of psychopathology (symptoms and disorders) in boys and girls. We are able to test for associations of pubertal timing effects across a wide range of disorders including major depression, anxiety, disruptive behavior, substance use, and eating disorders. Because timing effects have been demonstrated over a range of subclinical problems, we also examine several dimensions of psychosocial dysfunction. On the basis of the previous literature, it is hypothesized that for girls early maturation will be associated with psychopathology, whereas for boys late maturation will be associated with psychopathology.

The current investigation makes use of data from the Oregon Adolescent Depression Project (OADP). The OADP is a large epidemiological study of psychopathology in high school students (aged 14 through 18 years) who were assessed at two waves, 1 year apart. Previous publications have reported on the prevalence and incidence of mental disorders, the psychosocial correlates of depression, and continuity of psychopathology (Lewinsohn et al., 1993, 1994; Orvaschel et al., 1995). This is the first report in which we examine the relationship between timing of puberty and a spectrum of psychosocial functioning.

METHOD

Participants

Three cohorts of adolescents were drawn from nine senior high schools in urban and rural western Oregon (total population of 10,200 students). Sampling within schools was proportional to size of school, size of grade within school, and proportion of boys and girls within grade to obtain a final sample of 1,709 adolescents that was representative of the larger population of students. Although adolescents were seen 1 year later for a follow-up assessment, only information from the first year was used in this study.

Prior publications from the OADP have described the representativeness of the sample and the comparison of adolescents who did and did not participate in the study (see Lewinsohn et al., 1993, for details). The demographic characteristics of the sample were as follows: mean age was 16.6 years (SD = 1.2); 52.1% were girls; 8.9% were nonwhite; 71.3% lived with two parents; 53.2% lived with both biological parents; 14.9% were in 9th, 27.2% were in 10th, 26.3% were in 11th, and 31.6% were in 12th grade, and 12.3% had repeated a grade. Parents' occupational status consisted of 2.5% unskilled, 8.0% semiskilled, 21.2% skilled, 57.9% minor professional, and 10.3% professional.

Diagnostic Interview

Adolescents were interviewed with the Schedule for Affective Disorders and Schizophrenia for School-Age Children (K-SADS) adapted from K-SADS-E (Epidemiologic version) (Orvaschel et al., 1982) and K-SADS-P (Present Episode version). Items were added to derive diagnoses of past and current psychiatric disorders as out-lined in *DSM-III-R* (American Psychiatric Association, 1987), the version of the *DSM* in usage at the time of assessment. Interviewer reliability as indicated by the κ statistic was substantial to nearly perfect (Landis and Koch, 1977), with most equal to or greater than .80 with the exception of a few diagnoses (Lewinsohn et al., 1993).

Diagnoses were collapsed into five primary categories of disorder: (1) major depressive disorder; (2) anxiety, which was composed of panic disorder, agoraphobia, social phobia, simple phobia, obsessive-compulsive disorder, separation anxiety, and overanxious disorder; (3) disruptive behavior, which was composed of attention-deficit hyperactivity, conduct, and oppositional disorders; (4) substance use, which was composed of substance abuse and dependence disorders; and (5) eating disorder, which included anorexia and bulimia nervosa.

Psychosocial Constructs

An extensive questionnaire battery tapping all psychosocial variables known or hypothesized to be related to depression was administered (materials available upon request). Measures were shortened for administration (Andrews et al., 1993) and reduced to 20 composite scores (see Lewinsohn et al., 1993, for details). All variables were scored such that higher values indicated more problematic functioning.

Stress: Daily Hassles ($\alpha = .79, r = .55$) consisted of 20 items from the Unpleasant Events Schedule (Lewinsohn et al., 1985).

Stress: Major Life Events ($\alpha = .78, r = .52$) consisted of 14 events from the Schedule of Recent Experiences (Holmes and Rahe, 1967) and the Life Events Schedule (Sandler and Block, 1979).

Current Depression (mean interscale $r = .54$, $\alpha = .82$, $r = .40$) consisted of the 20-item Center for Epidemiologic Studies-Depression Scale (Radloff, 1977); the 21-item Beck Depression Inventory (Beck et al., 1961); a single item assessing depression level during the preceding week; and the interviewer-rated 14-item Hamilton Rating Scale for Depression (Hamilton, 1960).

Internalizing Behavior Problems (mean interscale $r = .25$, $\alpha = .72$, $r = .55$) assessed the tendency to worry (5 items; Maudsley Obsessional Compulsive Inventory) (Hodgson and Rachman, 1977); hypomanic behavior (12 items; General Behavior Inventory) (Depue et al., 1981); State Anxiety (10 items) (Spielberger et al., 1970); sleep patterns (8 items); and hypochondriasis (8 items) (Pilowsky, 1967).

Externalizing Behavior Problems (mean interscale $r = .32$, $\alpha = .71$, $r = .42$) consisted of current K-SADS symptoms for attention-deficit hyperactivity (15 items), conduct (17 items), and oppositional disorders (11 items) and an unpublished scale assessing conduct problems (6 items).

Depressotypic Negative Cognitions (mean interscale $r = .29$, $\alpha = .61$, $r = .61$) consisted of the Frequency of Self Reinforcement Attitude Questionnaire (10 items) (Heiby, 1982); the Subjective Probability Questionnaire (5 items) (R. F. Muñoz and P. M. Lewinsohn, unpublished); the Dysfunctional Attitude Scale (9 items) (Weissman and Beck, 1978); and perceived control over one's life (3 items) (Pearlin and Schooler, 1978).

Depressotypic Attributional Style ($\alpha = .63$, $r = .55$) consisted of the Kastan Attributional Style Questionnaire for Children (48 items) (Kaslow et al., 1978).

Self-Consciousness ($\alpha = .74$, $r = .54$) consisted of the Self-Consciousness Scale (nine items) (Fenigstein et al., 1975).

Self-Esteem (mean interscale $r = .33$, $\alpha = .59$, $r = .62$) consisted of the Body Parts Satisfaction Scale (three items) (Berscheid et al., 1973); the Physical Appearance Evaluation Subscale (three items) (B.A. Winstead and T.F. Cash, unpublished); and the Rosenberg Self-Esteem Scale (three items) (Rosenberg, 1965).

Self-Rated Social Competence (mean interscale $r = .60$, $\alpha = .75$, $r = .64$) consisted of the Social Subscale of Perceived Competence Scale (five items) (Harter, 1982) and seven additional items (Lewinsohn et al., 1980).

Emotional Reliance ($\alpha = .83$, $r = .54$) consisted of the Emotional Reliance Scale (10 items) (Hirschfeld et al., 1976) assessing interpersonal sensitivity and the desire for support and approval from others.

Future Goals were assessed in three domains—Family (five items; $\alpha = .61$, $r = .58$); Occupational (three items; $\alpha = .63$, $r = .48$); and Academic (five items; mean interscale $r = .39$, $\alpha = .72$, $r = .74$)—using an adapted form of the Importance Placed on Life Goals Scale (Bachman et al., 1985).

Coping Skills ($\alpha = .76$, $r = .55$) consisted of 17 items from the Self-Control Scale (Rosenbaum, 1980), the Antidepressive Activity Questionnaire (Rippere, 1977), and the Ways of Coping Questionnaire (Folkman and Lazarus, 1980).

Social Support: Family (mean interscale $r = .30$, $\alpha = .77$, $r = .64$) consisted of the Conflict Behavior Questionnaire (11 items) (Prinz et al., 1979); the Parent Attitude Research Instrument (6 items) (Schaefer, 1965); the Cohesion subscale of the Family Environment

Scale (3 items) (Moos, 1974); the Competence scale of the Youth Self-Report (2 items) (Achenbach and Edelbrock, 1987); and an adaptation of the Arizona Social Support Interview Schedule (Barrera, 1986).

Social Support: Friends (mean interscale $r = .28, \alpha = .72, r = .60$) consisted of the Social Competence Scale (two items) (Harter, 1982); the UCLA Loneliness Scale (eight items) (Russell et al., 1980); the Competence scale of the Youth Self-Report (three items); and the number of friends providing social support (from the Arizona Social Support Interview Schedule).

Interpersonal: Conflict With Parents ($\alpha = .81$, $r = .51$) was based on occurrence and intensity of conflicts in the preceding 2 weeks using the Issues Checklist (45 items) (Robin and Weiss, 1980).

Interpersonal: Attractiveness ($\alpha = .94$, $r = .22$) consisted of the interviewer-rated Interpersonal Attraction Measure (17 items) (McCroskey and McCain, 1974).

Physical Illness (mean interscale $r = .25, \alpha = .51, r = .46$) consisted of number of visits to a physician, days spent in bed as a result of illness, and the occurrence of 88 physical symptoms in the previous year.

Miscellaneous Measures. Measures that did not rationally fit into a general cluster or did not load significantly on a component (i.e., $<.40$) included death of a parent before age 13; social desirability (6 items, $\alpha = .53$, $r = .54$; Marlowe-Crowne Social Desirability Scale) (Crowne and Marlowe, 1960); hypomanic personality style (15 items, $\alpha = .68$, $r = .55$; Hypomanic Personality Scale) (Eckblad and Chapman, 1986); and vocabulary level (10 items, $\alpha = .72$, $r = .72$; the Shipley Institute of Living Scale) (Shipley, 1940). Single-item measures of self-reported academic performance included grade point average (GPA), satisfaction with GPA, perceived parental satisfaction with GPA, number of missed school days in the previous 6 weeks, number of times late for school in the previous 6 weeks, frequency of failure to complete homework, and repeated a grade in school. Two health measures were included: self-rated health (4-point scale) and the lifetime occurrence of 88 physical symptoms. Finally, three K-SADS items were included: ever used tobacco (yes or no), current rate of tobacco use (6-point scale), and ever attempted suicide (yes or no).

Physical Maturation. Adolescents reported their height and weight and completed an adapted version of the Pubertal Development Scale (Petersen et al., 1988). As adolescents were in senior high school (14 through 18 years of age), most reported pubertal development that was at the mid to advanced level. Adolescents also indicated whether their physical growth and development was early, on time, or late in comparison with that of most teenagers their age ($n = 1,669$). Stability of response to this item over a 1-year period was assessed. Finally, adolescents were asked to indicate the ages when hair first appeared on their bodies and when they experienced the most rapid change in growth. These responses were compared to the perceived timing measure. Because these additional questions ask adolescents to recollect a specific age for events of unknown personal salience, the question directly assessing perceived timing is considered the most reliable report for this construct.

RESULTS

Reliability of Perceived Pubertal Timing

A series of analyses examined the reliability and validity of the self-reported pubertal timing measure. Analyses first tested the consistency of self-reported pubertal timing with self-reported weight and height. Weight was associated with gender ($F[1, 1{,}657] = 371.11$, $p < .001$) and perceived pubertal timing ($F[2, 1{,}657] = 31.78$, $p < .001$) such that boys were heavier than girls and early maturers were heavier than late maturers; on-time maturers reported weights between the other two timing groups (comparing within gender) as would be expected. There was a gender by timing group interaction for height ($F[2, 1{,}657] = 3.90$, $p < .05$), along with main effects for gender ($F[1, 1{,}657] = 1{,}094.99$, $p < .001$) and pubertal timing ($F[2, 1{,}657] = 16.48$, $p < .001$). Again, as would be expected, boys were significantly taller than girls. The interaction effect occurred because there were differences in height by timing group for boys but not for girls such that early- and on-time-maturing boys were significantly taller than late-maturing boys. These findings are in line with the literature on pubertal development in that girls complete growth spurt in height earlier than boys and have growth in height slightly earlier than growth in weight (e.g., Marshall and Tanner, 1986). Comparisons of timing with self-reported ages for fastest change in growth and first appearance of body hair were again consistent with expectations from the literature on puberty; specific findings are not reported.

Test-retest reliability of the perceived timing item (over a 1-year interval) was within acceptable ranges for boys and girls. Specifically, the percentage agreement and κ statistics over a 1-year period were 83% agreement and $\kappa = .61$ for girls and 77% agreement and $\kappa = .48$ for boys. Less than 2% of adolescents changed their ratings by more than one category; agreements are slightly better than those reported by Dubas et al. (1991b). Overall, results suggested reasonable confidence in the validity and reliability of self-reported pubertal timing.

Demographic Characteristics

Differences between the three pubertal timing groups with regard to gender, age, ethnicity, parental education, and whether the adolescent resided with both biological parents were examined. A statistically significant difference was obtained for gender ($\chi^2[2, N = 1{,}669] = 25.28$, $p < .001$); the proportions within the early, on-time, and late groups were .20, .71, and .09 for girls and .14, .70, and .16, for boys, respectively. Previous research has also found that about two thirds of adolescents perceive themselves to be on time in their pubertal development (Dubas et al., 1991b), although gender differences in perceptions of pubertal timing have not been previously reported. None of the other demographic measures differed significantly ($p < .05$) between the three timing groups.

Association Between Pubertal Timing and Psychiatric Disorders

The associations between the three perceived pubertal timing groups and the lifetime and current prevalence rates of major depression, anxiety, substance abuse/dependence, disruptive behavior disorders, and any disorder were examined using contingency table analysis and logistic regression. In addition, the association between the pubertal timing groups and the lifetime prevalence of eating disorders was examined for girls; the current prevalence rate of eating disorders among girls was too low ($n = 3$), as was the lifetime prevalence among boys ($n = 1$), to make group comparisons. Given the interest in gender-specific associations, all analyses were conducted separately for girls and boys. For each analysis, two planned contrasts were tested: (1) the early group versus the on-time group and (2) the late group versus the on-time group. Adolescent's age was entered as a covariate in the logistic regression analyses to control for potential confounding effects; hence, the Wald tests reported are adjusted for age.

The lifetime and current rates of psychiatric disorders for the three pubertal timing groups by gender are shown in Table 1. Compared with on-time girls, early-maturing girls had significantly elevated lifetime rates of major depression (30.2% versus 22.1%), substance abuse/dependence (14.5% versus 6.7%), disruptive behavior disorders (9.9% versus 3.0%), eating disorders (3.5% versus 0.8%), and any psychiatric disorder (52.9% versus 37.8%). Notably, early-maturing girls had a lifetime history of substance abuse and disruptive behavior disorders at twice the rate experienced by either on-time or late-maturing girls. Late-maturing girls also had a significantly elevated lifetime rate of major depression compared with the on-time girls (33.8% versus 22.1%). With regard to current diagnoses, early-maturing girls had a significantly higher rate of disruptive behavior disorders compared with their on-time counterparts (2.9% versus 0.5%). For boys, the only significant contrast was obtained for the lifetime rate of substance abuse/dependence; late-maturing boys had significantly lower rates than did on-time boys (3.2% versus 8.4%).

Association Between Pubertal Timing and Psychosocial Measures

The associations between the three pubertal timing groups and the psychosocial measures were examined separately by gender using analysis of covariance (controlling for age) for continuous variables and logistic regression analysis for the dichotomous measures. Planned contrasts between the on-time group versus the early and late groups were conducted. Standardized scores (with mean = 0 and SD = 1.0) were computed within gender for the numeric measures. (See Table 2 for means, adjusted for age, and proportions for the respective psychosocial measures.)

For the 35 psychosocial measures, 12 (34%) significant associations ($p < .05$) were obtained for the contrasts between early-maturing and on-time girls. Compared with on-time girls, early-maturing girls reported significantly elevated levels of depression symptoms, externalizing behavior problems, and depressotypic attributional style; had lower self-esteem, poorer coping skills, and less support from family and friends; had more days missed at school, poorer self-rated health, and higher rates of ever having used tobacco and current tobacco use; and had a higher rate of suicide attempts. Only 3 (9%) of the planned contrasts between late-maturing and on-time girls were significant. Late-maturing girls reported more self-consciousness, higher future academic goals, and more conflict with parents.

For boys, 8 (23%) significant associations were obtained for the contrasts between early-maturing and on-time boys. Compared with on-time boys, early-maturing boys reported

TABLE 1
Pubertal Timing Group Rates of Psychiatric Disorders Separately for Girls and Boys

	Girls					Boys				
	Group			Planned Contrasts		Group			Planned Contrasts	
Disorder	Early ($n = 172$)	On Time ($n = 629$)	Late ($n = 77$)	Early vs. On Time	Late vs. On Time	Early ($n = 108$)	On Time ($n = 559$)	Late ($n = 124$)	Early vs. On Time	Late vs. On Time
Lifetime (%)										
Major depression	30.2	22.1	33.8	5.01*	4.71*	13.0	10.0	13.7	0.95	0.94
Anxiety	14.5	10.3	9.1	2.35	0.11	5.6	5.7	5.6	0.00	0.05
Substance use	14.5	6.7	5.2	10.42**	0.27	10.2	8.4	3.2	0.47	4.47*
Disruptive behavior	9.9	3.0	5.2	13.18***	1.04	11.1	9.5	9.7	0.27	0.00
Eating	3.5	0.8	1.3	6.09*	0.18	—	—	—	—	—
Any	52.9	37.8	49.4	12.69***	3.52	36.1	29.7	31.5	1.93	0.02
Current (%)										
Major depression	2.3	3.5	3.9	0.59	0.04	2.8	1.6	0.8	0.72	0.50
Anxiety	4.7	4.0	3.9	0.14	0.00	0.9	1.4	2.4	0.14	0.30
Substance use	1.7	1.9	3.9	0.02	1.29	3.7	2.1	1.6	1.04	0.30
Disruptive behavior	2.9	0.5	1.3	5.95*	0.80	3.7	2.5	1.6	0.46	0.26
Any	13.4	10.2	13.0	1.38	0.63	9.3	7.3	6.5	0.53	0.23

Note: Age-adjusted Wald tests via logistic regression analysis are reported for the planned contrasts. The lifetime prevalence of eating disorders among male subjects ($n = 1$) was too low for analysis.
$^{*}p < .05$; $^{**}p < .01$; $^{***}p < .001$.

more major life events, a higher level of depression, more emotional reliance on others, higher future family goals, more physical illness, an elevated hypomanic personality style, a greater lifetime number of physical symptoms, and a higher current rate of tobacco use. In contrast, 13 (37%) significant associations were obtained for the contrasts between late-maturing and on-time boys. Late-maturing boys reported more daily hassles, higher level of depression, more internalizing behavior problems, more negative cognitions, more depressotypic attributional style, more self-consciousness, more emotional reliance on others, poorer coping skills, more conflict with parents, elevated hypomanic personality style, more parental dissatisfaction with grades, more tardiness at school, and lower homework completion.

Multivariate Analyses

For the set of psychiatric disorders and psychosocial measures that were found to be significantly associated with pubertal timing, logistic regression analysis was used to determine which of the variables were uniquely related to pubertal timing. Age was also included among the set of predictor variables. For each gender, two models were computed; one model predicted early versus on-time maturation and the other model predicted late versus on-time maturation. The likelihood ratio backward elimination procedure ($p < .05$) was used to determine which of the variables should remain in the equation for each model.

For the model predicting early versus on-time maturation in girls, lifetime history of major depression, substance abuse/dependence, disruptive behavior disorders, and eating disorders and the 12 significant psychosocial variables were included. The aggregate variable of any lifetime disorder and the current disruptive behavior disorders variable were not included in the model given their overlap with the other psychiatric variables. The final equation retained the following variables: lifetime history of eating (Wald test = 5.07, $p < .05$) and disruptive behavior (Wald test = 8.67, $p < .01$) disorders, low self-esteem (Wald test = 10.98, $p < .001$), and history of a suicide attempt (Wald test = 9.21, $p < .01$).

For the model predicting late versus on-time maturation in girls, lifetime history of major depression, self-consciousness, low academic goals, and conflict with parents were included. Self-consciousness (Wald test = 11.55, $p < .001$) and high academic goals (Wald test = 5.32, $p < .05$) were the only variables retained in the final equation.

For the model predicting early versus on-time maturation in boys, the eight significant psychosocial variables were included. Retained in the final equation were emotional reliance (Wald test = 4.91, $p < .05$), higher future family goals (Wald test = 4.05, $p < .05$), physical illness (Wald test = 5.36, $p < .05$), and current rate of tobacco use (Wald test = 5.61, $p < .05$).

For the model predicting late versus on-time maturation in boys, lifetime history of substance abuse/dependence and the 13 significant psychosocial measures were included. The variables retained in the final equation were low rate of substance abuse/dependence (Wald test = 6.34, $p < .05$), internalizing behavior problems (Wald test = 5.47, $p < .05$), emotional reliance (Wald test = 4.88, $p < .05$), and failure to complete homework (Wald test = 5.37, $p < .05$).

TABLE 2
Pubertal Timing Group Means for the Psychosocial Variables Separately for Girls and Boys

	Girls					Boys				
	Group			Planned Contrasts		Group			Planned Contrasts	
Variable	Early	On Time	Late	Early vs. On Time	Late vs. On Time	Early	On Time	Late	Early vs. On Time	Late vs. On Time
Daily hassles	.09	−.05	.16	1.63	1.74	.06	−.05	.18	1.01	2.29*
Major life events	.13	−.03	−.03	1.83	0.05	.17	−.05	.06	2.07*	1.07
Current depression	.18	−.05	.03	2.63**	0.64	.14	−.07	.18	2.03*	2.58**
Internalizing behavior problems	.11	−.04	.09	1.78	1.06	.09	−.09	.28	1.80	3.95***
Externalizing behavior problems	.23	−.08	−.05	3.58***	0.19	.05	−.04	.04	0.90	0.83
Negative cognitions	.11	−.03	.04	1.67	0.61	.04	−.05	.14	0.90	2.00*
Attributional style	.14	−.03	.05	2.02*	0.67	−.08	−.03	.19	−0.44	2.28*
Self-consciousness	.05	−.05	.35	1.11	3.34***	−.08	−.03	.29	−0.41	3.26**
Low self-esteem	.31	−.05	−.23	4.18***	−1.54	−.06	−.01	.05	−0.50	0.63
Emotional reliance	.09	−.03	.07	1.47	0.83	.21	−.11	.28	3.03**	4.00***
Low future goals: academic	.12	−.01	−.26	1.53	−2.14*	.06	−.01	−.03	0.72	−0.20
Low future goals: family	−.01	.01	−.03	−0.21	−0.29	−.20	.04	−.03	−2.29*	−0.69
Poor coping skills	.19	−.04	−.12	2.68**	−1.71	−.07	−.03	−.18	−0.39	2.06*

Low social support: family	.17	−.06	.07	2.69**	1.13	−.04	−.03	.06	−0.14	0.89
Low social support: friends	.13	−.04	.07	2.02*	0.93	−.07	.02	−.01	−0.86	−0.31
Interpersonal: conflict with parents	.00	−.02	.22	0.16	2.00*	.01	−.05	.19	0.53	2.34*
Physical illness	.10	−.03	−.02	1.47	0.04	.24	−.07	.12	2.91**	1.85
Hypomanic personality style	.07	−.03	.02	1.12	0.42	.15	−.09	.17	2.32*	2.61**
Dissatisfaction with grades[a]	.49	.44	.42	1.70	0.08	.57	.48	.57	3.02	3.82*
Parental dissatisfaction with grades[a]	.27	.28	.25	0.05	0.29	.46	.38	.48	2.16	4.64*
Days missed at school	.16	−.05	−.04	2.40*	0.02	.12	−.06	.12	1.81	1.92
Late for school	.04	−.01	.08	0.63	0.81	.13	−.06	.16	1.76	2.23*
Failure to complete homework	.12	−.03	−.05	1.75	−0.20	.06	−.05	.21	1.08	2.64**
Poor self-rated health	.19	−.04	−.11	2.63**	−0.61	.06	.00	−.06	0.56	−0.52
Lifetime No. of physical symptoms	.10	−.05	.19	1.78	1.96	.20	−.06	.11	2.47*	1.71
Ever used tobacco[a]	.53	.44	.39	4.23*	0.90	.57	.48	.52	3.12	0.53
Current rate of tobacco use	.18	−.04	−.09	2.50*	−0.43	.23	−.03	−.11	2.52*	−0.85
Ever attempted suicide[a]	.19	.08	.10	19.36***	0.72	.04	.03	.06	0.16	1.49

Note: T values are reported for the planned contrasts on the numeric measures; Wald tests are reported for the planned contrasts on the dichotomous measures. All tests are adjusted for age.

[a]Dichotomous measure.

$^{*}p < .05$; $^{**}p < .01$; $^{***}p < .001$.

DISCUSSION

To our knowledge, this is one of the first epidemiological investigations of adolescent psychopathology to examine links between timing of puberty and disorders. This investigation addressed the magnitude and pervasiveness of the effects of the timing of puberty on psychopathology during this period of life. As hypothesized, adolescents' perception that their pubertal development was off-time in comparison with peers (i.e., early for girls or late for boys) was associated with serious mental health outcomes during adolescence. Furthermore, early-maturing girls had the poorest current and lifetime history of adjustment problems. A range of psychopathologies, but especially depression, may be related to earlier or later maturation. These findings emphasize the importance of including information about pubertal timing in clinical assessments with adolescents and may serve as one form of screening device for early detection of psychopathology. Knowledge of this aspect of development should help in understanding the context in which the problems occur and may have direct implications for treatment in that off-time maturers may need to cope with the unique developmental challenges facing them due to social "deviance" (e.g., Brooks-Gunn et al., 1985).

Our findings confirm previous findings on subclinical symptoms and correlates of psychopathology for girls (Caspi and Moffitt, 1991; Graber et al., 1994; Stattin and Magnusson, 1990) and extend the risk to encompass the upper range of the continuum of psychopathology as suggested by recent work by Hayward et al. (1997). As gender differences in depression emerge in adolescence (12 through 14 years of age), the identification of early pubertal development as a source of individual differences within girls is particularly important for understanding girls' mental health. Early maturation was also associated with lifetime history of eating disorders, again in line with prior studies on eating symptoms (Attie and Brooks-Gunn, 1989; Graber et al., 1994).

Of note is the risk for not only internalizing (i.e., depression and anxiety) but also externalizing behaviors that is conferred to girls via early maturation. Rates of current and lifetime disruptive behavior disorders and lifetime substance abuse for these girls were comparable with the rates experienced by boys. Perhaps most alarming was the finding that early-maturing girls were the most likely to have attempted suicide. The finding of significantly poorer concurrent coping skills for early-maturing girls lends support to the hypothesis that they not only were less able to meet the challenges placed on them during puberty but that they still have deficits in coping that have not been ameliorated in the recent postpubertal years. Cultural pressures for thinness may be particularly strong for early-maturing girls because they gain weight when other girls are still thin. Societal definitions of appropriate adult behavior may also place pressure on these girls to engage in behaviors appropriate to their appearance rather than experience and coping.

Altering school environments may help combat cultural and societal pressures on early-maturing girls. Prior research has suggested that single-gender schools reduce conduct problems for early-maturing girls (Caspi et al., 1993) and that fewer school changes (e.g., staying in the same school from kindergarten through eighth grade) may promote better self-esteem for these girls (Simmons and Blyth, 1987). An alternative approach to restructuring schools would be better educational programs for parents and children such that families receive more comprehensive information about pubertal development. It is unlikely that parents are aware of the risks of early maturation for girls and that they are prepared to assist their daughters in regulating the emotional and social demands conveyed on them through their maturation and younger involvement with boys (Stattin and Magnusson, 1990). That boys who developed off time also exhibited some psychopathology further suggests that many adolescents and families would benefit from such public health information.

For boys, early and late maturation conferred several similar adjustment problems such as higher levels of current depression symptoms, higher emotional reliance on others, and more hypomanic personality style than on-time maturers. Fewer studies have examined pubertal timing in boys than in girls. Prior research identified positive effects of early maturation for boys in social interactions (Jones, 1965) but did not examine psychopathology as extensively as our investigation. Thus, deleterious effects of early maturation for boys may be the result of different methodologies or historical change; this investigation cannot address these possibilities.

Late-maturing boys reported greater self-consciousness, more conflict with parents, and more trouble in school as indicated by parental dissatisfaction over grades. Our findings are consistent with prior studies that have linked late maturation in boys with less social competence, more internalizing tendencies, and more problems around school (Dubas et al., 1991a; Jones, 1965). In contrast, late-maturing girls actually seemed to be doing better in school. It has been suggested that these girls may spend more time studying to compensate for fewer heterosocial activities (Dubas et al., 1991a).

Because our investigation was cross-sectional, we are unable to consider whether these associations have implications for psychopathology in adolescence only or for longer-term adjustment. It could be argued that off-time adolescents experienced severe disturbance that was confined to the pubertal period and that present elevated symptoms merely indicate that they have not fully recovered. The participants in the OADP are being recontacted for a follow-up study of mental health in young adulthood (age 24) at which time some of these issues can be clarified.

This investigation is also limited by the reliance on self-report for assessing pubertal timing. Reliability of this report was good across several analyses and was in line with other studies of objective and perceived timing (Dubas et al., 1991b), but it is unlikely that the perception of timing would match identically with an objective measure of timing. On the other hand, perceptions of timing have been found to be a better predictor of feelings about puberty and body image than timing based on an objective measure (Dubas et al., 1991b).

The relationship between pubertal timing and psychopathology needs further investigation. Prospective, longitudinal studies that begin before children enter puberty and follow them through adolescence are needed to understand how off-time development confers risk to youth for psychiatric and developmental problems. Recent reports of racial differences in pubertal timing among girls (NHLBI Growth and Health Study Research Group, 1992) also suggest that future studies should consider whether pubertal timing is experienced similarly across subgroups of adolescents.

REFERENCES

Achenbach TM, Edelbrock CS (1987), *Manual for the Youth Self-Report and Profile.* Burlington: University Vermont Department of Psychiatry

American Psychiatric Association (1987), *Diagnostic and Statistical Manual of Mental Disorders, 3rd edition-revised (DSM-III-R).* Washington, DC: American Psychiatric Association

Andersson T, Magnusson D (1990), Biological maturation in adolescence and the development of drinking habits and alcohol abuse among young males: a prospective longitudinal study. *J Youth Adolesc* 19:33–41

Andrews JA, Lewinsohn PM, Hops H, Roberts RE (1993), Psychometric properties of scales for the measurement of psychosocial variables associated with depression in adolescence. *Psychol Rep* 73:1019–1046

Attie I, Brooks-Gunn J (1989), Development of eating problems in adolescent girls: a longitudinal study. *Dev Psychol* 25:70–79

Bachman JG, Johnston J, O'Malley PM (1985), Some recent trends in the aspirations, concerns, and behaviors of American young people. Paper presented at the 40th Annual Conference of the American Association for Public Opinion Research, McAfee, NJ

Barrera M Jr (1986), Distinctions between social support concepts, measures, and models. *Am J Community Psychol* 14:413–445

Beck AT, Ward CH, Mendelson M, Mock J, Erbaugh J (1961), An inventory for measuring depression. *Arch Gen Psychiatry* 4:561–571

Berscheid E, Walster E, Bohrnstedt G (1973), The happy American body: a survey report. *Psychol Today* 7:119–131

Bird HR, Canino G, Rubio-Stipec M et al. (1988), Estimates of the prevalence of childhood maladjustment in a community survey in Puerto Rico: the use of combined measures. *Arch Gen Psychiatry* 45:1120–1126

Brooks-Gunn J, Graber JA, Paikoff RL (1994), Studying links between hormones and negative affect: models and measures. *J Res Adolesc* 4:469–486

Brooks-Gunn J, Petersen AC, Eichorn D (1985), The study of maturational timing effects in adolescence. *J Youth Adolesc* 14:149–161

Caspi A, Lynam D, Moffitt TE, Silva PA (1993), Unraveling girls' delinquency: biological, dispositional, and contextual contributions to adolescent misbehavior. *Dev Psychol* 29:19–30

Caspi A, Moffitt TE (1991), Individual differences are accentuated during periods of social change: the sample case of girls at puberty. *J Pers Soc Psychol* 61:157–168

Crowne DP, Marlowe D (1960), A new scale of social desirability independent of psychopathology. *J Consult Psychol* 24:349–354

Depue RA, Slater JF, Wolfsetter-Kausch H, Klein D, Goplerud E, Farr D (1981), A behavioral paradigm for identifying persons at risk for bipolar depressive disorder: a conceptual framework and five validation studies. *J Abnorm Psychol* 90:381–437

Dubas JS, Graber JA, Petersen AC (1991a), The effects of pubertal development on achievement during adolescence. *Am J Educ* 99:444–460

Dubas JS, Graber JA, Petersen AC (1991b), A longitudinal investigation of adolescents' changing perceptions of pubertal timing. *Dev Psychol* 27:580–586

Eckblad M, Chapman LJ (1986), Development and validation of a scale for hypomanic personality. *J Abnorm Psychol* 95:214–222

Fenigstein A, Scheier MF, Buss AH (1975), Public and private self-consciousness: assessment and theory. *J Consult Clin Psychol* 43:522–527

Folkman S, Lazarus RS (1980), An analysis of coping in a middle-aged community sample. *J Health Soc Behav* 21:219–239

Graber JA, Brooks-Gunn J, Paikoff RL, Warren MP (1994), Prediction of eating problems: an eight year study of adolescent girls. *Dev Psychol* 30:823–834

Hamilton M (1960), A rating scale for depression. *J Neurol Neurosurg* 23:56–61

Harter S (1982), The Perceived Competence Scale for Children. *Child Dev* 53:87–97

Hayward C, Killen JD, Wilson DM et al. (1997), Psychiatric risk associated with early puberty in adolescent girls. *J Am Acad Child Adolesc Psychiatry* 36:255–262

Heiby EM (1982), A self-reinforcement questionnaire. *Behav Res Ther* 20:397–401

Hirschfeld RMA, Klerman GL, Chodoff P, Korchin S, Barrett J (1976), Dependency, self-esteem, and clinical depression. *J Am Acad Psychoanal* 4:373–388

Hodgson RJ, Rachman S (1977), Obsessional-compulsive complaints. *Behav Res Ther* 15:389–395

Holmes TH, Rahe RH (1967), *Schedule of Recent Experiences*. Seattle: University of Washington School of Medicine

Jones MC (1965), Psychological correlates of somatic development. *Child Dev* 56:899–911

Kaslow N, Tannenbaum R, Seligman M (1978), *The KASTAN: A Children's Attributional Style Questionnaire*. Philadelphia: University of Pennsylvania

Landis JR, Koch GG (1977), The measurement of observer agreement of categorical data. *Biometrics* 33:159–174

Lewinsohn PM, Hops H, Roberts RE, Seeley JR, Andrews JA (1993), Adolescent psychopathology, I: prevalence and incidence of depression and other *DSM-III-R* disorders in high school students. *J Abnorm Psychol* 102:133–144

Lewinsohn PM, Mermelstein RM, Alexander C, MacPhillamy D (1985), The Unpleasant Events Schedule: a scale for the measurement of aversive events. *J Clin Psychol* 41:483–498

Lewinsohn PM, Mischel W, Chaplin W, Barton R (1980), Social competence and depression: the role of illusory self-perceptions. *J Abnorm Psychol* 89:203–212

Lewinsohn PM, Roberts RE, Seeley JR, Rohde P, Gotlib IH, Hops H (1994), Adolescent psychopathology, II: psychosocial risk factors for depression. *J Abnorm Psychol* 103:302–315

Marshall WA, Tanner JM (1986), Puberty. In: *Human Growth*, Vol 2: *Postnatal Growth Neurobiology*, Falkner F, Tanner JM, eds. New York: Plenum, pp 171–209

McCroskey JC, McCain TA (1974), The measurement of interpersonal attraction. *Speech Monogr* 41:261–266

McGee R, Feehan M, Williams S, Partridge F, Silva PA, Kelly J (1990), *DSM-III* disorders in a large sample of adolescents. *J Am Acad Child Adolesc Psychiatry* 29:611–619

Moos RH (1974), *Family Environment Scale*. Palo Alto, CA: Consulting Psychologists Press

NHLBI Growth and Health Study Research Group (1992), Obesity and cardiovascular disease risk factors in black and white girls: the NHLBI Growth and Health Study. *Am J Public Health* 82:1613–1620

Orvaschel H, Lewinsohn PM, Seeley JR (1995), Continuity of psychopathology in a community sample of adolescents. *J Am Acad Child Adolesc Psychiatry* 34:1525–1535

Orvaschel H, Puig-Antich J, Chambers WJ, Tabrizi MA, Johnson R (1982), Retrospective assessment of prepubertal major depression with the Kiddie-SADS-E. *J Am Acad Child Psychiatry* 21:392–397

Pearlin LI, Schooler C (1978), The structure of coping. *J Health Soc Behav* 19:2–21

Petersen AC, Crockett L, Richards M, Boxer A (1988), A self-report measure of pubertal status: reliability, validity, and initial norms. *J Youth Adolesc* 17:117–133

Petersen AC, Sarigiani PA, Kennedy RE (1991), Adolescent depression: why more girls? *J Youth Adolesc* 20:247–271

Pilowsky I (1967), Dimensions of hypochondriasis. *Br J Psychiatry* 113:89–93

Prinz RJ, Foster S, Kent RN, O'Leary KD (1979), Multivariate assessment of conflict in distressed and nondistressed mother–adolescent dyads. *J Appl Behav Analysis* 12:691–700

Radloff LS (1977), The CES-D Scale: a self-report depression scale for research in the general population. *Appl Psychol Meas* 1:385–401

Rippere V (1977), Some cognitive dimensions of antidepressive behavior. *Behav Res Ther* 15:57–63

Robin AL, Weiss JG (1980), Criterion-related validity of behavioral and self-report measures of problem-solving communication skills in distressed and nondistressed parent–adolescent dyads. *Behav Assess* 2:339–352

Rosenbaum M (1980), A schedule for assessing self-control behaviors: preliminary findings. *Behav Ther* 11:109–121

Rosenberg M (1965), *Society and the Adolescent Self-Image*. Princeton, NJ: Princeton University Press

Russell D, Peplau LA, Cutrona CE (1980), The Revised UCLA Loneliness Scale: concurrent and discriminant validity evidence. *J Pers Soc Psychol* 39:472–480

Sandler IN, Block M (1979), Life stress and maladaptation of children. *Am J Community Psychol* 7:425–439

Schaefer ES (1965), Children's reports of parental behavior: an inventory. *Child Dev* 36:413–424

Shipley WC (1940), A self-administering scale for measuring intellectual impairment and deterioration. *J Psychol* 9:371–377

Simmons RG, Blyth DA (1987), *Moving Into Adolescence: The Impact of Pubertal Change and School Context*. New York: Aldine

Spielberger CD, Gorsuch RL, Lushene RE (1970), *Manual for the State-Trait Anxiety Inventory*. Palo Alto, CA: Consulting Psychologists Press

Stattin H, Magnusson D (1990), *Pubertal Maturation in Female Development*. Hillsdale, NJ: Erlbaum

Weissman AN, Beck AT (1978), Development and validation of the Dysfunctional Attitude Scale. Presented at the Annual Meeting of the Association for the Advancement of Behavior Therapy, Chicago

7

Psychiatric Outcomes in Low-Birth-Weight Children at Age 6 Years: Relation to Neonatal Cranial Ultrasound Abnormalities

Agnes H. Whitaker, Ronan Van Rossem, and Judith F. Feldman
Columbia University, New York, New York
Irvin Sam Schonfeld
City College of the City University of New York, New York, New York
Jennifer A. Pinto-Martin
University of Pennsylvania, Philadelphia, Pennsylvania
Carolyn Torre and David Shaffer
Columbia University, New York, New York
Nigel Paneth
Michigan State University, East Lansing, Michigan

Background: *This study examined the relation of neonatal cranial ultrasound abnormalities to psychiatric disorder at age 6 years in a regional birth cohort of low-birth-weight children.* **Methods:** *Neonatal cranial ultrasound abnormalities were classified as (1) isolated germinal matrix and/or intraventricular hemorrhage (suggestive of injury to glial precursors) or (2) parenchymal lesions and/or ventricular enlargement (suggestive of white matter injury) with or without germinal matrix–intraventricular hemorrhage. Psychiatric disorders by DSM-III-R at age 6 years were assessed by means of a structured parent interview. Children with severe mental retardation were excluded. Analyses were conducted first in the entire sample and then in children with

---

Reprinted with Permission from *Archives of General Psychiatry*, 1997, Vol. 54, 847–856.

This work was supported by the John Merck Fund, the March of Dimes Birth Defects Foundation (grant 12-261), and the National Institute of Mental Health (grant 5-R01 MH4583-04). We thank the children and families who made this study possible. We also thank Janet Baxendale and Dawn McCulloch, MS, for their contributions to data collection; Suzannah Blumenthal and Mary Rojas, PhD, for their contributions to data management and analysis; Prudence Fisher, MS, for assistance with the diagnostic interview; and Jim Johnson, PhD (deceased), Mark Davies, MPH, Michael Parides, PhD, Daniel Pine, MD, and Claudia Holzman, DVM, PhD, for their valuable suggestions.

normal intelligence. **Results:** *Twenty-two percent of the cohort had at least 1 psychiatric disorder, the most common being attention deficit hyperactivity disorder (15.6%). In the entire sample, parenchymal lesions and/or ventricular enlargement increased risk relative to no abnormality, independently of other biological and social predictors, for any disorder (odds ratio [OR], 4.4; 95% confidence interval [CI], 1.8-10.3; P* < .001), *attention deficit hyperactivity disorder (OR, 3.4; CI, 1.3-8.7; P* = .02), *and tic disorders (OR, 8.7; CI, 1.3-57.7; P* = .02). *In children of normal intelligence, parenchymal lesions/ventricular enlargement independently increased risk for any disorder (OR, 4.8; CI, 1.6-12.0; P* < .01), *attention deficit hyperactivity disorder (OR, 4.5; CI, 1.3-16.0; P* = .02), *and separation anxiety (OR, 5.3; CI, 1.1-24.8; P* = .03). *These effects were not ameliorated by female sex or social advantage. Isolated germinal matrix/intraventricular hemorrhage was not related to psychiatric disorder at age 6 years.* **Conclusion:** *Neonatal cranial ultrasound abnormalities suggestive of white matter injury significantly increased risk for some psychiatric disorders at age 6 years in low-birth-weight children.*

INTRODUCTION

In the early 1980s, of ultrasonography (US) as a noninvasive means of imaging the brain in low-birth-weight (LBW; <2.5 kg) newborns brought an unprecedented opportunity to study the sequelae of perinatal brain injury. While a substantial body of literature now exists on the motor and cognitive sequelae of neonatal cranial US abnormalities in LBW infants,[1-3] the relation of these abnormalities to childhood psychiatric disorders has been relatively neglected. Such research is timely because the balance of evidence suggests that behavior problems,[4-8] in particular those found in attention deficit hyperactivity disorder (ADHD),[9-17] are an important aspect of the morbidity found among schoolage LBW survivors, whose numbers continue to grow as a result of improved techniques of newborn intensive care.[18] Such research is important because an estimated 6.5% of children who will become of school age in the United States in 1997 were LBW infants (Nigel Paneth, MD, written communication, August 1996), and because term infants of normal birth weight may sustain similar types of brain injury during the late second and early third trimesters.[19,20]

In LBW neonates, perinatal brain injury is most commonly subcortical, reflecting site-specific vulnerabilities of the developing fetal brain in the late second and early third trimesters.[21,22] One site of vulnerability is the germinal matrix. The germinal matrix proliferates neuroblasts and glioblasts during early and middle gestation and provides the protomap for the columnar organization of the cortex; it then involutes by 34 weeks of gestation. In response to metabolic and hemodynamic stress, the fragile capillaries of the germinal matrix can easily bleed, sometimes into the adjacent ventricle. Such hemorrhage occurs in up to 40% of very LBW (VLBW) neonates during the perinatal period.[23]

A second site of vulnerability is the developing subcortical white matter, which is especially sensitive to ischemic injury and metabolic insults before 32 weeks of gestation because of both vascular and cellular factors. From a vascular standpoint, the deep white matter has but a single arterial supply[24,25] and thus may be especially susceptible to injury from hypoperfusion. From a cellular standpoint, the immature oligodendroglia that form myelin appear to be extremely sensitive to oxidative stress and injury from free radical formation.[26] Perinatal white matter injury, which occurs in 5% to 10% of VLBW infants,[26] is frequently found in association with, and often on the same side as, germinal matrix hemorrhage (GMH) and/or intra-ventricular hemorrhage (IVH) but probably represents a distinct pathophysiological process.[25] On postmortem examination, perinatal white matter lesions are correlated with ventricular enlargement[25,27] and with ischemic/infarctive lesions of the basal ganglia, brainstem, and cerebellum.[25,27] In premature neonates, unlike full-term neonates, cortical gray matter is limited in extent,[19] and distinct lesions of cortical gray matter are infrequently reported. However, cortical development might be adversely affected in preterms by both GMH/IVH and ischemic white matter injury because of their effects on late migration, organization and myelination.[28]

Thus far, only 4 studies have examined the relation of neonatal cranial US abnormalities to behavioral outcomes at school age in LBW children; all used relatively small samples from individual hospitals. While 3 of these studies[29-31] found no relation of US abnormalities to behavior, a fourth found that attention problems and/or hyperactivity were related to those types of US abnormalities suggestive of white matter injury.[32] However, this last study did not control for other behavioral predictors, and none of these studies examined the possible moderating role of sex or social disadvantage on the relation of US status to behavioral outcome.

The present study examines the relation of neonatal cranial US abnormalities to psychiatric disorder at age 6 years in a large, regional LBW cohort. A range of child psychiatric diagnoses was assessed by means of a structured diagnostic interview of the parent, and detailed information was collected on other predictors and outcomes. The following questions are addressed: Which, if any, types of US abnormalities are related independently of other predictors to psychiatric disorder at age 6 years? Is the relation diagnostically specific? Does the relation differ by sex or social disadvantage? Does any relation remain when the sample is restricted to children of normal intelligence?

SUBJECTS AND METHODS

Birth Cohort and Attrition

Birth cohort. Participants were members of the Neonatal Brain Hemorrhage Study birth cohort.[25,33] That study prospectively enrolled 1105 consecutive infants with birth weights of 501 to 2000 g who were cared for in the neonatal intensive care units of 3 New Jersey hospitals between September 1, 1984, and June 30, 1987. Enrollees accounted for 83% of all neonates weighing less than 2000 g and for about 90% of all those weighing less than 1500 g born in 3 New Jersey counties during that period. According to a protocol described elsewhere,[33] the cohort was screened with cranial US scans obtained at 4 hours, 24 hours, and 7 days of life; 98% of the cohort was scanned at least 1 of these times and 47% were also scanned between the third and fifth hospital weeks and/or before discharge. Scans were read independently by at least 2 radiologists who were unaware of all clinical information except birth weight and were submitted to a third reader in cases of disagreement. In 94% of cases, diagnostic agreement by 2 readers was obtained.[33] A maternal interview and systematic chart abstraction provided other important prenatal, perinatal, and neonatal information.[33] At about 2 years of age, 86% of survivors were assessed for major neurodevelopmental impairments[2] and for behavior problems, by means of a standardized parent questionnaire, the Child Behavior Checklist for 2- to 3-year-olds (CBCL/2-3).[34]

Age 6 years. By age 6 years, 207 infants had died, leaving 898 children eligible for follow-up, of whom 685 (76%) participated in the study at age 6 years. Of the 213 nonparticipants, 45 families (5% of those eligible) refused, 143 (16%) could not be located, and 25 children (3%) had been adopted. While nonparticipants had higher scores on an index of maternal social disadvantage[3] (mean risk count, 1.8 vs 0.9; $P < .001$), they did not differ from participants in birth characteristics, including US status, or on behavior problems at age 2 years (CBCL/2-3 Total Problem Score).[34] Of the 685 participants, 597 (87%) were assessed at home visits, representing 66.5% of the eligible sample; the remainder were assessed by telephone (85 subjects) or mail (3 subjects). Birth characteristics, maternal social disadvantage, and total behavior problems at 2 and 6 years of age (as measured with the CBCL for 4- to 18-year-olds)[35] did not differ by mode of assessment.

The present report was limited to the 564 children seen at home for whom the psychiatric diagnostic interview was obtained and considered valid. The interview was not obtained on 12 children because of time constraints or other factors and was considered invalid for 21 children too severely disabled to be tested with the Stanford-Binet Intelligence Scale, Fourth Edition (SB).[36] These latter 21 children had a mean (±SD) composite score on the Vineland Adaptive Behavior Scale[37] of 39.4 ± 8.5, indicating that they were truly disabled rather than uncooperative. There were no sociodemographic differences between the children having psychiatric interview data and the 33 children without it.

Procedures

All procedures were approved by the New York State Psychiatric Institute institutional review board. A pediatric nurse practitioner (C.T.) and a psychologist, both unaware of US status, conducted the home visits after obtaining written informed consent. The nurse obtained parental reports on child psychiatric disorder, behavior problems and adaptive functioning, family functioning, and parental mental health. She examined the child for motor problems and rated the child's level of socioemotional impairment and the home environment. The psychologist administered the child cognitive assessments and rated the child's behavior during testing. Teacher report on behavior problems was also requested.

Predictors

Neonatal cranial US status. Ultrasound abnormalities are defined as follows. A GMH was defined by focal echodensity in the thalamocaudate groove, just lateral to the frontal horns of the lateral ventricles. An IVH was defined by an echodense focus or foci within the lateral, third, or fourth ventricles separate from, and at least as echodense as, the choroid plexus. A parenchymal lesion (PL) was defined by focal or confluent echodense and/or echolucent areas in the parenchyma. A ventricular enlargement (VE) was defined by at least moderate enlargement, as judged by the radiologist, of at least 1 lateral ventricle on the final scan obtained.

On postmortem examination, both GMH and IVH are associated with destruction of the germinal matrix and its glial precursor cells,[38,39] while PLs and VEs are associated with evidence of ischemic injury to white matter.[26,27] Thus, 3 mutually exclusive groups, more consistent with pathological findings than the widely used Papile classification,[40] were formed: (1) no abnormality (NA); (2) isolated GMH and/or IVH (GMH/IVH); and (3) PL and/or VE, with or without GMH or IVH (PL/VE).

Non-US predictors. Prenatal factors included maternal social disadvantage, defined by a composite index described elsewhere[3]; maternal tobacco use, measured by the average number of cigarettes smoked per day during this pregnancy (log transformed); and maternal alcohol consumption during pregnancy, scored as a 3-category variable (none; mild [1-6 drinks a week and <3 drinks on any occasion]; and severe [≥7 drinks a week or ≥3 drinks on any occasion]).[41] *Perinatal factors* included sex, 5-minute Apgar score, gestational age, and fetal growth ratio (birth weight relative to the median of the weight-for-gestational-age distributions compiled by Williams et al[42]). *Neonatal complications of prematurity* were indexed by fraction of inspired oxygen at the end of 24 hours,[43,44] and *neonatal chronic illness* by days receiving mechanical ventilation.[3] *Social disadvantage at age 6* was measured by means of 2 composite indexes. One index, "distal social disadvantage" (mean ± SD, −0.02 ± 0.68), was calculated as the sum of the standardized scores of the following variables: single-parent family, mother's education (reversed), household income (reversed), any income from welfare, and the Four Factor Index of Social Status (A. B. Hollingshead, PhD, unpublished data, 1975; scale reversed); if any of these variables were missing, the mean of the remaining variables was substituted. The second index, "proximal social disadvantage" (mean ± SD, −0.03 ± 0.69), was calculated similarly by means of the HOME[45] total score (reversed), the General Health Questionnaire,[46] and the Family Dysfunction Scale of the Family Health and Activity Questionnaire.[47]

Child Outcomes

Psychiatric diagnoses at age 6 years. The Diagnostic Interview Schedule for Children–Parent version 2.1P (DISC 2.1P)[48] is a structured interview that assesses *DSM-III-R*[49] psychiatric disorders. The child version was not used because of the unreliability of self-report at this age.[50] The DISC 2.1P has been shown to have good sensitivity for rare disorders[48] and adequate test-retest reliability for common disorders in older children.[51]

In the present sample, DISC 2.1P diagnoses showed reasonable agreement with standardized assessments of behavior problems. For example, children with ADHD, when compared with children with other diagnoses, had higher ratings of attention problems from parents on the CBCL/4-18[35] (mean ± SD T score, 65.4 ± 8.8 vs 57.7 ± 6.2; $t[121] = 4.79$, $P < .001$) and from teachers on the Teacher's Report Form[52] (mean ± SD T score, 61.8 ± 8.8 vs 57.2 ± 11.1; $t[83] = 2.08$, $P = .04$). Moreover, children with ADHD were more likely to be rated as inattentive (31.0%) or hyperactive (42.9%) by the study psychologist on the Test Behavior Checklist[53] than were children with other diagnoses (5.9% [$P < .01$] and 17.6% [$P = .01$], respectively) (additional data available on request).

Table 1 shows the specific disorders assessed, grouped into diagnostic clusters consistent with *DSM-III-R*. Some *DSM-III-R* disorders were not assessed because of their rarity at

TABLE 1
Prevalence of DISC 2.1P Diagnoses Overall and by Ultrasound Status*

Diagnosis	Entire Sample (N = 562-564)	Ultrasound Status NA (n = 453-454)	Ultrasound Status GMH/IVH (n = 77-78)	Ultrasound Status PL/VE (n = 31-32)
Any disorder	22.0	20.3	21.8	46.9†
Any disruptive disorder	17.2	15.9	19.2	31.3‡
Attention deficit hyperactivity disorder	15.6	14.3	16.7	31.3‡
Oppositional defiant disorder	6.0	5.7	7.7	6.3
Conduct disorder	1.4	1.3	1.3	3.1
Any anxiety disorder	10.3	9.9	10.3	15.6
Obsessive-compulsive disorder	6.6	6.8	3.8	9.4
Separation anxiety	4.1	3.7	3.8	9.4
Overanxious disorder	1.4	0.9	2.6	6.3‡
Simple phobia	0.7	0.7	1.3	0.0
Avoidant disorder	0.4	0.4	0.0	0.0
Panic disorder	0.0	0.0	0.0	0.0
Any elimination disorder	7.1	6.6	7.7	12.5
Nocturnal enuresis	6.0	5.7	7.7	6.3
Diurnal enuresis	1.2	1.1	1.3	3.1
Encopresis	1.2	1.3	0.0	3.1
Any tic disorder	2.0	1.8	0.0	9.4‡
Transient tics	0.4	0.4	0.0	0.0
Motor tics	0.9	0.7	0.0	6.3‡
Vocal tics	0.4	0.2	0.0	3.2
Tourette syndrome	0.4	0.4	0.0	0.0
Other disorders				
Major depressive disorder	0.2	0.2	0.0	0.0
Elective mutism	0.4	0.4	0.0	0.0
Pica	0.4	0.2	0.0	3.1
Any disorder other than attention deficit hyperactivity disorder and tic disorders	17.2	16.5	16.7	28.1

*Prevalence is given as the percentage of the group having the relevant diagnosis. The effective number for each group varies by diagnosis because occasionally the answer to a question required for the assignment of a particular diagnosis was missing for a child. Missing answers were most common for transient tics, for which the effective numbers for the entire sample, and for groups with no abnormality (NA), germinal matrix hemorrhage/intraventricular hemorrhage (GMH/IVH), and parenchymal lesions and/or ventricular enlargement (PL/VE) were, respectively, 554, 448, 78, and 28. DISC 2.1P indicates Diagnostic Interview Schedule for Children–Parent Version 2.1P.

† $P < .01$ vs the NA group.

‡ $P < .05$ vs the NA group.

this age. "Any disorder" was defined as any 1 of the 19 disorders listed. Diagnoses were derived by means of algorithms (available on request) that implemented diagnostic inclusion criteria in the *DSM-III-R*.[49] Psychiatric exclusion criteria were not used; developmental exclusion criteria were used for the elimination disorders. Consistent with other studies,[54,55] a diagnosis of disorder was not assigned on the basis of symptoms alone. It was also necessary to have at least mild psychosocial impairment (defined by a nurse's rating of <71 on the Children's Global Clinical Assessment Scale).[55] The diagnosis of ADHD, for example, was assigned only if the child had at least 8 of 14 possible symptoms of ADHD, each symptom had been present most of the time for at least 6 months, and the overall Children's Global Clinical Assessment Scale score was less than 71.

Other child characteristics. Intelligence at 6 years of age was defined as the composite score on the SB, and motor problems as the total score on the Riley Motor Problems Inventory.[56]

Statistical Analysis

The bivariate relations of US status to psychiatric outcomes were examined by means of logistic regression with 2 dummy variables as predictors, each encoding the comparison of 1 of the 2 US abnormality groups (GMH/IVH or PL/VE) with the NA group. The log odds of psychiatric disorder vs no disorder were the dependent variables. The bivariate relations of US status to other (non-US) predictors and the relations of diagnoses of disorders to non-US predictors and other child outcomes (eg, intelligence) were examined by means of χ^2 or Fisher exact tests for categorical variables and 1-way analyses of variance for continuous ones; the strength of these relations was assessed with correlations (ϕ, point-biserial, and product-moment, as appropriate).

Throughout this article, 2-tailed 5% significance levels were used. For the multivariate analysis, only diagnoses and diagnostic clusters having a bivariate relation to US status with a significance level of $P < .10$ were considered. When the number of cases of a given diagnosis was less than 10, the related diagnostic cluster was used instead, as long as it also showed a bivariate relation to US status. When the relation of a diagnostic cluster to US status was due primarily to 1 disorder in the cluster, that disorder was used. Explanatory variables were entered in 2 steps: first the US status variables and then the complete set of all non-US predictors. This strategy allowed evaluation of the robustness of the effect of US status when controlling for other potential risk factors. A subsequent logistic regression analysis included, in a third step, multiplicative terms representing the interaction of US status with sex and distal and proximal social disadvantage. Separate sets of logistic regressions were run for each interaction. The change in the −2 log likelihood (L^2) was used to evaluate the contribution of the interactions to the prediction of the outcome.[57] These analyses were repeated for a subsample of children with normal intelligence (SB composite scores $\geq$85) and for a subsample that excluded all children diagnosed at age 2 years with disabling cerebral palsy.[2]

To conserve cases and power, missing values were substituted with the sample mean or mode, while dummy-coded missing value indicators were added to equations.[58] None of the missing value indicators related significantly to any outcome.

RESULTS

Sample Description

Of the 564 children in the present sample, 454 (80.5%) had no US abnormalities, 78 (13.8%) had GMH/IVH, and 32 (5.7%) had PL/VE. Of those with PL/VE, 15 also had GMH/IVH. Fifty-one percent (287/564) of the sample were male, 21% (119/564) were black, 16% (89/559) lived in single-parent households, 7% (39/564) had a caretaker who received welfare benefits, and 9% (48/555) of the mothers had not finished high school. The mean (±SD) age at follow-up was 6.3 ± 0.28 years (range, 5.2-8.7 years). Many of the children were in kindergarten (58% [325/564]) or first grade (32% [181/564]). Consistent with most LBW samples,[59] general intellectual functioning (mean ± SD, 102.3 ± 13.4 on the SB) was close to the national average, while nearly 21% (116/564) had excessive motor problems as defined by scores in the top second percentile of the Riley Motor Problems Inventory standardization sample. As noted earlier, children too severely disabled to be psychometrically tested were excluded, but 14 children in the present sample had some type of impairment: 9 had mental retardation (4 mild and 5 moderate) as defined in a previous report[3]; 9 required assistance with walking because of disabling cerebral palsy as diagnosed at age 2 years[2]; and 4 children had both conditions.

Prevalence of Psychiatric Disorder

As shown in Table 1, slightly more than one fifth of the sample (22%) had at least 1 psychiatric disorder, the most common being ADHD (15.6%). More than two thirds of those with any disorder had more than 1. Boys were more likely than girls to have any disorder (28.9% vs 14.8%; $P < .001$), any disruptive disorder (23.8% vs 10.5%; $P < .001$), ADHD (22.0% vs 9.0%; $P < .001$), oppositional defiant disorder (8.0% vs 4.0%; $P < .001$), obsessive-compulsive disorder (8.7% vs 4.3%; $P = .04$), and nocturnal enuresis (9.4% vs 2.5%; $P < .001$).

Relation of US Status to Psychiatric Disorders

The prevalences of several disorders and clusters of disorders were greater in the PL/VE than in the NA group, namely, any disorder (unadjusted odds ratio [OR], 3.5; 95% confidence interval [CI], 1.7-7.2; $P < .001$), any disruptive disorder (OR, 2.4; 95% CI, 1.1-5.3; $P = .03$), ADHD (OR, 2.7; 95% CI, 1.2-6.0; $P = .01$), overanxious disorder (OR, 7.5; 95% CI, 1.3-42.6; $P = .02$), any tic disorder (OR, 5.8; 95% CI, 1.4-22.9; $P = .01$), and motor tics (OR, 10.0; 95% CI, 1.6-62.15; $P = .01$); all $P < .05$. The GMH/IVH group did not differ significantly from the NA group for any psychiatric outcome. Of the disorders and clusters listed, 3 did not meet criteria for further consideration (see "Statistical Analysis" section): any disruptive disorder (because its relation to PL/VE was due primarily to ADHD) and overanxious disorder and motor tics (because of their low prevalence). For any disorder other than ADHD or tics, the comparison between the PL/VE and NA groups was nearly

TABLE 2
Nonultrasound Predictors by Ultrasound Status*

		Ultrasound Status		
Predictors	Total (N = 564)	NA (n = 454)	GMH/IVH (n = 78)	PL/VE (n = 32)
Prenatal factors				
Social disadvantage at birth	0.9 ± 1.2	0.9 ± 1.2	0.8 ± 1.2	1.0 ± 1.3
Cigarettes per day (ln)	0.7 ± 1.2	0.8 ± 1.2	0.4 ± 0.9	0.9 ± 1.2
No.	491	397	64	30
Alcohol consumption				
No.	476	384	62	30
Mild	45.8 (218)	45.6 (175)	50.0 (31)	40.0 (12)
Severe	2.7 (13)	2.3 (9)	3.2 (2)	6.7 (2)
Perinatal factors				
Sex (male)	50.9 (287)	50.2 (228)	50.0 (39)	62.5 (20)
Fetal growth ratio†	0.9 ± 0.2	0.9 ± 0.2	1.0 ± 0.2	1.0 ± 0.2
No.	563	454	77	32
Gestational age,† d	221.7 ± 21.6	224.5 ± 21.0	211.4 ± 20.7	206.0 ± 18.2
Apgar score (5 min)†	7.9 ± 1.4	8.0 ± 1.3	7.6 ± 1.5	7.1 ± 1.4
No.	547	440	76	31
Neonatal complications of prematurity				
Fraction of inspired O_2, %†‡	37.4 ± 19.5	35.3 ± 17.7	41.4 ± 23.5	48.6 ± 21.6
Neonatal chronic illness				
Days receiving ventilator assistance†	5.6 ± 13.4	4.6 ± 12.7	7.8 ± 14.1	13.9 ± 17.8
Social disadvantage (measured at age 6 y)				
Distal	0.0 ± 0.7	0.0 ± 0.7	0.0 ± 0.6	0.2 ± 0.7
Proximal	0.0 ± 0.7	0.0 ± 0.7	0.0 ± 0.7	0.1 ± 0.8
No.	563	453	78	32

*The data are presented as percentage (number) for categorical variables and as mean ± SD for continuous variables. NA indicates no abnormality; GMH/IVH, germinal matrix hemorrhage and/or intraventricular hemorrhage; PL/VE, parenchymal lesions and/or ventricular enlargement; and ln, natural legarithm.
†F or χ^2, $P < .001$ for a comparison among the 3 groups.
‡Valid only for children receiving oxygen.

significant (OR, 2.0; 95% CI, 0.9-4.4; $P = .10$). Thus, the 4 outcomes considered further are any disorder, ADHD, tic disorders, and any disorder other than ADHD or tics.

Relation of Non-US Predictors to US Status

As shown in Table 2, the US groups did not differ by sex, by social disadvantage at birth or at age 6 years, or by maternal alcohol use during pregnancy. In general, the NA group tended to be at less perinatal and neonatal risk, having greater gestational age, higher 5-minute Apgar scores, lower fractions of inspired oxygen, and fewer ventilator days than either the GMH/IVH or PL/VE group. The lower fetal growth ratio in the gestationally more

TABLE 3
Adjusted ORs and Confidence Intervals for Selected Disorders: Full Model*

Predictors	Any Disorder (N = 564)		ADHD (N = 563)		Tic Disorders (N = 563)		Any Disorder Other Than ADHD or Tic Disorders (N = 564)	
	OR	95% Confidence Interval	OR	95% Confidence Interval	OR	95% Confidence Interval	OR	95% Confidence Interval
US status								
GMH/IVH	1.4	0.7-2.7	1.5	0.7-3.3	0.0	0.0-∞	1.1	0.5-2.2
PL/VE	4.4†	1.8-10.3	3.4‡	1.3-8.7	8.7‡	1.3-57.7	2.1	0.8-5.3
Prenatal factors								
Social disadvantage at birth	1.0	0.8-1.2	0.9	0.7-1.2	0.4	0.1-1.1	1.1	0.9-1.4
Cigarettes per day (ln)	1.5†	1.2-1.8	1.5†	1.2-1.9	2.0‡	1.0-3.8	1.3‡	1.0-1.6
Alcohol consumption (mild)	0.6	0.4-1.1	0.5‡	0.3-1.0	0.3	0.0-2.0	0.8	0.5-1.4
Alcohol consumption (severe)	1.4	0.4-4.9	0.2	0.0-1.7	3.4	0.2-54.4	1.7	0.4-6.3
MVI alcohol consumption	0.0	0.0-∞	0.0	0.0-∞	0.0	0.0-∞	0.0	0.0-∞
MVI smoking	664.9	0.0-∞	911.0	0.0-∞	5456.2	0.0-∞	436.1	0.0-∞
Perinatal factors								
Sex (male)	2.6†	1.7-4.2	3.4†	2.0-5.8	2.9	0.6-13.6	2.4†	1.5-4.0
Fetal growth ratio	0.8	0.2-3.4	0.6	0.1-3.0	0.1	0.0-5.1	0.8	0.2-3.7

Gestational age	1.0	1.0-1.0	1.0	1.0-1.0	0.9‡	0.9-1.0	1.0	1.0-1.0
Apgar (5 min)	1.0	0.8-1.2	1.0	0.8-1.3	1.5	0.8-2.7	1.1	0.9-1.3
MVI Apgar	2.6	0.5-13.9	2.7	0.3-22.5	109.4	0.3-35 205.9	3.7	0.5-26.8
Neonatal complications of prematurity								
Fraction of inspired O_2	1.0	1.0-1.0	0.6	1.0-1.0	1.0	0.9-1.0	1.0	1.0-1.0
MVI fraction of inspired O_2	0.7	0.4-1.2	1.0	0.6-1.8	1.7	0.3-9.2	0.7	0.4-1.2
Neonatal chronic illness								
Days receiving ventilatory assistance	1.0§	1.0-1.0	1.0	1.0-1.0	1.0	1.0-1.0	1.0	1.0-1.0
Social disadvantage (measured at age 6 y)								
Distal	0.8	0.5-1.3	0.9	0.5-1.5	1.7	0.4-8.0	0.7	0.5-1.2
Proximal	2.3†	1.6-3.3	2.1†	1.4-3.1	1.1	0.3-3.7	2.2†	1.5-3.1
MVI proximal	2128.6	0.0-∞	7808.8	0.0-∞	0.0	0.0-∞	4072.9	0.0-∞
Constant	0.0‡	0.0-0.4	0.0	0.0-1.5	86 933.6	0.0-∞	0.0	0.0-1.4

*ADHD indicates attention deficit hyperactivity disorder; OR, odds ratio; US, ultrasound; GMH/IVH, germinal matrix hemorrhage and/or intraventricular hemorrhage; PL/VE, parenchymal lesions and/or ventricular enlargement; and MVI, missing value indicator. The infinity sign (∞) stands for an extremely large number.

† $P < .001$.

‡ $P < .05$.

§ $P < .01$.

mature NA group, as compared with the other 2 groups, results from using birth weight to define the sample.[60]

Psychiatric Outcomes—Multivariate Analysis

Effects of US status on psychiatric disorder controlling for non-US predictors. Table 3 presents the results of regression analysis with all non-US predictors included. The adjusted ORs comparing the PL/VE with the NA group were strikingly similar to the unadjusted ones given above. The presence of PL/VE still significantly increased the risk for any disorder, ADHD, and tic disorders, while GMH/IVH again did not affect risk for any psychiatric outcome.

Effects of non-US predictors on psychiatric disorder. Several of the non-US predictor variables were related independently to the 4 psychiatric outcomes of interest. Maternal smoking elevated risk for all 4 outcomes. Male sex and proximal (but not distal) social disadvantage predicted 2 of the outcomes: any disorder and ADHD. For both, the odds of disorder increased by a little more than 2 times for each unit increase in the scale for proximal social disadvantage. Days receiving mechanical ventilation, maternal alcohol use, and gestational age were each related to a single outcome.

Moderating effect of sex and distal and proximal social disadvantage on the relation of US abnormalities to psychiatric outcomes. Neither sex nor proximal social disadvantage modified the effect of US status on any psychiatric outcome. However, distal social disadvantage actually reduced the risk for ADHD associated with PL/VE (OR, 0.2; Wald $\chi^2 = 5.0$; $df = 1$; $P = .05$).

Relation of US status to psychiatric disorder among children of normal intelligence. In the sample as a whole, intelligence was negatively related to psychiatric disorder (point-biserial $r = -0.35$, $P < .001$, for any disorder with the SB composite). Intelligence was also associated with US status; as reported elsewhere,[3] children in the PL/VE group had significantly lower SB composite scores than children in the NA group.

To address the possibility that the association between US status and psychiatric disorder might be influenced by the children with low intelligence in the sample, all analyses were repeated with the sample restricted to children of at least normal intelligence. In this subsample (n = 521), as in the full sample, GMH/IVH (n = 72) was not related to any psychiatric outcome. Also as in the full sample, PL/VE (n = 20) was significantly related to any disorder (unadjusted OR, 3.0; 95% CI, 1.2-7.7; $P = .02$). Now, PL/VE was also significantly related to separation anxiety disorder (unadjusted OR, 4.9; 95% CI, 1.3-18.4; $P = .02$) but not to tic disorders. While the bivariate relation of PL/VE to ADHD was not significant, it did meet the .10 criterion for further examination (unadjusted OR, 2.5; 95% CI, 0.9-7.1; $P = .09$).

With all other predictors controlled, PL/VE was related to any disorder (adjusted OR, 4.8; 95% CI, 1.6-12.0; $P < .01$), ADHD (adjusted OR, 4.5; 95% CI, 1.3-16.0; $P = .02$), and separation anxiety disorder (adjusted OR, 5.3; 95% CI, 1.1-24.8; $P = .03$). Non-US predictors were related to any disorder and to ADHD among the children with normal IQ in essentially the same way as in the sample as a whole (data available on request). Also as in the intact sample, distal social advantage reduced the risk associated with PL/VE for ADHD

(OR, 0.04; Wald $\chi^2 = 5.6$; $df = 1$; $P = .04$). No other significant interactions between US status and sex or social disadvantage were found. When the sample was restricted to those who had not been diagnosed (at age 2 years) as having disabling cerebral palsy (n = 530), the results were essentially identical to those obtained in this subsample of children with normal IQ.

COMMENT

This study examined the relation of perinatal brain injury, as detected on neonatal cranial US, to psychiatric disorder in LBW children at early school age. The study has several methodological strengths: children with neonatal US abnormalities were prospectively identified based on screening of a large regional birth cohort; a structured parent interview was used to diagnose a range of child psychiatric disorders at age 6 years; and detailed information was available on other social and biological predictors and other child outcomes.

Although the study has some limitations, these do not pose major threats to the validity of the findings. While our pathological studies[27] as well as those of others[61] have shown that US is not completely sensitive to milder forms of white matter injury, this limitation would lead to an underestimation of the effects of PL/VE on outcomes. Although the sample was limited to children seen on home visits, comprising only two thirds of those eligible to be seen at age 6 years, the effective sample remained reasonably representative, as discussed in the section on the birth cohort and attrition. Finally, although psychiatric diagnoses were based solely on parental interviews, parent, teacher, and psychologist ratings of behavior were in reasonable agreement.

The finding that isolated GMH/IVH did not increase risk for psychiatric disorder at age 6 years was surprising given that in most LBW infants, the germinal matrix is still proliferating (primarily glioblasts) at the time of birth.[62] It must be underscored that isolated GMH/IVH may have behavioral effects at age 6 years that are not captured by diagnosable psychiatric disorder or may be related to disorders that typically emerge later.

By constrast, PL/VE, which is indicative of ischemic injury to white matter,[27] increased by 4-fold the risk for having at least 1 psychiatric disorder, even after control for other predictors. However, the relation of PL/VE to any disorder was accounted for by its relation to specific disorders, most strongly and consistently ADHD. This study extends an earlier finding[32] to a rigorously diagnosed and population-based sample, while controlling for other predictors. As in other schoolage LBW cohorts[11,13,15] and among 6-year-olds in the general population,[63] ADHD was the most common disorder. The relation of PL/VE to ADHD was unlikely to have resulted from its greater frequency, however, because some other common disorders (eg, oppositional defiant disorder) were not related to PL/VE. Neither birth weight nor gestational age increased risk for ADHD independent of US status, suggesting that recent reports of elevated rates of ADHD in LBW cohorts[11,13,15] may reflect the higher rates of PL/VE likely to have been present in such groups.

Here, as in other other recent studies,[64-66] maternal smoking during pregnancy adversely affected childhood behavior; the present study shows this effect to be independent of PL/VE and social disadvantage. A recent review[66] of the effects of nicotine on the fetal brain points to functional alteration of receptors within the basal ganglia as a possible mechanism for this effect.[67] However, postnatal maternal smoking, a factor not assessed here, might also have played a role.

As in other population-based studies of childhood psychiatric disorder,[63] male sex independently predicted increased risk for ADHD, a finding that has been attributed to sex differences in the development of the dopaminergic system.[68-70] The advantage of female sex was constant across brain injury groups, however, and was not particularly pronounced in the presence of perinatal brain injury.

In the present study, proximal social disadvantage was an independent predictor of ADHD; previous studies on this point have been inconsistent.[71] Distal social disadvantage actually reduced the risk of ADHD among children with PL/VE; findings from a recent study[72] raise the possibility that this effect may result from selective mortality among LBW infants born to severely disadvantaged mothers.

From a theoretical standpoint, the findings of the present study are not consistent with the widely accepted interactional model of biological and social risk.[73-75] According to that model, among children who are not severely disabled, higher rates of psychiatric disorder would be expected with greater social disadvantage, and perinatal brain injury per se would have an effect only among socially disadvantaged children. Among advantaged children, inherent "self-righting tendencies" would counteract any adverse effects of perinatal risk factors,[73] including presumedly those of perinatal brain injury. Instead, in this study both PL/VE and social disadvantage raised the risk of psychiatric disorder independently of one another, and social advantage did not protect children with PL/VE from increased risk for psychiatric disorder. Of course, an interaction suggesting a protective effect of social advantage in the presence of some other aspects of perinatal risk might still exist. However, it does appear from the present results that the relation of PL/VE to psychiatric disorder at age 6 years is more consistent with a main effects model than an interactional model.

Consistent with modern neurodevelopmental models of psychiatric disorders, such as that proposed by Weinberger for schizophrenia,[76] the effects of PL/VE on ADHD, tic disorders, and separation anxiety disorder at age 6 years may reflect an effect of perinatal ischemic injury on brain maturational events that occurs at this age, in particular maturation of the striatum (caudate and putamen) of the basal ganglia. Maturation of the striatum is thought to play an important role in the improvement of behavioral inhibition that normally occurs in middle childhood[77] but is notably deficient in ADHD, tic disorders, and anxiety disorders.[78,79] In a postmortem study in this cohort,[25] ischemic/infarctive white matter lesions were statistically associated with ischemic/infarctive lesions of the basal ganglia, probably because they share with deep white matter the distinction of having only 1 arterial supply and thus are especially vulnerable to hypoperfusion.[24] Structural and functional brain imaging studies of children with ADHD[80-83] and tic disorders[84,85] have found abnormalities in the basal ganglia, specifically the corpus striatum (caudate and putamen), while subtle motor impairments in a subset of children with anxiety disorders[86] also suggest basal ganglia abnormalities. The striatum receives substantial dopaminergic input from the substantia nigra,[87] and dysregulation of the dopaminergic system has been implicated in both ADHD[78,88] and tic disorders.[78,89] Alterations of the dopaminergic system have been shown to accompany ischemic brain injury in human neonates[90] and in rats.[91] The striatal dopaminergic system appears to be more vulnerable to ischemic injury than other striatal neurotransmitter systems (eg, serotonin),[92] perhaps because, in the striatum, dopamine synapses are closely juxtaposed with glutamate synapses,[93] which are thought to play a key role in mediating the neurotoxic effects of ischemia.[94] As the cohort undergoes puberty, which is accompanied by cortical maturation[95] and synaptic pruning,[96-99] it is possible that PL/VE will increase risk for disorders that typically have a later onset and in which abnormalities of cortical–basal ganglionic circuits have been implicated, such as mood disorders,[100] obsessive-compulsive disorder,[101] and schizophrenia.[93,100,102,103] Certainly, further longitudinal follow-up of this cohort will be of great interest.

REFERENCES

1. Levene MI. Cerebral ultrasound and neurological impairment: telling the future. *Arch Dis Child.* 1990;65:469-471.
2. Pinto-Martin JA, Riolo S, Cnaan A, Holzman C, Susser MW, Paneth N. Cranial ultrasound prediction of disabling and non-disabling cerebral palsy at age two in a low birthweight population. *Pediatrics.* 1995;95:249-254.
3. Whitaker AH, Feldman JF, Van Rossem R, Schonfeld IS, Pinto-Martin JA, Torre C, Blumenthal SR, Paneth NS. Neonatal cranial ultrasound abnormalities in LBW infants: relation to cognitive outcomes at age six. *Pediatrics.* 1996;98:719-729.
4. Breslau N, Klein N, Allen L. Very low birthweight: behavioral sequelae at nine years of age. *J Am Acad Child Adolesc Psychiatry.* 1988;27:605-612.
5. Klein NK. Children who were very low birthweight: cognitive abilities and class-room behavior at five years of age. *J Spec Educ.* 1988;22:41-54.
6. Rose SA, Feldman JF, Rose SL, Wallace IF, McCarton C. Behavior problems at 3 and 6 years: prevalence and continuity in full-terms and preterms. *Dev Psychopathol.* 1992;4:361-374.
7. Ross G, Lipper EG, Auld PAM. Social competence and behavior problems in premature children at school age. *Pediatrics.* 1990;86:391-397.
8. McCormick M, Workman-Daniels K, Brooks-Gunn J. The behavioral and emotional well-being of school-age children with different birthweights. *Pediatrics.* 1996;97:18-25.
9. Marlow N, Roberts BL, Cooke RWI. Motor skills in extremely low birthweight children at the age of 6 years. *Arch Dis Child,* 1989;64:839-847.
10. McCormick MC, Gortmaker SL, Sobol AM. Very low birth weight children: behavior problems and school difficulty in a national sample. *J Pediatr.* 1990;117:687-693.
11. Szatmari P, Saigal S, Rosenbaum P, Campbell D, King S. Psychiatric disorders at five years among children with birthweights <1000 g: a regional perspective. *Dev Med Child Neurol.* 1990;32:954-962.
12. Scottish Low Birthweight Study Group. The Scottish Low Birthweight Study, II: language attainment, cognitive status, and behavioural problems. *Arch Dis Child.* 1992;67:682-686.
13. Szatmari P, Saigal S. Rosenbaum P, Campbell D. Psychopathology and adaptive functioning among extremely low birthweight children at eight years of age. *Dev Psychopathol.* 1993;5:345-357.
14. Pharoah POD, Stevenson CJ, Cooke RWI, Stevenson RC. Prevalence of behavior disorders in low birthweight infants. *Arch Dis Child.* 1994;70:271-274.

15. Breslau N, Brown GG, DelDotto JE, Kumar S., Ezthuthachan S, Andreski P, Hufnagle KG. Psychiatric sequelae of low birth weight at six years of age. *J Abnorm Child Psychol.* 1996;24:385-400.
16. Breslau N. Psychiatric sequelae of low birth weight. *Epidemiol Rev.* 1995;17:96-106.
17. Buka SL, Lipsitt LP, Tsuang MT. Emotional and behavioral development of low-birthweight infants. In: Friedman SL, Sigman MD, eds. *The Psychological Development of Low-Birthweight Children.* Norwood, NJ: Ablex Publishing Corp;1992:187-214.
18. Hack M, Klein NK, Taylor HG. Long-term developmental outcomes of low birth weight infants. In: Behrman R, ed. *Low Birth Weight.* Los Altos, Calif: Center for the Future of Children, The David and Lucile Packard Foundation;1995:176-196.
19. Truwit CL, Barkovich AJ, Koch TK, Ferriero DM. Cerebral palsy: MR findings in 40 patients. *Am J Neuroradiol.* 1992;13:67-78.
20. Niemann G, Wakat JP, Krageloh-Mann I, Grodd W, Michaelis R. Congenital hemiparesis and periventricular leukomalacia: pathogenic aspects on magnetic resonance imaging. *Dev Med Child Neurol.* 1994;36:943-950.
21. Volpe JJ. Intracranial hemorrhage: germinal matrix–intraventricular hemorrhage of the premature infant. In: Volpe JJ, ed. *Neurology of the Newborn.* Philadelphia, Pa: WB Saunders Co; 1994:403-446.
22. Johnston MV. Neurotransmitters and vulnerability of the developing brain. *Brain Dev.* 1995;17:301-306.
23. Paneth N, Pinto-Martin J. The epidemiology of germinal matrix–intraventricular hemorrhage. In: Kiely J, ed. *Reproductive and Perinatal Epidemiology.* Boca Raton, Fla: CRC Press; 1991:371-399.
24. Moody DM, Bell MA, Challa VR. Features of the cerebral vascular pattern that predict vulnerability to perfusion or oxygenation deficiency: an anatomic study. *Am J Neuroradiol.* 1991;11:431-439.
25. Paneth N, Rudelli R, Kazam E, Monte W. *Brain Damage in the Preterm Infant.* London, England: MacKeith Press; 1994.
26. Leviton A, Paneth N: White matter damage in preterm newborns: an epidemiologic perspective. *Early Hum Dev.* 1990;24:1-22.
27. Paneth N, Rudelli R, Monte W, Rodriguez E, Pinto J, Kairam R, Kazam E. White matter necrosis in very low birth weight infants: neuropathologic and ultrasonographic findings in infants surviving six days or longer. *J Pediatr.* 1990;116:975-984.
28. Evrard P, Gressens P, Volpe JJ. New concepts to understand the neurological consequences of subcortical lesions in the premature brain. *Biol Neonate*, 1992;61:1-3.
29. Weisglas-Kuperus N, Baerts W, Fetter WPF, Sauer PJJ. Neonatal cerebral ultrasound, neonatal neurology and perinatal conditions as predictors of neurodevelopmental outcome in very low birthweight infants. *Early Hum Dev.* 1992;31:131-148.
30. Roth SC, Baudin J, McCormick DC, Edwards AD, Townsend J, Stewart AL, Reynolds EOR. Relation between ultrasound appearance of the brain of very preterm infants and neurodevelopmental impairment at eight years. *Dev Med Child Neurol.* 1993;35:755-768.
31. Sostek AM. Prematurity as well as intraventricular hemorrhage influence developmental outcome at 5 years. In: Friedman SL, Sigman MD, eds. *The Psychological Development of Low-Birthweight Children.* Norwood, NJ: Ablex Publishing Corp; 1992:259-274.

32. Fawer CL, Calame A. Significance of ultrasound appearances in the neurological development and cognitive abilities of preterm infants at 5 years. *Eur J Pediatr*. 1991;150:515-520.

33. Pinto-Martin J, Paneth N, Witomski T, Stein I, Schonfeld S, Rosenfeld D, Rose W, Kazam E, Kairam R, Katsikiotis V. The Central New Jersey Neonatal Brain Haemorrhage Study: design of the study and reliability of ultrasound diagnosis. *Paediatr Perinat Epidemiol*. 1992;6: 273-284.

34. Achenbach TM. *Manual for the Child Behavior Checklist/2-3 and 1992 Profile*. Burlington, Vt: University of Vermont Department of Psychiatry; 1992.

35. Achenbach TM. *Manual for the Child Behavior Checklist/4-18 and 1991 Profile*. Burlington, Vt: University of Vermont Department of Psychiatry; 1991.

36. Thorndike RL, Hagen EP, Sattler JM. *The Stanford-Binet Intelligence Scale: Fourth Edition—Guide for Administration and Scoring*. Chicago, Ill: Riverside Publishing Co; 1986.

37. Goodman S, Alegria M, Hoven C, Leaf P, Narrow W. *Core Service Utilization and Risk Factors (SURF) Modules: NIMH Multi-site Methodologic Survey of Child and Adolescent Populations Field Trials*. Rockville, Md: National Institute of Mental Health; 1992.

38. Larroche JC. Intraventricular hemorrhage in the premature neonate. In: Korobkin R, Guilleminault C, eds. *Advances in Perinatal Neurology*. New York, NY: SP Medical and Scientific Books; 1979:115-141.

39. Rorke LB. *Pathology of Perinatal Brain Injury*. New York, NY: Raven Press; 1982.

40. Papile LA, Burstein J, Burstein R. Incidence and evolution of subependymal and intraventricular hemorrhage. *J. Pediatr*. 1978;92:529-534.

41. Holzman C, Paneth N, Little R. Pinto-Martin J. Perinatal brain injury in premature infants born to mothers using alcohol in pregnancy. *Pediatrics*. 1995;95:66-73.

42. Williams RL, Creasy RK, Cunningham GC, Hawes WE, Norris FD, Tashiro M. Fetal growth and perinatal viability in California. *Obstet Gynecol*. 1982;59:624-632.

43. Tarnow-Mordi W, Ogston S, Wilkinson AR, Reid E, Gregory J, Saeed M, Wilke R. Predicting death from initial disease severity in very low birthweight infants: a method for comparing the performance of neonatal units. *BMJ*. 1990;300:1611-1614.

44. Cimma R, Risemberg H, White JJ. A simple objective system for early recognition of overwhelming neonatal respiratory distress. *J Pediatr Surg*. 1980;15:581-585.

45. Caldwell BM, Bradley RH. *Administration Manual—Home Observation for Measurement of the Environment*. Little Rock, Ark: University of Arkansas at Little Rock; 1984.

46. Goldberg DP. *The Detection of Psychiatric Illness by Questionnaire: A Technique for the Identification and Assessment of Non-psychotic Psychiatric Illness*. London, England: Oxford University Press; 1972.

47. Byles J, Byrne C, Boyle MH, Offord DR. Ontario Child Health Study: reliability and validity of the General Functioning Subscale of the McMaster Family Assessment Device. *Fam Process*. 1988;27:97-101.

48. Fisher PW, Shaffer D, Piacentini JC, Lapkin J, Kafantaris V, Leonard H, Herzog DB. Sensitivity of the Diagnostic Interview Schedule for Children, 2nd Edition (DISC-2.1) for specific diagnoses of children and adolescents. *J Am Acad Child Adolesc Psychiatry*. 1993;32:666-673.

49. American Psychiatric Association, Committee on Nomenclature and Statistics. *Diagnostic and Statistical Manual of Mental Disorders, Revised Third Edition*. Washington, DC: American Psychiatric Association; 1987.

50. Schwab-Stone M, Fallon T, Briggs T, Crowther B. Reliability of diagnostic reporting for children aged 6-11 years: a test-retest study of the Diagnostic Interview Schedule for Children–Revised. *Am J Psychiatry*. 1994;151:1048-1054.
51. Jensen P, Roper M, Fisher P, et al. Test-retest reliability of the Diagnostic Interview Schedule for Children (Version 2.1): parent, child and combined algorithms. *Arch Gen Psychiatry*. 1995;52:61-71.
52. Achenbach TM. *Manual for the Teacher's Report Form and 1991 Profile*. Burlington, Vt: University of Vermont Department of Psychiatry; 1991.
53. Aylward GP. *Test Behavior Checklist*. Brandon, Vt: Clinical Psychology Publishing Co Inc; 1986.
54. Bird H, Canino GJ, Rubio-Stipec M, Ribera JC. Further measures of the psychometric properties of the Children's Global Assessment Scale. *Arch Gen Psychiatry*. 1987;44:821-824.
55. Shaffer D, Gould MS, Brasic J, Ambrosini P, Fisher P, Bird H, Aluwahlia S. A. Children's Global Assessment Scale (CGAS). *Arch Gen Psychiatry*. 1983;40:1228-1231.
56. Riley GD. *Riley Motor Problems Inventory—Manual*. Los Angeles, Calif: Western Psychological Services; 1976.
57. Fleiss JL. *Statistical Methods for Rates and Proportions*. New York, NY: John Wiley & Sons Inc; 1981.
58. Cohen J, Cohen P. *Applied Multiple Regression/Correlation Analysis for the Behavioral Sciences*. Hillsdale, NJ: Lawrence Erlbaum Assoc; 1983.
59. Ornstein M, Ohlsson A, Edmonds J, Asztalos E. Neonatal follow-up of very low birthweight/extremely low birthweight infants to school age: a critical overview. *Acta Scand Paediatr*. 1991;80:741-748.
60. Arnold CC, Kramer MS, Hobbs CA, McLean FH, Usher RH. Very low birth weight: a problematic cohort for epidemiologic studies of very small or immature neonates. *Am J Epidemiol*. 1991;134:604-613.
61. Hope PL, Gould SJ, Howard S, Hamilton PA, Costello AM, Reynolds EOR. Precision of ultrasound diagnosis of pathologically verified lesions in the brains of very preterm infants. *Dev Med Child Neurol*. 1988;30:457-471.
62. Volpe JJ. Neuronal proliferation, migration, organization, and myelination. In: Volpe JJ, ed. *Neurology of the Newborn*. Philadelphia, Pa: WB Saunders Co; 1995:43-85.
63. Offord DR, Boyle MH, Szatmari P, Rae-Grant MI, Links PS, Cadman DT, Byles JA, Crawford JW, Blum HM, Byrne C, Thomas H, Woodward CA. Ontario Child Health Study, II: six-month prevalence of disorder and rates of service utilization. *Arch Gen Psychiatry*. 1987;44:832-836.
64. Nichols PL, Chen TC. *Minimal Brain Dysfunction: A Prospective Study*. Hillsdale, NJ: Lawrence Erlbaum Assoc; 1981.
65. Fergusson DM, Horwood LJ, Lynskey MT. Maternal smoking before and after pregnancy: effects on behavioral outcomes in middle childhood. *Pediatrics*. 1993;92:815-822.
66. Weitzman M, Gortmaker S, Sobol A. Maternal smoking and behavior problems of children. *Pediatrics*. 1992;90:342-349.
67. Cairns NJ, Wonnacott S. 3H nicotine binding sites in fetal human brain. *Brain Res*. 1988;475:1-7.
68. Shaywitz BA, Cohen DJ, Leckman JF, Young JG, Bowers MB. Ontogeny of dopamine and serotonin metabolites in the cerebrospinal fluid of children with neurological disorders. *Dev Med Child Neurol*. 1980;22:748-754.

69. Wong DF, Wagner HN, Dannals RF, et al. Effects of age, dopamine and serotonin receptors measured by positron tomography in the living human brain. *Science*. 1984;226:1393-1396.
70. Seeman P, Bzowej NH, Guan HC, Bergeron C, Reynolds GP, Bird ED, Riederer P, Jellinger K, Watanabe S, Tourtellote W. Human dopamine receptors in children and aging adults. *Synapse*. 1987;1:399-405.
71. Szatmari P, Offord DR, Boyle MH. Correlates, associated impairments and patterns of service utilization of children with attention deficit disorder: findings from the Ontario Child Health Study. *J Child Psychol Psychiatry*. 1989;30:205-217.
72. National Center for Health Statistics. *Perinatal Mortality in the United States, 1985-91*. Washington, DC: National Center for Health Statistics; 1995;922-927.
73. Sameroff AJ, Chandler MJ. Reproductive risk and the continuum of caretaking casualty. In: Horowitz FD, ed. *Review of Child Development Research*. Chicago, III: University of Chicago Press; 1975:187-244.
74. Rubin RA, Balow B. Perinatal influences on behavior and learning problems of children. In: Lahey BB, Kazdin AE, eds. *Advances in Clinical Child Psychology*. New York, NY: Plenum Press; 1977:119-160.
75. Horowitz FD. The concept of risk: a reevaluation. In: Friedman SL, Sigman MD, eds. *The Psychological Development of Low-Birthweight Children*. Norwood, NJ: Ablex Publishing Corp; 1992:61-88.
76. Weinberger D. Schizophrenia as a neurodevelopmental disorder. In: Hirsch S, Weinberger D, ed. *Schizophrenia*. Cambridge, Mass: Blackwell Science; 1995:293-323.
77. Ornitz E. Developmental aspects of neurophysiology. In: Lewis M, ed. *Child and Adolescent Psychiatry: A Comprehensive Textbook*. Philadelphia, Pa: Williams & Wilkins; 1991:38-51.
78. Rogeness GA, Javors GA, Pliszka SR. Neurochemistry and child and adolescent psychiatry. *J Am Acad Child Adolesc Psychiatry*. 1996;31:765-781.
79. Gray JA, McNaughton N. The neuropsychology of anxiety: a reprise. In: Hope DA, ed. *Perspectives on Anxiety, Panic, & Fear*. Lincoln, Neb: University of Nebraska Press; 1996:61-134.
80. Lou HC, Henriksen L, Bruhn P, Borner H, Nielsen JB. Striatal dysfunction in attention deficit and hyperkinetic disorder. *Arch Neurol*. 1989;46:48-52.
81. Lou NC, Henriksen L, Bruhn P. Focal cerebral hypoperfusion in children with dysphasia and/or attention deficit disorder. *Arch Neurol*. 1984;41:825-829.
82. Castellanos FX, Giedd JN, Eckburg P, Marsh WL, Vaituzis C, Kaysen D, Hamburger SD, Rapoport JL. Quantitative morphology of the caudate nucleus in attention deficit hyperactivity disorder. *Am J Psychiatry*. 1994;151:1791-1796.
83. Hynd GW, Hern LK, Novey ES, Eliopulos D, Marshall R, Gonzalez JJ, Voeller KK. Attention deficit-hyperactivity disorder and asymmetry of the caudate nucleus. *J Child Neurol*. 1993;8:339-347.
84. Singer HS, Reiss AL, Brown JE, Aylward EH, Shih B, Chee E, Harris EL, Reader MJ, Chase GA, Bryan RN. Volumetric MRI changes in basal ganglia of children with Tourette's syndrome. *Neurology*. 1993;43:950-956.
85. Peterson B, Riddle MA, Cohen DJ. Reduced basal ganglia volumes in Tourette's syndrome using three-dimensional reconstruction techniques from magnetic resonance imaging. *Neurology*. 1993;43:941-949.
86. Pine D, Shaffer D, Schonfeld IS. Persistent emotional disorder in children with neurological soft signs. *J Am Acad Child Adolesc Psychiatry*. 1993;32:1229-1236.

87. Kitai ST, Kocsis JD, Preston RJ, Sugimori M. Monosynaptic inputs to caudate neurons identified by intracellular injection of horseradish peroxidase. *Brain Res.* 1976;109:601-606.
88. Castellanos FX, Rapoport JL. Etiology of attention-deficit hyperactivity disorder. *Child Adolesc Psychiatr Clin North Am.* 1992;1:373-384.
89. Singer HS. Neurobiological issues in Tourette syndrome. *Brain Dev.* 1994;16:353-364.
90. Blennow M, Zeman J, Dahlin I, Lagercrantz H. Monoamine neurotransmitters and metabolites in the cerebrospinal fluid following perinatal asphyxia. *Biol Neonate.* 1995;67:407-413.
91. Dell'Anna ME, Luthman J, Lindqvist E, Olson L. Development of monoamine systems after neonatal anoxia in rats. *Brain Res Bull.* 1993;32:159-170.
92. Gordon K, Statman D, Johnston MV, Robinson TE, Becker JB, Silverstein FS. Transient hypoxia alters striatal catecholamine metabolism in immature brain: an in vivo microdialysis study. *J Neurochem.* 1990;54:605-611.
93. Freed WJ. The therapeutic latency of neuroleptic drugs and nonspecific postjunctional supersensitivity. *Schizophr Bull.* 1988;14:269-277.
94. Johnston MV, Trescher WH, Taylor GA. Hypoxic and ischemic central nervous system disorders in infants and children. *Adv Pediatr.* 1995;42:1-45.
95. Fuster JM. *The Prefrontal Cortex.* New York, NY: Raven Press; 1989.
96. Huttenlocher PR. Synaptic density in human frontal cortex: developmental changes and effects in aging. *Brain Res.* 1979;163:195-205.
97. Feinberg I. Schizophrenia: caused by a fault in programmed synaptic elimination during adolescence? *J Psychiatr Res.* 1982;17:319-334.
98. Huttenlocher PR, deCourten C, Garey LJ, Van Der Loos H. Synaptogenesis in human visual cortex: evidence for synapse elimination during normal development. *Neurosci Lett.* 1982;33:247-252.
99. Purves D, Lichtman JW. Elimination of synapses in the developing nervous system. *Science.* 1980;210:153-157.
100. Swerdlow NR, Koob GF. Dopamine, schizophrenia, mania, and depression: toward a unified hypothesis of cortico-striato-pallido-thalamic function. *Behav Brain Sci.* 1987;10:197-245.
101. Brody AL, Saxena S. Brain imaging in obsessive-compulsive disorder: evidence for the involvement of frontal-subcortical circuitry in the mediation of symptomatology. *CNS Spectrums Int J Neuropsychiatr Med.* 1996;1:27-41.
102. Pettegrew JW, Keshavan MS, Minshew NJ. ^{31}P nuclear magnetic resonance spectroscopy: neurodevelopment and schizophrenia. *Schizophr Bull.* 1993;19:35-53.
103. Jernigan TL, Zisook S, Heaton RK, Moranville JT, Hesselink JR, Braff DL. Magnetic resonance imaging abnormalities in lenticular nuclei and cerebral cortex in schizophrenia. *Arch Gen Psychiatry.* 1991;49:238-243.

8

Cognitive Deficits in Parents From Multiple-Incidence Autism Families

Joseph Piven and Pat Palmer
University of Iowa College of Medicine, Iowa City

This study compares parents of two autistic children with parents of a Down syndrome (DS) proband, on tests of intelligence, reading and spelling, and executive function. Autism parents performed significantly worse than DS parents on performance IQ, a test of executive function, and some reading measures (e.g. passage comprehension and rapid automatized naming). These results suggest that cognitive deficits may be an expression of the underlying genetic liability for autism and that these characteristics may contribute to a more broadly defined autism phenotype.

Autism is a severe neuropsychiatric disorder defined by the presence of social deficits, communication abnormalities, stereotyped-repetitive behaviors, and a characteristic course. Results from family and twin studies indicate that the etiology of this disorder is mainly genetic (Piven & Folstein, 1994). The recurrence risk for autism (i.e. the frequency of autism in subsequently born siblings) is estimated at 6–8%, or up to 200 times the risk in the general population (Ritvo et al., 1989). Three twin studies of geographically defined populations have detected pairwise concordance rates of approximately 65% (the average over the three studies) and 0% in monozygotic and dyzygotic pairs respectively, producing a heritability estimate of over 90% (Bailey et al., 1995; Folstein & Rutter, 1977; Steffenburg, Gillberg, & Holmgren, 1989). There is, furthermore, no convincing evidence that perinatal factors play an important role in the etiology of most cases of autism (reviewed in Piven et al., 1993).

Although there is now general agreement about the importance of genetic factors in autism, the definition of the phenotype for use in genetic studies has continued to be the subject of debate. In the first twin study of autism, in addition to finding a pairwise concordance rate for autism of 36% among 11 monozygotic pairs, Folstein and Rutter (1977)

Reprinted with permission from the *Journal of Child Psychology and Psychiatry*, 1997, Vol. 38(8), 1011–1021.

The authors wish to acknowledge Sally Ozonoff, PhD, Frank Woods, PhD, Susan Folstein, MD, and Polly Nichols, PhD for their helpful comments on this manuscript, and Stephan Arndt, PhD for his assistance in the analyses.

This research was supported by National Institute of Mental Health Grants MH51217 and MH01028 (JP).

reported an even higher (82%) concordance rate for a more broadly defined cognitive impairment that included autism, mental retardation, language delay, reading disorder, spelling disorder, and/or articulation disorder. August, Stewart, and Tsai (1981) reported further possible evidence to support the relationship of cognitive disorders to autism, showing the familial aggregation of these disorders in the siblings of autistic probands on direct examination. However, these investigators questioned whether the aggregation of cognitive disorders in autism families was confounded by the co-occurrence of severe mental retardation, detected in the majority (7/8) of the autistic probands showing familial aggregation of cognitive disorders. Bailey et al. (1995) reported an 88% concordance rate for a history of a cognitive abnormality in monozygotic twins compared to a 9% rate in dyzygotic twins, replicating the previous results reported in the twin study by Folstein and Rutter (1977). Family history studies by Bolton et al. (1994) and Piven et al. (1990) also reported high rates of cognitive deficits in first-degree relatives of autistic probands, although the study by Piven et al. (1990) did not include a control group. In these studies (Bailey et al., 1995; Bolton et al., 1994; Piven et al., 1990), familial aggregation of cognitive deficits was largely due to academic and language-related disorders, with no evidence for the familial aggregation of mental retardation.

In addition to these studies of IQ, academic, and language-related deficits, Ozonoff, Rogers, Farnham, and Pennington (1993) reported significantly worse performance on the Tower of Hanoi, a measure of executive function, in siblings of high-functioning autistic probands compared to controls. No differences were detected on the Wisconsin Card Sort Test, another measure of executive function ability. Hughes, Leboyer, and Bouvard (1997) compared parents of children with autism to parents of both normally developing children and children with learning disabilities. Three measures of executive function were administered: the Tower of London planning task, the Intradimensional–Extradimensional set-shifting task, and a working memory task. Significant differences on all three executive function measures were found, with parents of individuals with autism performing less well than parents of normal children or children with mental retardation. Executive function deficits have consistently been reported in individuals with autism (Hughes, Russell, & Robbins, 1994; Ozonoff, Pennington, & Rogers, 1991; Ozonoff, Strayer, McMahon, & Filloux, 1994; Prior & Hoffman, 1990; Rumsey & Hamburger, 1988), supporting the validity of this finding in siblings and parents. Furthermore, executive function abilities are relatively independent of IQ (Welsh, Pennington, & Groisser, 1991), suggesting that high rates of at least some cognitive deficits in relatives of autistic probands are not secondary to their familial association with mental retardation in the proband.

Except for the studies by August et al. (1981) and Ozonoff et al. (1993), employing direct examination of siblings, and the study by Hughes et al. (1997) directly examining parents, the evidence suggesting familial aggregation of cognitive disorders in relatives of autistic probands has been based entirely on data obtained using the family history method. In contrast to these results, several other studies employing direct testing have concluded that cognitive disorders do not aggregate in families of individuals with autism. Freeman et al. (1989) used the Shipley–Hartford Test, a self-administered measure of intelligence, and the Wide Range Achievement Test, a measure of academic ability, with 122 parents and 153 siblings of 62 autistic probands. School-aged siblings were given an age-appropriate Wechsler Intelligence Scale rather than the Shipley–Hartford Test. Significantly lower scores were detected on the Shipley–Hartford Test in fathers; however, the scores of mothers and siblings did not differ significantly from available published norms. Szatmari et al. (1993) compared the parents and siblings of 52 probands with DSM–III–R Pervasive Developmental Disorders (PDD) (i.e. autistic disorder or pervasive developmental disorder, not otherwise specified) with the parents and siblings of 33 Down Syndrome (DS) and low birthweight probands. Parents were examined on five subtests of the Wechsler Adult Intelligence Revised (WAIS–R) (i.e. digit span, vocabulary, comprehension, block design, and digit-symbol coding); siblings were examined on the Stanford–Binet Intelligence Test, Wisconsin Card Sort Test, and Wide Range Achievement Test. No differences were detected between parent or sibling groups on any of the measures. More recently Szatmari et al. (1995) also failed to find a higher rate of cognitive deficits in relatives of PDD probands using the family history method.

Although the studies of Freeman et al. (1989) and Szatmari et al. (1993) suggest that cognitive deficits may not be detectable in relatives of autistic probands, there are several limitations to these studies that warrant comment. Both the Freeman et al. and Szatmari et al. studies employed narrow cognitive protocols in adults. The Freeman et al. study was also limited by the absence of a control group. Probands in the Szatmari et al. study met criteria for PDD including individuals with autism and pervasive developmental disorder not otherwise specified, a less severe and more prevalent disorder than autism. The use of PDD probands may have defined a sample of relatives with reduced genetic liability for a broader autism phenotype compared to the sample of relatives that would have been ascertained through an autistic proband only.

As a result of the conflicting findings of these studies, controversy continues over whether cognitive deficits in relatives constitute an expression of the underlying genetic liability for autism. Resolution of this issue has implications for future genetic research in autism. Delineation of a broader autism phenotype may prove to be important for use in genetic studies by increasing the power to detect linkage in autism where there is minimal to no vertical transmission and small family size. Clarification of the cognitive aspects of the broader autism phenotype may also provide insight into the fundamental neuropsychological deficits in autism.

In this paper, we directly examine cognitive abilities in parents ascertained through two siblings with autism (i.e. multiple-incidence autism families) and parents ascertained through a Down syndrome child using a comprehensive battery including assessment of IQ, a variety of reading-related measures, and examination of executive function. Rates of cognitive deficits have not previously been examined in multiple-incidence autism families and may be useful in delineating some manifestations of a broader autism phenotype. Probands in multiple-incidence autism families are less likely than single-incidence probands to have autism as a result of nongenetic causes (Piven & Folstein, 1994) and are therefore likely to represent a more etiologically homogeneous sample than those ascertained through a single autistic or PDD proband. In addition, relatives ascertained through multiple-incidence autism probands may have a higher genetic liability for autism and the genetically related broader autism phenotype than relatives ascertained through single-incidence autism or PDD probands. For these reasons, relatives in multiple-incidence autism families provide a potentially important study group for exploring the boundaries of the phenotype in autism.

METHODS

Sample

Families with at least two children with autism were ascertained for this study through a systematic attempt to identify all multiple-incidence autism families in Iowa ($N = 18$) and from multiple-incidence autism families known, at the start of this study, to two tertiary evaluation centres for autism in the Midwest ($N = 7$). Iowa families were ascertained through three sources: (1) medical record review of patients seen over the last 24 years in the Child Psychiatry Clinic at the University of Iowa and currently living in Iowa; (2) systematic screening of all primary care physicians in Iowa; and (2) systematic screening of all public schools in Iowa. Families of autistic probands were eligible for this study if two children (age 4–30 years) met algorithm criteria for autistic disorder of the Autism Diagnostic Interview (LeCouteur et al., 1989) and neither autistic proband had evidence of a significant co-occurring medical condition thought possibly to be etiologically related to autism, such as tuberous sclerosis, neurofibromatosis, phenylketonuria, significant CNS injury, Fragile X syndrome, or other chromosomal anomalies (Piven & Folstein, 1994) identified on direct physical examination, medical record review, and/or cytogenetic screening. The final sample consisted of parents from 25 multiple-incidence autism families and included 42 male and 8 female autistic probands ranging in age from 4 to 28 years.

Thirty families with a child with Down syndrome secondary to a non-disjunction of chromosome 21 constitute the comparison group in this study. Down syndrome families were ascertained through public schools ($N = 9$) and randomly selected from a list of the families of newborns diagnosed with Down syndrome at the University of Iowa who live within a 150-mile radius of the University ($N = 21$). An attempt was made to obtain equal numbers of families in each of three proband age groups: 4–12, 13–18, and 18 + years. The rationale for choosing this comparison group was based on our need to control for the effect of caring for a handicapped child on the emotional and social functioning of parents and siblings. Also, relatives of a Down syndrome child would not be expected to have an increased genetic liability, over the general population, for social or communication deficits, or stereotyped behaviors—the behavioral variables of interest in this study. The final sample consisted of parents from 30 Down syndrome families and included 13 male and 17 female probands ranging in age from 2–27 years. Further details on the ascertainment of both the autism and Down syndrome families are reviewed in a previous paper presenting family history data on these same individuals (Piven, Palmer, Jacobi, Childress, & Arndt, 1997). Twenty-five mothers and 23 fathers from 25 multiple-incidence autism families and 30 mothers and 30 fathers from 30 Down syndrome families were eligible to participate in this study. An autism parent was included in the analysis only if he or she were the parent of two children with autism. Two mothers had autistic children with two different fathers, resulting in only 23 autism fathers being eligible. Neither father's age ($t = 0.76$; $df = 51$; $p > .45$) or level of education ($\chi^2 = 1.39$; $df = 4$; $p = .85$) or mother's age ($t = 0.29$; $df = 53$; $p = .77$) or level of education ($\chi^2 = 6.95$; $df = 4$; $p = .14$) differed significantly between cases and controls. Father's occupational level, as specified by the *British manual of the classification of occupations* (Office of Population Censuses and Surveys, 1980), also did not differ

TABLE 1
Education and Occupational Levels in Autism and Down Syndrome Parents

	Autism N (%)	Down syndrome N (%)
Education		
<12 years	2 (4)	2 (3)
High school degree	19 (40)	19 (32)
2 year/partial college	8 (17)	21 (35)
University degree	12 (25)	12 (20)
Graduate degree	7 (15)	6 (10)
Father's occupation[a]		
Professional/intermediate	6 (26)	7 (23)
Non-manual skilled	4 (17)	7 (23)
Manual skilled	5 (22)	11 (37)
Partly skilled/unskilled	4 (17)	5 (17)
Chronically unemployed	4 (17)	0

[a]For purposes of comparison, fathers were assumed to be the primary wage earners in the family.

significantly between the two groups ($\chi^2 = 6.2$; $df = 4$). Frequencies of education and occupational levels appear in Table 1. Of the 48 autism and 60 Down syndrome parents eligible to participate in this study, 47 (98%) and 53 (88%) respectively were available and agreed to participate in the cognitive testing.

Assessment of Autistic Probands

Parental informants for all autistic subjects were interviewed regarding the subject's diagnosis with the Autism Diagnostic Interview (LeCouteur et al., 1989). An algorithm constructed for use with the Autism Diagnostic Interview has been shown to discriminate autistic from nonautistic IQ-matched controls (LeCouteur et al., 1989) adequately. Acceptable inter-rater agreement (Kappa > .90) on the Autism Diagnostic Interview-algorithm (using 10 videotaped interviews) for a diagnosis of autism was established by all raters prior to the start of data collection. In addition, probands were directly assessed using the Autism Diagnostic Observation Schedule (Lord et al., 1989), a structured observation and interview schedule developed to aid in the diagnosis and assessment of autistic individuals. The information from the Autism Diagnostic Observation Schedule functioned as a check on the probands' current behaviour as reported by parents on the Autism Diagnostic Interview.

All subjects were evaluated by a screening neurodevelopmental examination for evidence of significant neurological impairment or medical conditions thought to be etiologically related to autism (see earlier). In addition, almost all subjects had previously been screened through a medical evaluation at a tertiary care center and were not found to have evidence of any exclusion criteria for this study. No subject was excluded on the basis of our additional neurodevelopmental screening examination. At least one proband in each of the 25 multiplex sibships had been previously tested cytogenetically for Fragile X, or was tested as part of this study. All subjects were negative for the Fragile X anomaly.

Adequate performance IQ estimates were available on 46 of 50 probands from the medical record. The following IQ measures, if obtained by a psychologist, were considered adequate for estimation of performance IQ: the Wechsler Intelligence Scale for Children–Revised (Wechsler, 1974), the Wechsler Intelligence Scale for Children–III (Wechsler, 1991), the Wechsler Adult Intelligence Scale–R (Wechsler, 1981), the Leiter International Performance Scales (Arthur, 1952), or the Merrill–Palmer Scales (Stutsman, 1952). When multiple tests were available, the test (in the order of priority listed above) obtained closest to age 12 years was used for estimating performance IQ. Fifty percent of subjects had performance IQs in the 70 + range, 24% were in the 50–69 range, and 26% were in the 30–49 range; none scored less than 30. Four individuals were thought not to have had adequate testing at the time this study was undertaken, due either to an inappropriate test having been used or to difficulties with test administration. Resources were not available to attempt further testing of these four individuals.

Cognitive Assessment of Parents

Wechsler Adult Intelligence Scale–Revised (*WAIS–R*) (*Wechsler, 1981*). Because of time constraints, the initial protocol for estimation of verbal and performance IQ included only four subtests of the WAIS–R: vocabulary, similarities, block design, and object assembly. After the start of the study, it was determined that additional subtests could comfortably be added to the protocol. The comprehension and picture completion subtests of the WAIS–R were therefore also administered to a subset of subjects (all Down syndrome parents and 75% of autism parents). Reliability of the verbal and performance IQ scores of the WAIS–R has been shown to be very high, although reliability data for prorated estimates, as used in the present study, are unavailable (Wechsler, 1981).

Woodcock Johnson Tests of Achievement–Psychoeducational Battery–Revised (*WJ*) (*Woodcock & Johnson, 1991*). Several reading outcome measures including letter-word identification, word attack, passage comprehension, and dictation were employed from the WJ battery. In letter-word identification, the subject must identity upper- and lower-case letters printed in various typefaces (e.g. roman, italic) and read lists of isolated words of increasing difficulty. The word attack subtest requires untimed sounding-out of nonsense words or words of such low frequency that they are unlikely to be familiar to the subject. This latter task assesses phonological awareness, a deficit commonly found in poor readers and thought to be a central process affected in dyslexia. Problems with phonological awareness have also been shown to be a sensitive measure for detecting adults with a history of childhood dyslexia (Pennington, Van Orden, Smith, Green, & Haith, 1990). The passage comprehension subtest of the WJ utilizes a modified cloze procedure in which the subject silently reads a short passage and then identifies a missing word from the text. Dictation is essentially a test of spelling ability. Raw scores for all tests were converted to standard scores with a mean of 100 ($SD = 15$). Average test reliability in adults for the four tasks of the WJ employed in this study is very high ($r > .9$) (Woodcock & Mathers, 1989).

Rapid Automatized Naming Test (RAN) (Denckla & Rudel, 1976). In this task, subjects are asked to name, in sequence and as rapidly as possible, items (i.e. numbers, letters, objects, and colors) presented visually on a chart. The total number of seconds required to name each set of stimuli was the dependent variable of interest; thus, lower scores represent more rapid naming. This task has been shown to be associated with dyslexia in children (Denckla & Rudel, 1976); to identify adults with a childhood history of reading problems (Felton, Naylor, & Wood, 1990); and to predict later reading deficits in very young children (e.g. predicting 8th grade deficits from 2nd grade scores) (Meyer, Wood, Hart, & Felton, in press).

Tower of Hanoi (TOH) (Borys, Spitz, & Dorans, 1982; Piaget, 1976). This ring-transfer task requires subjects to plan a sequence of moves that transforms an initial configuration of rings into a "tower," in which the rings are arranged by size on a designated peg, thereby duplicating the examiner's configuration. This type of planning behavior has been shown to be deficient in adults with injury to the prefrontal cortex (Shallice, 1982). The dependent variable is a planning efficiency score, which reflects the number of trials required to solve problems of different move lengths and difficulty. Both the 3-ring (TPH3) and 4-ring (TPH4) versions of the task were administered. Following Borys et al. (1982), a maximum of six points was assigned to a problem solved in the first two trials, point totals decreasing with the number of trials required for solution (see Borys et al., 1982, for more detail on the scoring procedure).

Analysis

Sample characteristics (e.g. parental age, education level) and cognitive measures were compared using simple statistics (Student's t-test and chi-square). Nonparametric analyses were performed using the Mann–Whitney test. The intercorrelations of scores were examined using the Pearson Product–Moment Correlation. Tests were considered significant if they passed the $p < .05$ level of significance (two-tailed). Adjustments for multiple comparisons were made using the Bonferroni correction.

RESULTS

Table 2 presents the results of a comparison of the mean scores for autism and Down syndrome parents on each of the cognitive measures employed. Autism parents did not differ significantly from Down syndrome parents on verbal IQ on the WAIS–R but performed significantly worse on performance IQ. When compared to Down syndrome parents, autism parents also showed a significantly greater mean verbal-performance discrepancy ($t = 2.94$, $df = 96$; $p < .004$). To further examine the performance IQ differences, mean subtest scores were compared. Autism parents showed significantly worse performance than Down syndrome parents on the picture completion and object assembly subtests. Comparison of results on the TOH revealed that autism parents performed significantly worse than Down syndrome parents on the four-ring task. A similar trend was detected for the three-ring task. Autism parents took significantly longer to complete two of the four RAN tasks, color and object naming, and performed significantly worse on passage

TABLE 2
Mean Scores on Cognitive Measures in Multiple-incidence Autism and Down Syndrome Parents

	Autism		DS				
	Mean	(*SD*)	Mean	(*SD*)	t[a]	(*df*)	*p*
Wechsler Adult Intelligence Scale–Revised							
Verbal IQ	108.30	(19.4)	111.40	(18.2)	0.82	(96)	n.s.
Performance IQ	99.10	(17.7)	112.00	(16.8)	3.71	(97)	.0001*
Picture completion[b]	9.65	(3.2)	11.80	(3.3)	3.07	(86)	.003*
Block design	9.80	(3.2)	10.80	(2.7)	1.73	(97)	n.s.
Object assembly	8.23	(3.2)	10.10	(2.8)	3.07	(96)	.003*
Tower of Hanoi							
Three ring	33.30	(3.5)	34.50	(2.4)	1.99[c]	(79)	.050
Four ring	7.98	(4.8)	10.34	(5.0)	2.29	(89)	.024
Rapid Automatized Naming Task[d]							
Color	29.80	(5.6)	25.50	(6.2)	3.64	(98)	.0001*
Number	19.50	(3.9)	18.60	(5.3)	0.92	(98)	n.s.
Object	39.50	(6.6)	35.20	(8.0)	2.94	(98)	.004
Letter	19.50	(3.2)	20.10	(6.9)	0.52	(98)	n.s.
Woodcock Johnson Psycho-educational Battery[e]							
Word attack	110.50	(21.4)	112.50	(20.1)	0.48	(95)	n.s.
Letter word	110.30	(22.0)	105.40	(19.0)	1.16	(95)	n.s.
Passage comprehension	106.60	(20.1)	116.20	(22.1)	2.24	(97)	.027
Dictation	96.30	(20.0)	99.60	(17.5)	0.83	(90)	n.s.

[a]Two-tailed Student's t-test.
[b]Added to the cognitive battery after the start of the study.
[c]Separate variance estimate.
[d]Latencies in seconds.
[e]Scaled scores.
*Significant at $p < .05$ after Bonferroni correction for multiple comparisons.

comprehension of the Woodcock Johnson Psychoeducational Battery (WJ). No differences were detected on the word attack, letter-word identification, or dictation tasks of the WJ. After Bonferroni correction for multiple comparisons, differences on performance IQ, picture completion, object assembly, and the RAN color task continued to be significant. Results of all parametric analyses were consistent with nonparametric analyses with the exception that, on nonparametric analysis, significant differences were noted on comparison of autism and Down syndrome parents on the TOH three-ring task ($Z = 2.18$, $p < .03$). Subject age and sex were not significantly correlated with scores on the cognitive variables examined.

In a previous report by our group on family history data from this sample, there was a suggestion that communication deficits occurred more commonly in autism parents compared to Down syndrome parents and that this difference was mostly a result of higher rates of communication deficits in autism mothers (Piven et al., 1997). To examine whether the pattern of differences in cognitive measures differed between male and female groups, we compared autism fathers with Down syndrome fathers and autism mothers with Down syndrome mothers on performance IQ, TOH4, RAN color, RAN object, and passage comprehension. Except for RAN object, where significant differences were present between mean scores for autism mothers (mean = 39.4) and Down syndrome mothers (mean = 32.9) ($t = 4.27$; $df = 52$; $p < .0001$) but not for autism fathers (mean = 37.9) and Down syndrome fathers (mean = 39.6) ($t = 0.67$; $df = 44$), the pattern of differences across the two gender groups was identical and paralleled the findings in the total sample.

Table 3 presents the intercorrelations of the cognitive measures in the autism and Down syndrome parent groups. In the Down syndrome group, the four RAN tasks are highly intercorrelated. They are also significantly correlated with the WJ reading tasks and with verbal

TABLE 3
Intercorrelation of Scores on Cognitive Measures in Autism and Down Syndrome Parents

	Down syndrome ($N = 41$)									
	1	2	3	4	5	6	7	8	9	10
1. Color										
2. Number	**.75**									
3. Object	**.79**	**.74**								
4. Letter	**.66**	**.87**	**.69**							
5. TOH4	.22	.13	.04	.02						
6. Passage comp	**.43**	**.47**	**.58**	**.58**	.05					
7. Word attack	**.41**	**.53**	**.57**	**.57**	.22	**.75**				
8. Letter-word	**.52**	**.51**	**.55**	**.55**	.19	**.52**	**.63**			
9. Dictation	**.60**	**.60**	**.66**	**.67**	.16	**.59**	**.59**	**.68**		
10. Verbal IQ	**.56**	**.42**	**.53**	**.58**	.24	**.59**	.30	**.42**	**.62**	
11. Performance IQ	.12	.04	.06	.05	.32	.20	.03	.03	.07	.33
	Autism ($N = 45$)									
	1	2	3	4	5	6	7	8	9	10
1. Color										
2. Number	**.41**									
3. Object	.20	.02								
4. Letter	.35	**.74**	.11							
5. TOH4	.05	.02	.01	.10						
6. Passage comp	.13	.05	.13	.22	.06					
7. Word attack	.06	.19	.05	**.46**	.17	**.45**				
8. Letter-word	.02	.12	.07	.01	.10	**.64**	**.56**			
9. Dictation	.23	.07	.19	.38	.04	**.74**	**.62**	**.64**		
10. Verbal IQ	.21	.10	.13	.19	.20	**.81**	**.46**	**.67**	**.67**	
11. Performance IQ	.27	.27	.13	.10	.33	**.53**	.26	**.39**	**.48**	**.59**

Bold figures: $p < .01$.

IQ. In the autism parents, however, the four RAN tasks do not appear to be significantly correlated with either the WJ reading tasks or with verbal IQ.

DISCUSSION

Comparison to Other Family Studies of Autism

In this study, familial aggregation of a variety of cognitive deficits was detected in the parents of multiple-incidence autism probands. In general, these results are consistent with the finding of high rates of cognitive deficits in first-degree relatives of autistic individuals reported in a number of family history studies (Bailey et al., 1995; Bartak, Rutter, & Cox, 1975; Bolton et al., 1994; Folstein & Rutter, 1977; Piven et al., 1990). Both the method of data collection (i.e. family history versus direct assessment) and the definition of the cognitive deficits employed, however, differed between those reports and the present study. In previous autism family studies where cognitive abilities were directly assessed, the use of different study designs and assessment instruments makes comparison to the present study problematic. For the most part, studies employing direct assessment (August et al., 1981; Freeman et al., 1989; Szatmari et al., 1993) have not detected reading deficits at higher rates than expected. Previous studies, however, have only examined single word reading (i.e. using the Wide Range Achievement Test) as opposed to the present study where reading deficits were detected only in a complex comprehension task but not in tasks of single letter-word identification or spelling.

Whereas different instruments were used to assess reading in this and previous studies, performance IQ has been examined previously using the same scale (Wechsler Intelligence Scale) employed in this study, and differences of the type we report have not been reported. In the study by August et al. (1981), separate verbal and performance IQs were not reported. Minton, Campbell, Green, Jennings, and Samit (1982) compared the siblings of autistic probands to population norms and found that, in general, verbal scores were lower than performance scores. Although these results appear to be inconsistent with those of the present study, a comparison of the results from studies of siblings with those of parents is problematic. Parents, as in the present study, are by definition selected for parenthood, and therefore are likely to be less impaired than siblings who are unselected for social and cognitive abilities. In another family study, Freeman et al. (1989) assessed parental IQ using the Shipley–Hartford Test, a self-administered measure of IQ that produces a single quotient that is not easily compared to the Wechsler performance IQ and verbal IQ. Fathers in that study were found to have significantly lower scores than expected when compared to population norms, whereas mothers did not differ from population norms. The study by Szatmari et al. (1993) was the only study to employ portions of the Wechsler test as a measure of IQ in parents. However, performance IQ scores were prorated on the basis of only two subtests, digit-symbol and block design. These two performance subtests would not necessarily be expected to detect the performance IQ deficits we report in autism parents using the picture completion, object assembly, and block design subtests. In addition, as mentioned previously, another key difference between the design of the present study and that conducted by Szatmari et al. (1993) is that in the latter study parents were ascertained through either Pervasive Developmental Disorder Not Otherwise Specified or through autistic probands.

In the one study available for direct comparison, Santangelo and Folstein (1996) administered the complete WAIS–R to 166 parents of 90 individuals with autism and 75 parents of 40 controls with Down syndrome. Proband inclusion and exclusion criteria (except for the ascertainment of single-incidence autism families) were identical to the present study, and parent groups did not differ significantly on age, number of years of education, or parent's occupational level. As in the present study, in the Santangelo and Folstein (1996) study, autism parents did not differ from Down syndrome parents on verbal IQ but performed significantly worse on performance IQ. Autism parents also showed significantly worse performance on the picture completion subtest of the WAIS–R but did not differ from Down syndrome parents on the object assembly task. The results of this study on a large sample of parents from single-incidence autism families are consistent with the findings we report here in parents from multiple-incidence autism families.

In the present study we report deficits in autism parents on a measure of executive function, the Tower of Hanoi. This finding is consistent with a previous report by Ozonoff et al. (1993) where significant differences were detected on the TOH between siblings of autistic individuals and siblings of controls. In that study, no differences were reported between sibling groups on the Wisconsin Card Sort Test, another measure of executive function. In addition, the findings from our study replicate the recent report by Hughes et al. (1997) showing executive function deficits in parents of autistic probands compared to parents of normal and learning-disabled controls. Within those abilities thought to comprise executive function, the TOH is thought to be a measure of planning and working memory, whereas the Wisconsin Card Sort test is thought to be more a measure of cognitive flexibility (Ozonoff & McEvoy, 1994). In the study by Szatmari et al. (1993), no differences were detected between PDD and control sibling groups on the Wisconsin Card Sort Test. The implications of these differences in autistic individuals have been discussed in detail by Ozonoff and McEvoy (1994).

Potential Limitations

As in all epidemiologic studies, the possibility that a bias of ascertainment or other confounding factors (e.g. familial aggregation of cognitive deficits with mental retardation in the autistic proband) underlie the results obtained must be considered. The significant differences we observed between cognitive scores for autism and Down syndrome parents may simply reflect above-average performance of the Down syndrome parents secondary to an unknown bias of ascertainment, rather than lower performance in autism parents, as we have speculated. Several factors, however, suggest to us that a bias of ascertainment is unlikely to be responsible for the findings of this study. First, substantial effort was put into ascertaining families in a systematic manner, including epidemiologic ascertainment of autism families in Iowa. Second, whereas a bias of ascertainment could conceivably account for the finding of lower performance IQ in multiple-incidence autism parents, it is unlikely that autism families were systematically selected for having a significant verbal-performance split (not present in Down syndrome parents) as well as a pattern of intercorrelations among the cognitive scores that differed from those observed in the Down syndrome parents. Third, autism and Down syndrome parent groups were, in fact, comparable on age, level of education, and occupation, and age was not correlated with scores on any of the cognitive tasks. Finally, using identical methods, the results of this study replicate the IQ findings in the Baltimore Autism Family Study (Santangelo & Folstein, 1996) and the findings by Ozonoff et al. (1993) and Hughes et al. (1997) regarding deficits in executive function. It is unlikely that the same systematic ascertainment bias was present in these separately conducted studies.

Relationship to Cognitive Deficits in Autism

The meaning of the cognitive deficits we detected in parents is not easily interpreted in comparison to other family studies of autism because of the absence of comparable study designs; however, the comparison to cognitive patterns that have been identified in individuals with autism is useful. Because of their genetic relationship to their children with autism, parents might be expected to show a milder version of the pattern of cognitive deficits in IQ, reading, and executive function than have been reported in individuals with autism. Traditionally, performance IQ has been seen as being higher than verbal IQ in autism, reflecting a relative strength in visuospatial abilities for most children with autism (Green, Fein, Joy, & Waterhouse, 1995). This would speak against the validity of the findings of this study. A closer look at the cognitive profiles of individuals with autism published in previous studies, however, reveals that even within the performance domain there are areas of relative strength (e.g. block design) and areas of relative weakness (e.g. picture arrangement) (Lincoln, Courchesne, Kilman, Elmasian, & Allen, 1988). Complicating this issue further are some studies showing deficits in performance IQ relative to verbal IQ in individuals with high-functioning autism and in individuals with Asperger's syndrome. Rumsey and Hamburger (1990), in a study comparing men with high-functioning autism and subjects with dyslexia, found no differences on verbal IQ between the two groups but noted that the subjects with autism had lower mean performance IQ than did those with dyslexia. In particular, men with autism appeared to do relatively worse on the picture arrangement and picture completion subtests. Rumsey and Hamburger concluded that the Wechsler profiles in their study suggested that individuals with autism have both verbal and performance deficits. Szatmari, Tuff, Finlayson, and Bartolucci (1990) noted that studies in autism showing deficits in verbal abilities and strength in visual-perceptual function have generally been performed on children with lower-functioning autism. In their study of PDD individuals, the pattern of cognitive deficits appears to vary by overall IQ. Comparing high-functioning (full scale IQ > 85) and lower-functioning (full scale IQ 70–85) PDD individuals, they found that in the high IQ group, verbal IQ was significantly greater than performance IQ, whereas the reverse was true in the lower IQ group. Several recent studies report similar findings of higher verbal IQ and lower performance IQ in individuals with Asperger's syndrome (Goodman, 1989; Klin, Volkmar, Sparrow, Cichetti, & Rourke, 1995; Volkmar et al., 1994). Other studies of individuals with Asperger's syndrome and high-functioning autism, however, have not found this pattern of differences (Minshew, Goldstein, Muenz, & Payton, 1992; Ozonoff, Rogers, & Pennington, 1991).

The findings from the present study on the WJ reading measures, showing deficits on passage comprehension but no differences on letter-word identification, phonological processing (word attack), or spelling (dictation), are consistent with what might be expected based on previous studies of reading in autistic individuals. Frith and Snowling (1983) were the first to report decreased comprehension with intact decoding skills in children with autism versus controls. This dissociation of decoding skills and comprehension, differing from the typical profile seen in dyslexia where comprehension, phonological processing (word attack), and single word reading are all deficient, was also noted by Minshew, Goldstein, Taylor, and Siegel (1994). Their study showed no differences between individuals with high-functioning autism and controls on the Woodcock Johnson word attack and letter-word identification tests, but significantly worse performance in individuals with autism on passage comprehension. Findings consistent with these results were also reported by Welsh, Pennington, and Rogers (1987) in a study of hyperlexic children with autism and by Rumsey and Hamburger (1990) in a comparison of men with high-functioning autism and dyslexia.

Rapid-naming abilities, as assessed by the RAN, have consistently been found to be deficient in poor readers (Denckla & Rudel, 1976; Felton & Wood, 1989; Wolf, Bally, & Morris, 1986); however, the significance of finding decreased rapid-naming ability in autism parents is unclear. A comparison of the RAN color plus object scores in parents from this study to available norms on 180 adults (>45 years of age) from an ongoing study at the Bowman–Gray School of Medicine revealed the mean score for autism parents to be at the 15th percentile of the normative sample, whereas the mean score for Down syndrome parents was at the 50th percentile (F. Woods, personal communication). This reference to a population norm lends further validity to the differences we report between autism and Down syndrome parents. Although these deficits may be related to some aspect of reading ability and are consistent with previous reports of a higher than expected rate of reading problems by history in relatives of autistic individuals (Bailey et al., 1995; Bolton et al., 1994; Folstein & Rutter, 1977), it is notable that in autism parents, as compared to Down syndrome parents, significant correlations were not detected between the RAN tasks and reading abilities as assessed on the WJ.

The meaning of our finding of significant differences on the color and object RAN tasks, but not the number and letter RAN tasks, is also not clear. Meyer et al. (in press) note that numbers and letters are orthographic symbols whereas colors and objects are nonsymbolic, concrete objects or attributes. One possible explanation for the dissociation of RAN tasks found in this study is that compensatory skills in number and letter naming may have developed as a result of autism parents' exposure to print, whereas compensatory skills in color and object naming did not benefit from this experience. To further explore the significance of the RAN findings in autism parents, future studies should examine autistic individuals for similar deficits in color-object naming.

Overlap with the Nonverbal Learning Disability Syndrome

In a recent paper by Klin et al. (1995), it was suggested that the neuropsychological characteristics of individuals with Asperger's syndrome were related to the characteristics of the Nonverbal Learning Disabilities Syndrome (NVLD) as proposed by Rourke (1989).

Although there is not a one-to-one correspondence (e.g. verbal deficits identified by the RAN are not considered to be components of the NVLD syndrome), the pattern of deficits identified in autism parents has some overlapping features in common with this syndrome that warrant mention. Individuals with NVLD typically score below average on the performance scale of the Wechsler test but score average or higher on the verbal scale (Rourke, 1989). Both autism parents and NVLD individuals have strengths in the area of mechanical reading, phonetic analysis, and spelling with relative weaknesses in reading comprehension and pragmatic language (Landa, Folstein, & Issacs, 1991; Landa et al., 1992; Rourke, 1989). In the area of personality and psychiatric symptoms, both have been thought to have social deficits (Bailey et al., 1995; Bolton et al., 1994; Piven et al., 1994, 1997; Rourke, 1989; Santangelo & Folstein, 1995), an aversion to novel, complex situations (i.e. rigidity) (Piven et al., 1997; Rourke, 1989), and high rates of anxiety and depressive symptoms (Piven et al., 1991; Rourke, 1989; Smalley, McCracken, & Tanguay, 1995). The presence of an existing theoretical framework for NVLD as well as the overlap of the characteristics identified as part of the NVLD syndrome with those found in the present study lends further support to the emerging descriptions of a broader autism phenotype.

Implications for Future Studies

The findings of this study have several implications for genetic studies of autism. First, although several studies have documented the general features of a broader autism phenotype, other than in the reports by Ozonoff et al. (1993) and Hughes et al. (1997) of deficits in executive function in relatives of autistic individuals, neuropsychological measures that may contribute to the definition of this phenotype have not previously been reported. Neuropsychological measures, such as those used in the present study, are generally easy to administer and, in the case of the WAIS–R and WJ, their reliabilities are widely accepted. These features make them appealing for potential use in future family and genetic analytic studies of autism.

Second, although the findings of this study offer some potential insights into the cognitive aspects of a broader autism phenotype, further work defining their interrelationships is warranted. The pattern of intercorrelations between scores on the cognitive tasks we examined appears to differ in autism and Down syndrome parents, suggesting the possibility of a different underlying factor structure for these abilities in these two groups. Given the diverse and often dissociated neuropsychological findings in autism (e.g. decoding skills and comprehension), it is not surprising that a single core cognitive factor could not be identified. Indeed, Goodman (1989) has proposed that autism may be a syndrome of multiple primary deficits, and Minshew et al. (1992) have suggested that autism is the result of a generalized abnormality in complex information processing rather than a deficit in a single, localized neural mechanism. Related to this, the absence of significant intercorrelations on the cognitive tasks in autism parents may indicate that they are applying different strategies and employ different neural pathways for solving some of these cognitive tasks than do Down syndrome parents. Functional imaging of autism relatives, using cognitive activation tasks similar to those employed in this study, may provide additional insights into neural pathways in autism. This may be a particularly useful strategy in autism given the difficulties in conducting functional imaging studies in individuals with autism (such as their younger age and frequent lack of cooperation).

Third, future family studies in autism should examine the relationship of the cognitive deficits reported in this study to behavioral characteristics (e.g. social and communication abnormalities) that have been suggested to define the broader autism phenotype. Once potential aspects of the broader phenotype are identified consistently, it will be important to consider how they should be conceptualized for genetic analysis. Related to this issue is whether aspects of the extended autism phenotype that have been suggested by this and other studies (e.g. executive function deficits, deficits in rapid naming, speech abnormalities, social deficits in personality) should be viewed as an expression of a single underlying genetic factor, such as in previous conceptualizations of Tourette syndrome (Pauls & Leckman, 1986), or as expressions of different genes contributing to the autistic phenotype. The possibility that autism is the result of multiple interacting genes (i.e. an oligogenic disorder) has been suggested (Pickles et al., 1995). Examination of the components of the broader autism phenotype in relatives may allow us to disentangle genetically meaningful but distinct aspects of the autistic phenotype that segregate independently but together can combine to produce autism. This approach may be more fruitful for genetic analyses than employing syndromic-like definitions, where an algorithm is proposed that includes a number of conceptually unrelated aspects that together define the broader phenotype (Santangelo & Folstein, 1996). Current efforts at detecting genes in dyslexia, where separate linkages have been demonstrated to distinct reading tasks (e.g. phonological awareness and single word reading), suggest that this may be a useful approach for detecting genes of moderate effect in genetically heterogeneous, oligogenic disorders (Grigorenko et al., 1996).

The results of this study and those of others that suggest the existence of genetically related cognitive deficits in nonautistic relatives of individuals with autism indicate the need for further detailed studies, employing direct assessment of relatives, to clarify further the range and type of characteristics that define an extended phenotype for this disorder. The results we report, as well as those of future studies of cognitive deficits in relatives, may also provide insights into the fundamental neuropsychological deficits in autism by demonstrating the forme fruste of the disorder in individuals (i.e. nonautistic relatives) unselected for having autism.

REFERENCES

Arthur, G. (1952). *The Arthur Adaptation of the Leiter International Performance Scale.* Chicago, IL: The Psychological Services Press.

August, G. J., Stewart, M. A., & Tsai, L. (1981). The incidence of cognitive disabilities in the siblings of autistic children. *British Journal of Psychiatry, 138,* 416–422.

Bailey, A., Le Couteur, A., Gottesman, I., Bolton, P., Simonoff, E., Yuzda, E., & Rutter, M. (1995). Autism as a strongly genetic disorder: Evidence from a British twin study. *Psychological Medicine, 25,* 63–77.

Bartak, L., Rutter, M., & Cox, A. (1975). A comparative study of infantile autism and specific developmental receptive language disorders. *British Journal of Psychiatry, 126,* 127–145.

Bolton, P., MacDonald, H., Pickles, A., Rios, P., Goode, S., Crowson, M., Bailey, A., & Rutter, M. (1994). A case-control family study of autism. *Journal of Child Psychology and Psychiatry, 35*, 877–990.

Borys, S. V., Spitz, H. H., & Dorans, B. A. (1982). Tower of Hanoi performance of retarded young adults and nonretarded children as a function of solution length and goal state. *Journal of Experimental Child Psychology, 33*, 87–110.

Denckla, M., & Rudel, R. (1976). Naming of object-drawings by dyslexic and other learning disabled children. *Brain Language, 3*, 1–15.

Felton, R., Naylor, C., & Wood, F. (1990). Neuropsychological profile of adult dyslexics. *Brain Language, 39*, 485–497.

Felton, R., & Wood, F. (1989). Cognitive deficits in reading disability and attention deficit disorder. *Journal of Learning Disabilities, 22*, 3–13.

Folstein, S. E., & Rutter, M. L. (1977). Infantile autism: A genetic study of 21 twin pairs. *Journal of Child Psychology and Psychiatry, 18*, 297–321.

Freeman, B. J., Ritvo, E. R., Mason-Brothers, A., Pingree, C., Yokota, A., Jensen, W. R., McMahon, W. M., Petersen, P. B., Mo, A., & Schroth, P. (1989). Psychometric assessment of first-degree relatives of 62 autistic probands in Utah. *American Journal of Psychiatry, 146*, 361–364.

Frith, U., & Snowling, M. (1983). Reading for meaning and reading for sound in autistic and dyslexic children. *British Journal of Developmental Psychology, 1*, 329–342.

Goodman, R. (1989). Infantile autism: A syndrome of multiple primary deficits. *Journal of Autism and Developmental Disorders, 19*, 409–424.

Green, L., Fein, D., Joy, S., & Waterhouse, L. (1995). Cognitive functioning in autism: An overview. In E. Schopler & G. Mesibov (Eds.), *Learning and cognition* (pp. 200–215). New York: Plenum Press.

Grigorenko, E. L., Wood, F. B., Meyer, M. S., Hart, L. A., Speed, W. C., Shuster, A., & Pauls, D. L. (1996). Susceptibility loci for distinct components of developmental dyslexia on chromosomes 6 and 15. *American Journal of Human Genetics, 60*, 27–39.

Hughes, C., Leboyer, M., & Bouvard, M. (1997). Executive function in parents of children with autism. *Psychological Medicine, 27*, 209–220.

Hughes, C., Russell, J., & Robbins, T. W. (1994). Evidence for executive dysfunction in autism. *Neuropsychologica, 32*, 477–492.

Klin, A., Volkmar, F., Sparrow, S., Cichetti, D., & Rourke, B. (1995). Validity and neuropsychological characterization of Asperger syndrome: Convergence with nonverbal learning disabilities syndrome. *Journal of Child Psychology and Psychiatry, 36*, 1127–1140.

Landa, R., Folstein, S., & Issacs, C. (1991). Spontaneous narrative discourse performance of parents of autistic individuals. *Journal of Speech and Hearing Research, 34*, 1339–1345.

Landa, R., Piven, J., Wzorek, M., Gayle, J., Chase, G., & Folstein, S. (1992). Social language use in parents of autistic individuals. *Psychological Medicine, 22*, 245–254.

LeCouteur, A., Rutter, M., Lord, C., Rios, P., Roberson, S., Holdgrafer, M., & McLennan, J. (1989). Autism Diagnostic Interview: A standardized investigator-based instrument. *Journal of Autism and Developmental Disorders, 19*, 363–387.

Lincoln, A. J., Courchesne, E., Kilman, B. A., Elmasian, R., & Allen, M. (1988). A study of intellectual abilities in high-functioning people with autism. *Journal of Autism and Developmental Disorders, 8*, 505–523.

Lord, C., Rutter, M., Goode, S., Heemsbergen, J., Mawhood, L., & Schopler, E. (1989). Autism diagnostic observation schedule: A standardized observation of communicative and social behavior. *Journal of Autism and Developmental Disorders, 19*, 185–212.

Meyer, M., Wood, F., Hart, L., & Felton, R. (in press). Predictive value of rapid automatized naming for later reading. *Journal of Learning Disorders.*

Minshew, N., Goldstein, G., Muenz, L., & Payton, J. (1992). Neuropsychological functioning in nonmentally retarded autistic individuals. *Journal of Clinical and Experimental Neuropsychology, 14*, 749–761.

Minshew, N., Goldstein, G., Taylor, H., & Siegel, D. (1994). Academic achievement in high functioning autistic individuals. *Journal of Clinical and Experimental Neuropsychology, 16*, 261–270.

Minton, J., Campbell, M., Green, W., Jennings, S., & Samit, C. (1982). Cognitive assessment of siblings of autistic children. *Journal of the American Academy of Child and Adolescent Psychiatry, 3*, 256–261.

Office of Population Censuses and Surveys. (1980). *British manual of the classification of occupations.* London: HMSO.

Ozonoff, S., & McEvoy, R. (1994). A longitudinal study of executive function and theory of mind in autism. *Development and Psychopathology, 6*, 415–431.

Ozonoff, S., Pennington, B., & Rogers, S. (1991). Executive function deficits in high functioning autistic individuals: Relationship to theory of mind. *Journal of Child Psychology and Psychiatry, 32*, 1081–1105.

Ozonoff, S., Rogers, S., Farnham, J., & Pennington, B. (1993). Can standard measures identify subclinical markers of autism? *Journal of Autism and Developmental Disorders, 23*, 429–444.

Ozonoff, S., Rogers, S., & Pennington, B. (1991). Asperger's syndrome: Evidence of an empirical distinction from high-functioning autism. *Journal of Child Psychology and Psychiatry, 32*, 1107–1122.

Ozonoff, S., Strayer, D., McMahon, W., & Filloux, F. (1994). Executive function abilities in autism and Tourette syndrome: An information processing approach. *Journal of Child Psychology and Psychiatry, 35*, 1015–1032.

Pauls, D., & Leckman, J. (1986). The inheritance of Gilles de la Tourette Syndrome and associated behaviors. *New England Journal of Medicine, 315*, 993–997.

Piaget, J. (1976). *The grasp of consciousness.* Cambridge, MA: Harvard University Press.

Pennington, B., Van Orden, G., Smith, S., Green, P., & Haith, M. (1990). Phonological processing skills and deficits in adult dyslexics. *Child Development, 61*, 1753–1778.

Pickles, A., Bolton, P., Macdonald, H., Bailey, A., LeCouteur, A., Sim, C.-H., & Rutter, M. (1995). Latent-class analysis of recurrence risks for complex phenotypes with selection and measurement error: A twin and family history study of autism. *American Journal of Human Genetics, 57*, 717–726.

Piven, J., & Folstein, S. (1994). The genetics of autism. In M. L. Bauman & T. L. Kemper (Eds.), *The neurobiology of autism* (pp. 18–44). Baltimore, MD: Johns Hopkins University Press.

Piven, J., Gayle, J., Chase, G., Fink, B., Landa, R., Wzorek, M., & Folstein, S. (1990). A family history study of neuropsychiatric disorders in the adult siblings of autistic individuals. *Journal of the American Academy of Child and Adolescent Psychiatry, 29*, 177–183.

Piven, J., Landa, R., Gayle, J., Cloud, D., Chase, G., & Folstein, S. (1991). Psychiatric disorders in the parents of autistic individuals. *Journal of the American Academy of Child and Adolescent Psychiatry, 30*, 471–478.

Piven, J., Palmer, P., Jacobi, D., Childress, D., & Arndt, S. (1997). The broader autism phenotype: Evidence from a family history study of multiple-incidence autism families. *American Journal of Psychiatry, 154*, 185–190.

Piven, J., Simon, J., Chase, G., Wzorek, M., Landa, R., Gayle, J., & Folstein, S. (1993). The etiology of autism: Pre-, peri- and neonatal factors. *Journal of the American Academy of Child and Adolescent Psychiatry, 32*, 1256–1263.

Piven, J., Wzorek, M., Landa, R., Lainhart, J., Bolton, P., Chase, G. A., & Folstein, S. (1994). Personality characteristics of the parents of autistic individuals. *Psychological Medicine, 24*, 783–795.

Prior, M., & Hoffman, W. (1990). Brief report: Neuropsychological testing of autistic children through an exploration with frontal lobe tests. *Journal of Autism and Developmental Disorders, 20*, 581–590.

Ritvo, E. R., Jorde, L. B., Mason-Brothers, A., Freeman, B. J., Pingree, C., Jones, M. B., McMahon, W. M., Petersen, P. B., Jensen, W. R., & Mo, A. (1989). The UCLA–University of Utah epidemiologic survey of autism: Recurrence risk estimates and genetic counseling. *American Journal of Psychiatry, 146*, 1032–1036.

Rourke, B. (1989). *Nonverbal learning disabilities: The syndrome and the model*, New York: Guilford Press.

Rumsey, J., & Hamburger, S. (1988). Neuropsychological findings in high-functioning men with infantile autism, residual state. *Journal of Clinical and Experimental Neuropsychology, 10*, 201–221.

Rumsey, J. M., Hamburger, S. D. (1990). Neuropsychological divergence of high-level autism and severe dyslexia. *Journal of Autism and Developmental Disorders, 20*, 155–167.

Santangelo, S. L., & Folstein, S. E. (1995). Social deficits in the families of autistic probands. *American Journal of Human Genetics, 57*, Supplement, 89.

Santangelo, S. L., & Folstein, S. E. (1996). An empirical definition of the broader autism phenotype. Abstract. *Psychiatric Genetics, 6*, 156.

Shallice, T. (1982). Specific impairment of planning. In D. E. Broadbent & Weiskrantz (Eds.), *The neuropsychology of cognitive function* (pp. 199–209). London: The Royal Society.

Smalley, S. L., McCracken, J., & Tanguay, P. (1995). Autism, affective disorders, and social phobia. *American Journal of Medical Genetics, Neuropsychiatric Genetics, 60*, 19–26.

Steffenburg, S., Gillberg, C., & Holmgren, L. (1989). A twin study of autism in Denmark, Finland, Iceland, Norway, and Sweden. *Journal of Child Psychology and Psychiatry, 30*, 405–416.

Stutsman, R. (1952). Guide for administering the Merrill–Palmer Scale of Mental Tests. In L. M. Terman (Ed.), *Mental measurement of preschool children* (pp. 78–83). New York: Harcourt, Brace & World.

Szatmari, P., Jones, M. B., Fisman, S., Tuff, L., Bartolucci, G., Mahoney, W. J., & Bryson, S. E. (1995). Parents and collateral relatives of children with pervasive developmental disorders: A family history study. *American Journal of Medical Genetics, 60*, 282–289.

Szatmari, P., Jones, M. B., Tuff, L., Bartolucci, G., Fisman, S., & Mahoney, W. (1993). Lack of cognitive impairment in first-degree relatives of pervasive developmental disorder probands. *Journal of the American Academy of Child and Adolescent Psychiatry, 32*, 1264–1273.

Szatmari, P., Tuff, L., Finlayson, A., & Bartolucci, G. (1990). Asperger's syndrome and autism: Neurocognitive aspects. *Journal of the American Academy of Child and Adolescent Psychiatry, 29*, 130–136.

Volkmar, F., Klin, A., Siegel, B., Szatmari, P., Lord, C., Campbell, M., Freeman, B. J., Cicchetti, D., Rutter, M., Kline, W., Buitelaar, J., Hattab, Y., Fombonne, E., Fuentes, J., Werry, J., Stone, W., Kerbeshian, J., Hoshino, Y., Bregman, J., Loveland, K., Szymanski, L., & Towbin, K. (1994). Field trial for autistic disorder in DSM-IV. *American Journal of Psychiatry*, 151, 1361–1367.

Wechsler, D. (1974). *Wechsler Intelligence Scales for Children–Revised.* New York: Psychological Corporation.

Wechsler, D., (1981). *Wechsler Adult Intelligence Scale–Revised.* New York: Harcourt Brace Jovanovich.

Wechsler, D. (1991). *Wechsler Intelligence Scale for Children–Third Edition.* San Antonio, TX: Psychological Corporation.

Welsh, M. C., Pennington, B. F., & Groisser, D. B. (1991). A normative-developmental study of executive function: A window on prefrontal function in children. *Developmental Neuropsychology, 7*, 131–149.

Welsh, M., Pennington, B., & Rogers, S. (1987). Word recognition and comprehension in hyperlexic children. *Brain Language, 32*, 76–96.

Wolf, M., Bally, H., & Morris, R. (1986). Automaticity, retrieval processes, and reading: A longitudinal study in average and impaired readers. *Child Development, 57*, 988–1000.

Woodcock, R. W., & Johnson, M. (1991). *Woodcock-Johnson Tests of Achievement Psychoeducational Battery-Revised. Form B.* Allen, TX: DLM Teaching Resources.

Woodcock, R. W., & Mathers, N. (1989). WJ-R Tests of Achievement: Examiner's manual. In R. W. Woodcock & M. B. Johnson, *Woodcock-Johnson Psycho-Educational Battery-Revised* (pp. 110–123). Allen, TX: DLM Teaching Resources.

9

Pharmacology of the Selective Serotonin Reuptake Inhibitors in Children and Adolescents

Henrietta L. Leonard
Brown University, Providence, Rhode Island
John March
Duke University Medical Center, Durham, North Carolina
Kenneth C. Rickler
Brown University, Providence, Rhode Island
Albert John Allen
University of Illinois, Chicago, Illinois

Objective: *To review the pharmacology of a new class of medications, the potent selective serotonin reuptake inhibitors (SSRIs), what is known about their metabolism in children and adolescents, and the practical clinical implications of such.* **Method:** *Articles were retrieved through* Index Medicus *searches for articles published during the past 10 years on the SSRIs and on pediatric pharmacology.* **Results:** *More than 300 articles were reviewed. Pharmacological data, derived from relevant adult literature, were summarized and extrapolated to children and from the limited pediatric literature. The SSRIs represent a new class of antidepressants with distinct advantages in their side effect profile and their broad therapeutic index over that seen with the tricyclic antidepressants. Their advantage of few anticholinergic side effects and limited cardiovascular toxicities are particularly relevant for the pediatric population. The SSRIs are metabolized via the hepatic cytochrome isoenzyme P450 system, and potential drug-drug interactions are reviewed.* **Conclusions:** *The SSRIs appear to offer advantages over the tricyclic antidepressants. Unfortunately, pharmacokinetic data are lacking, and systematic studies of safety and efficacy in the pediatric age group are limited. Preliminary reports are encouraging, but further study is required.*

Reprinted with permission from the *Journal of the American Academy of Child and Adolescent Psychiatry*, 1997, Vol. 36(6), 725–736.

The recent introduction of the selective serotonin reuptake inhibitors (SSRIs) has made available an entirely new class of medications with exciting applications and has been a pivotal advance in pharmacotherapy. Despite the similar primary mechanism, the SSRIs differ in their specific pharmacokinetic and pharmacodynamic parameters, which have an impact on the practical issues of prescribing, monitoring, and predicting drug-drug interactions. These differences among the SSRIs are challenging enough when prescribing for adults, but the child psychiatrist must also consider their use in children and adolescents of varying ages, sizes, and pubertal status. The pediatric physician is specifically disadvantaged, since these new medications seemingly offer benefits over older agents, yet there are few pharmacokinetic, efficacy, or safety data for younger age groups.

This report will review the pharmacology of the SSRIs, what is known about their metabolism in children and adolescents, and the practical clinical implications of such.

PHARMACOKINETICS

Inhibition of Serotonin Reuptake: Potency and Selectivity

The SSRIs that are currently available in the United States include fluoxetine (Prozac®), sertraline (Zoloft®), paroxetine (Paxil®), and fluvoxamine (Luvox®). Clomipramine (Anafranil®) is the only tricyclic antidepressant (TCA) that significantly inhibits serotonin reuptake, but it is not selective inasmuch as it also inhibits noradrenergic reuptake; therefore, it is not an SSRI.

The SSRIs were named for their effect of the selective inhibition of serotonin reuptake into the presynaptic terminal, the resultant increase in serotonin concentration at the synaptic cleft, and their limited effect on other monamines. However, these acute effects probably do not explain the therapeutic effects seen several weeks later, which are hypothesized to involve neuroadaptive changes of a specific receptor subtype, perhaps the delayed desensitization of serotonin autoreceptors, and other adaptive changes (Hyman and Nestler, 1996).

The SSRIs with the most potent serotonergic reuptake inhibition are (in order of decreasing potency) paroxetine, fluvoxamine, sertraline, clomipramine, and fluoxetine (Tulloch and Johnson, 1992). However, it is not necessarily true that "more is better," as more potency has not been shown to correlate directly with clinical antidepressant and antiobsessional efficacy.

Although very selective for serotonin, at higher dosages all the SSRIs will inhibit the reuptake of norepinephrine and to a smaller degree dopamine. Paroxetine is more selective (noradrenaline-to-serotonin reuptake ratio) than sertraline, fluvoxamine, fluoxetine, and clomipramine (descending order) (Nemeroff, 1993; Tulloch and Johnson, 1992). Unlike the others, sertraline has more reuptake inhibition of dopamine than of norepinephrine (Koe, 1990; Tulloch and Johnson, 1992). Although the selectivity profile between the SSRIs has not been found to be related to the clinical efficacy, it may affect potential side effects and drug interactions. Unlike the TCAs, the SSRIs have a low affinity for cholinergic, noradrenergic, and histaminic receptors; thus they cause relatively few such adverse effects (e.g., anticholinergic, postural hypotension, and sedation), which is a distinct advantage of this class (Warrington, 1992).

METABOLISM

Developmental Issues for the Pediatric Population

Much less is known about the pharmacokinetics of psychotropic medications in children than in adults. Generally, drug response may vary with age, weight, sex, disease state, absorption, distribution, metabolism, and excretion; thus developmental factors that influence these are important to consider.

Although the extent of drug absorption for most medications is similar in children and adults, the rate of absorption may be faster in children, and peak levels are reached earlier (Bourin et al., 1992). This should be of less conern for drugs with long absorption times, such as the SSRIs. In addition, absorption is dependent on how the drug is compounded (thus it may differ among manufacturers) as well as the form in which the drug is administered (i.e., liquid versus tablet).

All of the SSRIs are metabolized primarily in the liver. Generally speaking, hepatic metabolism is highest during infancy and childhood (1 to 6 years), approximately twice the adult rate in prepuberty (6 to 10 years), and equivalent to adult values by age 15 (Bourin et al., 1992). This is clinically important, as younger children may require higher milligram-per-kilogram dosages of hepatically metabolized medications than older children or adults (Wilens et al., 1992). In addition, a transient decrease in metabolism for some medications has been reported in the few months before puberty, which is believed to be due to the competition for hepatic enzymes with sex hormones (Hughes and Preskorn, 1989). The association among serum levels, clinical response, and side effects is not well studied, and studies are needed to determine maturationally related changes of bioavailability, metabolism, and clearance.

Protein binding and volume of distribution affect the pharmacokinetics of medications. These parameters differ somewhat between children and adults and have practical clinical implications, such as the fraction of drug that is active (unbound) (Paxton and Dragunow, 1993). Change in protein binding or the volume of distribution, whether due to illness or concomitant medications, could potentially lead to change in plasma drug concentrations and toxicity.

Fat distribution varies across childhood, rising during year 1, then gradually falling until puberty, and increasing with obesity. Substantial fat stores slow elimination of highly liposoluble drugs from the body. With fluoxetine, for example, this property has been labeled as both a disadvantage (because of long-lasting side effects) and an advantage (because of lower likelihood of immediate relapse), and this may need to be considered in individual patients.

T_{max} *in the General Population*

The time that it takes to reach maximum concentration in the blood (T_{max}) may prove particularly clinically important when interpreting side effects. The SSRIs have a longer T_{max} (4 to 8 hours) compared with clomipramine. Side effects reported shortly after ingestion (i.e., nausea) would more likely be mediated by difficulties with gastric absorption than by central biochemical mechanisms (Preskorn, 1993), whereas sedation or stimulation seen 4 to 8 hours after dosage would most likely be explained by central effects and might warrant changing the time of the dosage (Preskorn, 1993). However, because of the long half-life of fluoxetine and its metabolite, changing the time of dosage to minimize side effects may not prove helpful, as there is little change in plasma drug concentration after each dose (Preskorn, 1993).

Active Metabolites and Half-Life

It is important to consider the clinical activity and the half-life of the parent compound and its metabolites. In some cases, a metabolite may be equipotent but have different pharmacokinetics. For example, if the metabolite were clinically active and had a long half-life (i.e., such as norfluoxetine), it would take a long time to reach steady state and to wash out the medication. Thus, the extended half-life of parent and metabolite compounds needs to be considered in titrating dose, interpreting side effects, and evaluating its effect on metabolism of other drugs.

Norfluoxetine, the primary metabolite of fluoxetine, is at least as potent an inhibitor of serotonin as its parent compound (Stokes, 1993). Norfluoxetine has a very long half-life (up to 15 days) in adults. Fluoxetine, the parent compound, also has a long half-life (1 to 4) days compared with other SSRIs (DeVane, 1992; Strokes, 1993). It takes several weeks for steady concentration to be reached, and fluoxetine remains in the system for up to 6 to 8 weeks after discontinuation (DeVane, 1992). This is important to consider, particularly if another medication is initiated in this time interval.

Paroxetine's metabolites appear to lack the ability to inhibit serotonin and monoamine reuptake (DeVane, 1992). The half-life of the parent compound has been reported to be about 24 hours in adult studies, but there is great interindividual variability. Steady state is achieved in about 7 to 14 days in adults (Nemeroff, 1993). With a short half-life of the parent compound and a clinically inactive metabolite, its presence after discontinuation is short-lived and could potentially make switching to another medication easier, although there may be an increased risk for a withdrawal syndrome in SSRIs with a relatively short half-life for the parent compound and a clinically inactive metabolite (Barr et al., 1994).

Desmethylsertraline, the principal metabolite of sertraline, has a long half-life compared with the parent compound (66 versus 24 hours in adult studies). The metabolite is 5 to 10 times less potent than sertraline and is not believed to produce clinically significant pharmacological effects (Heym and Koe, 1988; Nemeroff, 1993). Steady state is reached in about 7 days.

The metabolites of fluvoxamine have not been reported to be active (DeVane, 1992). In adult studies, the half-life of the parent compound is about 12 to 24 hours and steady state is reached in about 10 days (Palmer and Benfield, 1994).

Dose-Plasma Concentrations

Fluoxetine and paroxetine can inhibit their own metabolism; consequently, their half-lives lengthen with increased dosage (Preskorn, 1993). This inhibition of their own metabolism will be reflected in a nonlinear relationship between dose and plasma concentration; an increase in dosage will result in a disproportionate (nonlinear) increase in plasma concentration and side effects (Preskorn, 1993). In contrast, this does not appear to be true for sertraline or fluvoxamine (at usual therapeutic dosages), and they exhibit a linear relationship (Heym and Koe, 1988; Preskorn, 1993).

Dose-Response Curve

The highest dosage may not always impart a greater therapeutic response, and adaptive changes to long-term therapy (weeks and months), rather than the immediate effects on serotonin reuptake, may be responsible for eventual clinical response (Hyman and Nestler, 1996). Fluoxetine, paroxetine, sertraline, and fluvoxamine have a flat dose-response curve, suggesting that maximal clinical response usually is achieved at the minimum effective dose (Altamura et al., 1988; Dunner and Dunbar, 1992; Murdoch and McTavish, 1992; Palmer and Benfield, 1994). Generally speaking, allowing adequate time to obtain a clinical response is preferable to increasing dosage in order to avoid excessive side effects.

Metabolism and Cytochrome P450

Most of the psychotropic medications are metabolized by, or inhibit, at least one of the hepatic cytochrome P450 isoenzymes, of which more than 30 enzymes have been identified (Nemeroff et al., 1996). Identifying the substrates and inhibitors of the P450 isoenzymes is critical to understanding potential drug interactions. The SSRIs are metabolized by the cytochrome P450 system, and they are also potent inhibitors of several different isoenzymes (Nemeroff et al., 1996). In addition, some of the cytochrome P450 isoenzymes are subject to genetic polymorphism, which will result in significant variations in metabolism between individuals.

Cytochrome P450-2D6, one of the subfamilies of enzymes, has received significant attention as it is involved in the metabolism of the majority of psychotropics, including all of the SSRIs. Five percent to 10% of the Caucasian population are "slow" or "poor metabolizers" and are thought to have a deficiency in the cytochrome P450-2D6 isoenzyme activity, as a result of a specific genetic variant (Coutts, 1994). Slow metabolizers are found in other populations, but slow metabolism has not been well studied in other ethnic groups (Coutts, 1994; Shimoda et al., 1993). Slow metabolizers are at risk for developing toxic side effects, at what would normally be therapeutic dosages, because the prolonged elimination half-life and greater bioavailability result in higher plasma concentrations (von Moltke et al., 1994). Thus, they require much lower dosages than would be normally expected. Although slow metabolizers can be identified by metabolic probe studies and confirmed by genetic testing (Coutts, 1994), the diagnosis should be considered for any individual with significant side effects and/or an unusually high plasma level for the dosage. (Of note, "rapid metabolizers" are a variant of normal and are not thought to represent a genetic polymorphism.) A "normal" ("extensive") metabolizer may essentially be converted to a "poor metabolizer" (not a true genetic polymorphism) when medications that inhibit the P450-2D6 system are coadministered with those that are metabolized by P450-2D6.

Clinically, all patients should be treated as if they were poor metabolizers, when two such medications are prescribed.

Three other subfamilies (P450-1A2, 2C, 3A4) have been well described, and medications that are metabolized by and inhibit them are detailed subsequently. Genetic polymorphisms have been determined for P450-2C, but not for P450-1A2 or 3A4 (Nemeroff et al., 1996). Further study is needed for in vivo interaction studies and ex vivo inhibition studies to predict significant drug interactions (Nemeroff et al., 1996).

CLINICAL IMPLICATIONS

Drug Interactions

With increasing knowledge about the potential for drug-drug interactions, and with limited information about the unique vulnerabilities of children, caution should be exercised in prescribing concomitant medications. Several factors increase the possibility of clinically significant drug-drug interactions; these include drugs (1) that induce or inhibit hepatic microsomal enzymes, (2) that have a low therapeutic index, (3) that have multiple pharmacological actions, and (4) that may be metabolized differently by high-risk populations (Callahan et al., 1993). Agents with a narrow therapeutic window and for which high levels have significant adverse reactions merit special consideration, such as the type IC antiarrhythmics and the TCAs.

It should be noted that each SSRI has its own individual pattern of metabolism and inhibition, and often more than one system is involved. There is potentially an interaction between any medication metabolized by a P450 enzyme and another that inhibits that enzyme. The potential for interaction needs to be considered individually for each medication.

2D6. The cytochrome P450-2D6 metabolizes many different agents, including antidepressants (desipramine, nortriptyline, clomipramine, fluoxetine, paroxetine, sertraline, and venlafaxine), some antipsychottic agents (perphenazine and thioridazine), type IC antiarrhythmic agents, β-adrenergic–blocking agents, codeine, and dextromethorphan (Coutts, 1994; Nemeroff et al., 1996; von Moltke et al., 1994). Medications that inhibit cytochrome P450-2D6 include all of the SSRIs (except fluvoxamine), some antipsychotics (fluphenazine, haloperidol, and thioridazine), and some TCAs (amitriptyline, desipramine, and clomipramine) (Nemeroff et al., 1996). For example, two cases of children with near-toxic levels of imipramine when taken concomitantly with propranolol were reported, and the authors concluded that competitive inhibition resulted in the decreased clearance and a prolonged half-life (Gillette and Tannery, 1994).

Fluoxetine, paroxetine, and sertraline can potentially inhibit the metabolism of one another, as well as other medications metabolized by this system (Crewe et al., 1992). Potentially significant drug interactions may be seen with the administration of fluoxetine, sertraline, or paroxetine, with TCAs, some antipsychotics, and type IC antiarrhythmics. There are numerous case reports, in both children and adults, of increased plasma concentrations and potential toxicity when combining an SSRI and a TCA, as well as combining an SSRI with another SSRI. Concomitant use of a TCA and fluoxetine or sertraline has resulted in 2- to 10-fold increase in TCA levels (Brosen et al., 1993; Lydiard et al., 1993; March et al.,

1990; Maskall and Lam, 1993; Preskorn et al., 1994), so this requires careful monitoring, including of plasma TCA levels and electrocardiograms (ECGs).
1A2. Unlike the other SSRIs, fluvoxamine is a potent inhibitor of cytochrome P450-1A2 subfamily. Coadministration of fluvoxamine with agents metabolized by the 1A2 system (amitriptyline, clomipramine, clozapine, haloperidol, imipramine, or theophylline), may lead to elevated plasma levels of the other agent (Brosen et al., 1993; Nemeroff et al., 1996; Sperber, 1991).
2C. Fluoxetine, sertraline, and fluvoxamine may inhibit cytochrome P450-2C isoenzymes, and therefore they might interfere with the metabolism of agents metabolized by that system (amitriptyline, diazepam, imipramine, phenytoin, tolbutamide, and warfarin) (Nemeroff et al., 1996; Perucca et al., 1994; Shader et al., 1994; Skjelbo and Brosen, 1992).
3A4. This 3A subfamily is involved in the biotransformation of several benzodiazepines (alprazolam, triazolam, and midazolam), carbamazepine, clomipramine, erythromycin, lidocaine, and the antihistamines terfenadine (Seldane®) and astemizole (Hismanal®) (Nemeroff et al., 1996; von Moltke et al., 1994). In vitro studies suggest that all the SSRIs inhibit the P450-3A3 system, although clinical reports exist for concomitant treatment with fluvoxamine, fluoxetine, and sertraline (Fleishaker and Hulst, 1994; Joblin, 1994; Nemeroff et al., 1996; Pearson, 1990). Thus, caution should be used when administering the SSRIs with any of the above agents.

Coadministration of terfenadine with either ketoconazole or erythromycin has been reported to cause cardiac conduction abnormalities, and even fatal arrhythmias (Honig et al., 1992, 1993). Acute distress (shortness of breath, irregular heart rate, and orthostasis) developed in an adult who was taking fluoxetine and terfenadine (Swims, 1993); the author suggested that a similar risk may exist for the SSRIs. Combined use of astemizole or terfenadine with either fluvoxamine or nefazodone is contraindicated (prescribing information for fluvoxamine and nefazodone, 1996), and this concern may exist for other SSRIs, particularly fluoxetine. Conservative practice would suggest that an SSRI should not be prescribed within 2 months of astemizole and within 1 week of terfenadine treatment and that their concurrent use should be avoided.

It is incumbent on the prescribing physician to inquire about all prescription drugs, over-the-counter medications, and illicit drugs that the patient may be taking, to avoid potentially toxic combinations. One adolescent taking phenylpropanolamine (as an appetite suppressant) and fluoxetine (20 mg/day) experienced dizziness, "hyper" feelings, and palpitations (Walters, 1992). Visual hallucinations have been reported in an adult when fluoxetine and dextromethorphan were combined (Achamallah, 1992). A 21-year-old student who was taking fluoxetine 20 mg/day experienced mania with psychosis after smoking marijuana over a 36-hour period. The authors cautioned that this is a potentially hazardous interaction and hypothesized that marijuana may potentiate the action of fluoxetine at central serotonergic neurons (Stoll et al., 1991).

Therapeutic Drug Monitoring and Protein Binding

The extent of protein binding is a factor that should be considered when prescribing concomitant medications. The plasma protein binding of fluvoxamine is low (77%); thus displacement drug interactions are not likely. In contrast, fluoxetine, sertraline, and paroxetine are all highly bound (>95%), and they can displace other bound drugs from protein sites, so interactions can potentially occur. The extent of protein binding is particularly important if the coadministered drug is highly protein bound and has a low therapeutic index (i.e., valproic acid, phenytoin, warfarin) (Callahan et al., 1993). This process has not been well studied, but it should be considered when another medication is added, as dosage changes may be required.

Understanding the extent of protein binding is relevant to interpreting plasma drug levels. Plasma levels measure total (bound and unbound) drug; if there were high protein binding, active (unbound) drug might actually be a small fraction of the total. Plasma levels are not routinely obtained or typically used in the therapeutic monitoring of the SSRIs. Plasma levels are provided by laboratories, but their relationship to side effects and efficacy is not well studied. One might consider obtaining an SSRI and other plasma level in a child if there were a specific concern about concomitant medications or toxicity or to consider the issue of "slow (although this would not be diagnostic).

Hematology and chemistry testing is not routinely ordered for children who are receiving the SSRIs, and it would be ordered only if there were a specific medical concern.

ADVERSE REACTIONS

General Side Effects

The SSRIs offer the advantage of having fewer anticholinergic and antihistaminic side effects, in comparison with those seen with the TCAs. For example, pediatric clomipramine treatment trials reported the expected anticholinergic and antihistaminic side effect profile seen with a TCA. The most common side effects reported include (in order of decreasing frequency): dry mouth, somnolence, dizziness, fatigue, tremor, headache, constipation, anorexia, abdominal pain, dyspepsia, and insomnia (Leonard et al., 1989). Patients seemed most concerned by the annoyance of a dry mouth, the tremors interfering with writing, and the idiosyncratic combination of daytime sedation and nighttime (middle) insomnia.

Generally speaking, the SSRI side effect profile of fewer anticholinergic effects, less sedation, less weight gain, and fewer ECG changes, in comparison with the TCAs, seems to offer advantages. However, the SSRIs may not actually be associated with fewer side effects. In meta-analyses of studies of adults taking TCAs or SSRIs, dropout rates owing to adverse reactions were not significantly different between the two groups (Song et al., 1993). The most common side effects reported in association with the SSRIs include gastrointestinal difficulties (nausea, diarrhea, vomiting), CNS effects (agitation, disinhibition, jitteriness, headache, insomnia), and tremor. Rates of side effects differ among the individual SSRIs, although large, direct-comparison trials have not been done. In addition, differences between the rates of specific side effects experienced by adults, in comparison with those experienced by children and adolescents, have not been determined.

The common adverse effects reported for fluoxetine from adult studies include complaints of nausea, headache, nervousness, agitation, insomnia, diarrhea, anorexia, dizziness, tremor, and drowsiness (Stokes, 1993). In the limited pediatric trials of fluoxetine, it has been generally well tolerated, with side effects similar to those in adults; gastrointestinal upset, insomnia, and behavioral activation have been reported (Birmaher et al., 1994; Dummit et al., 1996; Geller et al., 1995; Jain et al., 1993; Riddle et al., 1992). Of specific note, behavioral activation and agitation are reported across the studies; it is not clear whether there is an increased risk for this in the younger ages, but it remains of concern. Motor restlessness and insomnia were reported in half of the patients in one study, although dosages were initiated at 20 to 40 mg/day (Riddle et al., 1991). In a retrospective chart review, 21% (8 of 38) of the children and adolescents experienced behavioral activation/dyscontrol during treatment, although 39% (15 of 38) had no side effects (Geller et al., 1995). As a matter of caution, children should be started at a low dosage, with the dosage increased slowly. In particular, with the long-half life of fluoxetine and its primary metabolite, side effects may not be experienced for several weeks.

In adults, sertraline's side effect profile is reported to include nausea, headache, diarrhea/loose stools, dry mouth, insomnia, sexual dysfunction (male), somnolence, dizziness, tremor, and fatigue (Murdoch and McTavish, 1992). From limited clinical experience with sertraline in children and adolescents, similar side effects have been noted, with gastrointestinal distress (stomachache, loose stools, gas) and mild sedation being the most common. Despite the limited, although increasing, pediatric experience, sertraline is frequently prescribed when a less activating SSRI is sought, although direct comparisons have not been done. In general, it appears to be well tolerated and may be a particularly logical choice if daytime agitation and/or nighttime insomnia is a complaint prior to initiating medication or if concomitant medications would suggest a likelihood of competitive inhibition.

Paroxetine's side effect profile in adults is reported to include nausea, tiredness, dry mouth, headache, asthenia, constipation, dizziness, and insomnia (Dunbar, 1989). In general, it appears to be somewhat similar to the profile seen with sertraline. Although systematic studies in children and adolescents are ongoing, there are none for review, and there is less anecdotal experience from which to draw.

Fluvoxamine's side effect profile in adults has been reported to include nausea, somnolence, asthenia, headache, dry mouth, insomnia, and abdominal pain (Palmer and Benfield, 1994). In a general sense, its side effect profile falls between that of clomipramine (most sedating) and fluoxetine (most activating). In a systematic pediatric trial (ages 8 to 17 years) for obsessive-compulsive disorder (OCD), it was generally well tolerated, with insomnia, agitation, hyperkinesia, somnolence, and dyspepsia being the most commonly reported side effects (Apter et al., 1994; Riddle et al., 1996).

Cardiovascular Effects

There are fewer cardiovascular concerns with the SSRIs, which is one of their major advantages over the TCAs in the pediatric age group. The literature on cardiovascular effects of TCAs in children has reported the "quinidine-like" effect, which can result in slower intracardiac conduction and increased heart rate (Bartels et al., 1991). No clinically significant ECG changes have been reported in several SSRI trials in adults; specifically, they do not appear to be associated with conduction abnormalities, anticholinergic effects, or changes in blood pressure or pulse (Fisch, 1985; Nemeroff, 1993; Palmer and Benfield, 1994).

The coadministration of an SSRI with other pharmacological agents merits specific consideration. Significant bradycardia developed in several adults receiving fluoxetine combined with either pimozide (Ahmed et al., 1993), clonazepam (Feder, 1991), or a β-adrenergic blocker (Walley et al., 1993). In one report, the authors hypothesized that bradycardia may have been due to fluoxetine inhibiting the metabolism of the lipophilic β-blockers, since when a hydrophilic β-blocker (sotalol) was used, it did not recur (Walley et al., 1993). A 9-year-old boy with a preexisting shifting cardiac pacemaker tolerated fluoxetine (5 mg/day) without bradycardia or ECG changes (Edleman et al., 1994). Thus, fluoxetine and the other SSRIs appear to have cardiovascular advantages over the TCAs, but periodic monitoring of vital signs, particularly if the child is taking combinations of medications, would be the conservative management (Edleman et al., 1994).

Neurological Side Effects

Headache. Headaches are commonly reported as a side effect of treatment with all the SSRIs, with an incidence up to 15% (Stokes, 1993). The literature does not distinguish between new-onset headaches and exacerbation of previously established headache syndromes. Exacerbation of preexisting migraine headaches has been reported during initiation and discontinuation of clomipramine therapy (Leonard et al., 1991). Practically speaking, a clinician should inquire into a family and personal history of migraines before initiating SSRI therapy and should consider a lower initial dosage for those with such a history.

Seizures. The SSRIs are less likely to lower the seizure threshold than are the TCAs, which is one of their advantages. Although there are rare case reports of an adult having a seizure while being treated with an SSRI, most were taking a concurrent medication, which may have increased plasma level (Prasher, 1993). Thus, patients with a previous seizure, underlying neurological vulnerability, or concomitant medications prescribed should receive consideration for this issue.

Serotonin syndrome. A "serotonin syndrome" with symptoms ranging from fever and myoclonus to confusion, hyperthermia, rigidity, tachycardia, hypotension, coma, and, in its most severe form, death (Sternbach, 1991) has been reported in adults taking either fluoxetine or sertraline combined with either a monoamine oxidase inhibitor (MAOI) or L-tryptophan (an amino acid supplement) (Ciraulo and Shader, 1990; Steiner and Fontaine, 1986). It is not known whether a family history of antidepressant-induced myoclonus may increase one's risk (Lejoyeux et al., 1992).

Thus, none of the SSRIs should be combined with an MAOI or L-tryptophan in children or adolescents. One might be cautious if combining an SSRI with other serotonergic agents, although this combination has not been well studied. Initiation of an MAOI after fluoxetine therapy should be done only after a long wash-out period (5 to 8 weeks) and after plasma fluoxetine and norfluoxetine levels are either low or no longer present.

Movement disorders. Extrapyramidal symptoms (EPS), including akathisia, parkinsonism, dyskinesia, and dystonia, are potential adverse reactions for patients taking any of the SSRIs, and they are probably underrecognized (Choo, 1993; Coulter and Pillans, 1995; George and Trimble, 1993; Shihabuddin and Rapport, 1994). Although EPS can occur on an SSRI alone, the risk is increased by concomitant administration with a dopamine-blocking agent, either by direct action of either medication or by increased drug levels via metabolic competitive inhibition (Coulter and Pillans, 1995; Ketai, 1993).

There is no evidence that children are more vulnerable to developing EPS while receiving SSRI therapy, and there are numerous case reports of such occurring. A 12-year-old girl who had no prior exposure to neuroleptic medication had acute dystonia on her third day of fluoxetine therapy, after recently discontinuing nortriptyline therapy and illicit amphetamine abuse (Jones-Fearing, 1996). A 9-year-old with Tourette's syndrome had an acute oculogyric crisis while taking paroxetine and pimozide (Horrigan and Barnhill, 1994), and a 11-year-old with Tourette's syndrome experienced acute dystonia while taking paroxetine and haloperidol (Budman et al., 1995). In conclusion, clinicians should assess patients for EPS at baseline and during SSRI therapy, and particular consideration should be made when prescribing an SSRI with a dopamine-blocking agent.

Fluoxetine is generally well tolerated, and frequently prescribed, in children and adolescents with tic disorders (Birmaher et al., 1994; Riddle et al., 1992). Only three cases of tics developing in patients taking fluoxetine were located, and two of these patients were receiving concomitant medications (Cunningham et al., 1990). In an atypical case, a 12-year-old boy with "some anxiety and a rigid personality" developed motor tics 6 months after being treated with fluoxetine (20 mg/day) as the sole medication (Eisenhauer and Jermain, 1993); other causative agents must also be considered. A 37-year-old man with Tourette's syndrome experienced marked worsening of his tics while taking fluoxetine, and fluoxetine was discontinued (Gatto et al., 1994).

Similarly, other SSRIs have also been implicated. A 14-year-boy with OCD (and no history of tics) had an abrupt onset of tics during treatment with loxapine (40 mg/day) and fluvoxamine (75 mg/day) (Fennig et al., 1994). Coadministration of medications may increase the risk, and further study is needed.

Neuropsychiatric/Behavioral Effects

Initial worsening of symptoms. The development of anxiety, restlessness, and agitation while taking antidepressants (including the SSRIs) has been described as "part of the complex and poorly self-described syndrome of akathisia" (Kalda, 1993). The "jitteriness syndrome," characterized by excess energy, irritability, restlessness, shakiness, agitation, and restless legs, has also been described (Pohl et al., 1988). Although the distinction between the phenomena is not entirely clear, "jitteriness syndrome" is most frequently described in the first 10 days of a medication trial for patients with panic disorder, after which it resolves (Pohl et al., 1988). Similarly, some patients with OCD may experience a worsening of their obsessive-compulsive symptoms in the initial 10 days of an SSRI trial. Typically, the exacerbation subsides and a positive clinical response ensues.

There is a behavioral activation, which is described differently among reports as akathisia, jitteriness, disinhibition, activation, or agitation, and it may represent different phenomena. This is an area of specific concern for children, as some studies report motor restlessness in nearly half of patients (Riddle et al., 1991) and excitement/disinhibition in 20% of patients (Dummit et al., 1996; Geller et al., 1995).

Mania. Mania and hypomania can result from treatment with any of the antidepressants, including the SSRIs (Dorevitch et al., 1993). There are reports of at least nine cases of children or adolescents in whom mania developed during fluoxetine therapy; some had a family history of affective disorder (Achamallah and Decker, 1991; Hersh et al., 1991; Jafri and Greenberg, 1991; Jerome, 1991; Venkataraman et al., 1992). Similarly, there are four case reports of mania in children or adolescents receiving sertraline (Ghaziuddin, 1994; Heimann and March, 1996; Kat, 1996). In conclusion, children and adolescents receiving SSRI therapy should be monitored for the development of hypomanic or manic symptoms, as studies attempt to delineate other risk factors.

Apathy and frontal lobe syndromes. A frontal lobe syndrome characterized by apathy, indifference, loss of initiative, and/or disinhibition has developed in some adults during SSRI therapy (Hoehn-Saric et al., 1990). In each case, the patient had a significant change in behavior, which included becoming indifferent toward work performance, exhibiting impulsive and disinhibited behavior, or developing poor concentration and forgetful behavior (Hoehn-Saric et al., 1991).

Although a frontal lobe syndrome may be rare, it is important to consider, as its symptoms could be easily misinterpreted. Apathy and indifference could be mistakenly attributed to depressive symptoms or sedation; impaired judgment and disinhibition could be attributed to hypomania-induced behavior. Although this has not been specifically described in the pediatric population, it merits consideration.

Self-injurious behavior. Since the initial report of six adults who experienced intense suicidal ideation during fluoxetine therapy (Teicher et al., 1990), the issue of a possible association has drawn interest and concern. However, the cause-and-effect relationship of this reported association is uncertain, as studies of the incidence of suicidal ideation and self-harm among patients receiving fluoxetine did not find an increase (Beasley et al., 1991).

There have been several case reports of suicidal ideation or self-injurious behavior (SIB) in children and adolescents during fluoxetine treatment. King and colleagues (1991) reported six cases of patients, aged 10 to 17 years, whose self-injurious ideation or behavior developed de novo, or intensified, during fluoxetine pharmacotherapy for OCD. The cases are varied and complex; onset of SIB ranged from weeks to 7 months, comorbidity was common, and three of the children had previously attempted suicide. The SIB ranged from bumping into things or pinching oneself, to marked suicidal behavior with suicide attempts. The relationship between medication and SIB is not clear, and the SSRIs are actually used to treat SIB. However, the development of or exacerbation of SIB would require assessment.

Memory impairment. Memory impairment was reported in a 20-year-old student with an eating disorder and OCD who was taking fluoxetine 60 mg/day and rivotril 1 mg at bedtime (rivotril is a benzodiazepine not available in the United States) (Bradley, 1993). The impairment in retaining information resolved after discontinuation of medication and did not recur when fluoxetine treatment was reinitiated at a lower dosage. It is not known whether this was due directly to one of the medications, or a combination thereof, since fluoxetine can increase benzodiazepine levels.

Sleep. All the SSRIs potentially can alter sleep architecture and decrease sleep efficiency, which may manifest as daytime sedation or impaired performance and/or as nighttime insomnia (Winokur and Reynolds, 1994). In addition, a change in sleep architecture can also be due to an undiagnosed, preexisting sleep disorder, which is often not considered in children, as well as due to the psychiatric illness itself, which is associated with sleep disturbances (Reynolds and Kupfer, 1987).

Fluoxetine, the most extensively studied SSRI, has been reported to decrease total sleep time and duration of rapid eye movement (REM) sleep and to increase awake activity and stage 1 (drowsy) sleep (Nicholson and Pascoe, 1988). Similar findings have been reported with paroxetine (Saletu et al., 1991) and sertraline (Winokur et al., 1991), but how the individual SSRIs differ from one another remains to be clarified. Thus, even if a patient has described a full night of sleep, the clinician should consider that daytime sedation or impaired concentration could be secondary to decreased nighttime sleep efficiency.

WITHDRAWAL SYNDROMES AND OVERDOSE TOXICITY

Overdose Toxicity

One of the major advantages of the SSRIs is their lack of serious systemic toxicity and their wide therapeutic index. A review of overdoses of fluoxetine concluded that they are usually without serious cardiovascular or neurological complication, and deaths caused solely by fluoxetine overdose are extremely rare (Stokes, 1993). In fact, one adult recovered without sequelae after taking 3,000 mg of fluoxetine (Stokes, 1993). A review of fluvoxamine overdoses in 171 adults noted that other agents were also taken in the majority of cases and that acute toxicity was rarely severe (Garnier et al., 1993). No deaths have been attributed to overdose with paroxetine or sertraline alone (Nemeroff, 1993).

There is limited information available about overdoses in the younger population. Riddle and colleagues (1989) reported the case of a 13-year-old boy who ingested ninety-four 20-mg capsules of fluoxetine and was treated with ipecac 45 to 75 minutes after ingestion. Subsequently, he had a generalized tonic-clonic seizure and ECG changes (ST depression), all of which resolved within a few days. Although the margin of safety for fluoxetine may be better than that for the TCAs, fluoxetine and its metabolites are not eliminated quickly (even with dialysis) because of their high protein binding.

Withdrawal Syndromes

Abrupt discontinuation of TCAs has been reported to result in a cholinergic rebound syndrome characterized by gastrointestinal disturbances, headache, malaise, and insomnia (Dilsaver and Greden, 1984). Unlike the TCAs, fluoxetine does not appear to have a withdrawal syndrome, and because of its long half-life there is no recommendation to taper (Stokes, 1993). Sertraline, paroxetine, and fluvoxamine do not have long halflives, and thus they should not be stopped abruptly (Barr et al., 1994; Black et al., 1993). Although there is little information about the discontinuation of SSRIs in children, it would seem prudent to taper them off these medications, as well.

Toxicity in Pre-, Peri-, and Postnatal Period

Prescribing medications to pregnant and lactating women raises issues to consider for the baby pre- and postnatally. The SSRIs are transferred across the placenta because of their high lipid solubility (Spencer, 1993), and they are transferred through lactation (Burch and Wells, 1992), although less than from transplacental transfer. Much study is needed in this area, and the reader is directed to several recent reports (Altshuler et al., 1996; Chambers et al., 1996).

CONCLUSION

The SSRIs offer a different pharmacological profile from TCAs and have distinct advantages with fewer anticholinergic side effects, limited cardiovascular toxicities, and wide therapeutic index. However, they do have a distinct pattern of adverse reactions characterized by gastrointestinal and CNS effects. It is not known whether this rate is increased in the pediatric age group. In addition, the increased potential for drug-drug interaction necessitates that the physician be cognizant of their pharmacology. Further study of their pharmacokinetics, pharmacodynamics, efficacy, and safety in the pediatric ages is necessary.

REFERENCES

Achamallah NS (1992), Visual hallucinations after combining fluoxetine and dextromethorphan (letter). *Am J Psychiatry* 149:1406

Achamallah NS, Decker DH (1991), Mania induced by fluoxetine in an adolescent patient. *Am J Psychiatry* 148:1404

Ahmed I, Dagincourt PG, Miller LG, Shader RI (1993), Possible interaction between fluoxetine and pimozide causing sinus bradycardia. *Can J Psychiatry* 38:62–63

Altamura AC, Montgomery SA, Wernicke JF (1988), The evidence for 20 mg a day of fluoxetine as the optimal dose in the treatment of depression. *Br J Psychiatry* 53 (suppl 3):109–112

Altshuler LL, Cohen L, Szuba MP, Burt VK, Gitlin M, Mintz J (1996), Pharmacologic management of psychiatric illness during pregnancy: dilemmas and guidelines. *Am J Psychiatry* 153:592–606

Apter A, Ratzoni G, King RA et al. (1994), Fluvoxamine open-label treatment of adolescent inpatients with OCD or depression. *J Am Acad Child Adolesc Psychiatry* 33:342–348

Barr LC, Goodman WK, Price L (1994), Physical symptoms associated with paroxetine discontinuation (letter). *Am J Psychiatry* 151:289

Bartels MG, Varley CK, Mitchell J, Stamm SJ (1991), Pediatric cardiovascular effects of imipramine and desipramine. *J Am Acad Child Adolesc Psychiatry* 30:100–103

Beasley CM, Dornseif BE, Bosomworth JC et al. (1991), Fluoxetine and suicide: a meta-analysis of controlled trials of treatment of depression. *Br Med J* 303:685–691

Birmaher B, Waterman GS, Ryan N et al. (1994), Fluoxetine for childhood anxiety disorders. *J Am Acad Child Adolesc Psychiatry* 33:993–999

Black DW, Wesner R, Gabel J (1993), Abrupt discontinuation of fluvoxamine in patients with panic disorder. *J Clin Psychiatry* 54:146–149

Bourin M, Couetoux D, Tertre A (1992), Pharmacokinetics of psychotropic drugs in children. *Clin Neuropharmacol* 15 (suppl): 114–225

Bradley SJ (1993), Fluoxetine and memory impairment. *J Am Acad Child Adolesc Psychiatry* 32:1078–1079

Brosen K, Hansen JG, Nielsen KK, Sindrup SH, Gram LF (1993), Inhibition by paroxetine of desipramine metabolism in extensive but not in poor metabolizers of sparteine. *Eur J Clin Pharmacol* 44:349–355

Brosen K, Skjelbo E, Rasmussen BB, Pousen HE, Loft S (1993), Fluvoxamine is a potent inhibitor of cytochrome P4501A2. *Biochem Pharmacol* 45:1211–1214

Budman CL, Sherlin M, Bruun RD (1995), Combined pharmacotherapy risk (letter). *J Am Acad Child Adolesc Psychiatry* 34:263–264

Burch KJ, Wells BG (1992), Fluoxetine/norfluoxetine concentrations in human milk. *Pediatrics* 89:676–677

Callahan AM, Fava M, Rosenbaum JF (1993), Drug interactions in psychopharmacology. *Psychiatr Clin North Am* 16:647–671

Chambers CD, Johnson KA, Dick L, Felix R, Jones KL (1996), Birth outcomes in pregnant women taking fluoxetine. *N Engl J Med* 335:1010–1015

Choo V (1993), Paroxetine and extrapyramidal reactions. *Lancet* 341:624

Ciraulo DA, Shader RI (1990), Fluoxetine drug-drug interactions, I: antidepressants and antipsychotics. *J Clin Psychopharmacol* 10:48–50

Coulter DM, Pillans PI (1995), Fluoxetine and extrapyramidal side effects. *Am J Psychiatry* 152:122–125

Coutts RT (1994), Polymorphism in the metabolism of drugs, including antidepressant drugs: comments on phenotyping. *J Psychiatr Neurosci* 19:30–44

Crewe HK, Lennard MS, Tucker GT, Woods FR, Haddock RE (1992), The effect of selective serotonin re-uptake inhibitors on cytochrome P4502D6 activity in human liver microsomes. *Br J Clin Pharmacol* 34:262–265

Cunningham M, Cunningham K, Lydiard RB (1990), Eye tics and subjective hearing impairment during fluoxetine therapy. *Am J Psychiatry* 147:947–948

DeVane C (1992), Pharmacokinetics of the selective serotonin reuptake inhibitors. *J Clin Psychiatry* 53 (suppl): 13–20

Dilsaver SC, Greden JF (1984), Antidepressant withdrawal phenomena. *Biol Psychiatry* 19:237–252

Dorevitch A, Frankel Yehuda, Bar-Halperin A, Aronzon R, Zilberman L (1993), Fluvoxamine associated manic behavior: a case series. *Ann Pharmacother* 27:1455–1457

Dummit ES, Klein RG, Tancer NK, Asche B, Martin J (1996), Fluoxetine treatment of children with selective mutism: an open trial. *J Am Acad Child Adolesc Psychiatry* 35:615–621

Dunbar GC (1989), An interim overview of the safety and tolerability of paroxetine. *Acta Psychiatr Scand* 80 (suppl 350):135–137

Dunner DL, Dunbar GC (1992), Optimal dose regimen for paroxetine. *J Clin Psychiatry* 53 (suppl 2):21–26

Edleman RJ, Pfeffer CR, Ehlers KH (1994), Cardiac effects and fluoxetine (letter). *J Am Acad Child Adolesc Psychiatry* 33:591–592

Eisenhauer G. Jermain DM (1993), Fluoxetine and tics in an adolescent. *Ann Pharmacother* 27:725–726

Feder R (1991), Bradycardia and syncope induced by fluoxetine (letter). *J Clin Psychiatry* 52:139

Fennig S, Naisberg-Fenning S, Pato M, Weitzman A (1994), Emergence of symptoms of Tourette's syndrome during fluvoxamine treatment of obsessive-compulsive disorder. *Br J Psychiatry* 164:839–841

Fisch C (1985), Effect on fluoxetine on the electrocardiogram. *J Clin Psychiatry* 46:42–44

Fleishaker JC, Hulst KL (1994), A pharmacokinetic and pharmacodynamic evaluation of the combined administration of alprazolam and fluvoxamine. *Eur J Clin Pharmacol* 46:35–39

Garnier R, Azoyan P, Chataigner D, Taboulet P, Dellattre D, Efthymiou ML (1993), Acute fluvoxamine poisoning. *J Int Med Res* 21:197–208

Gatto G, Pikielny R, Micheli F (1994), Fluoxetine in Tourette's syndrome. *Am J Psychiatry* 151:946–947

Geller DA, Biederman J, Reed ED, Spencer T, Wilens TE (1995), Similarities in response to fluoxetine in the treatment of children and adolescents with obsessive-compulsive disorder. *J Am Acad Child Adolesc Psychiatry* 34:36–44

George MS, Trimble MR (1993), Dystonic reaction associated with fluvoxamine. *J Clin Psychopharmacol* 13:220–221

Ghaziuddin M (1994), Mania induced by sertraline in a prepubertal child (letter). *Am J Psychiatry* 151:944

Gillette DW, Tannery LP (1994), Beta blocker inhibits tricyclic metabolism. *J Am Acad Child Adolesc Psychiatry* 33:223–224

Heimann SW, March JS (1996), SSRI-induced mania (letter). *J Am Acad Child Adolesc Psychiatry* 35:4–5

Hersh CB, Sokol, Pfeffer CR (1991), Transient psychosis with fluoxetine. *J Am Acad Child Adolesc Psychiatry* 30:851–852

Heym J, Koe BK (1988), Pharmacology of sertraline: a review. *J Clin Psychiatry* 49 (suppl):40–45

Hoehn-Saric R, Harris GJ, Pearlson GD, Cox SC, Machlin ST, Camargo EE (1991), A fluoxetine-induced frontal lobe syndrome in an obsessive compulsive patient. *J Clin Psychiatry* 52:131–133

Hoehn-Saric R, Lipsey JR, McLeod DR (1990), Apathy and indifference in patients on fluvoxamine and fluoxetine. *J Clin Psychopharmacol* 10:343–345

Honig PK, Woosley RL, Zamani K, Conner DP, Cantilena R (1992), Changes in the pharmacokinetics and electrocardiographic pharmacodynamics of terfenadine with concomitant administration of erythromycin. *Clin Pharmacol Ther* 52:231–238

Honig PK, Wortham DC, Zamani K, Conner DP, Mullin JC, Cantilena LR (1993), Terfenadine-ketoconazole interaction. *JAMA* 269:1513–1518

Horrigan JP, Barnhill LJ (1994), Paroxetine-pimozide drug interaction (letter). *J Am Acad Child Adolesc Psychiatry* 33:1060–1061

Hughes C, Preskorn SH (1989), Depressive syndromes in children and adolescents: diagnosis and treatment. *Ann Clin Psychiatry* 1:109–118

Hyman SE, Nestler EJ (1996), Initiation and adaptation: a paradigm for understanding psychotropic drug action. *Am J Psychiatry* 153:151–162

Jafri AB, Greenberg WM (1991), Fluoxetine side effects. *J Am Acad Child Adolesc Psychiatry* 30:852

Jain U, Birmaher B, Garcia M, Al-Shabbout M, Ryan N (1993), Fluoxetine: a chart review of efficacy and adverse effects. *J Child Adolesc Psychopharmacol* 2:259–265

Jerome L (1991), Hypomania with fluoxetine. *J Am Acad Child Adolesc Psychiatry* 30:850–851

Joblin M (1994), Possible interaction of sertraline with carbamazepine (letter). *NZ Med J* 107:43

Jones-Fearing KB (1996), SSRI and EPS with fluoxetine (letter). *J Am Acad Child Adolesc Psychiatry* 35:1107–1108

Kalda R (1993), Media- or fluoxetine induced akathisia (letter)? *Am J Psychiatry* 150:531–532

Kat H (1996), More on SSRI-induced mania (letter). *J Am Acad Child Adolesc Psychiatry* 35:975–976

Ketai R (1993), Interaction between fluoxetine and neuroleptics (letter). *Am J Psychiatry* 150:836–837

King RA, Riddle MS, Chappell PB et al. (1991), Emergence of self-destructive phenomena in children and adolescents during fluoxetine treatment. *J Am Acad Child Adolesc Psychiatry* 30:179–186

Koe BK (1990), Preclinical pharmacology of sertraline: a potent and specific inhibitor of serotonin reuptake. *J Clin Psychiatry* 51 (suppl B):13–17

Lejoyeux M, Fineyre F, Ades J (1992), The serotonin syndrome. *Am J Psychiatry* 149:1410–1411

Leonard HL, Lenane MC, Swedo SE, Rettew DC, Rapport JL (1991), A double-blind comparison of clomipramine and desipramine treatment of severe onychophagia (nail-biting). *Arch Gen Psychiatry* 48:828–833

Leonard HL, Swedo SE, Rapoport JL et al. (1989), Treatment of obsessive-compulsive disorder with clomipramine and desipramine in children and adolescents: a double-blind crossover comparison. *Arch Gen Psychiatry* 46:1088–1092

Lydiard RB, Anton R, Cunningham T (1993), Interactions between sertra-line and tricyclic antidepressants (letter). *Am J Psychiatry* 150:1125–1126

March JS, Moon RL, Johnston H (1990), Fluoxetine-TCA interaction (letter). *J Am Acad Child Adolesc Psychiatry* 29:986

Maskall DD, Lam RW (1993), Increased plasma concentration of imipramine following augmentation with fluvoxamine (letter). *Am J Psychiatry* 150:1566

Murdoch D, McTavish D (1992), Sertraline: a review of its pharmacodynamic and pharmacokinetic properties, therapeutic potential in depressive illness, and prospective role in the treatment of obsessive compulsive disorder. *Drugs* 44:604–624

Nemeroff CB (1993), Paroxetine: an overview of the efficacy and safety of a new selective serotonin reuptake inhibitor in treatment of depression. *J Clin Psychopharmacol* 13 (suppl):10–17

Nemeroff CB, DeVane CL, Pollock BG (1996), Newer antidepressants and the cytochrome P450 system. *Am J Psychiatry* 153:311–320

Nicholson AN, Pascoe P (1988): Studies on the modulation of the sleepwakefulness continuum in man by fluoxetine, a 5-HT uptake inhibitor. *Neuropharmacology* 27:597–602

Palmer KJ, Benfield P (1994), Fluvoxamine: an overview of its pharmacological properties and review of its therapeutic potential in non-depressive disorders. *CNS Drugs* 1:57–87

Paxton J, Dragunow M (1993), Pharmacology. In: *Practitioner's Guide to Psychoactive Drugs for Children and Adolescents*, Werry J, Aman M, eds. New York: Plenum, pp 34–46

Pearson HL (1990), Interaction of fluoxetine with carbamazepine (letter). *J Clin Psychiatry* 51:126

Perucca E, Gattu G, Cipolla G et al. (1994), Inhibition of diazepam metabolism by fluvoxamine: a pharmacokinetic study in normal volunteers. *Clin Pharmacol Ther* 56:471–476

Pohl R, Yeragani VK, Balon R, Lycaki H (1988), The jitteriness syndrome in panic disorder patients treated with antidepressants. *J Clin Psychiatry* 49:100–104

Prasher VP (1993), Seizures associated with fluoxetine therapy. *Seizure* 2:315–317

Preskorn S (1993), Pharmacokinetics of antidepressants: why and how they are relevant to treatment. *J Clin Psychiatry* 54 (suppl):14–34

Preskorn SH, Alderman J, Chung M, Harrison W, Messig M, Harris S (1994), Pharmacokinetics of desipramine coadministered with sertraline or fluoxetine. *J Clin Psychopharmacol* 14:90–98

Reynolds CF, Kupfer DJ (1987), Sleep research in affective illness: state of the art circa 1987. *Sleep* 10:199–215

Riddle MA, Brown N, Dzubinski D, Jetmalani AN, Law Y, Woolston JL (1989), Fluoxetine overdose in an adolescent. *J Am Acad Child Adolesc Psychiatry* 23:587–588

Riddle MA, Claghorn J, Gaffney G et al. (1996), Fluvoxamine for children and adolescents with OCD: a controlled multicenter trial. Presented at the 43rd Annual Meeting of the American Academy of Child and Adolescent Psychiatry, Philadelphia, October 25

Riddle MA, King RA, Hardin MT et al. (1991), Behavioral side effects of fluoxetine in children and adolescents. *J Child Adolesc Psychopharmacol* 1:193–198

Riddle MA, Scahill L, King RA et al. (1992), Double-blind, crossover trial of fluoxetine and placebo in children and adolescents with obsessive-compulsive disorder. *J Am Acad Child Adolesc Psychiatry* 31:1062–1069

Saletu B, Frey R, Krupka M, Anderer P, Grunberger J, See WR (1991), Sleep laboratory studies on the single-dose effects of serotonin reuptake inhibitors paroxetine and fluoxetine on human sleep and awakening qualities. *Sleep* 14:439–447

Shader RI, Greenblatt DJ, von Moltke LL (1994), Fluoxetine inhibition of phenytoin metabolism. *J Clin Psychopharmacol* 14:375–376

Shihabuddin L, Rapport D (1994), Sertraline and extrapyramidal side effects. *Am J Psychiatry* 151:288–289

Shimoda, Minowada T, Noguchi T, Takahashi S (1993), Interindividual variations of desmethylation and hydroxylation of clomipramine in an oriental psychiatric population. *J Clin Psychopharmacol* 13:181–188

Skjelbo E, Brosen K (1992), Inhibitors of imipramine metabolism by human liver microsomes. *Br J Pharmacol* 34:256–261

Song F, Freemantle N, Sheldon TA et al. (1993), Selective serotonin reuptake inhibitors: meta-analysis of efficacy and acceptability. *Br Med J* 306:683–687

Spencer MJ (1993), Fluoxetine hydrochloride (Prozac) toxicity in a neonate. *Pediatrics* 92:721–722

Sperber AD (1991), Toxic interactions between fluvoxamine and sustained release theophylline in an 11-year old boy. *Drug Saf* 6:460–462

Steiner W, Fontaine R (1986), Toxic reaction following the combined administration of fluoxetine and 1-tryptophan: five case reports. *Biol Psychiatry* 21:1067–1071

Sternbach H (1991), The serotonin syndrome. *Am J Psychiatry* 148:705–713

Stokes PE (1993), Fluoxetine: a five year review. *Clin Ther* 15:216–243

Stoll AL, Cole JO, Lukas SE (1991), A case of mania as a result of fluoxetine-marijuana interaction. *J Clin Psychiatry* 52:280–281

Swims MP (1993), Potential terfenadine-fluoxetine interaction (letter). *Ann Pharmacother* 27:1404

Teicher MH, Glod C, Cole J (1990), Emergence of intense suicidal preoccupation during fluoxetine treatment. *Am J Psychiatry* 147:207–210

Tulloch IF, Johnson AM (1992), The pharmacologic profile of paroxetine, a new selective serotonin reuptake inhibitor. *J Clin Psychiatry* 53(suppl):7–12

Venkataraman S, Naylor MW, King CA (1992), Mania associated with fluoxetine treatment in adolescents. *J Am Acad Child Adolesc Psychiatry* 31:276–281

von Moltke LL, Greenblatt DJ, Harmantz JS, Shader RI (1994), Cytochromes in psychopharmacology. *J Clin Psychopharmacol* 14:1–4

Walley T, Pirmohamed M, Proudlove C, Maxwell D (1993), Interaction of fluoxetine and metoprolol. *Lancet* 341:967–968

Walters AM (1992), Sympathomimetic-fluoxetine interaction (letter). *J Am Acad Child Adolesc Psychiatry* 31:565–566

Warrington SJ (1992), Clinical implications of the pharmacology of serotonin reuptake inhibitors. *Int Clin Psychopharmacol* 7:13–19

Wilens TE, Biederman J, Baldessarini RJ, Puopolo PR, Flood JG (1992), Developmental changes in serum concentrations of desipramine and 2-hydroxydesipramine during treatment with desipramine. *J Am Acad Child Adolesc Psychiatry* 31:691–698

Winokur A, Reynolds CF (1994), Effects of antidepressants on sleep physiology. *Primary Psychiatry* Nov/Dec, pp. 22–27

Winokur A, Sewitch, Phillips JL, Biniaur IV (1991), Sleep architecture and mood effects of sertraline in outpatients with major depression: a preliminary report (abstract). *Biol Psychiatry* 29:43.

10

Case Study: Ego-Dystonic Anger Attacks in Mothers of Young Children

Oommen Mammen, Katherine Shear, Kay Jennings, and Sally Popper
University of Pittsburgh, Pittsburgh, Pennsylvania

Parental anger can have detrimental effects on children and can contribute to physical abuse. Ego-dystonic anger attacks are an underrecognized psychiatric symptom that occurs in association with depression, with other psychiatric disorders, and in the absence of comorbid disorders. They are characterized by overwhelming anger and autonomic arousal occurring upon provocation viewed as trivial by the individual, and they respond well to treatment with serotonergic antidepressants. Consequently, they represent a readily treatable problem. Four cases of anger attacks in mothers of young children are described to illustrate the importance of recognizing and treating anger attacks.

High levels of parental anger can contribute to child physical abuse and can have detrimental effects on child behavior and development (Cummings and Davies, 1994; Kolko, 1996). Adult anger can affect child behavior by contributing to interparental conflict and by affecting parenting. Studies have shown that children are adversely affected by anger directed at the children themselves and also by witnessing anger expressed between adults (Cummings and Davies, 1994). Therefore, recognizing and treating problems of anger control in parents may be helpful for children.

Anger attacks are a form of anger dyscontrol recently described in clinical populations (Fava et al., 1993). They are characterized by a rapid onset of overwhelming anger and a crescendo of autonomic arousal that occurs upon provocation viewed as trivial by the individual. Anger attacks are clinically important because they are often associated with aggressive acts and tend to respond to treatment with serotonergic antidepressants (Fava et al., 1993; Gould et al., 1996). In one series of 56 depressed patients with anger attacks, during the anger attacks 93% felt like attacking others, 63% attacked others either verbally or physically, and 30% threw or destroyed objects (Fava et al., 1993). In two series, 13% to 15% of patients with anxiety or depressive disorder reported serious impairment (e.g., job

---

Reprinted with permission from the *Journal of the American Academy of Child and Adolescent Psychiatry,* 1997, Vol. 36(10), 1374–1377.
From Western Psychiatric Institute and Clinic, University of Pittsburgh.

loss, legal trouble, loss of friends) because of anger attacks (Gould et al., 1996). The anger experienced during anger attacks is ego-dystonic: patients report it is uncharacteristic of their usual personality, and the aggressive acts are followed by guilt and regret (Fava et al., 1993).

Anger attacks have been strongly related to current and past unipolar depression, but also occur in association with anxiety disorders, with personality disorders, and in the absence of other psychiatric disorders (Gould et al., 1996; Rubey et al., 1996). Fava and colleagues found that 34% to 44% of patients with unipolar depression experienced anger attacks (1993, 1995, 1996). There are no data examining rates of anger attacks in depressed parents, but likely they are a frequent problem in this group, too. Parental psychiatric disorders, especially depression, have been consistently associated with increased rates of child psychopathology. Though the precise mechanisms underlying this association remain unclear, genetic factors and various psychosocial variables contribute (Rutter, 1987). Cummings and Davies (1994) suggested that parental anger may contribute to the association between parental depression and child behavior problems. Because problems of anger control cut across psychiatric diagnoses (Rubey et al., 1996), anger may also be a factor in parental psychiatric disorders other than depression.

Anger attacks occur in both men and women (Fava et al., 1993). In this report we focus on mothers because the cases we describe below are of anger attacks in mothers and because mothers are most commonly the primary caregivers for young children.

Parental anger may affect young children in the following ways. It may cause arousal and dysregulation of emotions and behavior, and it may also model angry responses and aggressive acts for the child (Cummings and Davies, 1994). In addition, parental anger and irritability play a part in various aspects of the coercive cycles that maintain oppositional behavior (Patterson, 1982). Because of the intense demands of caregiving for young children, aversive events are ubiquitous for the mothers of young children (Patterson, 1982). There is no evidence that occasional episodes of anger are harmful to children. However, mothers with anger attacks are likely to respond to provocations with frequent and intense anger outbursts. These anger outbursts may escalate the child's provocative behavior and, when not backed up by consistent limits, may reinforce the oppositional behavior (Patterson, 1982). In addition, mothers experiencing anger attacks report avoiding their children to reduce the likelihood of becoming angry with them. The resulting paucity of mother–child interactions can motivate the child to persist in oppositional behavior as a means of engaging the mother.

Diagnosing anger attacks is of particular clinical importance because they tend to respond well to treatment with serotonergic reuptake inhibitors (Fava et al., 1993), and this may make a dramatic difference in mother–child interactions. Nevertheless we are not aware of reports describing parental anger attacks in the child psychiatric literature. Here we describe anger attacks in the mothers of four young children who presented to our clinic.

CASE STUDIES

The patients were seen in two clinics that work together closely: a psychiatric clinic for preschool children and a clinic for psychiatric disorders in pregnant and postpartum women.

Because maternal psychiatric illness and child psychopathology frequently coexist, mothers and children are often simultaneously treated in these two clinics.

Anger attacks in the mothers described below had the characteristics described by Fava and colleagues (1993): rapid onset of anger out of proportion to provocations viewed as mild by the individual, physiological arousal (e.g., rapid heart beat, sweating, hot flashes, trembling), guilt over the anger and aggressive acts, and feeling that the anger attacks are uncharacteristic of one's usual personality.

Case 1

Ms. A, a 38-year-old married white woman with two children, presented at 3 months postpartum because of inability to control her anger. Her baby was a much-wanted child, and she described her husband as supportive. She was especially distressed at responding to the minor misbehaviors of her 2-year-old daughter with explosive anger, uncontrollable shouting, and pounding on the floor. She exercised great restraint to avoid hitting her daughter and feared she might abuse this child. She was terrified at having hit her and pulled her hair. Ms. A's only solution had been to get away from the situation: she would go into the shower and scream until she had calmed down. Her postpartum anger attacks began a few days after delivery, and she had no other depressive or anxiety symptoms. She elected to try a course of psychotherapy focused on parenting, rather than try medication for the anger attacks. Because she was not helped after a month of working with an experienced therapist, Ms. A agreed to a trial of medication. The anger attacks stopped within days of starting sertraline 25 mg/day. She was left with premenstrual anger attacks that responded to increasing the dose of sertraline to 50 mg/day. There were no side effects, and she has done well for the past year.

Case 2

Ms. B, a 28-year-old divorced white woman with two children, came requesting help for her $2\frac{1}{2}$-year-old son's severe temper tantrums, physical aggression, and defiant behavior. Marital conflict, parental separation, and disruptions in early caregiving contributed to his problems. Ms. B believed that all boys are fated to have problems with anger and aggression, as did other males in her family. Treatment helped Ms. B change her feelings about having a son and improved the quality of their relationship. However, this attitudinal change, in addition to behavioral treatment for the oppositional behavior and medication trials for her son, did not help change his behavior. A year after treatment began, Ms. B disclosed problems controlling her own anger. She was having anger attacks with rage out of proportion to most of her son's behaviors. Although she did not have an active mood or anxiety disorder, she had experienced an episode of major depression when her son was 6 months old. Her anger attacks began during this depression and continued after the depression spontaneously resolved in 6 months. Ms. B started treatment with fluoxetine 10 mg/day, and the anger attacks diminished in frequency and intensity within days. With fluoxetine 20 mg/day, Ms. B reported a dramatic improvement in her ability to manage her son's behavior without becoming enraged, and she expressed regret about not having started her treatment earlier. These clinical effects have been maintained for the past 6 months, and her son's behavior problems have finally begun to show gradual improvement.

Case 3

Ms. C, a 31-year-old single African-American woman with two children, presented at the eighth week of an unintended pregnancy. She had a recurrence of major depression, and she also had anger attacks directed at her children and boyfriend. Her boyfriend observed that during the anger attacks, the volume of her voice, her facial expressions, verbalizations, and sheer rage caused her to look as though she was "going crazy." Ms. C reported needing to physically remove herself from the scene until she could clam down. She tearfully described becoming enraged by minor problems that she easily dealt with when not depressed. She was also concerned about her 5-year-old son, who was about lose his place in day care because of his aggressive behavior. At first Ms. C planned to pursue treatment for her son. However, feeling that his behavior might improve if she were in better control of herself, she decided to seek help for herself. Ms. C planned to terminate her pregnancy, and therefore she chose to immediately start treatment with fluoxetine in addition to psychotherapy. With treatment her anger attacks ceased, the depression improved, and she described a return to her usual self. Her son's behavior also improved, and Ms. C reported that he no longer required treatment.

Case 4

Ms. D, a 33-year-old married white woman with two children, presented for treatment at 3 months postpartum. She had major depression and anger attacks and stated that her most distressing symptom was her intense, angry responses to her 2-year-old son's demands. She reported avoiding her son to prevent having anger attacks directed at him. Ms. D chose to have her depression and anger attacks treated with cognitive and behavioral therapy. Two months later she and her husband started treatment focusing on their 2-year-old's behavior. As Ms. D's depression and anger attacks improved, she was able to institute the behavior management techniques without having angry outbursts. Also, as she began to be able to interact with her son without having anger attacks, she stopped avoiding him and was thus able to positively reinforce his prosocial behaviors.

DISCUSSION

In this report we have described ego-dystonic anger attacks among mothers in two clinical situations of great importance in the practice of child psychiatry: the potential for child abuse (case 1) and disruptive behavior disorders (cases 2, 3, and 4). The anger attacks responded well to treatment. Although we cannot infer causality, it appears that maternal treatment was associated with positive effects for the children. This suggests that maternal anger attacks may be a readily treatable problem within the context of emotional and behavior problems in early childhood and that in some cases this treatment may reduce the risk for child abuse.

Although this report is limited by the absence of data using standardized instruments to document patient reports of clinical improvement, the cases described here suggest it is important to identify and treat anger attacks in the mothers of young children brought to psychiatric clinics. The presence of major depression, as in cases 3 and 4, increases the likelihood that the mother will receive treatment. Antidepressant medication targeting the depression is likely to help with the anger attacks (Fava et al., 1993). Case 4 suggests that anger attacks may also improve in response to treatment with psychotherapy. When anger attacks occur in the absence of other psychiatric disorders, there are no comorbid disorders that would cause the clinician to suspect the presence of emotional problems in the mother. Cases 1 and 2 are examples of this pattern.

Case 1 is of interest because of the postpartum onset of anger attacks without comorbid mood or anxiety disorder. Postpartum women are known to be at risk for the onset and exacerbation of mood and anxiety disorders, but we are not aware of any reports of postpartum-onset anger attacks. Some postpartum women present for treatment worrying that they may hurt their child because of their angry responses to the exhausting demands of infants and toddlers. In such cases it may be worth assessing patients for anger attacks, because anger attacks may respond dramatically to serotonergic antidepressants. Data on the efficacy of other antidepressants for the treatment of anger attacks are limited.

Case 2 is of interest because in this mother anger attacks persisted after spontaneous recovery from major depression, and the anger attacks likely contributed to her son's behavior problems. This suggests that anger attacks may be present even in mothers who have recovered from depression.

Clinically, it is useful to keep in mind that problems of anger that do not have all of the characteristics of anger attacks may also respond to treatment with serotonergic antidepressants (Rubey et al., 1996). Eckhardt and Deffenbacher (1996) have provided useful descriptions of various ways in which problems of anger can manifest and have also discussed the relationship between anger and psychiatric disorders. A discussion of this and the differential diagnosis of anger attacks is beyond the scope of this brief report.

Anger has been a generally neglected topic in psychiatric research and practice (Rubey et al., 1996), and anger attacks are likely an underrecognized symptom. Underrecognition and undertreatment of conditions for which effective treatments exist is a well-known problem which even occurs with extensively studied conditions such as depressive disorders (Hirschfeld et al., 1997). The absence of published reports on anger attacks in parents of children presenting to child psychiatric clinics may represent another example of this problem. Another factor that may contribute to the underrecognition of anger attacks is that such problems are not specifically addressed by currently used diagnostic systems. This suggests the importance of targeting for treatment distressing or disabling symptoms (such as anger) rather than only treating disorders (such as depressive disorders and anxiety disorders) which may not even be present in some patients (as in cases 1 and 2).

Underrecognition of anger attacks may be a particular problem among mothers because women are socialized to deny and disavow anger (Bernardez-Bonesatti, 1978). Consequently, mothers may not volunteer that they have trouble controlling their anger. In cases 2, 3, and 4 of this report, mothers acknowledged having anger attacks only upon being directly questioned. In our experience, mothers with anger attacks typically do not disclose their problems with anger unless directly asked, even though they report experiencing great distress over the anger directed at their children.

Anger attacks may be a more common problem than is generally recognized. There are no data on the prevalence of anger attacks in community samples. However, in patients with unipolar depression, Fava and colleagues found that 34% to 44% of patients experienced anger attacks (1993, 1995, 1996). Epidemiological data suggest that depressive disorders are a common problem, with a lifetime prevalence of 15% in men and 24% in women (Hirschfeld et al., 1997). Although the generalizability of these findings to mothers of young children is not known, it is possible that a number of the mothers with a current or past history of depression may have anger attacks.

This report suggests the need for research on the prevalence, correlates, and etiology of parental anger attacks and their relationship to child psychopathology. In particular, it is important to know whether mothers of young children are especially vulnerable to this problem because of the stresses associated with caring for young children and also because of the hormonal changes associated with pregnancy and the postpartum period. Finally, although this report deals with anger attacks in mothers, research with fathers is also indicated.

REFERENCES

Bernardez-Bonesatti T (1978), Women and anger: conflicts with aggression in contemporary women. *J Am Med Wom Assoc* 33:215–219

Cummings E, Davies P (1994), Maternal depression and child development. *J Child Psychol Psychiatry* 33:73–112

Eckhardt C, Deffenbacher J (1996), Diagnosis of anger disorders. In: *Anger Disorders: Definition, Diagnosis, and Treatment,* Kassinove H, ed. Bristol, PA: Taylor and Francis, pp 29–48

Fava M, Alpert J, Nierenberg A et al. (1996), Fluoxetine treatment of anger attacks: a replication study. *Ann Clin Psychiatry* 8:7–10

Fava M, Nierenberg A, Quitkin F, Zisook S, Rosenbaum J (1995), A preliminary study on the efficacy of sertraline and imipramine on anger attacks in depression. *Psychopharmacol Bull* 31:567

Fava M, Rosenbaum J, Pava J, McCarthy M, Steingard R, Bouffides E (1993), Anger attacks in unipolar depression, part 1: clinical correlates and response to fluoxetine treatment. *Am J Psychiatry* 150:1158–1163

Gould R, Ball S, Kaspi S et al. (1996), Prevalence and correlates of anger attacks. *J Affect Disord* 39:31–38

Hirschfeld R, Keller M, Panico S et al. (1997). The National Depressive and Manic-Depressive Association Consensus Statement on the undertreatment of depression. *JAMA* 277:333–340

Kolko D (1996), Child physical abuse. In: *The ASPAC Handbook of Child Maltreatment,* Briere J, Berliner LJ, Bulkely J, Jenny C, Reid T, eds. Chicago: American Professional Society on Abuse of Children, pp. 21–50

Patterson G (1982), *Coercive Family Processes.* Eugene, OR: Castalia

Rubey R, Johnson M, Emmanuel N, Lydiard B (1996), Fluoxetine in the treatment of anger: an open clinical trial. *J Clin Psychiatry* 57:398–401

Rutter M (1987), Parental mental disorder as a psychiatric risk factor. *Annu Rev Psychiatry* 6:647–663

Part III

TREATMENT ISSUES

The papers in Part III focus attention on a range of biological, psychological, and psychosocial treatments for children and adolescents. In the first paper, Rey and Walter review the literature on the efficacy and safety of electroconvulsive therapy (ECT) in children and adolescents over the past 50 years. Although the indications for, efficacy of, and unwanted effects of ECT in adults have been subjects of intense study and scrutiny, the same is not true for their effects in children and adolescents. All studies, both those published in English and those published in other languages, on the use of ECT in persons 18 years of age or younger were systematically reviewed, yielding 60 reports describing ECT in 396 patients. Most (63%) were single-case reports. There were no controlled trials, and the quality of reports was generally poor. These limitations notwithstanding, rates of improvement across studies were 63% for depression, 80% for mania, 42% for schizophrenia, and 80% for catatonia. Serious complications were very rarely reported, but minor, transient side effects appeared to occur commonly. Rey et al. conclude that ECT appears similar in effectiveness and side effects to ECT in adults, but this conclusion is qualified by a lack of systematic evidence.

ECT should be used with caution in young people because of the relative lack of knowledge. Rey and Walter urge the establishment of registers to expand the database on the safety and efficacy of ECT in children and adolescents. Nevertheless, ECT should not be overlooked as a treatment alternative. Both the American Psychiatric Association (APA, 1990) and the Royal College of Psychiatrists (Freeman, 1995) offer guidelines for the use of ECT in young people. Rey and Walter urge that child psychiatrists considering ECT stop all nonessential medications during administration because of reports of increased length of seizure and post-ECT convulsions. They further suggest that consideration be given to determining the seizure threshold, to EEG monitoring, and possibly to EEG examinations before and after a course of ECT. Psychometric assessment before and some time after ECT might also be valuable. Consent issues require particular attention, with both parents and child involved whenever possible.

In the second paper in Part III, Swedo and colleagues present the result of a controlled trial of light therapy for the treatment of pediatric seasonal affective disorder (SAD). Winter SAD is a variant of recurrent affective disorder in which mood changes and atypical vegetative symptoms occur during the winter months, disappearing completely during the spring and summer. SAD has been well described in adults, but less is known about the clinical presentation and treatment of children with SAD. Nevertheless, recent epidemiological studies suggest that winter SAD may affect as many as 3%–4% of school-age children whose symptoms appear similar to those in adults.

The results of this placebo-controlled, double-blind crossover trial in 28 children who ranged in age from 7 to 17 years, living in two geographically distinct sites, suggest that bright-light therapy is an effective treatment for pediatric SAD. During the week of active treatment, which consisted of a combination of light-box therapy and dawn simulation, the children's depressive symptoms as assessed by the child version of the Structured Interview Guide for the Hamilton Depression Rating Scale, Seasonal Affective Disorders version, were significantly decreased from baseline as compared with both the placebo and washout phases. Scores on the parent version of the same instrument also decreased from baseline during active treatment.

Active treatment was not associated with a higher frequency of side effects than placebo, and it appeared to be well tolerated. The clinical responses of the children and their parents underscored the statistical results. In the posttreatment survey, the vast majority of the parents and children rated the active-treatment week as the phase during which they felt best. Nearly all of the children at both sites continued to use bright-light therapy after the study had finished.

Although only preliminary, the generalizability of the findings is strengthened by the fact that they were internally replicated at two geographically distinct sites, Boston and Washington, DC. Given the high prevalence of pediatric SAD, the need for a safe and effective treatment for this troublesome condition is clear. The results of this investigation suggest that bright-light therapy is such an intervention.

The next three papers in Part III address aspects of treatment of disruptive behavior disorders. Frankel, Myatt, Cantwell, and Feinberg direct attention to the troublesome problem of impaired social skills in children with disruptive behavior disorders, most particularly attention deficit–hyperactivity disorder (ADHD). Although peer rejection is a significant part of the clinical presentation of many children with ADHD, the results of social skills training programs designed to improve the skills of children who are rejected by their peers have not been encouraging. In summary, previous research has not found compelling evidence that social skills learned in treatment generalize to home, classroom, or playground. Noting the absence of parental involvement in social skills training programs, Frankel et al. hypothesized that generalization of gains made in an outpatient social skills training program would be enhanced when parents were specifically trained in skills relevant to their child's social adjustment.

In all, 35 children with ADHD and 14 children without ADHD attended 12 social skills training sessions (treatment group). Outcome was compared with 12 children with ADHD and 12 children without ADHD who were on a waiting list for treatment (waiting-list group). Nineteen children with oppositional defiant disorder (ODD) were in the treatment group and 5 were in the waiting list group. All children with ADHD were on stimulant medication. Formal parent sessions were held concurrently for the entire hour of all child sessions. Each parental group session consisted of both specifically targeted didactic presentations and socialization homework assignments. The results indicate that children with ADHD showed improvement comparable with that of children without ADHD on all teacher- and parent-reported measures of peer adjustment and social skills, with the exception of teacher-reported withdrawal. Children with ODD had outcomes comparable to those of children without ODD. Effect sizes ranged from 0.93 to 1.34, indicating that the average treatment group child was better off than 83% of waiting list children.

The results demonstrate that socially rejected children may benefit substantially from social skills training when their parents are trained to facilitate transfer of treatment effects. As Frankel et al. underscore, inclusion of parents in treatment is especially important as it is parents who typically arrange and monitor their children's peer interactions. This paper is of particular value in regard to the detail with which the social skills training curriculum for both children and parents is described. The careful presentation of session content will facilitate not only the conduct of replication research but, just as important, the direct incorporation of similar techniques into ongoing clinical practice.

Klein and colleagues report the clinical efficacy of methylphenidate in conduct disorder (CD) with and without ADHD. Although stimulants have long been recognized as an effective treatment in children with ADHD, they are generally not considered appropriate for children with CD. Klein et al. hypothesized that methylphenidate would not significantly improve symptoms of CD. Eighty-four children with CD who were between 6 and 15 years of age were randomly assigned to receive methylphenidate hydrochloride (up to 60 mg/d) or placebo for 5 weeks. Two thirds of the children also met criteria for ADHD. Behavior was evaluated by parent, teacher, and clinician reports and by direct classroom observation. The results indicated that, contrary to expectation, symptoms of CD were markedly responsive to short-term methylphenidate treatment at the doses used. Moreover, drug effects on multiple aspects of CD are not dependent on the severity of ADHD symptoms. Partialing out severity of ADHD symptoms did not alter the significant specific superiority of methylphenidate on CD ratings.

Although the effectiveness of methylphenidate is impressive, Klein et al. point out that clinical normalization almost never occurred in the study sample. Alone, stimulant treatment provided clinically meaningful but incomplete therapeutic impact. Also, the duration of the study was only 5 weeks, and CDs are chronic conditions. The true value of the intervention will depend on its stability over time, but long-term administration increases the likelihood of abuse. Abuse is a major concern associated with the administration of stimulants to antisocial individuals whose potential for abuse is well documented. The issue is one that requires careful consideration, although concerns about abuse may be somewhat tempered by the fact that oral administration is not associated with euphoric responses. In the Klein et al. study, no child reported experiencing "highs" with medication.

Although there is no obvious behavioral model to account for methylphenidate efficacy on symptoms of CD, it is plausible that impulsivity is a key pathologic abnormality in both CD and ADHD that is specifically reduced by stimulants. In children with CD, enhanced impulse control is likely to induce multiple positive secondary effects. On active medication, children were described by parents as more reasonable and tractable, which in turn might lead to improvement in some maladaptive social behaviors. Mechanisms aside, Klein et al.'s data suggest that the successful treatment of CDs may well include stimulant treatment as well as the combination of psychosocial measures discussed in the final paper in this section.

Although many different types of treatment have been applied to conduct-disordered youths, little outcome evidence exists for most of the techniques. Kazdin, in the last paper in Part III, reviews psychosocial treatment for CD. He has used the following criteria to identify and to select promising treatments from among the array of available interventions: conceptual underpinnings, basic research to support the conceptualization, preliminary outcome evidence, and process-outcome connections. Noting that currently no single treatment adequately meets all of these criteria, Kazdin has selected four treatments with the most promising evidence to date for detailed discussion and evaluation: problem-solving skills training, parent management training, functional family therapy, and multisystemic therapy.

Cognitive problem-solving skills training focuses on cognitive processes that underlie social behavior. Parent management training is directed at altering parent–child interactions in the home, particularly those interactions related to child-rearing practices and coercive interchanges. Functional family therapy uses principles of systems theory and behavior modification as the basis for altering interactions, communication, and problem solving among family members. Multisystemic therapy focuses on the individual, family, and extrafamilial systems and their interrelations as a way to reduce symptoms and to promote prosocial behavior.

Despite these promising beginnings, it is not yet possible to say that one particular intervention can ameliorate conduct disorder and overcome the poor long-term prognosis. However, much of what is practiced in clinical settings—including psychodynamically oriented treatment, general relationship counseling, family therapy, and group therapy with antisocial youths as members—has not been evaluated carefully in controlled trials. Although Kazdin acknowledges that the absence of evidence is not tantamount to ineffectiveness, he also points out that the promising treatments considered in this review rest on a much more substantial database. Perhaps, as Kazdin suggests, a special argument might be needed to administer treatments that have neither basic research on their conceptual underpinnings in relation to CD nor outcome evidence from controlled clinical trials on their behalf. This informative and provocative review provides much food for thought regarding the management and treatment of this frequently occurring and costly disorder of children and adolescents.

REFERENCES

American Psychiatric Association. (1990). *The practice of electroconvulsive therapy: Recommendations for treatment, training and privileging: A task force report of the American Psychiatric Association.* Washington, DC: Author.

Freeman, C. P. (1995). ECT in those under 18 years old. In C. P. Freeman (Ed.), *The ECT handbook* (pp. 18–21). London: Royal College of Psychiatrists.

11

Half a Century of ECT Use in Young People

Joseph M. Rey and Garry Walter
University of Sydney, Sydney, New South Wales, Australia

Objective: *Pharmacological treatments for certain psychiatric disorders in young people are often ineffective and may cause major side effects; thus, it is important to investigate other treatments. This article reviews the literature on the efficacy and safety of ECT in this age group and examines the evidence for the suggestion that it may be used inappropriately.* **Method:** *All studies published in English and other languages on the use of ECT in persons 18 years of age or younger were obtained. The reports were systematically reviewed and rated according to the quality of the information in several domains, yielding an overall quality score for each study. Individual cases from each report were then examined and grouped according to diagnosis and response to ECT.* **Results:** *Sixty reports describing ECT in 396 patients were identified; most (63%) were single case reports. The overall quality was poor but improved in the more recent studies. There were no controlled trials. Rates of improvement across studies were 63% for depression, 80% for mania, 42% for schizophrenia, and 80% for catatonia. Serious complications were very rare, whereas minor, transient side effects appeared common.* **Conclusions:** *ECT in the young seems similar in effectiveness and side effects to ECT in adults. However, this conclusion is qualified by the lack of systematic evidence. More research and education of professionals and the public are needed. It is suggested that ECT registers be set up, that surveys and controlled trials be conducted, and that seizure thresholds, the optimal anesthetic, effects of concurrent medications, and cognitive consequences of ECT in the young be investigated.*

There are several reasons for examining the use of ECT in young people. First, there is burgeoning interest in ECT, particularly in its application in the young (1, 2). Second, it is necessary to have information in order to accept or reject the criticisms of those who

---

Reprinted with permission from the *American Journal of Psychiatry*, 1997, Vol. 154(5), 595–602.

The authors thank K. Walter and M. Rozska for assistance in translating papers; M. Fairley, G.F.S. Johnson, and P. Mitchell for suggestions; and H.A. Robinson and F.N. Moise for providing information not available in their reports.

condemn or wish to ban the procedure for this age group (3, 4). Third, disorders that may potentially benefit from ECT are common, handicapping, and often resistant to alternative treatments. For example, depression in children and adolescents may be increasing in prevalence (5), it causes substantial morbidity and mortality (6), and it frequently does not improve with traditional antidepressants (7, 8). Finally, psychotropic drugs can produce severe side effects, and there is often a lag before the onset of action.

The indications for, efficacy of, and unwanted effects of ECT in adults have been subjects of intense study and scrutiny. There is good evidence that ECT is effective in the treatment of a variety of disorders and is a safe procedure, even in elderly, frail, or physically ill patients (9, 10). However, results obtained with adults are not necessarily applicable to children and adolescents, as experience with tricyclic antidepressants has shown (7, 8).

Is the reluctance to use ECT in young people justified? Are we irrationally depriving our young patients of an effective and safe treatment, or would we be exposing them to a futile and risky procedure? The aim of this study was to answer these questions by conducting a systematic review of the literature on the use, efficacy, and unwanted effects of ECT in patients aged 18 years or younger. While there have been previous reviews (e.g., reference 11), they were not comprehensive, and a number of new studies have been published in the last few years.

HISTORICAL NOTE

In April 1942, in the midst of the German occupation, Georges Heuyer and his colleagues (12) reported to the Société Médico-Psychologique of Paris the positive effects of ECT in two teenagers. The following year, Heuyer et al. (13) reported on a series of 40 children and adolescents with a variety of conditions who had been treated with the new procedure. They concluded that ECT was safe for this age group and that it was effective in the treatment of melancholia, less consistently successful in the treatment of mania, and not beneficial in the treatment of schizophrenia. The first mention of a child treated with ECT (a 3-year-old with epilepsy) had occurred in 1941 (14).

Effective treatments for mental disorders in children and adolescents were few in the 1940s. It is not surprising that psychiatrists were keen to embrace a new therapy. For example, in 1947 Lauretta Bender (15) reported on the efficacy of ECT in a series of 98 children under the age of 12 years treated at Bellevue Hospital in New York. She had diagnosed them as suffering from "childhood schizophrenia" (it is unlikely that many would have met current criteria for schizophrenia; the majority probably had disruptive behavior or developmental disorders [16]). The children received courses of 20 daily unmodified ECTs. Bender observed a "positive change in behavior following treatment" in all but two or three of them. At the same time she recognized that "remissions such as are seen in adults occurred in only a few children."

Despite these encouraging early results reported in France and the United States, there are suggestions that the use of ECT in young patients then diminished. Such decline was probably due to apprehension about possible harmful effects (17, 18) as well as to the advent of psychotropic drugs. ECT for children and adolescents became a "controversial treatment" (19) of "last resort" (20). There have been moves recently in England to prohibit ECT for this age group (3), while ECT has been outlawed for various groups of young people in several states in the United States (21).

QUALITY OF THE EVIDENCE

In order to focus on the use of ECT in children and adolescents, as opposed to adults, we chose a conservative cutoff age of 18 years. Systematic searches of medical and psychological databases (including publications in English and in other languages), reports quoted by other writers, and manual searches up to March 1996 yielded 60 reports (11–13, 15, 17–72) describing 396 patients. Works in which individuals younger than 19 years could not be identified (e.g., reference 73) were excluded. Publications in languages other than English were translated into English; eight were in French (12, 13, 22–27), four in German (28–31), and one in Polish (32). Restricting the scope of the review to studies published in English (11, 15, 17–21, 33–72) would have resulted in a considerable loss of information.

The largest series were those described in the 1940s by Bender (15) and Heuyer et al. (13), with 98 and 40 cases, respectively. However, the vast majority of reports were either of single cases (N = 38, 63%) (not all of these were single case reports; occasionally, a single case could be extracted from other series) or small, anecdotal collections of cases (N = 9, 15%). The largest recent series had 28 cases (60).

The quality of the reports was evaluated independently by each author, and the independent ratings were then compared. When there was disagreement, reports were jointly reexamined and consensus was reached. Aspects rated included the following: whether gender and age were given; the system used for case detection; diagnostic information; whether previous and concurrent treatments were described; whether electrode position and number and frequency of treatments were mentioned; and whether unwanted effects, immediate results, and longer-term outcome were reported. A quality score was obtained by adding up the ratings on these variables. The maximum possible score was 20.

Overall, the quality of the reports was poor (mean score = 8.9, SD = 3.2, range = 2–17); there were no controlled studies. The closest to a controlled study was the work by Kutcher and Robertson (56), which compared the outcome of a group of 16 patients (nine of them 19 years of age or older) who received ECT with the outcome of six patients who refused. This is also the only study that used a structured diagnostic interview.

Almost one-half of the studies (43%, N = 26) provided no diagnosis, or there was insufficient information on symptoms to make a diagnosis. Previous and concurrent treatments were not indicated in 23% (N = 14) and 68% (N = 41), respectively. Electrode position and number and frequency of ECTs were not mentioned in 62% (N = 37), 20% (N = 12), and 72% (N = 43), respectively. Unwanted effects were not reported in 63% (N = 38). Short-term outcome was poorly described in 35% (N = 21), while information on longer-term outcome (6 or more months after ECT) was provided in less than one-half (42%, N = 25) of the studies. Only two reports (45, 56) used quantitative measures of outcome.

To examine the quality of the studies over time, we divided the reports into those published before DSM-III and those published after. Studies published after 1980 had higher scores for quality (mean = 9.9, SD = 2.9, versus mean = 7.5, SD = 3.2; t = 3.06, df = 58, p = 0.003) and were more likely than earlier studies to supply better diagnostic information, to describe electrode placement, and to mention unwanted effects in more detail.

COLLATION OF INDIVIDUAL CASES

All individuals for whom there was sufficient information about diagnosis and outcome were coded in order to examine the response to ECT across reports. Patients from 15 studies (13, 15, 23, 25, 28, 30, 35, 38, 41, 44–46, 48, 57, 60) were excluded because diagnosis or outcome was not described or could not be identified individually. Information about diagnosis and outcome was available for 39% (N = 154) of the 396 reported cases.

Among the 98 patients for whom age was specified, the mean age was 15.4 years (SD = 2.2). The youngest patient was 7 years old, and only five were younger than 12 years. About one-half (47%, N = 55) of the 118 subjects whose gender was known were female. By contrast, female adults are more likely than male adults to be treated with ECT (74). This disparity is consistent with the smaller gender imbalance for mood disorders during childhood and adolescence.

Treatment prior to ECT was described for 57 patients; 35% (N = 20) had courses of both antipsychotic and antidepressant drugs, 9% (N = 5) received antidepressants alone, 26% (N = 15) received antipsychotics alone, and the rest had other treatments or a combination of treatments. The reasons for using ECT were given for 57 individuals; failure to respond to other treatments together with severity of symptoms were the most common (92%). Seeking a second opinion before the administration of ECT was mentioned for 11 patients.

The number of ECTs was given for 95 individuals. The mean of 9.6 (SD = 4.9, range = 1–23) is similar to what has been reported for adults (75, 76).

When electrode position was mentioned (61 patients), 38% (N = 23) had unilateral and 48% (N = 29) bilateral electrode placement; a further 15% (N = 9) had both. EEG monitoring of seizures was used in 38 cases from four studies (21, 49, 50, 67). The technique of "stimulus dosing" (77) was not mentioned in recent reports.

EFFECTIVENESS

The proportions of patients, according to diagnosis, who benefited from ECT are presented in table 1. Reliability of diagnosis was not reported in any of the studies. Cases in which there was clear evidence of bipolar disorder were included in two groups, the bipolar group and the depressed or manic group. To examine specifically the effectiveness of ECT in patients with catatonic symptoms (78), subjects with those symptoms (e.g., stupor) were included in a separate group (catatonia) irrespective of whether they had an affective, schizophrenic, or organic diagnosis. Twenty (24%) of the 85 patients in whom comorbidity could be ascertained had comorbid mental disorders, while 13 (15%) of the 85 had a comorbid physical illness.

Response to treatment was almost invariably described in an impressionistic, not quantitative, way. Consequently, we conservatively divided immediate outcome into two categories: patients who showed marked improvement or recovery and those who did not. This required a degree of inference in some cases. We divided outcome at 6 months into groups

TABLE 1
Initial Response to ECT and Longer-Term Outcome in Young Patients Described in the Literature, by Diagnosis

Diagnosis	Immediately After ECT: Number of Patients	Patients With Remission or Marked Improvement: N	%	6 Months After ECT[a]: Number of Patients	Patients With Good Functioning: N	%
Depression	40	25	63	18	13	72
Major	26	19	73	14	11	79
Psychotic	14	6	43	4	2	50
Manic episode	20	16	80	10	8	80
Bipolar disorder[b]	51	37	73	24	17	71
Schizophrenia	36	15	42	10	1	10
Schizoaffective disorder	2	1	50	—	—	—
Catatonia[c]	24	18	75	13	6	46
Neuroleptic malignant syndrome	4	2	50	2	1	50
Other disorders	28	4	14	6	2	33
Total[d]	154	81	53	59	31	53

[a]Most patients had other treatments after ECT.
[b]Includes manic, depressed, and catatonic.
[c]Includes mood disorder with catatonic features, catatonic schizophrenia, and catatonia associated with physical illness.
[d]Excludes bipolar disorder.

of patients who were described as functioning near or at the premorbid level and those who were not. Interpretation of these results warrants caution, for it is possible that published cases, especially single case studies, are biased.

Overall, 53% (N = 81) of the 154 patients for whom data on diagnosis and outcome were available showed marked improvement or remission of symptoms by the end of the course of ECT. If those who had a mild or moderate response are also counted, the proportion who benefited increases to 67%. The results presented in table 1 are broadly similar to those described for adult patients. For example, Mukherjee et al. (79) showed a marked improvement in mania of 80% across studies of ECT. These data also suggest that ECT in this age group is comparatively less effective for schizophrenia than for mood disorders. The main incongruence with data on adults (80) refers to psychotic depression: table 1 shows a lower response rate than that for other types of mood disorder and similar to that for schizophrenia. This may reflect difficulties in distinguishing between psychotic depression and schizophrenia in adolescents.

When all disorders were combined, there were no differences in the rates of improvement according to electrode placement (unilateral versus bilateral), age (younger [<16 years] versus older), or whether there was comorbidity. Cases from reports published after 1980 showed higher rates of response than earlier ones.

There was information in 22 cases about when improvement was first observed. This generally occurred early in the course of treatments, but in some cases it took up to 10 treatments (mean = 3.7, SD = 2.4, range = 1–10).

ADVERSE EVENTS

When we examined adverse events, all 60 reports were considered. No fatalities among the young as a consequence of ECT have been described. A 16-year-old girl with neuroleptic malignant syndrome and a stuporous state had eight ECTs without improvement (55). She died of cardiac failure 10 days after the last treatment. Her death is likely to have been due to the continued administration of neuroleptic medication in spite of her neuroleptic malignant syndrome.

Earlier studies that tended to use a large number of treatments or very frequent ECTs did not report long-term problems. For example, Bauer (17) noted the case of a 15-year-old girl with schizophrenia who received 200 ECTs in 1 year. Heuyer et al. (25) described a 16-year-old girl diagnosed as suffering from dementia praecox who was treated with 15 unmodified ECTs in 3 days. She developed an organic brain syndrome, with an abnormal EEG, which subsided over a period of 3 weeks.

The presence of physical illness does not appear to be a contraindication for ECT in most cases. Mansheim (59) described a patient with meningomyelocele, hydrocephalus with functioning shunt, and seizures who tolerated ECT well. Schneekloth et al. (67) reported on a patient with a kidney transplant who had no harmful effects from ECT. Warren et al. (70) described an individual with major depression and comorbid Down's syndrome who showed no unwanted effects.

Bender (15) reported one case of a fractured vertebra. This occurred before the introduction of modified ECT with muscle relaxants. Five patients were reported to have ended the course of ECT prematurely because of side effects (21, 26, 29, 30, 68). These included a depressed teenager who underwent a switch to mania after five ECTs (26); two whose treatment was discontinued because of increasing agitation (30, 68); one who showed marked confusion after two treatments (29); and an 18-year-old female patient with bipolar disorder who developed neuroleptic malignant syndrome following one ECT, after which the course was terminated (21). She had been given droperidol before and after ECT (F.N. Moise, personal communication).

Seizures

Prolonged seizures induced by ECT (lasting more than 180 seconds) (81) and post-ECT seizures have been described. Guttmacher and Cretella (49) reported prolonged convulsions in three cases. Two of these patients were taking concurrent medication (one was taking desipramine and one trifluoperazine). The third adolescent suffered from Tourette's disorder and pervasive developmental disorder and had had a seizure at the age of 11 years. Ghaziuddin et al. (45) also reported prolonged seizures in five of seven cases. However, details such as the actual length of the convulsion, whether the patients were taking concurrent medication, history of seizures, etc. were not given. Prolonged seizures were described in another three patients (2%) out of 142 treatments (21). It is not known whether they had concurrent medication.

Bender (15) reported one case of post-ECT seizures in a child who had had a convulsion at the age of 18 months. It is noteworthy that most (72%) of the children she described had abnormal EEGs prior to ECT. The EEG had worsened in only one of the 22 patients tested 6 months later (this was a child with petit mal before ECT), while the EEG had improved in eight (36%). Post-ECT seizures were described in another three patients (45, 63, 67). One of them, a mentally retarded boy, developed a nonconvulsive status epilepticus following the ninth ECT (63). He was also taking neuroleptics.

Although there is concern that the seizure threshold may be lower in children and adolescents (1), the evidence that young people are particularly at risk of having lengthy convulsions or of developing post-ECT seizures is not persuasive. The rate of lengthy seizures in the young does not seem to be greater than the rate of 1.1% cited for adults (82).

Other Adverse Events

Overall, the most common complaint was headache, reported in 16 cases. Subjective memory loss was described in nine patients (19, 26, 29, 39, 40) and manic symptoms in seven (23, 26, 29, 34, 62). Disinhibition was described in two subjects (40, 68) and hemifacial flushing in one (52).

The frequency of side effects was higher in recent studies that examined them systematically. Paillère-Martinot et al. (26) reported mild side effects in seven (78%) of nine patients, while Ghaziuddin et al. (45) reported headaches in their entire group. Kutcher and Robertson (56) reported mild, transient side effects following 28% of ECTs: headache, 15%; confusion, 5%; agitation, 3%; hypomanic symptoms, 2%; subjective memory loss, 2%; and vomiting, 1%. This suggests that minor, transient side effects have often been underreported or overlooked.

Cognitive Functioning

Cognitive functioning before and after ECT was seldom alluded to. The reason sometimes given was that children were too sick to undergo psychometric tests. Unfortunately, too, the few studies that have formally assessed cognitive functioning after ECT were conducted in the 1940s and 1950s (15, 83–85). Nevertheless, they reported no permanent ill effects. Bender (15) carried out "extensive psychometric examination . . . before shock, immediately following shock and at intervals thereafter whenever possible." Her data show no evidence of "a lasting effect on intellectual functioning." In another study (84), children were asked to draw human figures and perform the "visual motor gestalt test" before and after ECT. The abnormalities that occurred lasted up to 6 hours after each daily ECT and increased throughout the course, but they cleared approximately 36 hours after the last treatment. Using a battery of tests, Des Lauriers and Halpern (83) found that after ECT, children and adolescents showed a slight increase in IQ and greater ability to concentrate but no change in reasoning or judgment. Another study (85) reported that intellectual "efficiency" was reduced immediately after a course of treatment but recovered at follow-up 5–27 months later. Six individuals in other studies (12, 25, 26, 29) developed an organic brain syndrome that resolved quickly after cessation of treatment.

Overall, adverse events appear similar in type and frequency to those described for adults. Because the literature has limitations, it is not certain that more serious adverse events did not occur. Also, side effects were often not commented upon and were seldom scrutinized systematically.

USE AND MISUSE OF ECT

It was estimated that approximately 500 (1.5%) of 33,384 patients who received ECT in the United States in 1980 were in the 11- to 20-year age range (86). On average, eight patients under the age of 18 received ECT each year in California in 1977–1983, 0.3% of all persons treated with ECT during those 7 years (87). Over 12 years, 22 patients aged 16–19 were treated with ECT at the University Hospital, Stony Brook, N.Y. (1). Five patients (all female and aged 17 years) were given ECT in Edinburgh between 1982 and 1992 (41), while ECT was used for adolescents three times in 10 years at Bethlem Hospital in London (88). Seven adolescents aged 15–18 years received ECT at the Hôpital de la Salpêtrière in Paris between 1986 and 1988 (26). No patient younger than 19 years was given ECT at an acute unit in Sydney, Australia, between 1982 and 1988 (76). Therefore, rates of ECT use in young people are low.

These findings are consistent with results of practice surveys. All psychiatrists working in psychiatric facilities in New York reported occasionally treating adolescent patients with ECT (89). Of 433 British psychiatrists surveyed, 31 (7%) had used this treatment in patients younger than 16 (90). Lower age limits are set by certain hospitals and governments (21). For example, ECT was not administered to children under the age of 16 in the former Soviet Union (91).

Although concerns have been expressed about inappropriate use of ECT in young people (3, 4) there is little systematic information to help determine whether such practices actually exist. When the very early studies, which do not reflect current practice, are excluded, it can be inferred that ECT is hardly ever used to treat prepubertal children and very rarely to treat adolescents. When administered, it is almost always after other treatments have failed and when the patient's symptoms are very incapacitating or life-threatening. That is, ECT is used almost exclusively as a treatment of last resort. Bearing in mind the severity and complexity of illness of the patients treated with ECT and the mild, transient nature of most adverse events, a rate of improvement across disorders of 67% (or 53% if only marked improvement or complete remission is counted) is more than heartening. If anything, the collective data suggest that ECT may be underutilized.

These conclusions should be tempered by the fact that we do not know whether the published cases are biased; that is, cases in which there was poor response or severe adverse events might have been less likely to be reported. However, the results of a recent survey (unpublished work of Walter and Rey) suggest that published reports, as a whole, actually reflect what happens in practice (at least in Australia). In that study, all persons aged 18 years or under who received ECT between 1990 and 1996 in the Australian state of New South Wales were identified. Forty-two patients had a total of 49 courses comprising 450 ECTs, about 1% of all treatments. The youngest patients were 14 years old. Marked improvement or resolution of symptoms occurred in one-half of the completed courses. Side effects were mild and transient. Prolonged seizures occurred in 0.4% of the treatments.

DIRECTIONS FOR RESEARCH

It is evident that our knowledge about ECT in children and adolescents is deficient. Given the scarcity of studies, funding agencies and clinicians must give more priority to ECT research. Randomized, controlled trials of ECT versus sham ECT are needed to show conclusively whether ECT is effective or not in this age group. While serious ethical arguments to prevent such trials are lacking (1, 8), public opinion may impede that research. Fortunately, alternatives that will also increase our knowledge are available. For example, it would be valuable to compare the outcome of youngsters who undergo ECT with that of others who refuse or do not receive ECT, to confirm and extend the results reported by Kutcher and Robertson (56). These authors found that the hospital stay was shorter for patients who received ECT; use of ECT also more than halved the cost of treatment. Long-term follow-up of these patients may clarify whether ECT influences the course of the illness (11). If so, this may be relevant, since early onset appears to be associated with a worse course in some disorders (92).

Epidemiological information on the use of ECT is also necessary to show whether published reports are biased. Setting up registers to collect systematic data about ECT in the young could provide this information at low cost. Such registers could also be used to monitor adverse events and standards of practice.

Increasing our knowledge about the seizure threshold in children and adolescents should be a priority because of both the suggestion that these patients may be more likely to experience prolonged seizures and concerns about post-ECT seizures. Whether propofol results in shorter seizures (93) in young people than do other induction agents is also worth studying, as are the structural and psychometric effects of ECT. Finally, it is necessary that the quality of the published reports be improved.

IMPLICATIONS FOR EDUCATION AND CLINICAL PRACTICE

ECT should be used with caution in young people because of the relative lack of knowledge. However, it may also be overlooked as a treatment alternative (2, 78). Although a detailed discussion is beyond the scope of this review, it is worth speculating about why sections of the psychiatric profession and the community oppose the use of ECT in the young. One reason may be an antipathy toward ECT generally. This, in turn, has many determinants (94). The fear of adverse effects of ECT on the developing brain and the assumption that children and adolescents cannot fully understand—and thus cannot properly consent to—the treatment are often mentioned. Lack of knowledge of, or familiarity with, the procedure, particularly in the case of child psychiatrists, may also contribute to a negative perception of ECT. This is not surprising because of the low rates of utilization and the paucity of reports and because ECT is often ignored in textbooks on child and adolescent psychiatry (e.g., reference 95). Preliminary results of a survey of the majority (83%) of Australian and

New Zealand child and adolescent psychiatrists (unpublished work of Walter et al.) showed that 40% rated themselves as having no knowledge or negligible knowledge about ECT in the young, and only 31% had first-hand experience of it.

The American Psychiatric Association offers guidelines for the use of ECT in the young (81). Similar guidelines have been published recently by the Royal College of Psychiatrists (96). Other psychiatric associations should follow this lead.

Because of reports of increased length of seizure and post-ECT convulsions, clinicians are advised to stop all nonessential medications while administering ECT. Concurrent medications are used often and may be responsible for many of the adverse events. There is a case for determining the seizure threshold, for EEG monitoring, and possibly for EEG examinations before and after a course of ECT. Psychometric assessment before and some time after ECT would also be valuable.

Finally, consent issues require particular attention (81, 96). The parents and the child should be involved whenever possible and should be given adequate information. The opportunity to discuss ECT with other young people who have received it may be helpful (56).

CONCLUSIONS

"On February 10, 1977, electroconvulsive treatment was administered for the first time to a 16-year-old female who had not eaten, spoken or walked unaided for the past four months .... The first treatment produced an unclinching of the fists .... The second treatment produced consumption of small amounts of fluid .... The fifth was productive of eating and talking normally .... She was allowed to go home two days after the last treatment and for the past three months has been getting along nicely and doing all things previously done in a satisfactory fashion." This account by Perkins and Tanaka (18) of the dramatic effect of seven ECTs is hardly unique but illustrates vividly why we need to learn more about this treatment. It is sobering that our knowledge has grown so little beyond that which Heuyer and his colleagues acquired half a century ago (13).

REFERENCES

1. Fink M: Electroconvulsive therapy in children and adolescents. Convulsive Therapy 1993; 9:155–157
2. Fink M, Carlson GA: ECT and prepubertal children. J Am Acad Child Adolesc Psychiatry 1995; 34:1256–1257
3. Baker T: ECT and young minds (letter). Lancet 1994; 345:65
4. Miller JP: ECT and prepubertal children. J Am Acad Child Adolesc Psychiatry 1995; 34:1257–1258
5. Weissman MM, Bruce ML, Leaf PJ, Florio LP, Holzer C: Affective disorders, in Psychiatric Disorders in America. Edited by Robins LN, Regier DA. New York, Free Press, 1991, pp 53–80
6. Rao U, Weissman MM, Martin JA, Hammond RW: Childhood depression and risk of suicide: a preliminary report of a longitudinal study. J Am Acad Child Adolesc Psychiatry 1993; 32:21–27
7. Campbell M, Cueva JE: Psychopharmacology in child and adolescent psychiatry: a review of the past seven years: part II. J Am Acad Child Adolesc Psychiatry 1995; 34:1262–1272

8. Hazell P, O'Connell D, Heathcote D, Robertson J, Henry D: Efficacy of tricyclic drugs in treating child and adolescent depression: a meta-analysis. BMJ 1995; 310:897–890
9. Devanand DP, Dwork AJ, Hutchinson ER, Bolwig TG, Sackeim HA: Does ECT alter brain structure? Am J Psychiatry 1994; 151:957–970
10. Rice EH, Sombrotto LB, Markowitz JC, Leon AC: Cardiovascular morbidity in high-risk patients during ECT. Am J Psychiatry 1994; 151:1637–1641
11. Bertagnoli MW, Borchardt CM: A review of ECT for children and adolescents. J Am Acad Child Adolesc Psychiatry 1990; 29:302–307
12. Heuyer G, Bour, Feld: Electrochoc chez des adolescents. Ann Med Psychol (Paris) 1942; 2:75–84
13. Heuyer G, Bour, Leroy R: L'électrochoc chez les enfants. Ann Med Psychol (Paris) 1943; 2:402–407
14. Hemphill RE, Walter WG: The treatment of mental disorders by electrically induced convulsions. J Ment Sci 1941; 87:256–275
15. Bender L: One hundred cases of childhood schizophrenia treated with electric shock. Trans Am Neurol Soc 1947; 72:165–169
16. Clardy ER, Rumpf EM: The effect of electric shock treatment on children having schizophrenic manifestations. Psychiatr Q 1954; 28:616–623
17. Bauer W: Treatment of a 15-year-old hebephrenic girl in a community hospital. Dis Nerv Syst 1976; 37:474–476
18. Perkins IH, Tanaka K: The controversy that will not die is the treatment that can and does save lives: electroconvulsive therapy. Adolescence 1979; 14:607–616
19. Sokol MS, Pfeffer CR, Solomon GE, Esman A, Robinson G, Gold RL, Orr-Adrawes A: An abused psychotic preadolescent at risk for Huntington's disease. J Am Acad Child Adolesc Psychiatry 1989; 28:612–617
20. Berman E, Wolpert EA: Intractable manic-depressive psychosis with rapid cycling in an 18-year-old woman successfully treated with electroconvulsive therapy. J Nerv Ment Dis 1987; 175:236–239
21. Moise FN, Petrides G: ECT in adolescents. J Am Acad Child Adolesc Psychiatry 1996; 35:312–318
22. Constantidinis J: Etude clinique et psychologique de deux adolescents psychotiques jumeaux univitellins. Ann Med Psychol (Paris) 1969; 2:161–171
23. Fillastre M, Fontaine A, Depecker L, Degiovanni A: Cinq cas de syndrome de Cotard de l'adolescent et de l'adult jeune. Encephale 1992; 18:65–66
24. Heuyer G, Dauphin, Levovici S: La practique de l'électrochoc chez l'enfant. Zeitschrift fur Kinderspychiatrie (Bern) 1947; 14:60–64
25. Heuyer G, Lebovici S, Amado G: Les électrochocs en sommation. Ann Med Psychol (Paris) 1948; 1:205–208
26. Paillère-Martinot ML, Zivi A, Basquin M: Utilisation de l'ECT chez l'adolescent. Encephale 1990; 16:399–404
27. Revuelta E, Bordet R, Piquet T, Ghawche F, Destee A, Goudemand M: Catatonie aigue et syndrome malin des neuroleptiques: un cas au cours d'une psychose infantile. Encephale 1994; 20:351–354
28. Friederich MH, Leixnering W: Zur problematik der elektro-schocktherapie jugendlicher psychosen. Ideggyogyaszati Szemle 1980; 33:278–284
29. Hift C, Hift S, Spiel W: Ergebnisse der schockbedhandlungen bei kindlischen schizophrenien. Schweiz Arch Neurol Psychiatrie 1960; 86:256–272

30. Knitter H: Erfahrungen mit Elektrokrampftherapie bei Psychosen des Kindesalters. Padiatr Grenzgeb 1986; 25:449–452
31. Sauer H, Koehler KG, Funfgeld EW: Folgen unterlassener elektrokrampftherapie: ein kasuistischer beitrag. Nervenarzt 1985; 56:150–152
32. Bilikiewitz T: A case of apallic syndrome (inaccurately so called) in a child in the light of a 17-year follow-up. Psychiatr Pol 1978; 12:619–622
33. Addonizio G, Susman VL: ECT as a treatment alternative for patients with symptoms of neuroleptic malignant syndrome. J Clin Psychiatry 1987; 48:102–105
34. Andrade C, Gangadhar BN, Channabasavanna SM: Further characterization of mania as a side effect of ECT. Convulsive Therapy 1990; 6:318–319
35. Arajarvi T, Alanen YO, Viitamaki O: Psychoses in childhood. Acta Psychiatr Scand Suppl 1964; 174:1–93
36. Black DW, Wilcox JA, Stewart M: The use of ECT in children: case report. J Clin Psychiatry 1985; 46:98–99
37. Campbell JD: Manic depressive psychosis in children: report of 18 cases. J Nerv Ment Dis 1952; 116:424–439
38. Campbell M: Biological interventions in psychoses in childhood. J Autism Child Schizophr 1973; 3:347–373
39. Carr V, Dorrington C, Schrader G, Wale J: The use of ECT for mania in childhood bipolar disorder. Br J Psychiatry 1983; 143:411–415
40. Cizadlo BC, Wheaton A: Case study: ECT treatment of a young girl with catatonia. J Am Acad Child Adolesc Psychiatry 1995; 34:332–335
41. Cook A, Scott A: ECT for young people. Br J Psychiatry 1992; 161:718–719
42. Dinwiddie SH, Drevets WC, Smith DR: Treatment of phencyclidine-associated psychosis with ECT. Convulsive Therapy 1988; 4:230–235
43. Frances A, Susman VL: Managing an acutely manic 17-year-old girl with neuroleptic malignant syndrome. Hosp Community Psychiatry 1986; 37:771–772, 788
44. Gallinek A: Controversial indications for electric convulsive therapy. Am J Psychiatry 1952; 109:361–366
45. Ghaziuddin N, King C, Naylor M, Ghaziuddin M, Chaudhary N, Greden J: Electro-convulsive treatment (ECT) in refractory adolescent depression (abstract). Biol Psychiatry 1995; 37:593
46. Gillis A: A case of schizophrenia in childhood. J Nerv Ment Dis 1955; 121:471–472
47. Gujavarty K, Greenberg LB, Fink M: Electroconvulsive therapy and neuroleptic medication in therapy-resistant positive-symptom psychosis. Convulsive Therapy 1987; 3:185–195
48. Gutierrez-Esteinou R, Pope HG: Does fluoxetine prolong electrically induced seizures? Convulsive Therapy 1989; 5:344–348
49. Guttmacher LB, Cretella H: Electroconvulsive therapy in one child and three adolescents. J Clin Psychiatry 1988; 49:20–23
50. Guttmacher LB, Cretella H, Houghtalen R: ECT in children and adolescents. J Clin Psychiatry 1989; 50:106–107
51. Hassanyeh F, Davison K: Bipolar affective psychosis with onset before age 16 years: report of 10 cases. Br J Psychiatry 1980; 137:530–539
52. Idupuganti S, Mujica R: Hemifacial flushing during unilateral ECT (letter). Am J Psychiatry 1988; 145:1037–1038

53. Jeffries JJ, Lefebvre A: Depression and mania associated with Kleine-Levin-Critchley syndrome. Can Psychiatr Assoc J 1973; 18:439–444

54. Kaponen H, Repo E, Lepola U: Neuroleptic malignant syndrome. Biol Psychiatry 1988; 24:943–944

55. Kish SJ, Kleinert R, Minauf M, Gilbert J, Walter GF, Slimovitch C, Maurer E, Rezvani Y, Myers R, Hornykiewicz O: Brain neurotransmitter changes in three patients who had a fatal hyperthermia syndrome. Am J Psychiatry 1990; 147:1358–1363

56. Kutcher S, Robertson HA: Electroconvulsive therapy in treatment-resistant bipolar youth. J Child and Adolescent Psychopharmacology 1995; 5:167–175

57. Krinsky LW, Jennings RM: The management and treatment of the pseudopsychopathic schizophrenic in an adolescent pavilion. J Asthma Res 1968; 5:207–212

58. Levy S, Southcombe RH: Value of convulsive therapy in juvenile schizophrenia. Arch Neurol Psychiatry 1951; 65:54–59

59. Mansheim P: ECT in the treatment of a depressed adolescent with meningomyelocele, hydrocephalus, and seizures. J Clin Psychiatry 1983; 44:385–386

60. Otegui J, Lyford-Pike A, Zurmendi P, Savi P, Flores D, Castro G: Electroconvulsive therapy (ECT) in adolescents and children in private hospitals in Montevideo (Uruguay) (abstract). Convulsive Therapy 1995; 11:73

61. Pataki J, Zervas IM, Jandorf L: Catatonia in a university inpatient service (1985–1990). Convulsive Therapy 1992; 8:163–173

62. Powell JC, Silveira WR, Lindsay R: Pre-pubertal depressive stupor: a case report. Br J Psychiatry 1988; 153:689–692

63. Rao KMJ, Gangadhar BN, Janakiramaiah N: Nonconvulsive status epilepticus after the ninth electroconvulsive therapy. Convulsive Therapy 1993; 9:128–129

64. Ries RK, Schuckit MA: Catatonia and autonomic hyperactivity. Psychosomatics 1980; 21:349–350

65. Rosen A: Case report: symptomatic mania and phencyclidine abuse. Am J Psychiatry 1979; 136:118–119

66. Sands D: Acute psychotic disturbance and regression in an adolescent girl. Nurs Times 1978; 74:2055–2057

67. Schneekloth TD, Rummans TA, Logan KM: Electroconvulsive therapy in adolescents. Convulsive Therapy 1993; 9:159–166

68. Slack T, Stoudemire A: Reinstitution of neuroleptic treatment with molindone in a patient with a history of neuroleptic malignant syndrome. Gen Hosp Psychiatry 1989; 11:365–367

69. Warneke L: A case of manic-depressive illness in childhood. Can Psychiatr Assoc J 1975; 20:195–200

70. Warren AC, Holroyd S, Folstein MF: Major depression in Down's syndrome. Br J Psychiatry 1989; 155:202–205

71. Weeston TF, Constantino J: High-dose T4 for rapid-cycling bipolar disorder. J Am Acad Child Adolesc Psychiatry 1996; 35:131–132

72. Zorumski CF, Burke WJ, Rutherford JL, Reich T: ECT: clinical variables, seizure duration and outcome. Convulsive Therapy 1986; 2:109–119

73. Gralnick A, Rabiner EL, Del Castillo G, Zawel D: Treatment considerations in the adolescent inpatient. Dis Nerv Syst 1969; 30:833–842

74. Thompson JW, Weiner RD, Myers CP: Use of ECT in the United States in 1975, 1980, and 1986. Am J Psychiatry 1994; 151:1657–1661
75. Mills MJ, Pearsall DT, Yesavage JA, Salzman C: Electroconvulsive therapy in Massachusetts. Am J Psychiatry 1984; 141:534–538
76. Gassy JE, Rey JM: A survey of ECT in a general hospital psychiatry unit. Aust NZ J Psychiatry 1990; 24:385–390
77. Sackeim H, Decina P, Prohovik I, Malitz S: Seizure threshold in electroconvulsive therapy: effects of age, sex, electrode placement and number. Arch Gen Psychiatry 1987; 44:355–360
78. Fink M: Indications for the use of ECT. Psychopharmacol Bull 1994; 30:269–280
79. Mukherjee S, Sackeim HA, Schnur DB: Electroconvulsive therapy of acute manic episodes: a review of 50 years' experience. Am J Psychiatry 1994; 151:169–176
80. Parker G, Roy K, Hadzi-Pavlovic D, Pedic F: Psychotic (delusional) depression: a meta-analysis of physical treatments. J Affect Disord 1992; 24:17–24
81. The Practice of Electroconvulsive Therapy: Recommendations for Treatment, Training, and Privileging: A Task Force Report of the American Psychiatric Association. Washington, DC, APA, 1990
82. Greenberg LB: Detection of prolonged seizures during electroconvulsive therapy: a comparison of electroencephalogram and cuff monitoring. Convulsive Therapy 1985; 1:32–37
83. Des Lauriers A, Halpern F: Psychological tests in childhood schizophrenia. Am J Orthopsychiatry 1947; 17:57–67
84. Bender L, Keeler WR: The body image of schizophrenic children following electroshock therapy. Am J Orthopsychiatry 1952; 22:335–355
85. Gurevitz S, Helme WH: Effects of electroconvulsive therapy on personality and intellectual functioning of the schizophrenic child. J Nerv Ment Dis 1954; 120:213–226
86. Thompson JW, Blaine JD: Use of ECT in the United States in 1975 and 1980. Am J Psychiatry 1987; 144:557–562
87. Kramer BA: Use of ECT in California, 1977–1983. Am J Psychiatry 1985; 142:1190–1192
88. Steinberg D: Basic Adolescent Psychiatry. Oxford, England, Blackwell, 1987, p 243
89. Asnis GM, Fink M, Saferstein S: ECT in metropolitan New York hospitals: a survey of practice. Am J Psychiatry 1978; 135:479–482
90. Parmar R: Attitudes of child psychiatrists to electroconvulsive therapy. Psychiatr Bull 1983; 17:12–13
91. Bloch S: The political misuse of psychiatry in the Soviet Union, in Psychiatric Ethics, 2nd ed. Edited by Bloch S, Chodoff P. New York, Oxford University Press, 1991, pp 493–515
92. Lish JD, Dime-Meenan S, Whybrow PC, Price RA, Hirschfeld RMA: The National Depressive and Manic-Depressive Association (DMDA) survey of bipolar members. J Affect Disord 1994; 31:281–294
93. Fear CF, Littlejohns CS, Rouse E, McQuail P: Propofol anaesthesia in electroconvulsive therapy: reduced seizure duration may not be relevant. Br J Psychiatry 1994; 165:506–509
94. Durham J: Sources of public prejudice against ECT. Aust NZ J Psychiatry 1989; 23:453–460
95. Werry JS, Aman MG: Practitioner's Guide to Psychoactive Drugs for Children and Adolescents. New York, Plenum, 1993
96. Freeman CP: ECT in those under 18 years old, in The ECT Handbook. Edited by Freeman CP. London, Royal College of Psychiatrists, 1995, pp 18–21

PART III: TREATMENT ISSUES

12

A Controlled Trial of Light Therapy for the Treatment of Pediatric Seasonal Affective Disorder

Susan E. Swedo and Albert John Allen
National Institute of Mental Health, Bethesda, Maryland
Carol A. Glod
McLean Hospital, Belmont, Massachusetts
Catherine H. Clark
National Institute of Mental Health
Martin H. Teicher
McLean Hospital, Belmont, Massachusetts
Dan Richter, Cara Hoffman, Susan D. Hamburger, Sara Dow, Charlotte Brown, and Norman E. Rosenthal
National Institute of Mental Health, Bethesda, Maryland

Objective: *To evaluate the efficacy of light therapy for the treatment of pediatric seasonal affective disorder (SAD).* **Method:** *28 children (aged 7 to 17 years) at two geographically distinct sites were enrolled in a double-blind, placebo-controlled, crossover trial of bright-light treatment. Subjects initially entered a week-long baseline period during which they wore dark glasses for an hour a day. They were then randomly assigned to receive either active treatment (1 hour of bright-light therapy plus 2 hours of dawn simulation) or placebo (1 hour of clear goggles plus 5 minutes of low-intensity dawn simulation) for 1 week. The treatment phase was followed by a second dark-glasses phase lasting 1 to 2*

Reprinted with permission from the *Journal of the American Academy of Child and Adolescent Psychiatry*, 1997, Vol. 36(6), 816–821.

This research was supported in part by R01 MH48343 and donations from the Freund Foundation and Mr. and Mrs. Richard Simchas to Dr. Teicher. The authors thank Eric Turner, M.D., Joanna Pleeter, Chris Luetke, Ann Polcari, R.N., M.S.C.S., Cindy McGreenery, and Elizabeth Witowski for their assistance with data collection; Emily Yamada for her help with instrument development; and David Avery, M.D., for his advice regarding the use of dawn simulation. Thanks to the Sun Box Company for the loan of light boxes and to PsiSq for the donation of the dawn simulators.

weeks. After this phase, the children received the alternate treatment. Response was measured using the parent and child versions of the Structured Interview Guide for the Hamilton Depression Rating Scale, Seasonal Affective Disorders version (SIGH-SAD). **Results:** *Data were analyzed as change from baseline. SIGH-SAD-P total depression scores were significantly decreased from baseline during light therapy compared with placebo (one-way analysis of variance, p = .009), and no differences were found between the placebo and control phases. Subscores of atypical and typical depression were also significantly decreased during the active treatment (p = .004 and .028, respectively). A similar trend was noted with the SIGH-SAD-C, but this did not reach significance. At the end of the study, 78% of the parents questioned and 80% of the children questioned rated light therapy as the phase during which the child "felt best."* **Conclusion:** *Light therapy appears to be an effective treatment for pediatric SAD.*

Winter seasonal affective disorder (SAD) is a variant of recurrent affective disorder in which mood changes and atypical vegetative symptoms regularly occur during the winter months and disappear completely during the spring and summer (Rosenthal et al., 1984). Although SAD has been well described in adults (Rosenthal, 1993), less is known about the clinical presentation and treatment of children with SAD. Recent epidemiological studies suggest that winter SAD may affect as many as 3% to 4% of school-age children (Carskadon and Acebo, 1993; Swedo et al., 1995), and symptoms seem similar to those in adults. Rosenthal and colleagues (1986) described seven children who regularly experienced depressive symptoms during the winter months, particularly irritability, fatigue, sadness, sleep changes, and problems at school. After an open trial of bright-light therapy, all seven subjects experienced improvement in these symptoms, particularly school performance and mood. At 7-year follow-up, J. Giedd (written communication, 1994) found that all six of the children who could be reached still had seasonal symptoms and continued to use some form of light therapy during the winter.

Other reports suggest that pediatric SAD may be similar to the adult variant, not only in clinical presentation, but also in response to light therapy. Sonis et al. (1987) compared bright-light therapy to relaxation treatment in a double-blind, controlled study of five children with SAD. They found that light therapy, but not relaxation therapy, significantly decreased the severity of the SAD symptoms. Moreover, the benefits of light therapy appeared to be fairly specific to seasonal symptoms, since four children with nonseasonal major depression and five subjects with attention deficit disorder did not show similar improvement. On the basis of the adult literature and anecdotal pediatric experiences, we predicted that light therapy would be effective in reducing the symptoms of pediatric SAD.

Because little is known about the responsiveness of pediatric SAD patients to light therapy, and because other pediatric affective disorders appear to be relatively refractory to treatment (Ryan, 1992), we chose to maximize treatment effect by using both dawn simulation and afternoon bright-light therapy for the active-treatment phase. Inasmuch as both of these modalities have been reported to be effective for the treatment of adult SAD (Rosenthal, 1993; Rosenthal et al., 1984), we reasoned that the combination would be more effective than either modality alone.

METHOD

Study Criteria

Eligible subjects met all *DSM-III-R* criteria for recurrent major depression with a winter seasonal pattern (American Psychiatric Association, 1987), except that only two prior episodes of winter depression were required instead of three (in keeping with Rosenthal et al., 1986). To be accepted into the study, seasonal affective symptoms had to be present both at home and at school. Children who had a history of nonwinter depression were excluded, as were those who had had a prior trial of bright-light therapy.

Subjects

This study was conducted over two consecutive winters at two collaborating sites, one in the Washington, D.C., metropolitan area and the other in Boston. In the Washington, D.C., area, subjects were recruited using announcements in Parent-Teacher Association and school newsletters. These announcements generated 110 telephone calls, which produced 65 completed telephone interviews. From this group, 30 children and adolescents were identified as potential subjects and came into the outpatient clinic for an evaluation. All children were seen by two mental health professionals experienced in the diagnosis of pediatric SAD, one or both of whom were physicians. Evaluations included general medical and psychiatric interviews with one (or both) parents and the child, as well as the parent and child versions of the Structured Interview Guide for the Hamilton Depression Rating Scale, Seasonal Affective Disorders version (SIGH-SAD-P and SIGH-SAD-C) (Williams et al., 1994). In addition, potential subjects completed three self-report questionnaires: the Seasonal Pattern Assessment Questionnaire (SPAQ) (Kasper et al., 1989), a survey version of the SPAQ designed for children and adolescents, the Kiddie-SPAQ (Swedo et al., 1995), and the Seasonal Screening Questionnaire (Rosenthal et al., 1989). These structured assessments, in combination with the semistructured clinical interview, were used to make the diagnosis of SAD in the Washington, D.C., subjects. Of those evaluated, six children were excluded from the study, one because of a prior trial of light therapy and five because their symptoms did not meet criteria for pediatric SAD. Eighteen children were enrolled, the first starting in early November and the last completing the study in mid-March, with most subjects participating during January and February. Two patients withdrew during the course of the study (one because of surgery and one to seek active treatment).

In the Boston metropolitan area, subjects were also recruited by newspaper advertisements and self-referral. These referral sources generated 25 telephone calls, which produced 20 completed telephone screenings. Of the 20 screened, 15 were identified as potential SAD cases and were evaluated. Evaluations were completed by two mental health professionals experienced in the diagnosis of pediatric SAD and consisted of thorough medical and psychiatric interviews with one or both parents, including the Schedule for Affective Disorders and Schizophrenia for School-Age Children-Epidemiologic version (a semistructured questionnaire) (Orvaschel and Puig-Antich, 1987) and the SIGH-SAD-P. (The SIGH-SAD-C was not used in Boston.) Of the children evaluated, one failed to meet criteria and another declined to participate in the study in order to receive immediate, active treatment. Thus, 13 children were enrolled, the first starting the study in early December and the last finishing in early March, with most subjects participating during January and February. During the course of the study, one patient withdrew because of an extended vacation.

Study Design

A randomized, double-blind, crossover design was used in this treatment trial. The baseline consisted of a 1-week period during which subjects wore dark glasses (neutral gray with peripheral filters, with 10% light transmittance) for 1 hour between 4 and 8 P.M. when outside and not at school. The main purpose of the dark glasses was to attempt to create a double-blind. Subjects and their parents were told that the goal of the study was to compare the effectiveness of different frequencies of light for the treatment of SAD, and as a result the child would wear different pairs of light-filtering glasses during the different phases of the study. This explanation was based on studies which have reported that certain wavelengths of light may be more effective than others for the treatment of seasonal affective symptoms (Oren et al., 1991). Subjects wore the dark glasses at the same time of day that they would later wear the clear glasses or receive the active treatment. After the baseline dark-glasses phase, subjects were randomly assigned to receive either active or placebo treatment.

Active treatment consisted of 2 hours of dawn simulation to a maximum of 250 lux at 6:30 A.M., plus 1 hour of bright-light therapy (2,500 lux for children younger than 9 years old and 10,000 lux for those aged 9 or older) between 4 and 8 P.M. The decision to use a lower light intensity for the younger children was based on theoretical concerns about exposure of the children's eyes to high-intensity light sources (G.C. Brainard, personal communication, 1992), as well as clinical data suggesting that younger children respond to shorter durations and lower intensities of light (Rosenthal et al., 1986). Subjects were instructed to sit 18 inches in front of the light box and to glance at the light frequently while they played, read, or watched television. Placebo treatment consisted of 5 minutes of dawn simulation to a maximum of 2 lux, and 1 hour wearing clear glasses while doing sedentary activities (such as reading, watching television, etc.) at the same time of day that the child had received the active treatment. As with the dark glasses worn at baseline, subjects were told that the clear glasses might affect their SAD symptoms by filtering ambient light. The purpose of this explanation was to ensure that subjects had similar expectations for improvement before entering the placebo and active-treatment phases. Children and parents filled out comparative expectation ratings before each phase of the study to test the effectiveness of this explanation.

After a week of either placebo or active treatment, subjects entered a washout period (1 to 2 weeks) when they again wore the dark glasses. By design (and in accordance with institutional review board recommendations), the washout period could be terminated after the first week if the child demonstrated significant clinical deterioration. Six (38%) of the 16 children in Washington, D.C., and 7 (58%) of the 12 children in Boston had a 1-week washout. After washout, all subjects received the alternate treatment (placebo if they had had active treatment first or active treatment if they had already received placebo.)

Ratings and Outcome Measures

All ratings of symptom severity were obtained by separate individuals from those who provided the clinical care, to ensure that raters remained blind to treatment phase. In addition, to prevent accidental disclosure of the treatment, parents and children were specifically told not to discuss any aspect of their treatment with the raters. Ratings included a joint comparative expectations questionnaire, a side effects questionnaire, and the SIGH-SAD-C and SIGH-SAD-P. The SIGH-SAD-C and SIGH-SAD-P are modified versions of the widely used SIGH-SAD (Williams et al., 1994), a semistructured interview designed to measure severity of seasonal depressive symptoms (Terman et al., 1990, 1996). The SIGH-SAD-C and SIGH-SAD-P are similar to the adult version, but they contain additional items to measure symptoms that are unique to children: irritability, school performance/behavior, and concentration/attention. In addition, the language of the child interview was adjusted to approximately the second- to third-grade level, with the interviewer having some discretion over the language used with younger children. Both the SIGH-SAD-C and the SIGH-SAD-P can be scored to yield a total depression score or can be broken down into subscores of atypical or typical depression (instruments available upon request from the corresponding author).

In addition to these weekly ratings, at the end of the study, parents and children at one site were also asked to rank the phases in which the child "felt best," "felt second best," or "felt worst." Discussions of treatment effect were delayed until after these rankings to prevent physician opinion from biasing the patient's responses.

Statistical Analysis

No treatment-order effects were found at either site for any of the scales (analysis of variance [ANOVA]). However, significant site differences were found for baseline values of the SIGH-SAD-P, both for total depression scores ($p = .004$) and subscores of atypical and typical depression ($p = .009$ and .02, respectively). Therefore, subsequent statistical analyses were conducted on change scores. Scores were converted to change scores by subtracting phase scores from baseline scores for each subject. These change scores were then examined using one-way ANOVA for repeated measures with Bonferroni's post hoc testing. Additional analyses with *t* test and regression were used to determine whether there was any relationship between age or sex and baseline severity. All statistical analyses were done using SAS (SAS Institute, 1985). All reported *p* values are two-tailed.

RESULTS

Subjects

Table 1 summarizes the demographic information for the subjects in the two sites. Although the proportion of females to males differed in the two samples (Boston, 5:1; D.C., 1:2), no relation was found between gender and baseline severity on the SIGH-SAD-P. Age at onset and age at time of study were not significantly different between the sites, either. A regression analysis of age and baseline SIGH-SAD-P score did not show significant

TABLE 1
Patient Characteristics

	Washington, D.C. ($n = 16$)	Boston ($n = 12$)
Females: No. (%)	5 (31)	10 (83)
Males: No. (%)	11 (69)	2 (17)
Girls:boys	1:2	5:1
Age:yr (±SD)	12.2 (±2.7)	11.6 (±3.2)
Age at onset of SAD symptoms: yr (±SD)	7.8 (±2.7)	8.2 (±3.4)
No. of previous episodes of SAD (±SD)	4 (±2)	3 (±2)
Duration of previous episodes of SAD: months (±SD)	4.8 (±1.5)	5.0 (±1.3)

Note: SAD = seasonal affective disorder.

differences, suggesting that symptom severity was not related to the age of the subject. To further assess the impact of age on symptom severity, the group was divided into subgroups of children younger than 12 ($n = 13$) and those 12 or older ($n = 15$). The means were then compared using a t test, and again no differences were found. A t test comparing symptom severity of males ($n = 13$) versus females ($n = 15$) using the SIGH-SAD-P also found no significant differences.

Seasonal affective symptoms were similar to those reported previously (Rosenthal et al., 1984, 1986), with episodes of winter depression beginning around the end of October and extending until the end of March. The worst symptoms were noted in January.

Comorbid psychiatric diagnoses were found in 10 of 28 subjects: four children met diagnostic criteria for attention-deficit hyperactivity disorder (ADHD), two for a learning disorder, and one for both ADHD and a learning disorder; in addition, one child had a history of separation anxiety disorder and two met criteria for posttraumatic stress disorder.

Outcome

Data from the SIGH-SAD-P and the SIGH-SAD-C were analyzed as change from baseline using a one-way ANOVA (Table 2). As predicted, SIGH-SAD-P scores were significantly decreased from baseline during active treatment compared with both placebo and washout dark-goggles phases. No differences were found between the placebo and washout phases. This result was true for total depressive scores ($p = .009$), as well as subscores of atypical and typical depression ($p = .004$ and .028, respectively). While no significant differences were found with the SIGH-SAD-C, there was a trend toward greater improvement during active treatment than during the placebo phase (Table 2).

Because no diagnostic cutoff scores have been developed for the SIGH-SAD-P, it was not possible to determine the rate of clinical remission during active treatment. However, 20 (71%) of 28 subjects had at least a 50% decrease of symptoms during the active treatment,

TABLE 2
Improvement From Baseline for Children Treated With Bright-Light Therapy and Placebo

	Change Scores From Baseline[a]				
	Light Therapy	Placebo	Washout	F	p
SIGH-SAD-P ($n = 28$)					
Typical	7.07	3.00	2.89	4.0	.028[b]
Atypical	4.93	1.89	1.67	6.3	.004[b]
Total	12.0	4.96	4.56	5.4	.009[b]
SIGH-SAD-C[c] ($n = 16$)					
Typical	5.19	3.45	2.94	1.2	.31
Atypical	2.88	1.56	.63	2.8	.09
Total	8.06	5.00	3.56	2.1	.16

Note: SIGH-SAD-P and SIGH-SAD-C = parent and child versions of the Structured Interview Guide for the Hamilton Depression Rating Scale, Seasonal Affective Disorders version.
[a]All values were converted to change scores by subtracting subjects' scores in each phase from baseline score (larger score means greater change from baseline), and differences were analyzed by one-way analysis of variance for repeated measures.
[b]Light therapy > placebo.
[c]SIGH-SAD-C ratings were obtained at one site only ($n = 16$).

whereas only 7 (25%) of 28 had such a decrease during placebo. The effectiveness of the active treatment was confirmed in a posttreatment survey of the Washington, D.C., subjects, in which 78% of the parents (11/14) and 80% of the children (12/15) rated active treatment as the one in which the child "felt best" (one child and two parents did not complete the survey).

Reported expectations for improvement were not significantly different between the phases (as measured by the comparative expectations measure), suggesting that neither the children nor their parents were biased toward active treatment.

Data on side effects of treatment were obtained using structured questionnaires. Only one or two children in each phase noted any side effect (abdominal pains, dizziness, eyestrain, fatigue, feeling "wired," headaches, insomnia, muscle aches, nausea, sweaty palms, and disturbed vision were each reported), and there were no differences across phases.

To assess compliance, parents were asked about missed treatments, difficulties with setting the dawn simulator, and their children's wearing of the prescribed goggles. All reported that their children were able to comply fully with the wearing of the special glasses and sitting in front of the light box as directed. However, two families had some difficulty with the dawn simulation device initially (one during active phase, one during placebo) and therefore were not sure whether their children had received the appropriate light exposure during the first 2 days of the week-long trial.

DISCUSSION

The results of this placebo-controlled, double-blind, crossover trial suggest that bright-light therapy is an effective treatment for pediatric SAD. During the week of active treatment (a combination of light-box therapy and dawn simulation), the children's depressive symptoms on the SIGH-SAD-P were significantly decreased from baseline compared with both the placebo and washout phases. Scores on the SIGH-SAD-C were also decreased from baseline during active treatment, though this difference was not significant (perhaps because of the smaller sample size). Active treatment was not associated with a higher frequency of side effects than placebo, and it appeared to be well tolerated. The clinical responses of the children and their parents are perhaps of even greater importance than these statistical results, and in the posttreatment survey, the vast majority of the parents and children rated the active-treatment week as the phase during which they "felt best." Moreover, nearly all of the children at both sites continued to use bright-light therapy after the study had finished.

The following case is illustrative of the children's response to the light therapy trial: S.J., a 15-year-old female 10th-grader, reported a history of two major depressive episodes with seasonal variation beginning at age 12. Onset of her depressive symptoms typically began in late October and remission occurred in early to mid-April. At the time of the study, she described a moderate degree of depressed mood and irritability, increased appetite with a particular penchant for carbohydrates and sweets, a 3-hour/day increase in sleep duration, feeling fatigued throughout the day most days, and a moderate decrease in mood and energy in the late afternoons. Her baseline SIGH-SAD score was 32.

S.J. was randomly assigned to receive active treatment first. She responded with a dramatic reduction in symptoms, reporting that only a mild hyperphagia, slight fatigue, and a 2-hour increase in sleep remained. Her SIGH-SAD score had decreased to 6. She remarked, "It was like I was my old-self again—like I am in the summer. I felt like going out and doing fun things." After a 1-week washout, S.J.'s symptoms had returned (SIGH-SAD score = 23) and remained consistently worse during the placebo phase (SIGH-SAD score = 22.)

Both S.J. and her parent decided that she should continue the light therapy. They purchased a 10,000 lux light box. With daily light therapy, S.J. remained in remission throughout the remainder of the season. In contrast to prior years, she maintained an active social life and consistently good grades. She even researched the literature on SAD and presented a paper at her high school's science fair. She has continued light therapy each winter since her participation in the study and is now using her treatment during her freshman year in college.

As with all investigations, there are some limitations to these findings. First and foremost is the issue of the validity of pediatric SAD as a diagnosis. Although in the literature there are several reports of children with seasonal affective symptoms, the diagnosis of pediatric SAD has yet to be well established. In this study, all subjects were seen by a nurse or physician experienced in the diagnosis of childhood depression and all met criteria for major depressive disorder of a seasonal affective type. However, it is possible that some children may have had depressive symptoms that coincidentally worsened in the winter, in which case their disorder may have been misdiagnosed as SAD. The lack of summer symptoms in these children and their differential response to light therapy would speak against this.

The brevity of the treatment limits the generalizability of these findings. Although subjects improved significantly during the week of active treatment, no systematic information is available regarding their response to long-term treatment. For those subjects from whom follow-up information was received, light therapy continued to be of benefit. This is in keeping with a follow-up study by Giedd et al. (1994, written communication) in which six children with SAD sustained positive effects of light therapy over a 7-year period. Future studies could include follow-up data or could use a parallel design to determine whether the improvement produced by the light therapy is longlasting. In addition, the use of both dawn simulation and light-box therapy complicates the results because it is possible that either treatment might not be effective if used alone. Further studies will be needed to determine the differential efficacy of these two therapies.

These preliminary findings are strengthened by the fact that they were internally replicated at two geographically distinct sites (Boston and Washington, D.C.). At both sites, active treatment was superior to placebo treatment and patients demonstrated significant improvement from baseline. This is the first systematic controlled study to find significant improvement of seasonal affective symptoms in children using bright-light therapy. With new studies (Carskadon and Acebo, 1993; Swedo et al., 1995) reporting that the prevalence of pediatric SAD may be as high as 3% to 4%, there is clearly a need for effective treatment for this troublesome condition. The findings of this study require amplification and replication, but they suggest that bright-light therapy is an effective treatment for pediatric SAD.

REFERENCES

American Psychiatric Association (1987), *Diagnostic and Statistical Manual of Mental Disorders, 3rd edition-revised (DSM-III-R)*. Washington, DC: American Psychiatric Association

Carskadon MA, Acebo C (1993), Parental reports of seasonal mood and behavior changes in children. *J Am Acad Child Adolesc Psychiatry* 32:264–269

SAS Institute (1985), *Sas User's Guide: Statistics, Version 5*. Cary, NC: SAS Institute

Kasper S, Wehr TA, Bartko JJ, Gaist PA, Rosenthal NE (1989), Epidemiological findings of seasonal changes in mood and behavior: a telephone survey of Montgomery County, Maryland. *Arch Gen Psychiatry* 46:823–833

Oren DA, Brainard GC, Johston SH, Joseph-Vanderpool JR, Sorek E, Rosenthal NE (1991), Treatment of seasonal affective disorder with green light and red light. *Am J Psychiatry* 148:509–511

Orvaschel H, Puig-Antich J (1987), *Schedule for Affective Disorders and Schizophrenia for School-Age Children-Epidemiologic Version*. Philadelphia: Medical College of Pennsylvania, Eastern Pennsylvania Psychiatric Institute

Rosenthal NE (1993), Diagnosis and treatment of seasonal affective disorder. *JAMA* 270:2717–2720

Rosenthal NE, Carpenter CJ, James SP, Parry BL, Rogers SL, Wehr TA (1986), Seasonal affective disorder in children and adolescents. *Am J Psychiatry* 143:356–358

Rosenthal NE, Kasper S, Schulz PM et al. (1989), New concepts and developments in seasonal affective disorder. In: *Seasonal Affective Disorders*, Thompson C, Silverstone T, eds. London: CNS Publishers, pp 97–132

Rosenthal NE, Sack DA, Gillin JC et al. (1984), Seasonal affective disorder: a description of the syndrome and preliminary findings with light therapy. *Arch Gen Psychiatry* 41:72–80

Ryan ND (1992), The pharmacologic treatment of child and adolescent depression. *Psychiatr Clin North Am* 15:29–40

Sonis WA, Yellin AM, Garfinkel BD, Hoberman HH (1987), The antidepressant effect of light in seasonal affective disorder of childhood and adolescence. *Psychopharmacol Bull* 23:360–363

Swedo SE, Pleeter JD, Richter DM et al. (1995), Rates of seasonal affective disorder in children and adolescents. *Am J Psychiatry* 152:1016–1019

Terman JS, Terman M, Schlager D et al. (1990), Efficacy of brief, intense light exposure for treatment of winter depression. *Psychopharmacol Bull* 26:3–11

Terman M, Amira L, Terman JS, Ross DC (1996), Predictors of response and nonresponse to light treatment for winter depression. *Am J Psychiatry* 153:1423–1429

Williams JBW, Link MJ, Rosenthal NE, Amira L, Terman M (1994), *Structured Interview Guide for the Hamilton Depression Rating Scale, Seasonal Affective Disorders Version (SIGH-SAD)*, revised ed. New York: New York State Psychiatric Institute

13

Parent-Assisted Transfer of Children's Social Skills Training: Effects on Children With and Without Attention-Deficit Hyperactivity Disorder

Fred Frankel, Robert Myatt, Dennis P. Cantwell, and David T. Feinberg
University of California, Los Angeles, California

Objective: *Previous research has demonstrated that peer rejection is a significant part of the clinical presentation of many children with attention-deficit hyperactivity disorder (ADHD). Outcome studies of treatment interventions have typically failed to show generalization of treatment gains to the home and classroom. This has been especially true for children who have comorbid oppositional defiant disorder (ODD). The present study was intended to demonstrate generalization of an outpatient social skills training program when parents were trained in skills relevant to their child's social adjustment.* **Method:** *Thirty-five children with ADHD and 14 children without ADHD were given 12 sessions of treatment (treatment group). Outcome was compared with 12 children with ADHD and 12 children without ADHD who were on a waitlist for treatment (waitlist group). Nineteen children with ODD were in the treatment group and five in the waitlist. Stimulant medication was prescribed for all children with ADHD.* **Results:** *Subjects with ADHD showed improvement comparable with that of subjects without ADHD on all teacher- and parent-reported measures of peer adjustment and social skills, except teacher-reported withdrawal. Children with ODD had outcome comparable with that of children without ODD. Effect sizes ranged from 0.93 to 1.34, indicating that the average treatment group subject was better off than 83.4% of waitlist subjects on outcome measures.* **Conclusions:** *The present results suggest that children with ADHD are best helped by a combination of social skills training for themselves, collateral training for their parents, and stimulant medication.*

Children with attention-deficit hyperactivity disorder (ADHD) (*DSM-III-R*) (American Psychiatric Association, 1987) are at substantial risk for poor social relationships with

Reprinted with permission from the *Journal of the American Academy of Child and Adolescent Psychiatry*, 1997, Vol. 36(8), 1056–1064.

peers (Barkley, 1990; Frederick and Olmi, 1994; Pelham and Bender, 1982; Pope et al., 1989; Teeter, 1991; Whalen and Henker, 1985). Children with ADHD are more frequently nominated by peers as "liked least" than normal controls (Lahey et al., 1984). Peers characterize the child with ADHD as obnoxious, impulsive, or inconsiderate (Frankel et al., 1996; Landau and Moore, 1991). Social problems of children who have ADHD may continue into adolescence and adulthood (Weiss and Hechtman, 1986).

Biederman et al. (1991) note that many children with ADHD also meet criteria for oppositional defiant disorder (ODD) and that children with both ADHD and ODD are less responsive to treatment than children with ADHD alone. Some studies suggest that children with ADHD are more likely to be rejected by peers than children with other disruptive behavior disorders (Carlson et al., 1987; Pope et al., 1989). However, recent research suggests that peers are more likely to reject a child who is aggressive than a child displaying behaviors associated with ADHD (Hinshaw and Melnick, 1995).

Social skills training programs are designed to improve the skills of children who are rejected by their peers. The most common intervention setting has been the child's school. However, results of social skills training have not been encouraging. In a recent meta-analysis of social skills programs, Kavale et al. (1996) found that the mean effect size (effect size = [treatment group mean – control group mean]/control group SD) for all group studies was 0.199. This indicated that the average treated subject was better off than 58% of subjects receiving no training (an 8% improvement over no training). Researchers do not find compelling evidence that social skills learned in treatment generalize to home, classroom, or playground (DuPaul and Eckert, 1994).

The few studies of social skills training in outpatient clinic settings (Kolko et al., 1990; Michelson et al., 1983; Yu et al., 1986) have usually failed to demonstrate convincing evidence of success. One study (Yu et al., 1986) failed to replicate effects across two experimental groups of outpatient boys, each having small *n*'s. Another study (Michelson et al., 1983) demonstrated significant effects, but used measures with unknown discriminative or predictive validity with regard to peer adjustment.

Parent involvement has been notably absent from social skills training programs (Budd, 1986; Ladd and Asher, 1985; Sheridan et al., 1996). It is reasonable to expect that such involvement would enhance treatment generalization, especially since parents typically play a large role in scheduling and supervising children's play experiences (Frankel, 1996; Ladd et al., 1992; Lollis et al., 1992). Previous research (Frankel et al., 1995, 1996) demonstrated that a social skills program that included 1-hour parent sessions which were structured only during the last 10 minutes resulted in significant treatment gains reported by parents and generalization to the school setting. However, generalization to school was obtained only for children without the diagnosis of ODD. Frankel et al. (1995) hypothesized that children with ODD did not demonstrate improvement on teacher-reported measures because the basic program did not attempt to decrease disruptive and aggressive behavior likely to occur in the classroom (cf. Campbell et al., 1977). Frankel et al. also noticed that discussion during the unstructured portions of parent sessions occasionally wandered into areas that seemed counter-therapeutic (most frequently, parents would gripe about their child's noncompliant and oppositional behavior).

Cantwell et al. focused on the results of this treatment program for 70 boys and 18 girls with diagnosed ADHD (D. P. Cantwell, F. Frankel, R. Myatt, D. T. Feinberg, unpublished). Results for teacher-reported aggression indicated that the average child for whom stimulant medication was prescribed ($n = 61$) improved more than 83% of those for whom stimulant medication was not prescribed. These results support the contention by many authors (e.g., Cantwell, 1996; Cousins and Weiss, 1993) that multimodal intervention is necessary in order to bring about satisfactory outcome for children with ADHD.

The purpose of the present study was to demonstrate improved teacher-reported outcome for children with diagnosed ODD, while replicating previous results for teacher-reported outcome for children without ODD and parent-reported outcome for all subjects. The treatment program was revised in two ways. First, modules were added which addressed disruptive classroom behavior and aggression. Second, all parent session time was structured to focus parents on improving homework compliance and to teach parents relevant aspects of their child's friendship needs. Didactic presentations were made to parents on how accepted children enter groups and how their child should handle teasing by others and confrontations with adults. Parents were guided to praise their child's attempts at socialization, to provide appropriate consequences for physical fighting or defiance of adults, and to structure their child's play dates to avoid conflict. Preliminary comparison, using small *n*'s (Frankel et al., 1995), suggested improved outcome of the revised program over previous results.

The present study was designed to compare the results of children administered the revised training procedure with a waitlist control. It tested the following hypotheses, which were not tested in previous research: (1) The group receiving the revised treatment will show significantly greater improvement than will a waitlist control group. (2) Treatment gains will be evident for children with ADHD for whom stimulant medication was prescribed as well as for children without ADHD. (3) Children with ODD will benefit from the social skills training.

METHOD

Subjects

Subjects were 57 boys and 17 girls between the ages of 6 years 11 months (but attending at least second grade) and 12 years 11 months (but attending seventh grade or below) whose parents requested their participation in the UCLA Children's Social Skills Program. This program is a clinical service offered within the child outpatient clinic of a large university hospital. The most common parental complaint was that the subjects were having difficulty making and/or keeping close friends. Other frequent complaints were peer rejection and being teased by peers. Exclusionary criteria for the present study were (1) a diagnosis of ADHD without being prescribed stimulant medication and (2) placement in a special education class for children with developmental disabilities or psychosis or a previous chart diagnosis of a developmental or psychotic disorder. Children with a diagnosis of ADHD who did not have stimulant medication prescribed were not included in the study (but participated in treatment) because previous research (Cantwell et al., unpublished) indicated their response to treatment would be lower than that of children for whom medication was prescribed. Separate analysis of their data would complicate the design and analysis of the study.

Referral to the program was most commonly made by other professional staff at the hospital (32.5%), professionals in private practice (23.9%), the child's parents in response to publicity (24.1%), or personnel at the child's school (9.8%). In 9.7% of cases the source of referral was not recorded.

The treatment group was composed of 49 children (37 boys and 12 girls). Subjects received treatment in 16 small groups (including children not analyzed, mean group $n = 8.0$, range 6 to 9) over a span of 104 weeks. The age span within any group was not greater than $2\frac{1}{2}$ years. The waitlist group was composed of 24 children (19 boys and 5 girls) on the waitlist for treatment.

Table 1 presents the mean demographic characteristics for subjects in both groups and proportions of subjects in both groups receiving other treatment at the time of the study. In the treatment group, methylphenidate was prescribed for 41 ADHD subjects (mean daily dosage = 26.1 mg), dextroamphetamine for 5 (mean daily dosage = 21.6 mg), and pemoline

TABLE 1

Mean Measurement Intervals, Demographic Characteristics, and Baseline Raw Scores for Each Group

	Treatment		Waitlist		
	ADHD ($n = 35$)	NADHD ($n = 14$)	ADHD ($n = 12$)	NADHD ($n = 12$)	Dropout ($n = 11$)
Child age (years)	8.6	9.1	9.5	9.0	9.0
No. of girls	11	1	2	3	5
No. with ODD	17	2	7	2	3
% Other treatment	27	31	18	33	72.3
SES	58.7	56.9	53.3	49.1	50.9
Parent interval[a]	120	132	138	149	—
Teacher interval[b]	119	121	118	103	—
Self-Control	8.6	7.9	6.7	8.6	7.6
Assertion	12.1	10.3	12.0	11.8	11.0
Withdrawal	3.2	4.1	5.5	3.4	3.6
Likability	1.7	1.1	1.7	1.8	1.9
Aggression	3.2	3.3	1.8	2.4	2.5[c]
Hyperactivity	4.8	4.1	4.5	4.0	3.9[c]
Inattention	1.5	1.1	2.0	1.7	1.5[c]

Note: ADHD = attention-deficit hyperactivity disorder; NADHD = non-ADHD; ODD = oppositional defiant disorder; SES = socioeconomic status.

[a]Number of days between initial and final administration of the Social Skills Rating System to parents.

[b]Number of days between initial and final administration of the Pupil Evaluation Inventory to teachers.

[c]Data unavailable for one subject.

for 1 (daily dosage = 60 mg). In the waitlist group, methylphenidate was prescribed for 11 (mean daily dosage = 22.1 mg) and dextroamphetamine for 1 (daily dosage = 20 mg). Eleven subjects received other psychotropic medication (i.e., bupropion, carbamazepine, clonidine, fenfluramine, fluoxetine, lithium carbonate, sertraline, or valproic acid). No subjects changed medication status during the course of the study. Subjects who were involved in other treatments were usually in individual psychotherapy concurrent with the present study. Parent socioeconomic status (SES) was calculated using the procedure described by Hollingshead (1975). Racial composition was 63 white, 1 African-American, 3 Asian, 3 Latino, 1 each of mixed white and African-American or Latino ancestry.

In addition to the 74 subjects who participated in the study, an additional 11 subjects (6 boys and 5 girls) dropped out. Demographic characteristics of these subjects are also presented in Table 1. Racial composition was nine white, one Asian, and one Latino subject. Four subjects met criteria for ADHD. Three were taking methylphenidate and one was taking dextroamphetamine. Three subjects were taking fluoxetine. Demographic characteristics were similar to those of subjects persisting in the study, except that a higher proportion of subjects dropping out were in concurrent treatment (72.3% compared with 18% to 33% of persisting subjects).

Measures

Structured diagnostic interview. The ADHD Clinic Parent Interview (Barkley, 1991) is composed of a series of questions keyed to *DSM-III-R* criteria for ADHD, ODD, dysthymic disorder, major depressive disorder, separation anxiety disorder, and overanxious disorder. Both parents were interviewed when available, but usually only the mother was available. Interviewers were two staff social workers and one of the present authors (F.F.). The author (F.F.) trained clinic staff to use this interview and score diagnostic criteria.

To assign *DSM-III-R* child diagnoses, the ADHD Clinic Parent Interview was used as a starting point and complete charts were rated independently by two authors (F.F. and D.T.F.) for *DSM-III-R* criteria. Agreement between the two authors for child diagnosis was 87.9% for ADHD ($k = .80$), 89.5% for ODD ($k = .82$), and 50.0% for dysthymia/major depression ($k = .61$). Separation anxiety and overanxious disorder were uncommonly identified; one rater identified either one or the other in four children and the other rater in seven children. Because of low incidence and poor agreement for other diagnoses, only ADHD and ODD were considered further.

Diagnostic categories were constructed for analysis based on whether subjects had or did not have ODD and/or ADHD. The diagnoses for each subject in which raters initially disagreed ($n = 6$) was assigned by consensus after discussion by both raters. Table 1 shows the distribution of ADHD and ODD diagnoses across the groups.

Social skills rating system. The Social Skills Rating System (Gresham and Elliott, 1990) is a questionnaire consisting of 55 items rated as either "never," "sometimes," or "very often." The parent form was administered to the mother in the present study. Among the seven subscales that compose this instrument, only the Assertion and Self-Control subscales measure attributes relevant to friendships and will be considered further. The Assertion subscale measures making friends and playing well with them (e.g., "Makes friends easily").

The Self-Control subscale measures appropriate response to provocation by others (e.g., "Responds appropriately when hit or pushed by other children"). Mean raw baseline scores for these two subscales are presented in Table 1.

Pupil evaluation inventory. The Pupil Evaluation Inventory (PEI) (Pekarik et al., 1976) consists of 35 items, each rated as "describes child" or "does not describe child." Correlations between peer and teacher PEI ratings have exceeded .54 (Ledingham et al., 1982). The present study used the 42-item teacher-rated PEI presented by Pope et al. (1991) which contains the following scales: Withdrawal (9 items) assesses shyness (e.g., "Those who are too shy to make friends easily") and sadness (e.g., "Those who never seem to have a good time"); Likability (5 items) assesses very prosocial behavior (e.g., "Those who are especially nice"); Aggression (10 items) assesses teasing and physical aggression (e.g., "Those who start a fight over nothing"); Hyperactivity (15 items) assesses impulsive and disruptive behavior (e.g., "Those who want to show off in class"); and Inattention (6 items) assesses immaturity (e.g., "Those who act like a baby"). Teacher responses the to 42 PEI items were collected by telephone interview. Teachers were not informed of the treatment status of the children on which they were asked to report.

Frankel and Myatt (1994) have demonstrated that the Withdrawal and Likability scales tap a dimension of social competence, while the Aggression scale taps a dimension of externalizing behavior. Cantwell et al. (unpublished) report that mean Hyperactivity and Inattention scores were lower for children with ADHD who were receiving stimulant medication than for unmedicated ADHD children. Teacher and peer PEI assessments in first grade have been shown to be equally good predictors of antisocial behavior 7 years later (Tremblay et al., 1988). Mean raw baseline scores for each teacher-rated PEI scale are presented in Table 1.

Procedure

Parents inquiring about treatment for their child's socialization problems were told that the intervention was a class intended to teach their child to make and keep friends and that all of the children in the class had problems in this area. They were told that the other children were available to facilitate practice of skills during the class and that children were unlikely to make lasting friendships with others in the class (play dates between class members were prohibited until after the class was over). Parents were instructed in this way because (1) dropout due to parents viewing their child as less deviant than others in the class would be reduced, and (2) children and parents would be more apt to try new approaches because they would be not be concerned about having continuing relationships with class members.

Parents requesting treatment for their child were mailed a packet of questionnaires that included a biographical form (from which SES and marital status were derived), the Social Skills Rating System, and a release to obtain the PEI from the teacher. In all cases, the mother filled out the packet. Calls were made to the teacher to obtain the baseline PEI within 2 weeks before the start of the first session.

After return of completed packets, mothers (and fathers, when available) attended a 1-hour intake session during which the structured diagnostic interview was administered. Mothers were advised to inform the subject that the social skills class was intended to teach children how to make and keep friends. In cases in which the child did not appear willing to participate, mothers were told to contract for a specified reward for attending the first two sessions. Subjects were allowed to discontinue at this point and obtain the reward.

The intervention took place for 1 hour on each of 12 consecutive Thursdays (sessions were rescheduled for the following week if a holiday occurred). Concurrent child and parent sessions were conducted by two Ph.D. psychologists or a Ph.D. psychologist and an L.C.S.W. Up to two coaches were also available, who were undergraduate or graduate students. In all cases, the mothers attended concurrent sessions with the child, although fathers were also welcome. Post-testing of mothers occurred on the last scheduled session. Teachers were contacted for posttreatment PEIs within 3 weeks after the last session.

The treatment addressed previously identified social skill deficits in children rejected by their peers. The emphasis was placed on avoiding conflict through modification of strategies with which rejected children and their parents approach key peer situations (Frankel, 1996; Frankel et al., 1995).

Child sessions. Each child session (except for the first and last) was composed of four segments. During the first segment (10 minutes), children reported the results of the homework assignment given in the previous session. The second segment (15 minutes) consisted of a didactic presentation, behavioral rehearsal between children, and coaching. The third segment (25 minutes) consisted of coached play. In the fourth segment (10 minutes), parents and children were reunited and contracts for homework were finalized.

Subjects were taught conversational techniques (voice volume, smile, physical closeness) (Bierman and Furman, 1984; cf. Foster, 1983, for exclusion of eye contact from this list) and rehearsed them in the context of introductions to other class members. Subjects were instructed on how to "play detective" (Gottman et al., 1975) as an information-sharing and query technique with other class members in order to plan future play activities (Gottman, 1983; Gottman et al., 1975). They also rehearsed calling another class member on the telephone.

Techniques of group entry (Garvey, 1984; Putallaz, 1983; Putallaz and Gottman, 1981) were described. Subjects were instructed on good and bad times and places to make friends, how to watch a group of children in play to understand what the group was doing (Dodge et al., 1983b), and what the rules were to participate. They were also coached to make relevant comments or praise the children who were playing (e.g., "good shot") (Gottman et al., 1975) and to join by "helping them play their game" (Phillips et al., 1951). Subjects were cautioned not to ask questions, mention themselves or their feelings, or disagree with or criticize the children playing the game (Dodge et al., 1983a). Subjects were told to expect 50% rejection in their entry attempts (Corsaro, 1981). Reasons for rejection were discussed as well as what to do in each case.

Subjects listed things they could say to praise others during play. They were instructed on how to avoid "playing referee" (i.e., criticizing others) and to let others have fun (i.e., let them catch the ball, too). Techniques of persuasion and negotiation were taught to allow subjects to change activities when they lost interest (cf. Dodge et al., 1990; Gottman, 1983).

The "rules for a good host" were presented in order for children to avoid conflict on play dates: (1) the guest is always right (he or she gets to pick the games, take turns, etc.); (2) praise the guest's behavior (e.g., "nice try," "great shot"); (3) no refereeing (i.e., criticism of the guest); (4) if you are bored, make a deal with the guest for the next game; and (5) be loyal to your guest (play dates were to be with only one guest at a time, who was not to be left alone).

The main reason for teasing was reviewed (i.e., the teaser wants them to get upset) (Perry et al., 1990). Subjects were taught to react neutrally or humorously to teasing (Coie and Dodge, 1988) in the following manner: Each subject produced a tease they had recently heard and identified the perpetrator. The therapist modeled how to "make fun of the teasing" so that the perpetrator was teased about his or her inability to tease well (e.g., "I've heard that one before," "Can't you think of anything else to say?" "That's so old it's got dust on it" (cf. Perry et al., 1990). Subjects practiced "making fun of the teasing" in response to structured teasing from the class (Goodwin and Mahoney, 1975).

Handling confrontations with adults was reviewed: (1) do not answer back or give dirty looks, and (2) try to explain yourself only once. If this does not work, be quiet. Subjects were told that the group leaders may subsequently accuse them unfairly in order to practice this response. Subjects discussed how to avoid fights, which included avoiding "breaking up fights between other children."

Coached play. Coached play began during the second session. Coaches were prohibited from taking a direct part in subjects' play activities but watched, dispensed token and verbal reinforcement, and delivered consequences for misbehavior (Ladd and Golter, 1988).

Dyads were chosen from some subjects to play a game they brought from home. Subjects not chosen to be in a dyad practiced entry into playing dyads. They were prompted as necessary until they understood the game structure. Then they were prompted as necessary to join by making relevant comments and praising other children (Black and Hazen, 1990). Coaches praised and gave tokens for correct rule behavior, taking turns, letting other children have turns and praising other children's performance (Hartup et al., 1967). Coaches facilitated the subjects' suggesting and negotiating a change in activity or having a turn. Emphasis was placed on "helping others play" rather than "winning at all costs" (Ladd and Mize, 1983). Subjects were broken into dyads to practice being a good host (one was the "host" and one was the "guest" in each dyad).

Very competitive games (e.g., basketball, between three and five subjects per team) were introduced in session 9 (Gelb and Jacobson, 1988; Oden, 1986; Tryon and Keane, 1991). Coaches occasionally "accused" children unjustly in order to practice appropriate handling of confrontations with adults.

Discipline and rewards. During the didactic part of each session, subjects were given stars on the blackboard and verbal reinforcement for quietly listening in seat, raising hands before talking, and class participation. Rewards to the whole group were occasionally delivered. During coached play, coaches dispensed token and verbal reinforcement immediately after instances of good sportsmanship and demonstrated mastery of the social skills being taught (Bernhardt and Forehand, 1975). Coaches also provided consequences for misbehavior (Ladd and Golter, 1988). Disruptive behavior was given one warning. Upon reoccurrence of the behavior, the subject was given a 2-minute time-out outside the classroom or in the corner of the play area by the coach.

Parent sessions and child socialization homework. Formal parent sessions were held concurrently for the entire hour of all child sessions. Session 1 was devoted to parent orientation (with an accompanying handout) and arrangements for calling other class members. Sessions 2 to 11 were broken into four segments. During the first segment (15 minutes), the session leader reviewed parent and child performance on the previous socialization homework assignment. During the next segment (30 minutes), the parent handout was read with the parents and relevant questions were answered. In the third segment, the next socialization homework assignment was presented and specific problems anticipated by the parent were discussed. During the last 10 minutes of each session, parent and child were reunited and contracts were made between them for completion of the next socialization homework assignment.

The parent handouts covered the following areas: (1) Encouragement and discouragement of children's social behavior—The major purpose of this handout was to discourage parents from making negative comments about their child to others and especially in front of their child. (2) Parent support of social skills—This handout promoted discussion of the availability of physical (a place to play in the house away from siblings) and time (enough time for play dates) resources for play dates. Specific deficiencies for any subject in these resources were addressed. (3) Group entry and rejection—The handout reviewed the differences in group entry behavior between children who are accepted and those who are rejected from the group. It also made the point that children are refused entry to a group of children at play about 50% of the time. Far from being a crushing blow, this type of rejection is a normal part of children's play experiences. (4) The elements of effective praise—The handout presented components of developmentally appropriate parental praise and gave examples of how parents were to use praise in social situations with their children. (5) How to have a successful play date—The handout reviewed how parents were to help arrange the play date. It also provided guidelines for how to enforce the "rules of a good host." (6) How children "make fun of the tease"—The handout reviewed why children tease (because of the reaction of the victim) and gave examples of how group leaders taught subjects to "make fun of the tease." (7) Confrontations with adults—The handout reviewed how children should handle confrontations with adults. It gave guidelines for when and how the parent should assist. (8) How to decrease physical fighting—The handout gave guidelines for delivering immediate, brief consequences to decrease physical fights at school or home.

Socialization homework assignments were keyed to the didactic presentations and in-session practice. No assignment was made until its contents were practiced in the child sessions and presented to parents. Socialization homework assignments were as follows: (1) The subject was to telephone another member of the class (parents were to arrange the day and time of the call during sessions and were not to listen in at the time of the call) and practice information sharing and query (playing detective). (2) Children were to bring a nonviolent, interactive toy from home to all sessions. (3) Subjects were to practice joining a group of children at play. To increase their chances of gaining entry, they were encouraged to approach slightly younger children with whom they were unfamiliar (Furman et al., 1979; Tryon and Keane, 1991). Parents were to help the subject decide where and when this would be attempted. The parent was instructed to let the subject try this by himself or herself and not try to help in any way. (4) Parent and subject agreed on a child they would like to invite over to their house for 1 hour and possible times for this (Krappmann, cited in Parke and Bhavnagri, 1989; Ladd and Golter, 1988). The subject was to call this child and "play detective" to generate a list of possible games to play. The parent was to check with the invited child's parent to arrange the date, time, and length of the play date. At the time of the play date, the parent was to monitor the subject from within earshot (Ladd and Golter, 1988), to enforce the rules of a good host, and to praise the subject for compliance. (5) Subjects were to practice "making fun of the teasing" with a selected child who had teased the subject. Session 12 consisted of parent post-testing and a handout on maintenance of treatment gains which focused on maintaining weekly one-on-one play dates with other children.

Treatment fidelity. Treatment fidelity was ensured in three ways, suggested by Moncher and Prinz (1991): (1) The principal child trainer was a Ph.D.-level psychologist (author R.M.) with 7 years of experience in social skills training. The principal parent trainer was either a Ph.D.-level psychologist (author F.F.) or an L.C.S.W. with at least 1 year of experience in social skills training. (2) A manual was developed and followed which detailed the curriculum for each parent and child session. The therapist began each topic by reading from the manual. (3) An undergraduate observer, using a checklist for each session, verified that each topic in the manual was reviewed and that no topics were presented other than those in the manual.

RESULTS

Means for demographic variables, measurement intervals, and baseline raw scores for the outcome measures are presented in Table 1. Two-way 2 × 2 (group × ADHD status) fixed-effects analyses of variance revealed a significant main effect for SES ($F[1, 68] = 5.77$, $p < .05$). This indicated that the mean SES for the treatment group (58.2) was significantly higher than that of the waitlist group (51.2). The group × diagnosis interaction was significant for PEI Withdrawal baseline scores ($F[1, 67] = 6.73$, $p < .05$). Inspection of means in Table 1 revealed that ADHD subjects in the waitlist group tended to have a higher mean baseline score (5.5) than subjects in all other groups (range of means was 3.2 to 4.1). However, Newman-Keuls post hoc statistics (Winer, 1971) failed to confirm these differences (p values > .05). No other baseline variable, measurement interval, or demographic variable reached significance (p values > .05).

To simplify presentation, a difference score (baseline raw score − posttreatment raw score) was used for all measures except Likability, Assertion, and Self-Control. Difference scores (posttreatment raw score − baseline raw score) were used for these two measures. Positive values indicated improvement on all scales. (Subjects having "0" baseline scores on the PEI Withdrawal scale, Aggression, Hyperactivity, Inattention scales or subjects having Likability baseline scale scores greater than 1 were not included in the respective analyses.) Preliminary 2 × 2 (sex × group) analyses revealed no significant main effects or interactions. Low cell frequencies did not permit simultaneous factorial analyses that included both ODD and ADHD. Instead, outcome variables were submitted to 2 × 2 (group × diagnosis) fixed-effects analyses of variance, first using the presence of ODD as the diagnostic factor, next using the presence of ADHD. Since the Aggression scale of the PEI showed the only significant correlation with SES, this variable was submitted to a 2 × 2 (group × diagnosis) analysis of covariance with SES as a covariate.

TABLE 2
Effect Size and Percentage of Treatment Group Subjects Who Were Better Off Than the Average Waitlist Subject for Each Variable of the Present Study

Group	Effect Size	% Treatment Group Subjects
Withdrawal (NADHD)	0.99	83.9
Likability	0.93	82.4
Aggression	0.99	83.9
Self-Control	1.10	86.4
Assertion	1.34	91.0

Note: NADHD = non–attention-deficit hyperactivity disorder.

The analysis of the parent-reported Assertion and Self-Control subscales revealed significant main effects of treatment ($F[1, 50] = 11.12$, $p < .01$ and $F[1, 37] = 3.12$, $p < .05$, respectively). The treatment group (mean difference score for Assertion = +3.0; for Self-Control = +4.3) showed significantly greater improvement on both of these scales than the waitlist group (mean difference scores = +0.2 and +1.4, respectively).

The analysis of the Withdrawal scale revealed a significant group × diagnosis interaction, using the presence of ADHD as the diagnostic factor ($F[1, 63] = 5.84$, $p < .05$). Newman-Keuls post hoc statistics revealed that the treatment group without ADHD (mean difference score = +1.52, $n = 12$) was significantly better than the waitlist group without ADHD (mean difference score = −1.01, $n = 11$; $q = 9.56$, $p < .01$), but the treatment and waitlist groups with ADHD did not differ significantly (mean difference scores were −.15 and +.20, n's = 34 and 10, respectively, $p > .05$). The analysis of the Aggression scale revealed a significant main effect of group ($F[1, 47] = 5.29$, $p < .05$). Inspection of means revealed that the treatment group (mean difference score = 1.9) was significantly greater than the waitlist group (mean difference score = −0.9). No other main effects or interactions were significant for the above analyses ($p > .25$) and the analysis of the Likability scale ($p = .06$ for group main effect, all other p values > .25). The main effect and interactions with presence/absence of ODD were not significant.

Table 2 shows the effect sizes and percentages of the treatment group subjects who were better off than the mean waitlist group subjects for each outcome variable which produced at least marginally statistically significant results. The lowest effect size was obtained for the Likability scale, indicating that 82.4% of treatment group subjects showed greater positive change than the average waitlist group subject. The highest effect sizes were obtained on the two parent-reported measures, indicating that 86.4% of treatment group subjects showed greater positive change than the average waitlist subject.

DISCUSSION

The present study, using parents to aid in transfer of their child's social skills treatment, confirmed two of the three hypotheses. The treatment group was superior to the waitlist group on the Aggression and Withdrawal teacher-reported scales and on the Assertion and

Self-Control parent-reported subscales. The effect sizes for all scales except Hyperactivity and Inattention were large and indicated that at least 82.4% of treatment group children were better off than the average waitlist child after treatment. This confirmed the first hypothesis, that the intervention would produce significantly better outcome than the waitlist control group. The second hypothesis was partially confirmed: children with ADHD showed comparable gains on all measures except the PEI Withdrawal scale. The reasons for the lack of improvement are unclear. However, Cantwell et al. (unpublished) did not observe stimulants to facilitate improvement on the Withdrawal scale after social skills training.

The third hypothesis was confirmed. In contrast to previous research (Frankel et al., 1995), children with ODD showed treatment generalization comparable with that of children without ODD. Noncompliance, aggressive behaviors, and disruptive behaviors all characterize children with ODD and may have impaired transfer of training to the school setting in previous research (Frankel et al., 1995). Positive results of the present intervention on children with ODD may have been due to the following treatment components not present in previous research: (1) Parent session time was completely structured to help parents to increase child compliance with homework assignments. (2) Child and parent sessions focused on decreasing aggression and disruptive classroom behavior. Parents were instructed on how to work with the child's teacher to provide appropriate consequences for disruptive and aggressive behaviors. Disruption of the didactic components of the child sessions was also given immediate consequences.

The treatment group did not demonstrate significant advantage over the waitlist group on the Hyperactivity and Inattention scales. Cantwell et al. (unpublished) found that children with ADHD who were taking stimulant medication had lower means on these scales than unmedicated ADHD children, and neither group showed improvement on these two scales after social skills training. Mean baseline levels of both scales did not differ between medicated ADHD children and children without ADHD in the present study. Taken together, these results suggest that the beneficial effects of stimulants and social skills intervention are specific and different from each other. The beneficial effects of stimulants may be specific to hyperactive and inattentive behaviors. Children in the present study had low baseline levels on these two scales, either because they did not meet criteria for ADHD, or if they did, they were taking stimulant medication.

Several methodological issues arose during the course of the present study. First, the treatment and waitlist groups differed significantly in mean SES. It is not clear how this difference emerged, as no systematic selection process could be identified which could account for differential assignment of lower-SES children to the waitlist group. However, SES did not correlate with any outcome variable except Aggression. The results of the analysis of covariance for Aggression demonstrated that group differences were not due to differences in SES.

The second methodological issue was that the ADHD children of the present study were prescribed stimulant medication by their own private physicians prior to beginning the intervention. All parents indicated that they and/or school nurses administered medication as prescribed. Parent report seemed to be reliable in this regard, since treatment staff were not associated with the prescribing physician and parents lacked motivation to distort these reports. However, no attempt was made by the present authors to independently verify this or to verify that the prescribed dosage was optimal, in terms of the best therapeutic response for each child. The results of Cantwell et al. (unpublished) suggest that stimulants facilitate beneficial effects of social skills training. Previous research (Firestone, 1982) indicates that parents tend to decrease administration of prescribed stimulants as time elapses since the prescribing visit to the physician. It is likely that differences between treatment and waitlist groups would be larger if all medication was given as prescribed. Future research must explore this issue and determine whether there is an optimal dosage of stimulants to produce beneficial effects of social skills training.

The unavailability of peer sociometric assessment to more directly assess peer acceptance made it difficult to judge how improvements in teacher-reported measures translate to better peer acceptance. Collection of peer sociometrics might enable a clearer interpretation of the effect of diagnosis on outcome. The lack of measures of play date success make it difficult to judge how improvements reported by parents translate into better play dates and more success at making best friends. Future research must correct these deficiencies.

Conclusions

The present results demonstrated that socially rejected children may benefit substantially from social skills training when their parents are trained to facilitate transfer of treatment effects. Inclusion of parents in treatment is especially important, since parents today typically arrange and monitor the peer interactions of their children. The present results, together with those of Cantwell et al. (unpublished), suggest that children with ADHD are best helped by a combination of social skills training for themselves, training for their parents, and stimulant medication. Stimulants appear to have both direct and indirect benefits for children with ADHD who are socially rejected. Stimulants act directly to reduce hyperactive behavior and increase attention. Stimulants also act indirectly, by facilitating the beneficial effects of treatment for children with ADHD, particularly in reducing aggressive behavior.

REFERENCES

American Psychiatric Association (1987), *Diagnostic and Statistical Manual of Mental Disorders, 3rd edition-revised (DSM-III-R)*. Washington, DC: American Psychiatric Association

Barkley RA (1990), *Attention-Deficit Hyperactivity Disorder*. New York: Guilford

Barkley RA (1991), *ADHD Clinic Parent Interview*. Worcester: University of Massachusetts, School of Medicine

Bernhardt AJ, Forehand R (1975), The effects of labeled and unlabeled praise upon lower and middle class children. *J Exp Child Psychol* 19:536–543

Biederman J, Newcorn J, Sprich S (1991), Comorbidity of attention deficit hyperactivity disorder with conduct, depressive, anxiety and other disorders. *Am J Psychiatry* 148:564–577

Bierman KL, Furman W (1984), The effects of social skills training and peer involvement in the social adjustment of preadolescents. *Child Dev* 55:151–162

Black B, Hazen NL (1990), Social status and patterns of communication in acquainted and unacquainted preschool children. *Dev Psychol* 26:379–387

Budd KS (1986), Parents as mediators in the social skills training of children. In: *Handbook of Social Skills Training and Research,* L'Abate L, Milan MA, eds. New York: Wiley, pp 245–262

Campbell SB, Endman MW, Bernfeld G (1977), Three-year follow-up study of hyperactive preschoolers into elementary school. *J Child Psychol Psychiatry* 18:239–249

Cantwell DP (1996), Attention deficit disorder: a review of the past 10 years. *J Am Acad Child Adolesc Psychiatry* 35:978–987

Carlson CL, Lahey BB, Frame CL, Walker J, Hynd GW (1987), Sociometric status of clinically referred children with attention deficit disorders with and without hyperactivity. *J Abnorm Child Psychol* 15:537–547

Coie JD, Dodge KA (1988), Multiple sources of data on social behavior and social status. *Child Dev* 59:815–829

Corsaro WA (1981), Friendship in the nursery school: social organization in a peer environment. In: *The Development of Children's Friendships,* Asher SR, Gottman JM, eds. New York: Cambridge University Press, pp 207–241

Cousins LS, Weiss G (1993), Parent training and social skills training for children with attention-deficit hyperactivity disorder: how can they be combined for greater effectiveness? *Can J Psychiatry* 38:449–457

Dodge KA, Coie JD, Brakke NP (1983a), Behavioral patterns of socially rejected and neglected preadolescents: the roles of social approach and aggression. *J Abnorm Child Psychol* 10:389–410

Dodge KA, Coie JD, Petit GS, Price JM (1990), Peer status and aggression in boys' groups: developmental and contextual analysis. *Child Dev* 61:1289–1309

Dodge KA, Schlundt DC, Schocken I, Delugach JD (1983b), Social competence and children's sociometric status: the role of peer group entry strategies. *Merrill-Palmer Q* 29:309–336

DuPaul GJ, Eckert TL (1994), The effects of social skills curricula: now you see them, now you don't. *Sch Psychol Q* 2:113–132

Firestone P (1982), Factors associated with children's adherence to stimulant medication. *Am J Orthopsychiatry* 52:447–457

Foster S (1983), Critical elements in the development of children's social skills. In: *New Directions in Social Skills Training,* Ellis R, Whitington D, eds. New York: Methuen, pp 229–265

Frankel F (1996), *Good Friends Are Hard to Find: Help Your Child Find, Make, and Keep Friends.* Los Angeles: Perspective Publishing

Frankel F, Cantwell DP, Myatt R (1996), Helping ostracized children: social skills training and parent support for socially rejected children. In: *Psychosocial Treatments for Child and Adolescent Disorders: Empirically Based Approaches*, Hibbs ED, Jensen PS, eds. Washington, DC: American Psychological Association, pp 591–617

Frankel F, Myatt R (1994), A dimensional approach to the assessment of the social competence of boys. *Psychol Assess* 6:249–254

Frankel F, Myatt R, Cantwell DP (1995), Training outpatient boys to conform with the social ecology of popular peers: effects on parent and teacher ratings. *J Clin Child Psychol* 24:300–310

Frederick BP, Olmi DJ (1994), Children with attention-deficit/hyperactivity disorder: a review of the literature on social skills deficits. *Sch Psychol Rev* 31:288–296

Furman W, Rahe DF, Hartup WW (1979), Rehabilitation of socially withdrawn preschool children through mixed-age and same-age socialization. *Child Dev* 50:915–922

Garvey C (1984), *Children's Talk*. Cambridge, MA: Harvard University Press

Gelb R, Jacobson JL (1988), Popular and unpopular children's interactions during cooperative and competitive peer group activities. *J Abnorm Child Psychol* 16:247–261

Goodwin SE, Mahoney MJ (1975), Modification of aggression through modeling: an experimental probe. *J Behav Ther Exp Psychiatry* 6:200–202

Gottman JM (1983), How children become friends. *Monogr Soc Res Child Dev* 48(Serial No. 201)

Gottman JM, Gonso J, Rasmussen B (1975), Social interaction, social competence and friendship in children. *Child Dev* 46:709–718

Gresham FM, Elliott SN (1990), *Social Skills Rating System: Manual*. Circle Pines, MN: American Guidance Service

Hartup WW, Glazer JA, Charlesworth R (1967), Peer reinforcement and sociometric status. *Child Dev* 38:1017–1024

Hinshaw SP, Melnick SM (1995), Peer relationships in boys with attention deficit hyperactivity disorder with and without comorbid aggression. *Dev Psychopathol* 7:627–647

Hollingshead AB (1975), *Four Factor Index of Social Status*. New Haven, CT: Yale University

Kavale KA, Mathur SR, Forness SR, Rutherford RB Jr, Quinn MM (1996), Effectiveness of social skills training for students with behavior disorders: a meta-analysis. In: *Advances in Learning and Behavioral Disabilities*, Vol. 11, Scruggs T, Mastropieri M, eds. Greenwich, CT: JAI Press

Kolko DJ, Loar LL, Sturnick D (1990), Inpatient social-cognitive skills training with conduct disordered and attention deficit disordered children. *J Child Psychol Psychiatry* 31:737–748

Ladd GA, Asher SR (1985), Social skill training and children's peer relations. In: *Handbook of Social Skills Training and Research*, L'Abate L, Milan MA, eds. New York: Wiley, pp 219–244

Ladd GW, Golter BS (1988), Parents' management of preschoolers peer relations: is it related to children's social competence? *Dev Psychol* 24:109–117

Ladd GW, Mize J (1983), A cognitive-social learning model of social skill training. *Psychol Bull* 90:127–157

Ladd GW, Profilet SM, Hart CH (1992), Parent's management of children's peer relations: facilitating children's activities in the peer culture. In: *Family-Peer Relationships: Modes of Linkage*, Parke RD, Ladd GW, eds. Hillsdale, NJ: Erlbaum, pp 215–253

Lahey BB, Schaughency EA, Strauss CC, Frame CL (1984), Are attention deficit disorders with and without hyperactivity similar or dissimilar disorders? *J Am Acad Child Psychiatry* 24:613–616

Landau S, Moore L (1991), Social skill deficits in children with attention-deficit hyperactivity disorder. *Sch Psychol Rev* 20:235–251

Ledingham JE, Younger A, Schwartzman A, Bergeron G (1982), Agreement among teacher, peer and self-ratings of children's aggression, withdrawal and likability. *J Abnorm Child Psychol* 10:363–372

Lollis SP, Ross HS, Tate E (1992), Parents' regulation of children's peer interactions: direct influences. In: *Family-Peer Relationships: Modes of Linkage*, Parke RD, Ladd GW, eds. Hillsdale, NJ: Erlbaum, pp 255–281

Michelson L, Mannarino AP, Marchione KE, Stern M, Figeroa J, Beck S (1983), A comparative outcome study of behavioral social-skills training, interpersonal-problem-solving, and non-directive control treatments with child psychiatric outpatients. *Behav Res Ther* 21:545–556

Moncher FJ, Prinz RJ (1991), Treatment fidelity in outcome studies. *Clin Psychol Rev* 11:247–266

Oden S (1986), Developing social skills instruction for peer interaction and relationships. In: *Teaching Social Skills to Children: Innovative Approaches*, 2nd ed, Cartledge G, Milburn JF, eds. New York: Pergamon, pp 187–218

Parke RD, Bhavnagri NP (1989), Parents as managers of children's peer friendships. In: *Children's Social Networks and Social Supports*, Belle D, ed. New York: Wiley, pp 241–259

Pekarik E, Prinz R, Liebert D, Weintraub S, Neil J (1976), The Pupil Evaluation Inventory: a sociometric technique for assessing children's social behavior. *J Abnorm Child Psychol* 4:83–97

Pelham WE, Bender ME (1982), Peer relationships in hyperactive children: description and treatment. In: *Advances in Learning and Behavioral Disabilities*, Vol 1, Gadow KD, Bialer I, eds. Greenwich, CT: JAI Press, pp 365–436

Perry DG, Williard JC, Perry LC (1990), Peer perceptions of the consequences that victimized children provide aggressors. *Child Dev* 61:1310–1325

Phillips EL, Shenker S, Revitz P (1951), Assimilation of the new child into the group. *Psychiatry* 14:319–325

Pope AW, Bierman KL, Mumma GH (1989), Relations between hyperactive and aggressive behavior and peer relations at three elementary grade levels. *J Abnorm Child Psychol* 17:253–267

Pope AW, Bierman KL, Mumma GH (1991), Aggression, hyperactivity, and inattention-immaturity: behavior dimensions associated with peer rejection in elementary school boys. *Dev Psychol* 27:663–671

Putallaz M (1983), Predicting children's sociometric status from their behavior. *Child Dev* 54:1417–1426

Putallaz M, Gottman JM (1981), An interactional model of children's entry into peer groups. *Child Dev* 52:986–994

Sheridan SM, Dee CC, Morgan JC, McCormick ME, Walker D (1996), A multimethod intervention for social skills deficits in children with ADHD and their parents. *Sch Psychol Rev* 25:57–76

Teeter PA (1991), Attention deficit hyperactivity disorder: a psychoeducational paradigm. *Sch Psychol Rev* 20:266–280

Tremblay RE, LeBlanc M, Schwartzman AE (1988), The predictive power of first-grade peer and teacher ratings of behavior: sex differences in antisocial behavior and personality at adolescence. *J Abnorm Child Psychol* 16:571–583

Tryon AS, Keane SP (1991), Popular and aggressive boys' initial social interaction patterns in cooperative and competitive settings. *J Abnorm Child Psychol* 19:395–406

Weiss G, Hechtman LT (1986), *Hyperactive Children Grown Up*. New York: Guilford

Whalen CK, Henker B (1985), The social worlds of hyperactive children. *Clin Psychol Rev* 5:1–32

Winer BJ (1971), *Statistical Principles in Experimental Design*. New York: McGraw-Hill

Yu P, Harris GE, Solovitz BL, Franklin JL (1986), A social problem-solving intervention for children at high risk for later psychopathology. *J Clin Child Psychol* 15:30–40.

14

Clinical Efficacy of Methylphenidate in Conduct Disorder With and Without Attention Deficit Hyperactivity Disorder

Rachel G. Klein, Howard Abikoff, Emily Klass, David Ganeles, Laura M. Seese, Simcha Pollack

Long Island Jewish Medical Center, New Hyde Park, New York

Background: *Stimulants are not considered appropriate for the treatment of children with conduct disorders (CDs). The postulated differences in stimulant effect between children with attention deficit hyperactivity disorder (ADHD) and CD led to the hypothesis that methylphenidate hydrochloride, which is effective in ADHD, would not significantly improve symptoms of CD.* **Methods:** *We randomly assigned 84 children with CD, between the ages of 6 and 15 years, to receive methylphenidate hydrochloride (up to 60 mg/d) or placebo for 5 weeks. Behavior was evaluated by parent, teacher, and clinician reports and by direct classroom observations. Two thirds of the children also met criteria for ADHD.* **Results:** *Contrary to prediction, ratings of antisocial behaviors specific to CD were significantly reduced by methylphenidate treatment. The magnitude of methylphenidate effect indicated meaningful clinical benefit. Partialling out severity of ADHD did not alter the significant superiority of methylphenidate on CD ratings specifically ($P < .001$).* **Conclusions:** *Methylphenidate has short-term positive effects on children and adolescents with CD. Key aspects of antisocial adjustment appear to be treatment responsive. This effect was independent of severity of the children's initial ADHD symptoms.*

The *DSM-III* was criticized for establishing arbitrary diagnostic distinctions.[1] One of the contentious issues concerned diagnostic refinements among disruptive disorders. One view, especially salient in the United Kingdom, holds that symptoms of attention deficit hyperactivity disorder (ADHD) are nonspecific correlates of behavior disorders[2-5] and argues against isolating ADHD symptoms into a distinct diagnosis, except in rare cases.[6] In keeping

---

Reprinted with permission from Archives of General Psychiatry, 1997, Vol. 54, 1074–1080.

This study was supported in part by Public Health Service grant MH-35779 from the National Institute of Mental Health, Rockville, Md.

with this argument, the frequent ADHD diagnosis in the United States has been shown to correspond largely to conduct disorder (CD) in the United Kingdom.[7] A counter view, especially prevalent in the United States, holds that the disorders are distinct. Inevitably, these contrasting diagnostic approaches have therapeutic implications. The rationale for the present clinical trial rested on this diagnostic controversy. To elucidate the diagnostic distinction between CD and ADHD, a study was initiated in the late 1980s to investigate the efficacy of methylphenidate hydrochloride in children with CD, free of ADHD[8-10] (the current acronym is used in this report). Although treatment studies do not provide conclusive proof of diagnostic distinctions, they are suggestive when interventions have differential impact on subtypes within a diagnostic class.[11] In this vein, a study was undertaken, with the strategy of pharmacological dissection, to test the validity of distinguishing between ADHD and CD.

Although the treatment literature on CD, which goes back several decades, is rich in reports of short-term interventions, psychopharmacotherapy does not figure as an option. This neglect is probably related to the fact that the existing literature on stimulant treatment of CD is scant and fails to provide clearly defined outcomes. Two placebo-controlled studies found dextroamphetamine superior to placebo in delinquents.[12,13] Problematically, the effect was not described and reductions in antisocial symptoms per se cannot be inferred. One study of methylphenidate in the treatment of delinquents was negative[14]; another[15] included recently hospitalized patients with CDs who received a placebo and 3 methylphenidate doses, each for 4 days. Improvement in oppositional behavior was obtained at the highest dose only. It is not clear that CD symptoms were reduced; however, it would be difficult to detect such effects during a 4-day trial, especially since overt antisocial acts are typically infrequent in new admissions.

These few drug studies have had no impact on the field. For example, chapters on CD in major texts[16,17] ignore medication as a potential treatment, as do most reviews of child psychopharmacology.[18,19] Some state explicitly that stimulants have no role in the treatment of children and adolescents with CD.[20-23] The only mention of stimulant treatment in CD[24] notes efficacy for aggression, but not for other CD symptoms.

A sizable literature documents positive stimulant effects on aggression in children with ADHD.[25-34] Conduct "problems" in ADHD also respond to stimulants, but these symptoms refer to aversive behaviors that differ from cardinal signs of CD. Aggression and oppositionality are common among the latter but are only part of a broad range of destructive, antisocial behavior that includes deliberate rule breaking and destructive, malicious antisocial acts (eg, stealing, cruelty to animals). Distinguishing between symptoms of CD and conduct problems, which are part of ADHD and respond to stimulants, is critical to appropriate diagnostic and therapeutic inference. Although treatment findings obtained in aggressive or oppositional children with ADHD have incontrovertible clinical importance, they do not inform on CD specifically.

In sum, the efficacy of stimulant medications in ADHD was well established when the study was initiated, but the huge literature did not address treatment of antisocial behaviors; in addition, there was no clinical consensus, and little empirical evidence, concerning stimulant efficacy in CD. In turn, the few studies in CD do not address the possible contribution of ADHD to positive drug effects. We hypothesized that children with CD, without comorbid ADHD, would fail to derive benefit from stimulant treatment,[35] a view shared by others.[36]

A clinical pattern emerged early that altered the thrust of the study. Children referred with CD mostly presented with comorbid ADHD. The plan to study children with CD only, ie, pure CD, appeared unfeasible. More important, the study's original question regarding methylphenidate efficacy in pure CD did not appear relevant to the clinical population. Therefore, the trial was modified to address whether symptoms of CD specifically respond favorably to methylphenidate. To our knowledge, no study has addressed this issue. A second goal was to examine whether drug-induced improvement, if any, was dependent on ADHD severity.

SUBJECTS AND METHODS

Subjects

Referrals were solicited from schools and juvenile probation offices via fliers and direct contact. Children, aged 6 to 15 years, had to be attending school. Families were given a full explanation of procedures. Children older than 12 years and all parents gave signed consent. Younger children gave assent.

The study was initiated before *DSM-III-R*[9] was finalized; *DSM-III* criteria for CD, requiring 1 symptom, were used with slight modification: lying could not qualify for the diagnosis. Child psychiatrists evaluated children and parents with specific inquiry for CD and ADHD, and a social worker or psychologist (E.K.) interviewed parents with the DICA[37] for these disorders. Both clinicians had to agree on a diagnosis of CD, coupled with impairment. Consensus was reached on disagreements.

There was no validated scale for assessing severity of CD. An accommodation was made by using the Iowa Aggression Scale,[38,39] which reflects defiant behavior. A minimum score of 7 by teachers, previously established as a clinical threshold,[38] was required (range, 0-15). For children in junior high school and high school, we averaged ratings from 3 teachers. Moderate to severe impairment ratings by teachers or parents were required on an overall severity scale.

In addition, children had to have IQs above 70,[40] be medically healthy, and be nonpsychotic. Substance disorders were excluded, but not occasional illicit drug use.

Standards for establishing ADHD (which initially were exclusionary) were similar to those in previous studies[41,42] and were consistent with *DSM-IV*[10] criteria. Children had to have *cross-situational* hyperactivity and receive means of at least 1.5 on the Conners Teacher Rating Scale hyperactivity factor.[39] Applying these criteria, 69% of children were comorbid for ADHD.

Existing instruments were inadequate for assessing the symptomatic repertoire of CD. Therefore, a rating scale was generated by adding, to the Conners Teacher Rating Scale, subscales of the Quay Revised Behavior Problem Checklist[43] and global estimates of severity of behavioral and academic problems.[44] Parents and teachers completed identical ratings.

Classroom Observations

Classroom observations have been found to differentiate children with ADHD and normal children[45] as well as to be sensitive to stimulant treatment. To characterize the treatment response, observations were undertaken in elementary schools. These were judged unfeasible in later grades.

Procedures were adapted from previous studies[46] that used the Classroom Observation Code.[47] Observers were trained by an expert until reliability was established. During instructional classes, the observers, unaware of the study design and children's diagnostic and treatment status, recorded the code behaviors of patients and "average" children, nominated by teachers as having unremarkable adjustment. In addition, observers recorded "absence of behavior," indicating that no code behavior had occurred. Interobserver reliability was monitored throughout the study.

At the end of their observations, observers completed the Conners Teacher Rating Scale,[39] which is sensitive to stimulant effects in ADHD[42] when used as a direct observational measure.

Other Measures

Some negative mood in children with ADHD has been reported with single dextroamphetamine administration.[48] Mood changes have not been assessed with longer stimulant exposure and seemed important because negative mood effects might influence the treatment's cost-benefit ratio. Therefore, the Mood Scale[48] was administered.

Children were administered standardized measures of academic achievement: Wide-Range Achievement Test[49] (reading and arithmetic) and Gilmore Reading Test[50] (reading and reading comprehension).

Treatment

Children were randomly assigned to matching placebo or methylphenidate hydrochloride for 5 weeks via a table of random numbers. Treatment was double-blind. Provided significant adverse effects did not occur, a preset titration was applied, up to 60 mg/d, in 2 divided doses. Children and parents were seen weekly by psychiatrists who adjusted dosage on the basis of adverse effects[51] and clinical response, which was based on parents', children's, and teachers' reports (obtained weekly by telephone).

Parents received weekly supportive counseling. No psychosocial therapy was given to the child.

Posttreatment Assessments

Rating scales and global improvement ratings were obtained at the end of treatment, and 3 classroom observations were conducted.

Data Analyses

Group differences before treatment examined Student *t* tests for independent means. Phi coefficients were computed for reliability of classroom observations. To evaluate treatment effects, analyses of covariance—controlling for pretreatment values—were applied to continuous measures; χ^2 to categorical measures.

Several analytical procedures were implemented to examine the relationship between ADHD and drug-induced improvement. First, we correlated global improvement ratings with hyperactivity ratings obtained before treatment: (1) teachers' Iowa inattentive/overactive factor, (2) clinician rating of ADHD in school and (3) at home, and (4) observed "interference" and "off-task" in school. Second, to control for potential impact of ADHD on global improvement with methylphenidate, pretreatment ADHD scores were removed from global improvement ratings by means of analyses of covariance. Third, drug effects on CD ratings were analyzed controlling for the above ADHD measures. Fourth, interactions between treatment effects and ADHD measures were obtained. All analyses were planned.

RESULTS

Subjects and Treatment Characteristics

During the 3-year study period, 297 patients were referred; 62 parents did not pursue treatment (of these, 20 [6.7% of the total] explicitly refused medication); and 151 children failed to meet criteria. The remaining 84 entered the study. One child withdrew before treatment. Of the remaining 83, 41 were randomized to receive methylphenidate and 42 to placebo. As a whole, children did not come from the most disadvantaged circumstances, as evidenced by the relatively high proportion of children living in 2-parent homes (Table 1).

Four children taking methylphenidate and 5 taking placebo left the study. Seventy-four (88%) completed the study, 37 in each group. Criteria for CD were met in school *and* home in 55%; only at home in 10%; and only in school in 34% (rounded percentages). All but 2 children (97.6%) had at least 3 symptoms of CD, consistent with *DSM-IV*. Criteria for ADHD were met by 51 (69%) of 74 children.

At study end, the average methylphenidate hydrochloride dose was 41.3 mg/d (1.0 mg/kg). Morning and noon doses were virtually identical. When dissimilar, they differed by only 5 mg. After 5 treatment weeks, adverse effects occurred in 84% (31/37) of children taking methylphenidate vs 46% taking placebo. Only a few instances of delayed sleep with medication were severe.

Treatment Outcome

Children taking methylphenidate were rated as significantly better by teachers on all CD measures, except socialized aggression (Table 2); this measure reflects severe delinquent behavior, such as gang membership, which was rare. As anticipated, methylphenidate had positive significant impact on teacher ratings of ADHD symptoms. Specific aspects of CD were significantly affected by methylphenidate, eg, obscene language, attacks others, destroys property, and deliberately cruel.

Favorable significant methylphenidate effects were also obtained on parent factors, except for socialized aggression (Table 3). In the case of parents, as well, specific CD ratings were ameliorated significantly by treatment (eg, cruel to others, bad companions, steals outside home).

TABLE 1
Sample Characteristics*

	Methylphenidate Hydrochloride ($n = 41$)	Placebo ($n = 42$)
Age, y (mean ± SD)	10.2 ± 2.3	10.2 ± 2.5
Sex, No. (%) M	36 (88)	38 (90)
Sibship size, No. (%)		
1-2 children	31 (75)	36 (86)
3 children	7 (17)	2 (5)
≥4 children	3 (6)	4 (9)
SES (mean ± SD)†	3.2 ± 1.1	3.5 ± 1.1
WISC-R IQ (mean ± SD)		
Full-Scale IQ (74-136)	101.2 ± 14.3	95.4 ± 12.5
Verbal IQ	102.4 ± 15.4	95.6 ± 12.5
Performance IQ	99.9 ± 14.2	96.2 ± 14.5
Gilmore Reading Test, stanine (mean ± SD)		
Accuracy	4.4 ± 1.7	4.4 ± 1.8
Comprehension	4.8 ± 1.8	4.2 ± 1.9
Race, No. (%)		
White	26 (63)	28 (67)
African American	12 (29)	12 (29)
Hispanic	3 (7)	2 (5)
Child lives with, No. (%)		
Both parents	13 (32)	21 (50)
Parent and stepparent	8 (20)	5 (12)
One parent	17 (41)	14 (33)
Other relative	2 (5)	2 (5)

*Percentages are rounded. SES indicates socioeconomic status; WISC-R, Wechsler Intelligence Scale for Children–Revised. Verbal IQ, $P < .05$; all other contrasts nonsignificant.

†Hollingshead and Redlich Index of Social Position.[52] Range, 1 to 5; higher value represents lower status.

Global improvement was dichotomized between improved (ie, improved, much improved, completely well) and unimproved (slightly improved, worse). Compared with the placebo group, significantly more children taking methylphenidate were viewed as improved by all informants. Respective improvement rates for children taking methylphenidate and placebo were as follows: teachers, 59% vs 9%; mothers, 78% vs 27%; and psychiatrists, 68% vs 11% ($P < .001$ for all).

Observations were obtained for 51 elementary school–aged children at baseline, but 4 were missing at the posttest evaluation. Interrater reliability ranged from 0.69 to 0.87 (average, 0.76). Significant reductions were found with methylphenidate on motor activity ($P < .05$ and .01), off-task ($P < .02$s), and interference (disruptive behavior) ($P < .000$). In addition, methylphenidate treatment was associated with a significantly lower rate of physical aggression ($P < .03$). The rate of problem-free behavior was significantly higher in the

TABLE 2
Teacher Ratings of Children Before and After Treatment

Behavior	Before Treatment (Mean ± SD) ($N = 71$)	After Treatment (Mean ± SE)* Placebo ($n = 35$)	Methylphenidate Hydrochloride ($n = 36$)	P†
Factor scores				
Aggression (Iowa scale)‡	10.6 ± 3.3	9.9 ± 0.6	5.2 ± 0.6	<.001
Conduct problems§	2.1 ± 0.7	1.9 ± 0.1	1.0 ± 0.1	<.001
Conduct disorder‖	1.8 ± 0.6	1.7 ± 0.1	0.9 ± 0.1	<.001
Socialized aggression‖	0.5 ± 0.5	0.5 ± 0.1	0.3 ± 0.1	<.08
Inattentive/overactive (Iowa scale)	2.1 ± 0.6	2.0 ± 0.1	1.0 ± 0.1	<.001
Hyperactivity§	2.2 ± 0.7	2.0 ± 0.1	1.0 ± 0.1	<.001
Inattentive/passive§	1.6 ± 0.6	1.5 ± 0.1	1.0 ± 0.1	<.001
Overall rating				
Conduct problems	2.6 ± 0.7	2.3 ± 0.1	1.3 ± 0.1	<.001
Academic problems	1.9 ± 1.0	1.9 ± 0.1	1.5 ± 0.1	<.03

*Controlled for pretreatment values.
†Two-tailed.
‡Sum of 5 items (range, 0-15).
§Factors from the Conners Teacher Rating Scale[39] (range, 0-3).
‖Factors from Quay Revised Behavior Checklist[45] (range, 0-3) (numbers of subjects are reduced because of missing ratings: placebo, $n = 25$; methylphenidate, $n = 28$).

TABLE 3
Parent Ratings of Children Before and After Treatment

Behavior (Factor Scores)	Before Treatment (Mean ± SD) ($N = 74$)	After Treatment (Mean ± SE)* Placebo ($n = 37$)	Methylphenidate Hydrochloride ($n = 37$)	P†
Aggression (Iowa scale)‡	10.5 ± 3.4	8.3 ± 0.5	6.0 ± 0.5	<.003
Conduct problems§	1.9 ± 0.7	1.4 ± 0.1	1.0 ± 0.1	<.002
Conduct disorder‖	1.8 ± 0.6	1.4 ± 0.1	0.9 ± 0.1	<.001
Socialized aggression‖	0.4 ± 0.5	0.3 ± 0.1	0.2 ± 0.1	<.09
Inattentive/overactive (Iowa scale)	2.1 ± 0.7	1.7 ± 0.1	1.3 ± 0.1	<.02
Impulsive/hyperactive§	2.3 ± 0.7	1.9 ± 0.1	1.5 ± 0.1	<.02

*Controlled for pretreatment values.
†Two-tailed.
‡Sum of 5 items (range, 0-15).
§Factors from the Conners Parent Rating Scale[39] (range, 0-3).
‖Factors from Quay Revised Behavior Checklist[45] (range, 0-3).

TABLE 4
Behavior Scale Ratings by Classroom Observers Before and After Treatment

		After Treatment (Mean ± SE)*		
Behavior (Factor Scores)	Before Treatment (Mean ± SD) ($N = 47$)	Placebo ($n = 24$)	Methylphenidate Hydrochloride ($n = 23$)	P†
Aggression (Iowa scale)‡	3.5 ± 0.7	4.5 ± 0.5	2.5 ± 0.5	<.03
Conduct problems§	0.5 ± 0.6	0.6 ± 0.1	0.4 ± 0.1	<.11
Inattentive/overactive (Iowa scale)	1.4 ± 0.6	1.4 ± 0.1	0.8 ± 0.1	<.01
Hyperactivity§	1.3 ± 0.7	1.3 ± 0.4	0.8 ± 0.1	<.01
Global rating of conduct problems	1.5 ± 0.7	1.5 ± 0.1	0.8 ± 0.1	<.001

*Controlled for pretreatment values.
†Two-tailed.
‡Sum of 5 items (range, 0-15). Range of other factors, 0-3.
§Factors from the Conners Teacher Rating Scale.[39]

methylphenidate-treated group ($P < .005$). As shown in Table 4, significant improvement in those taking methylphenidate occurred on observer-rated conduct problem factors and overall conduct disturbance severity.

Self-ratings of negative mood were very low before treatment. However, our purpose was to detect deleterious drug effects, and low values maximized the likelihood of their detection. Methylphenidate significantly improved 8 of 28 mood items; none was worse.

No significant treatment differences occurred on reading (mean ± SD for methylphenidate and placebo groups, respectively: Wide-Range Achievement TestReading, 101.5 ± 10.0 vs 93.9 ± 10.0; Wide-Range Achievement Test Arithmetic, 97.2 ± 20.0 vs 89.6 ± 11.0; Gilmore (stanines), accuracy, 5.2 ± 2.0 vs 4.6 ± 2.0; comprehension, 5.7 ± 2.0 vs 5.3 ± 2.0).

Methylphenidate Effects Controlled for Initial Hyperactivity

No significant positive associations were found between the children's level of ADHD symptoms before treatment and overall improvement ratings with methylphenidate ($r = -0.34$ to 0.20). Table 5 presents global clinical improvement ratings after removal of the influence of initial ADHD in school and home. On all outcome measures, methylphenidate remained significantly superior to placebo. Similarly, drug-induced improvement on CD symptoms was significant after partialling for initial ADHD ratings. The control for ADHD did not alter the relative advantage of methylphenidate on any rating. No significant interaction between initial ADHD and treatment outcome was obtained, indicating that ratings of ADHD did not impact significantly on response to methylphenidate.

COMMENT

Two clinical findings emerged. One, symptoms of CD are markedly responsive to short-term methylphenidate treatment at the doses used. Two, drug effects on multiple aspects of CD are not dependent on the severity of ADHD symptoms.

TABLE 5

Mother, Teacher, and Clinician Mean Global Improvement Ratings* Adjusted for Initial ADHD

		Mother				Teacher				Psychiatrist			
ADHD Variable Controlled	Group	No.	Mean	*P*	95% CI	No.	Mean	*P*	95% CI	No.	Mean	*P*	95% CI
Global Improvement													
Iowa inattention/overactivity	PBO	37	4.3	.001	3.9-4.7	34	5.0	.001	4.6-5.5	37	4.8	.001	4.5-5.1
	MTP	36	3.0		2.6-3.4	37	3.4		2.9-3.8	34	3.1		2.8-3.4
ADHD in school	PBO	37	4.3	.001	3.9-4.7	34	5.0	.001	4.6-5.5	37	4.8	.001	4.5-5.1
	MTP	36	3.0		2.6-3.4	37	3.4		2.9-3.8	34	3.1		2.8-3.4
ADHD at home	PBO	37	4.3	.001	3.9-4.7	34	5.0	.001	4.6-5.5	37	4.8	.001	4.5-5.1
	MTP	36	3.0		2.6-3.4	37	3.4		3.0-3.8	34	3.1		2.8-3.4
Off-task	PBO	28	4.3	.001	3.9-4.7	26	4.9	.001	4.4-5.4	27	4.7	.001	4.4-5.1
	MTP	23	2.8		2.4-3.3	24	3.2		2.7-3.7	23	3.2		2.8-3.5
Conduct Disorder Symptom Scales													
ADHD ratings†	PBO	37	0.9	<.001	0.4–1.4	37	1.5	<.001	1.1–1.8	...	...	...	...
	MTP	36	0.2		0.0–0.7	34	0.6		0.3–1.0	...	...	...	...

*1 indicates completely well; 2, much improved; 3, improved; 4, slightly improved; 5, unchanged; 6 and 7, worse. ADHD indicates attention deficit hyperactivity disorder; CI, confidence interval; PBO, placebo; and MTP, methylphenidate hydrochloride. Iowa inattention/overactivity is teacher ratings: ADHD in school/home, clinician-rated symptoms; and off-task, classroom observations.

†Baseline score on Teacher Iowa inattention/overactivity factor+number of ADHD symptoms by clinician+off-task in school. The mother ratings are a mean of 7 items: fights constantly, physical fights with peers, attacks others, violent to others, bullies, cruel to others, and steals from outside home. The teacher ratings are a mean of 9 items: obscene language/swearing/curshing, incites or goads others into fighting, gets involved in physical fights with peers, attacks others, destroys property, acts violently to children or adults, deliberately cruel to others, cheats, and admires and seeks "rougher" peers.

Our clinical experience led us to expect the recruitment of children with pure CD. Yet, 69% had ADHD (a rate similar to that reported by others in clinic referrals [65%]).[53] Reviews by 2 National Institute of Mental Health committees composed of experts in child psychiatry did not question the stated plan, or the rarity of the targeted clinical population. What accounted for the erroneous expectation that pure CDs were the rule rather than the exception? We believe that this mistaken belief stemmed from traditional clinical practice of focusing on children's antisocial symptoms to the detriment of other symptoms, because they are so salient. As a result, other dysfunctions may be overlooked or conceptualized as nonspecific aspects of CD.[54] Consistent with this point is the observation that a vast literature on CD does not refer to ADHD at all. Until recently, research was polarized between ADHD and CD, and it is with the relatively recent advent of scale criteria for ADHD, of clinical diagnostic criteria, and of systematic clinical interviews that the comorbidity between ADHD and CD became evident and a focus of interest.

An alternative explanation for the diagnostic composition of the study sample is that comorbid cases are more likely to come for treatment than others, and that we failed to elicit referrals from the pool of children with CD who did not have ADHD. This possibility appears plausible in the light of epidemiological studies that have identified CDs free of ADHD. Yet, in a recent large British epidemiological study, CD in younger children *never* occurred without ADHD.[51] If accurate, this observation would account for the composition of our sample, especially since the study children had early onset of CD. Relying on rating scales exclusively, CD without ADHD has been identified.[55] Unfortunately, rating scales are neither sufficiently sensitive nor specific to substitute for clinical diagnoses, and the 2 approaches likely produce different diagnostic outcomes. The relationship between ADHD and CD is beyond the scope of this discussion, but the comprehensive critical review by Hinshaw[55] reports impressive documentation for distinct constructs of hyperactivity and aggression; however, it also shows that most attempts to identify specific diagnostic correlates have failed.

Our study results indicate significant diminution of a range of antisocial behavior with methylphenidate. More important, the reductions were substantial and clinically meaningful. Clear treatment effects occurred on specific symptoms of CD, even covert ones such as cheating and stealing. Teachers indicated broad and marked amelioration in children who received methylphenidate and little alteration for those taking placebo. The relative advantage of methylphenidate over placebo is similar for teachers and mothers, but mothers held a more favorable view of their children's progress regardless of the treatment. It is possible that counseling had credibility and may have influenced mothers' perceptions of change. Since teachers observe children in a standardized functional setting, their estimates of improvement with placebo are likely more valid. Unlike behavioral ratings by teachers and parents, classroom observations of ADHD symptoms and aggression are independent and not susceptible to halo effects. The direct classroom observations provide independent corroboration of methylphenidate efficacy.

Although the effectiveness of methylphenidate is impressive, several reservations concerning its impact are in order. Whereas clinical normalization is frequent among good responders with uncomplicated ADHD, it almost never occurred in this population. Alone, stimulant treatment provides clinically meaningful but incomplete therapeutic impact. Also, treatment was short term, and CDs are chronic conditions. The true value of the intervention will depend on its stability. Problematically, the recalcitrant attitude toward psychiatric treatment of many families of children with CD limits wide application of successful pharmacotherapy, as it does any long-term intervention. Moreover, results include multiple contrasts. However, every difference is consistent with methylphenidate efficacy.

Psychopharmacology has made a major contribution to our understanding of psychiatric disorders. Treatment outcome has been an informative tool, but only when clinical groups have differed in response pattern. Had methylphenidate been ineffective in CD, as we had predicted, it would have been an argument in support of its distinction from ADHD. That the medication is effective in both disorders does not invalidate their representing discrete diagnostic entities, but it is not supportive of the distinction.

The effect of methylphenidate on antisocial behavior was not a function of the severity of children's ADHD symptoms, since positive medication effects remained after controlling for them. Moreover, there was no relationship between ADHD severity and improvement. There appears to be an independent influence of methylphenidate on provocative, aggressive, mean behaviors. The magnitude of this effect may be appreciated by an examination of the "true ranges" of improvement (confidence intervals) for each treatment after the influence of ADHD symptoms is removed (Table 5). There is virtually no group overlap between ranges of improvement. This outcome highlights the clinical meaningfulness of the drug effect independently of ADHD.

Adverse effects with methylphenidate were typical of those reported in ADHD—the most common being decreased appetite and delay of sleep. Of note, 47% of the children taking placebo reported at least 1 adverse effect at the end of treatment. This finding underscores the need for placebo conditions for informative results on medication-related adverse effects. Abuse is the major concern associated with the administration of stimulants to antisocial individuals, whose potential for abuse is well documented. The likelihood of abuse in children and adolescents studied was minimized by the fact that those with a current substance use disorder were excluded and, as far as we know, none abused methylphenidate during the study. However, this issue is one that requires consideration with long-term usage. Concerns about risks of methylphenidate abuse may be tempered by the fact that oral administration is not associated with euphoric responses[54]; indeed, no child experienced "highs" with the medication. More important, methylphenidate efficacy was not at the cost of impairing mood, and based on our results, effective stimulant use in children with CD is not accompanied by dysphoria or other mood changes. In animals as well as humans, increased aggressive and violent behavior with stimulant administration has been reported.[56] This negative effect did not occur.

There is no obvious behavioral model to account for methylphenidate efficacy on symptoms of CD. What appears plausible is that impulsivity is a key pathologic abnormality in both CD and ADHD, and that it is specifically reduced by stimulant treatment. In children with CD, enhanced impulse control is likely to induce multiple positive secondary effects. With methylphenidate, children were described by parents as more reasonable and tractable. In turn, this change may lead to improvement in some maladaptive social behaviors, such as having "bad companions," which were significantly reduced. It would be most unlikely for medication to have a direct impact on such complex comportment.

Kazdin[57] has argued that successful treatment of CDs probably requires combined psychosocial approaches. Our results suggest that stimulant treatment is likely to be a factor in the therapeutic equation devised for modifying symptoms of CD.

The weight of the evidence supports a close association between hyperactivity and CDs.[58] This relationship has important public health implications, since children who are comorbid for ADHD and CD are at high relative risk for sustained antisocial behavior compared with those with CD only.[59] Successful treatment in this clinical population would represent an important advance in psychiatry.

REFERENCES

1. Rutter M, Shaffer D. *DSM-III:* a step forward or back in terms of the classification of child psychiatric disorders? *J Am Acad Child Psychiatry.* 1980;19:371-394.
2. Sandberg ST. The overinclusiveness of the diagnosis of hyperkinetic syndrome. In: Gittelman M, ed. *Strategic Interventions for Hyperactive Children.* Armonk, NY: ME Sharpe; 1981:8-38.
3. Sandberg ST, Rutter M, Taylor E. Hyperkinetic disorder in psychiatric clinic attenders. *Dev Med Child Neurol.* 1978;20:279-299.
4. Sandberg ST, Wieselberg M, Shaffer D. Hyperkinetic and conduct problem children in a primary school population: some epidemiological considerations. *J Child Psychol Psychiatry.* 1980;21:293-311.
5. Shaffer D, Greenhill L. A critical note on the predictive validity of 'the hyperkinetic syndrome.' *J Child Psychol Psychiatry.* 1979;20:61-72.
6. Rutter M, Tizard J, Whitmore K. *Education, Health and Behavior.* Huntington, NY: Krieger Publishing Co; 1981.
7. Prendergast M, Taylor E, Rapoport JL, Bartko J, Donnelly M, Zametkin A, Ahearn MB, Dunn G, Wieselberg HM. The diagnosis of childhood hyperactivity: a U.S.-U.K. cross-national study of *DSM-III* and *ICD-9. J Child Psychol Psychiatry.* 1988;29:289-300.
8. American Psychiatric Association. *Diagnostic and Statistical Manual of Mental Disorders, Third Edition.* Washington, DC: American Psychiatric Association; 1980.
9. American Psychiatric Association. *Diagnostic and Statistical Manual of Mental Disorders, Third Edition, Revised.* Washington, DC: American Psychiatric Association; 1987.
10. American Psychiatric Association. *Diagnostic and Statistical Manual of Mental Disorders, Fourth Edition.* Washington, DC: American Psychiatric Association; 1994.
11. Klein DF. The pharmacological validation of psychiatric diagnosis. In: Robins LN, Barrett J, eds. *Validity of Psychiatric Diagnosis.* New York, NY: Raven Press; 1989: 203-216.
12. Eisenberg L, Lachman R, Molling PA, Lockner A, Mizelle JD, Conners CK. A psychopharmacologic experiment in a training school for delinquent boys: methods, problems, findings. *Am J Orthopsychiatry.* 1963;33:431-447.
13. Maletsky BM. *d*-Amphetamine and delinquency: hyperkinesis persisting? *Dis Nerv Syst.* 1974;35:543-547.
14. Conners CK, Kramer R, Rothschild GH, Schwartz L, Stone A. Treatment of young delinquent boys with diphenylhydantoin sodium and methylphenidate. *Arch Gen Psychiatry.* 1971;24:156-160.

15. Brown RT, Jaffe SL, Silverstein J, Magee H. Methylphenidate and adolescents hospitalized with conduct disorder: dose effects on classroom behavior, academic performance, and impulsivity. *J Clin Child Psychol.* 1991;20:282-292.
16. Sheldrick EC. Treatment of delinquents. In: Rutter M, Hersov L, eds. *Child and Adolescent Psychiatry.* 2nd ed. Boston, Mass: Blackwell Scientific Publications; 1985:743-752.
17. Earls F. Oppositional-defiant and conduct disorders. In: Rutter M, Taylor E, Hersov L, eds. *Child and Adolescent Psychiatry: Modern Approaches.* 3rd ed. Oxford, England: Blackwell Scientific Publications; 1994:308-329.
18. Maletic V, March JS, Johnston HF. Child and adolescent psychopharmacology. *Psychiatr Clin North Am: Ann Drug Ther.* 1994;1:101-124.
19. Wilens TE, Biederman J. The stimulants. In: Shaffer D, ed. *Psychiatr Clin North Am.* 1992;15:191-222.
20. Jacobvitz D, Sroufe LA, Steward M, Leffert N. Treatment of attentional and hyperactivity problems in children with sympathomimetic drugs: a comprehensive review. *J Am Acad Child Adolesc Psychiatry.* 1990;29:677-688.
21. Kaplan CA, Hussain S. Use of drugs in child and adolescent psychiatry. *Br J Psychiatry.* 1995;166:291-298.
22. O'Donnell DJ. Conduct disorders. In: Wiener JM, ed. *Diagnosis and Psychopharmacology of Childhood and Adolescent Disorders.* New York, NY: Basic Books; 1985:249-287.
23. Werry J. Pharmacotherapy of disruptive behavior disorders. *Child Adolesc Psychiatr Clin North Am.* 1994;3:321-341.
24. Stoewe JK, Kruesi MJP, Lelio DF. Psychopharmacology of aggressive states and features of conduct disorder. In: Riddle MA, ed. *Child Adolesc Psychiatr Clin North Am.* 1995;4:359-379.
25. Hinshaw SP. Stimulant medication and the treatment of aggression in children with attentional deficits. *J Clin Child Psychol.* 1991;20:301-312.
26. Barkley RA, McMurray MB, Edelbrock CS, Robbins K. The response of aggressive and nonaggressive ADHD children to two doses of methylphenidate. *J Am Acad Child Adolesc Psychiatry.* 1989;28:873-881.
27. Cunningham CE, Siegel LS, Offord DR. A dose-response analysis of the effects of methylphenidate on the peer interactions and simulated classroom performance of ADD children with and without conduct problems. *J Child Psychol Psychiatry.* 1991;32:439-452.
28. Gadow KD, Nolan EE, Sverd J, Sprafkin J, Paolicelli L. Methylphenidate in aggressive-hyperactive boys, I: effects on peer aggression in public school settings. *J Am Acad Child Adolesc Psychiatry.* 1990;29:710-718.
29. Hinshaw SP, Henker B, Whalen CK, Erhardt D, Dunington RE Jr. Aggressive, prosocial, and nonsocial behavior in hyperactive boys: dose effects of methylphenidate in naturalistic settings. *J Consult Clin Psychol.* 1989;87:636-643.
30. Kaplan SL, Busner J, Kupietz S, Wassermann E, Segal B. Effects of methylphenidate on adolescents with aggressive conduct disorder and ADDH: a preliminary report. *J Am Acad Child Adolesc Psychiatry.* 1990;29:719-723.
31. Klorman R, Brumaghim JT, Salzman LF, Strauss J, Borgstedt AD, McBride MC, Loeb S. Effects of methylphenidate on attention-deficit hyperactivity disorder with and without aggressive/noncompliant features. *J Abnorm Psychol.* 1988;97:413-422.

32. Klorman R, Brumaghim JT, Fitzpatrick PA, Borgstedt AD, Strauss J. Clinical and cognitive effects of methylphenidate on children with attention deficit disorder as a function of aggression/oppositionality and age. *J Abnorm Psychol.* 1994;103:206-221.

33. Murphy DA, Pelham WE, Lang AR. Aggression in boys with attention deficit-hyperactivity disorder: methylphenidate effects on naturalistically observed aggression, response to provocation, and social information processing. *J Abnorm Child Psychol.* 1992;20:451-466.

34. Stewart JT, Myers WC, Burket RC, Lyles WB. A review of the pharmacotherapy of aggression in children and adolescents. *J Am Acad Child Adolesc Psychiatry.* 1990;29:269-277.

35. Klein DF, Gittelman R, Quitkin F, Rifkin A. *Diagnosis and Drug Treatment of Psychiatric Disorders: Adults and Children.* Baltimore, Md: Williams & Wilkins; 1980.

36. Werry J. Differential diagnosis of attention deficits and conduct disorders. In: Bloomingdale LM, Sergeant JA, eds. *Attention Deficit Disorder: Criteria, Cognition, Intervention.* New York, NY: Pergamon Press; 1988:83-96.

37. Herjanic B, Reich W. Development of a structured psychiatric interview for children: agreement between child and parent on individual symptoms. *J Abnorm Child Psychol.* 1982;10:307-324.

38. Loney J, Milich R. Hyperactivity, inattention, and aggression in clinical practice. In: Wolraich M, Routh DK, eds. *Advances in Developmental and Behavioral Pediatrics.* Greenwich, Conn: JAI Press; 1982;3:113-147.

39. Goyette CH, Conners CK, Ulrich RF. Normative data on revised Conners Parent and Teacher Rating Scales. *J Abnorm Child Psychol.* 1978;6:221-236.

40. Wechsler D. *Wechsler Intelligence Scale for Children–Revised.* New York, NY: Psychological Corp; 1974.

41. Abikoff H, Gittelman R. Hyperactive children treated with stimulants: is cognitive training a useful adjunct? *Arch Gen Psychiatry.* 1985;42:953-961.

42. Gittelman R, Abikoff H, Pollack E, Klein DF, Katz S, Mattes J. A controlled trial of behavior modification and methylphenidate in hyperactive children. In: Whalen C, Henker B, eds. *Hyperactive Children: The Social Ecology of Identification and Treatment.* New York, NY: Academic Press; 1980:221-243.

43. Quay HC. A dimensional approach to children's behavior disorder: the Revised Behavior Problem Checklist. *School Psychol Rev.* 1983;12:244-249.

44. Miller LS, Klein RG, Piacentini J, Abikoff H, Shah MR, Samoilov A, Guardino M. The New York Teacher Rating Scale for disruptive and antisocial behavior. *J Am Acad Child Adolesc Psychiatry.* 1995;34:359-370.

45. Klein RG, Abikoff H, Barkley RA, Campbell M, Leckman JF, Ryan ND, Solanto MV, Whalen CK. Clinical trials in children and adolescents. In: Prien RF, Robinson DS, eds. *Clinical Evaluation of Psychotropic Drugs: Principles and Guidelines.* New York, NY: Raven Press; 1994:501-546.

46. Abikoff H, Gittleman R, Klein DF. A classroom observation code for hyperactive children: a replication of validity. *J Consult Clin Psychol.* 1980;48:555-565.

47. Abikoff H, Gittelman R. Classroom observation code: a modification of the Stony Brook Code. *Psychopharmacol Bull.* 1985;21:901-909.

48. Rapoport JL, Buchsbaum MS, Weingartner H, Zahn TP, Ludlow C, Mikkelsen EJ. Dextroamphetamine: cognitive and behavioral effects in normal and hyperactive boys and normal males. *Arch Gen Psychiatry.* 1980;37:933-943.

49. Jastak S, Wilkinson GS. *Wide Range Achievement Test.* New York, NY: Psychological Corp; 1984.

50. Gilmore JV, Gilmore EC. *Gilmore Oral Reading Test.* New York, NY: Harcourt Brace & Jovanovich; 1968.

51. McArdle P, O'Brien G, Kolvin I. Hyperactivity: prevalence and relationship with conduct disorder. *J Child Adolesc Psychol Psychiatry.* 1995;36:279-303.

52. Myers JK, Bean LL. *A Decade Later: A Follow-up of Social Class and Mental Illness.* New York, NY: John Wiley & Sons Inc; 1968.

53. Stewart MA, Cummings C, Singer S, deBlois CS. The overlap between hyperactive and unsocialized aggressive children. *J Child Psychol Psychiatry.* 1981;22:35-45.

54. Klein RG, Wender P. The role of methylphenidate in psychiatry. *Arch Gen Psychiatry.* 1995;52:429-433.

55. Hinshaw SP. On the distinction between attentional deficits/hyperactivity and conduct problems/aggression in child psychopathology. *Psychol Bull.* 1987;101:443-463.

56. Miczek KA. The psychopharmacology of aggression. In: Iversen LL, Iversen SD, Snyder SH, eds. *Handbook of Psychopharmacology.* New York, NY: Plenum Press; 1987;19:183-328.

57. Kazdin AE. Treatment of conduct disorder: progress and directions in psychotherapy research. *Dev Psychopathol.* 1993;5:277-310.

58. Biederman J, Newcorn J, Sprich SE. Comorbidity of attention deficit hyperactivity disorder (ADHD). *Am J Psychiatry.* 1991;138:564-577.

59. Farrington DP, Loeber R, Van Kammen WB. Long-term criminal outcomes of hyperactivity-impulsivity-attention deficit and conduct problems in childhood. In: Robins LN, Rutter M, eds. *Straight and Devious Pathways From Childhood to Adulthood.* New York, NY: Cambridge University Press; 1990:62-81.

15

Practitioner Review: Psychosocial Treatments for Conduct Disorder in Children

Alan E. Kazdin
Yale University, New Haven, Connecticut

The present paper reviews promising treatments for conduct disorder among children and adolescents. The treatments include problem-solving skills training, parent management training, functional family therapy and multisystemic therapy. For each treatment, conceptual underpinnings, characteristics and outcome evidence are highlighted. Limitations associated with these treatments (e.g. paucity of long-term follow-up evidence and of evidence for the clinical significance of the change) are also presented. Broader issues that affect treatment and clinical work with conduct-disordered youths are also addressed, including retaining cases in treatment, what treatments do not work, who responds well to treatment, comorbidity, the use of combined treatments and the need for new models of treatment delivery.

Antisocial behaviors in children refer to a variety of acts that reflect social rule violations and that are actions against others. Behaviors such as fighting, lying and stealing are seen in varying degrees in most children over the course of development. For present purposes, the term conduct disorder will be used to refer to antisocial behavior that is clinically significant and clearly beyond the realm of "normal" functioning. The extent to which antisocial behaviors are sufficiently severe to constitute conduct disorder depends on several characteristics of the behaviors including their frequency, intensity and chronicity, whether they are isolated acts or part of a larger syndrome with other deviant behaviors, and whether they lead to significant impairment of the child as judged by parents, teachers or others.

Little in the way of effective treatment has been generated for conduct disorder. This is unfortunate in light of the personal tragedy that conduct disorder can represent to children and their families and others who may be victims of aggressive and antisocial acts. From

---

Reprinted with permission from the *Journal of Child Psychology and Psychiatry*, 1997, Vol. 38(2), 161–178.

Completion of this paper was supported by a Research Scientist Award (MH00353) and a grant (MH35408) from the National Institute of Mental Health. Support for this work is gratefully acknowledged.

a social perspective, the absence of effective treatments is problematic as well. Conduct disorder is one of the most frequent bases of clinical referral in child and adolescent treatment services, has relatively poor long-term prognosis and is transmitted across generations (see Kazdin, 1995b). Because children with conduct disorder often traverse multiple social services (e.g. special education, mental health, juvenile justice) the disorder is one of the most costly mental disorders in the United States (Robins, 1981).

There have been significant advances in treatment. The present paper reviews research for four psychosocial treatments that have shown considerable promise in the treatment of conduct disorder in children and adolescents. ("Children" will be used to refer to both children and adolescents, unless a particular distinction is made between the two.) The treatments were selected because they have been carefully evaluated in controlled clinical trials. The paper describes and evaluates the underpinnings, techniques and evidence on behalf of these treatments. Critical issues that are raised in providing treatment to conduct disorder children and their families are also examined.

OVERVIEW OF CHARACTERISTICS OF CONDUCT DISORDER

Before discussing treatment of conduct disorder, it is important to delineate the "problem" as it is often presented clinically. From a treatment perspective, conduct disorder represents a very broad domain involving child, parent, family and contextual conditions. Many of the factors that influence delivery and effectiveness of treatment are not encompassed by the central diagnostic features of the disorder. Next we will consider briefly some salient domains that are relevant to treatment.

Central Features

The overriding feature of conduct disorder is a persistent pattern of behavior in which the rights of others and age-appropriate social norms are violated. Isolated acts of physical aggression, destruction of property, stealing and firesetting are sufficiently severe to warrant concern and attention in their own right. Although these behaviors may occur in isolation, several of these are likely to appear together as a constellation or syndrome and form the basis of a clinical diagnosis. For example, in the *Diagnostic and Statistical Manual of Mental Disorders* (DSM–IV; American Psychiatric Association, 1994), the diagnosis of Conduct Disorder (CD) is reached if the child shows at least 3 of the 15 symptoms within in the past 12 months, with at least 1 symptom evident within the past 6 months. The symptoms include: bullying others, initiating fights, using a weapon, being physically cruel to others or to animals, stealing while confronting a victim, firesetting, destroying property, breaking into others' property, stealing items of nontrivial value, staying out late, running away, lying, deliberate firesetting and truancy.

It is important to retain the distinction between conduct disorder as a general pattern of behavior and the diagnosis of CD. The general pattern of conduct disorder behavior has been studied extensively using varied populations (e.g. clinical referrals and delinquent samples) and defining criteria (Kazdin, 1995b). There is widespread agreement and evidence that a constellation of antisocial behaviors can be identified and has correlates related to child, parent and family functioning. Moreover, antisocial behaviors included in the constellation extend beyond those recognized in diagnosis (e.g. substance abuse, associating with delinquent peers).

The Scope of Dysfunction

If one were to consider "only" the symptoms of conduct disorder and the persistence of impairment, the challenge of identifying effective treatments would be great enough. However, the presenting characteristics of children and their families usually raise a number of other considerations that are central to treatment. Consider next the characteristics of children, parents, families and contexts that are associated with conduct disorder, as a backdrop for later comments on treatment.

Child characteristics. Children who meet criteria for CD are likely to meet criteria for other disorders as well. The coexistence of more than one disorder is referred to as comorbidity. In general, diagnoses involving disruptive or externalizing behaviors (CD, Oppositional Defiant Disorder [ODD], and Attention Deficit / Hyperactivity Disorder [ADHD]) often go together. In studies of community and clinic samples, a large percentage of youth with CD or ADHD (e.g. 45–70%) also meet criteria for the other disorder (e.g. Fergusson, Horwood & Lloyd, 1991; Offord, Boyle & Racine, 1991). The cooccurrence of CD and ODD is common as well. Among clinic-referred youth who meet criteria for CD, 84–96% also meet concurrent diagnostic criteria for ODD (see Hinshaw, Lahey & Hart, 1993).[1] CD is sometimes comorbid with anxiety disorders and depression (Hinshaw et al., 1993; Walker et al., 1991).

Several other associated features of CD are relevant to treatment. For example, children with conduct disorder are also likely to show academic deficiencies, as reflected in achievement level, grades, being left behind in school, early termination from school and deficiencies in specific skill areas such as reading. Youths with the disorder are likely to evince poor interpersonal relations, as reflected in diminished social skills in relation to peers and adults and higher levels of peer rejection. Conduct disorder youths also are likely to show a variety of cognitive and attributional processes. Deficits and distortions in cognitive problem-solving skills, attributions of hostile intent to others, and resentment and suspiciousness, illustrate a few cognitive features associated with conduct disorder.

Parent and family characteristics. Several parent and family characteristics are associated with conduct disorder (see Kazdin, 1995b; Robins, 1991; Rutter & Giller, 1983). Criminal behavior and alcoholism are two of the stronger and more consistently demonstrated parental characteristics. Parent disciplinary practices and attitudes, especially harsh, lax, erratic and inconsistent discipline practices, often characterize the parents. Dysfunctional relations are also evident, as reflected in less acceptance of their children, less warmth, affection and emotional support, and less attachment, compared to parents of nonreferred youth. Less supportive and more defensive communications among family members, less participation

---

[1] In DSM–IV, if the child meets criteria for CD, ODD is not diagnosed, because the former is likely to include many symptoms of the latter. Yet, invoking and evaluating the criteria for these diagnoses ignoring this consideration has been useful in understanding the relation and overlap of these diagnoses.

in activities as a family and more clear dominance of one family member are also evident. In addition, unhappy marital relations, interpersonal conflict and aggression characterize the parental relations of antisocial children. Poor parental supervision and monitoring of the child and knowledge of the child's whereabouts are also associated with conduct disorder. *Contextual conditions.* Conduct disorder is associated with a variety of untoward living conditions such as large family size, overcrowding, poor housing, and disadvantaged school settings (see Kazdin, 1995b). Many of the untoward conditions in which families live place stress on the parents or diminish their threshold for coping with everyday stressors. The net effect can be evident in parent–child interaction in which parents inadvertently engage in patterns that sustain or accelerate antisocial and aggressive interactions (e.g. Dumas & Wahler, 1983; Patterson, Capaldi & Bank, 1991).

Quite often the child's dysfunction is embedded in a larger context that cannot be neglected in conceptual views about the development, maintenance and course of conduct disorder nor in the actual delivery of treatment. For example, at our outpatient clinical service (Yale Child Conduct Clinic), it is likely that a family referred for treatment will experience a subset of these characteristics: financial hardship (unemployment, significant debt, bankruptcy), untoward living conditions (dangerous neighborhood, small living quarters), transportation obstacles (no car or car in frequent repair, state provided taxi service), psychiatric impairment of one of the parents, stress related to significant others (former spouses, boyfriends or girlfriends) and adversarial contact with an outside agency (schools, youth services, courts). Conduct disorder is conceived as a dysfunction of children and adolescents. The accumulated evidence regarding the symptom constellation, risk factors, and course over childhood, adolescence and adulthood attests to the heuristic value of focusing on individual children. At the same time, there is a child-parent-family-context gestalt that includes multiple and reciprocal influences that affect each participant (child and parent) and the systems in which they operate (family, school) (Kazdin, 1993). For treatment to be effective, it is likely that multiple domains will have to be addressed.

PROMISING TREATMENT APPROACHES

Overview: Criteria for Identifying Promising Treatments

Many different treatments have been applied to conduct-disordered youths, including psychotherapy, pharmacotherapy, psychosurgery, home, school and community-based programs, residential and hospital treatment, and social services (see Brandt & Zlotnick, 1988; Dumas, 1989; Kazdin, 1985; United States Congress, 1991). Of the over 230 documented psychotherapies available for children and adolescents (Kazdin, 1988), the vast majority have not been studied. Among those that have, none has been shown to controvert conduct disorder and its long-term course. Many treatments might seem conceptually justified as interventions for conduct disorder. Conduct disorder is a dysfunction with pervasive features so that one can point to virtually any domain (e.g. psychodynamics, family interaction patterns, cognitive deficiencies) and find aberrations, deficits and deficiencies.

In our own work, we have relied on several criteria (please see Table 1) to identify and to select promising treatments among the array of available interventions. The initial

TABLE 1
Criteria for Identifying Promising Treatments

1. CONCEPTUALIZATION
   Theoretical statement relating the mechanism(s) (e.g. intrapsychic, intrafamilial) to clinical dysfunction
2. BASIC RESEARCH
   Evidence showing that the mechanism can be assessed and relates to dysfunction, independently of treatment outcome studies
3. PRELIMINARY OUTCOME EVIDENCE
   Evidence in analogue or clinical research showing that the approach leads to change on clinically relevant measures
4. PROCESS–OUTCOME CONNECTION
   Evidence in outcome studies showing a relationship between the change in processes alleged to be operative and clinical outcome

criterion is that the treatment should have some theoretical rationale that notes how the dysfunction, in this case conduct disorder, comes about and then how treatment redresses the dysfunction. Specification of the mechanisms leading to conduct disorder and leading to therapeutic change are required for this initial criterion.

The second criterion considers whether there is any basic research to support the conceptualization. Basic research in this context refers to studies that examine conduct problems and factors that lead to their onset, maintenance, exacerbation, amelioration or attenuation. An example would be studies of the family that demonstrate specific interaction patterns among parents and children that exacerbate aggression within the home (Patterson, Reid & Dishion, 1992). Such research would advance considerably the conceptual view that posited the significance of these patterns and provided a warrant for treatments that are aimed at these interaction patterns.

The third criterion is whether there is any outcome evidence that the treatment can effect change. In canvassing the literature, we tend to be very lenient for invoking this criterion; we are interested in any demonstration (e.g. so-called open trials, studies with mildly disturbed cases). Obviously, randomized controlled clinical trials are preferred. However, the vast majority of treatments available for children and adolescents have never been tested in any controlled or uncontrolled trial (Kazdin, 1988). Understandably, we are encouraged if there is a crumb of data showing that someone changed somewhere after exposure to treatment.

Finally, evidence from an outcome study that shows a relation between these processes hypothesized to be critical to therapeutic change and actual change would be very persuasive. Assessment of processes might be reflected in cognitions, family interaction or core conflicts and defenses. Therapeutic change would be shown to covary with the extent to which these processes were altered in treatment. This latter criterion is very demanding indeed and perhaps is better conceived as a goal toward which we strive rather than a point of departure for identifying promising treatments.

No single treatment among those available adequately traverses all of these criteria. Yet, a number of promising treatments have been identified for conduct disorder. Four treatment approaches with evidence on their behalf are illustrated next. In highlighting the approaches, the purpose is not to convey that only four promising treatments exist. However, these four are clearly among the most well developed in relation to the criteria highlighted here and the number of controlled clinical trials.[2]

Cognitive Problem-Solving Skills Training

Background and underlying rationale. Cognitive processes refer to a broad class of constructs that pertain to how the individual perceives, codes and experiences the world. Individuals who engage in conduct disorder behaviors, particularly aggression, have been found to show distortions and deficiencies in various cognitive processes. These deficiencies are not merely reflections of intellectual functioning. Although selected processes (recall, information processing) are related to intellectual functioning, their impact has been delineated separately and shown to contribute to behavioral adjustment and social behavior.

A variety of cognitive processes have been studied, such as generating alternative solutions to interpersonal problems (e.g. different ways of handling social situations), identifying the means to obtain particular ends (e.g. making friends) or consequences of one's actions (e.g. what could happen after a particular behavior); making attributions to others of the motivation of their actions; perceiving how others feel; expectations of the effects of one's own actions and others (see Shirk, 1988; Spivack & Shure, 1982). Deficits and distortion among these processes relate to teacher ratings of disruptive behavior, peer evaluations and direct assessment of overt behavior (e.g. Lochman & Dodge, 1994; Rubin, Bream & Rose-Krasnor, 1991).

As an illustration, aggression is not merely triggered by environmental events, but rather through the way in which these events are perceived and processed. The processing refers to the child's appraisals of the situation, anticipated reactions of others and self-statements in response to particular events. For example, attribution of intent to others represents a salient cognitive disposition critically important to understanding aggressive behavior. Aggressive youths tend to attribute hostile intent to others, especially in social situations where the cues of actual intent are ambiguous (see Crick & Dodge, 1994). Understandably, when situations are initially perceived as hostile, youths are more likely to react aggressively.

Although many studies have shown that conduct-disordered youths experience various cognitive distortions and deficiencies, fundamental questions remain to be resolved. Among these questions are the specificity of cognitive deficits among diagnostic groups and youths of different ages, whether some of the processes are more central than others, and how these processes unfold developmentally. Nevertheless, research on cognitive processes among aggressive children has served as an heuristic base for conceptualizing treatment and for developing specific treatment strategies.

Characteristics of treatment. Problem-solving skills training (PSST) consists of developing interpersonal cognitive problem-solving skills. Although many variations of PSST have been applied to conduct problem children, several characteristics are usually shared. First, the emphasis is on how children approach situations, i.e. the thought processes in which

---

[2] The rationale, empirical underpinnings, outcome research and treatment procedures cannot be fully elaborated for each of the techniques. References will be made to reviews of the evidence and to treatment manuals that elaborate each of the treatments.

the child engages to guide responses to interpersonal situations. The children are taught to engage in a step-by-step approach to solve interpersonal problems. They make statements to themselves that direct attention to certain aspects of the problem or tasks that lead to effective solutions. Second, behaviors that are selected (solutions) to the interpersonal situations are important as well. Prosocial behaviors are fostered (through modeling and direct reinforcement) as part of the problem-solving process. Third, treatment utilizes structured tasks involving games, academic activities and stories. Over the course of treatment, the cognitive problem-solving skills are increasingly applied to real-life situations. Fourth, therapists usually play an active role in treatment. They model the cognitive processes by making verbal self-statements, apply the sequence of statements to particular problems, provide cues to prompt use of the skills and deliver feedback and praise to develop correct use of the skills. Finally, treatment usually combines several different procedures including modeling and practice, role-playing, and reinforcement and mild punishment (loss of points or tokens). These are deployed in systematic ways to develop increasingly complex response repertoires of the child.

Overview of the evidence. Several outcome studies have been completed with impulsive, aggressive and conduct-disordered children and adolescents (see Baer & Nietzel, 1991; Durlak, Furhman & Lampman, 1991 for reviews). Cognitively based treatments have significantly reduced aggressive and antisocial behavior at home, at school and in the community. At follow-up, these gains have been evident up to one year later. Many early studies in the field (e.g. 1970s-80s) focused on impulsive children and nonpatient samples. Since that time, several studies have shown treatment effects with inpatient and outpatient cases (see Kazdin, 1993; Kendall, 1991; Pepler & Rubin, 1991).

There is only sparse evidence that addresses the child, parent, family, contextual or treatment factors that influence treatment outcome. Some evidence suggests that older children profit more from treatment than do younger children, perhaps due to their cognitive development (Durlak et al., 1991). However, the basis for differential responsiveness to treatment as a function of age has not been well tested. Conduct-disordered children who show comorbid diagnoses, academic delays and dysfunction and lower reading achievement, and who come from families with high levels of impairment (parent psychopathology, stress and family dysfunction) respond less well to treatment than youths with less dysfunction in these domains (Kazdin, 1995a; Kazdin & Crowley, in press). However, these child, parent and family characteristics may influence the effectiveness of several different treatments for conduct-disordered youths rather than PSST in particular. Much further work is needed to evaluate factors that contribute to responsiveness to treatment.

Overall evaluation. There are features of PSST that make it an extremely promising approach. Perhaps most importantly, several controlled outcome studies with clinic samples have shown that cognitively based treatment leads to therapeutic change. Second, basic research in developmental psychology continues to elaborate the relation of maladaptive cognitive processes among children and adolescents and conduct problems that serve as underpinnings of treatment (Crick & Dodge, 1994; Shirk, 1988). Third and on a more practical level, many versions of treatment are available in manual form (e.g. Feindler & Ecton, 1986; Finch, Nelson & Ott, 1993; Shure, 1992). Consequently, the treatment can be evaluated in research and explored further in clinical practice.

Fundamental questions about treatment remain. To begin, the role of cognitive processes in clinical dysfunction and treatment warrant further evaluation. Evidence is not entirely clear, showing that a specific pattern of cognitive processes characterizes youths with conduct problems rather than adjustment problems more generally. Also, although evidence has shown that cognitive processes change with treatment, evidence has not established that change in these processes is correlated with improvements in treatment outcome. This means that the basis for therapeutic change has yet to be established. Also, characteristics of children and their families and parameters of treatment that may influence outcome have not been carefully explored in relation to treatment outcome. Clearly, central questions about treatment and its effects remain to be resolved. Even so, PSST is highly promising because treatment effects have been replicated in several controlled studies with conduct-disordered youth.

Parent Management Training

Background and underlying rationale. Parent management training (PMT) refers to procedures in which parents are trained to alter their child's behavior in the home. The parents meet with a therapist or trainer who teaches them to use specific procedures to alter interactions with their child, to promote prosocial behavior and to decrease deviant behavior. Training is based on the general view that conduct problem behavior is inadvertently developed and sustained in the home by maladaptive parent–child interactions. There are multiple facets of parent–child interaction that promote aggressive and antisocial behavior. These patterns include directly reinforcing deviant behavior, frequently and ineffectively using commands and harsh punishment, and failing to attend to appropriate behavior (Patterson, 1982; Patterson et al., 1992).

It would be misleading to imply that the parent generates and is solely responsible for the child–parent sequences of interactions. Influences are bidirectional, so that the child influences the parent as well (see Bell & Harper, 1977; Lytton, 1990). Indeed, in some cases the children engage in deviant behavior to help prompt the interaction sequences. For example, when parents behave inconsistently and unpredictably (e.g. not attending to the child in the usual ways), the child may engage in some deviant behavior (e.g. whining, throwing some object). The effect is to cause the parent to respond in more predictable ways (see Wahler & Dumas, 1986). Essentially, inconsistent and unpredictable parent behavior is an aversive condition for the child; the child's deviant behavior is negatively reinforced by terminating this condition. However, the result is also to increase parent punishment of the child.

Among the many interaction patterns, those involving coercion have received the greatest attention (Patterson et al., 1992). Coercion refers to deviant behavior on the part of one person (e.g. the child) that is rewarded by another person (e.g. the parent). Aggressive children are inadvertently rewarded for their aggressive interactions and their escalation of coercive behaviors, as part of the discipline practices that sustain aggressive behavior. The critical role of parent–child discipline practices has been supported by correlational research, relating specific discipline practices to child antisocial behavior, and by experimental research, showing that directly altering these practices reduces antisocial child behavior (see Dishion, Patterson & Kavanagh, 1992).

The general purpose of PMT is to alter the pattern of interchanges between parent and child so that prosocial, rather than coercive, behavior is directly reinforced and supported within the family. This requires developing several different parenting behaviors, such as establishing the rules for the child to follow, providing positive reinforcement for appropriate behavior, delivering mild forms of punishment to suppress behavior, negotiating compromises and other procedures. These parenting behaviors are systematically and progressively developed within the sessions in which the therapist shapes (develops through successive approximations) parenting skills. The programs that parents eventually implement in the home also serve as the basis for the focus of the sessions in which the procedures are modified and refined.

Characteristics of treatment. Although many variations of PMT exist, several common characteristics can be identified. First, treatment is conducted primarily with the parent(s), who implement several procedures in the home. The parents meet with a therapist who teaches them to use specific procedures to alter interactions with their child, to promote prosocial behavior and to decrease deviant behavior. There is usually little direct intervention of the therapist with the child. With young children, the child may be brought into the session to help train both parent and child how to interact and especially to show the parent precisely how to deliver prompts (antecedents) and consequences (reinforcement, time out from reinforcement). Older youths may participate to negotiate and to develop behavior-change programs in the home. Second, parents are trained to identify, define and observe problem behaviors in new ways. Careful specification of the problem is essential for the delivery of reinforcing or punishing consequences and for evaluating if the program is achieving the desired goals. Third, the treatment sessions cover social learning principles and the procedures that follow from them including: positive reinforcement (e.g. the use of social praise and tokens or points for prosocial behavior), mild punishment (e.g. use of time out from reinforcement, loss of privileges), negotiation, and contingency contracting. Fourth, the sessions provide opportunities for parents to see how the techniques are implemented, to practise using the techniques, and to review the behavior-change programs in the home. The immediate goal of the program is to develop specific skills in the parents. As the parents become more proficient, the program can address the child's most severely problematic behaviors and encompass other problem areas (e.g. school behavior). Over the course of treatment, more complex repertoires are developed, both in the parents and the child. Finally, child functioning at school is usually incorporated into the program. Parent-managed reinforcement programs for child deportment and performance at school, completion of homework, activities in the playground and so on are often part of the behavior-change programs. If available, teachers can play an important role in monitoring or providing consequences for behaviors at school.

Overview of the evidence. PMT is one of the most well-researched therapy techniques for the treatment of conduct-disordered youth. Scores of outcome studies have been completed with youths varying in age and degree of severity of dysfunction (e.g. oppositional, conduct disorder, delinquent youth) (see Kazdin, 1993; Miller & Prinz, 1990; Patterson, Dishion & Chamberlain, 1993). Treatment effects have been evident in marked improvements in child behavior on a wide range of measures including parent and teacher reports of deviant behavior, direct observation of behavior at home and at school and institutional (e.g. school, police) records. The effects of treatment have also been shown to bring problematic behaviors of treated children within normative levels of their peers who are functioning adequately in the community. Follow-up assessment has shown that the gains are often maintained 1–3 years after treatment. Longer follow-up assessment rarely takes place, although one program reported maintenance of gains 10–14 years later (Forehand & Long, 1988; Long, Forehand, Wierson & Morgan, 1994).

The impact of PMT is relatively broad. The effects of treatment are evident for child behaviors that have not been focused on directly as part of training. Also, siblings of children referred for treatment improve, even though they are not directly focused on in treatment. This is an important effect because siblings of conduct-disordered youths are at risk for severe antisocial behavior. In addition, maternal psychopathology, particularly depression, has been shown to decrease systematically following PMT (see Kazdin, 1985). These changes suggest that PMT alters multiple aspects of dysfunctional families.

Several characteristics of the treatment contribute to outcome. Duration of treatment appears to influence outcome. Brief and time-limited treatments (e.g. <10 hours) are less likely to show benefits with clinical populations. More dramatic and durable effects have been achieved with protracted or time-unlimited programs extending up to 50 or 60 hours of treatment (see Kazdin, 1985). Second, specific training components, such as providing parents with in-depth knowledge of social learning principles and including time out from reinforcement in the behavior-change program (in addition to reinforcement) in the home, enhance treatment effects. Third, some evidence suggests that therapist training and skill are associated with the magnitude and durability of therapeutic changes, although this has yet to be carefully tested. Fourth, families characterized by many risk factors associated with childhood dysfunction (e.g. socioeconomic disadvantage, marital discord, parent psychopathology, poor social support) tend to show fewer gains in treatment than families without these characteristics and to maintain the gains less well (e.g. Dadds & McHugh, 1992; Dumas & Wahler, 1983; Webster-Stratton, 1985). Some efforts to address parent and family dysfunction during PMT have led to improved effects of treatment outcome for the child in some studies (e.g. Dadds, Schwartz & Sanders, 1987; Griest et al., 1982) but not in others (Webster-Stratton, 1994). Much more work is needed on the matter, given the prominent role of parent and family dysfunction among many youths referred for treatment.

One promising line of work has focused on implementation of PMT in community, rather than clinic, settings. The net effect is to bring treatment to those persons least likely to come to or remain in treatment. In one study, for example, when PMT was delivered in small parent groups in the community, the effectiveness surpassed what was achieved with clinic-based PMT and was considerably more cost effective (Cunningham, Bremner & Boyle, 1995).

Conceptual development of processes underlying parent–child interaction and conduct disorder continues (e.g. Patterson et al., 1992). Also, recent research on processes in treatment represents a related and important advance. A series of studies on therapist–parent interaction within PMT sessions has identified factors that contribute to parent resistance (e.g. parent saying, “I can’t,” “I won’t”). The significance of this work is in showing that parent reactions in therapy relate to their discipline practices at home, that changes in resistance during therapy predicts change in parent behavior and that specific therapist ploys (e.g. reframing, confronting) can help overcome or contribute to resistance (Patterson & Chamberlain, 1994). This line of work advances our understanding of PMT greatly by relating in-session interactions of the therapist and parent to child functioning and treatment outcome.

Overall evaluation. Perhaps the most important point to underscore is that no other technique for conduct disorder has probably been studied as often or as well in controlled trials as has PMT. The outcome evidence makes PMT one of the most promising treatments. The evidence is bolstered by related lines of work. First, the study of family interaction processes that contribute to antisocial behavior in the home and evidence that changing these processes alters child behavior provide a strong empirical base for treatment. Second, the procedures and practices that are used in PMT (e.g. various forms of reinforcement and punishment practices) have been widely and effectively applied outside the context of conduct disorder. For example, the procedures have been applied with parents of children with autism, language delays, developmental disabilities, medical disorders for which compliance with special treatment regimens is required and with parents who physically abuse or neglect their children (see Kazdin, 1994b). Third, a great deal is known about the procedures and the parameters that influence the reinforcement and punishment practices that form the core of PMT. Consequently, very concrete recommendations can be provided to change behavior and to alter programs when behavior change has not occurred.

A major advantage is the availability of treatment manuals and training materials for parents and professional therapists (e.g. Forehand & McMahon, 1981; Sanders & Dadds, 1993). Also noteworthy is the development of self-administered videotapes of treatment. In a programmatic series of studies with young conduct problem children (3–8 years), Webster-Stratton and her colleagues have developed and evaluated videotaped materials to present PMT to parents; treatment can be self-administered in individual or group format supplemented with discussion (e.g. Webster-Stratton, 1994; Webster-Stratton, Hollinsworth & Kolpacoff, 1989). Controlled studies have shown clinically significant changes at post-treatment and follow-up assessments with variations of videotaped treatment. The potential for extension of PMT with readily available and empirically tested videotapes presents a unique feature in child treatment.

Several limitations of PMT can be identified as well. First, some families may not respond to treatment. PMT makes several demands on the parents, such as mastering educational materials that convey major principles underlying the program, systematically observing deviant child behavior and implementing specific procedures at home, attending weekly sessions and responding to frequent telephone contacts made by the therapist. For some families, the demands may be too great to continue in treatment. Interestingly, within the approach several procedures (e.g. shaping parent behavior through reinforcement) provide guidelines for developing parent compliance and the desired response repertoire in relation to their children.

Second, perhaps the greatest limitation or obstacle in using PMT is that there are few training opportunities for professionals to learn the approach. Training programs in child psychiatry, clinical psychology, and social work are unlikely to provide exposure to the technique, much less opportunities for formal training. PMT requires mastery of social learning principles and multiple procedures that derive from them (Cooper, Heron & Heward, 1987;

Kazdin, 1994a). For example, the administration of reinforcement by the parent in the home (to alter child behavior) and by the therapist in the session (to change parent behavior) requires more than passing familiarity with the principle and the parametric variations that dictate its effectiveness (e.g. need to administer reinforcement contingently, immediately, frequently, to use varied and high quality reinforcers; prompting, shaping). The requisite skills in administering these within the treatment sessions can be readily trained but they are not trivial.

PMT has been applied primarily to parents of preadolescents. Although treatment has been effective with delinquent adolescents (Bank, Marlowe, Reid, Patterson & Weinrott, 1991) and younger adolescents with conduct problems who have not yet been referred for treatment (Dishion & Andrews, 1995), some evidence suggests that treatment is more effective with preadolescent youths (see Dishion & Patterson, 1992). Parents of adolescents may less readily change their discipline practices and also have higher rates of dropping out of treatment. The importance and special role of peers in adolescence and greater time that adolescents spend outside the home suggest that the principles and procedures may need to be applied in novel ways. At this point, few PMT programs have been developed specifically for adolescents, and so conclusions about the effects for youths of different ages must be tempered. On balance, PMT is one of the most promising treatment modalities. No other intervention for conduct disorder has been investigated as thoroughly as PMT.

Functional Family Therapy

Background and underlying rationale. Functional family therapy (FFT) reflects an integrative approach to treatment that has relied on systems, behavioral and cognitive views of dysfunction (Alexander, Holtzworth-Munroe & Jameson, 1994; Alexander & Parsons, 1982). Clinical problems are conceptualized from the standpoint of the functions they serve in the family as a system, as well as for individual family members. The assumption is made that problem behavior evident in the child is the only way some interpersonal functions (e.g. intimacy, distancing, support) can be met among family members. Maladaptive processes within the family are considered to preclude a more direct means of fulfilling these functions. The goal of treatment is to alter interaction and communication patterns in such a way as to foster more adaptive functioning. Treatment is also based on learning theory and focuses on specific stimuli and responses that can be used to produce change. Social-learning concepts and procedures, such as identifying specific behaviors for change and reinforcing new adaptive ways of responding, and empirically evaluating and monitoring change, are included in this perspective. Cognitive processes refer to the attributions, attitudes, assumptions, expectations and emotions of the family. Family members may begin treatment with attributions that focus on blaming others or themselves. New perspectives may be needed to help serve as the basis for developing new ways of behaving.

The underlying rationale emphasizes a family systems approach. Specific treatment strategies draw on findings that underlie PMT in relation to maladaptive and coercive parent–child interactions, discussed previously. FFT views interaction patterns from a broader systems view that also focuses on communication patterns and their meaning. As an illustration of salient constructs, research underlying FFT has found that families of delinquents show higher rates of defensiveness in their communications, both in parent–child and parent–parent interactions, blaming and negative attributions, and also lower rates of mutual support compared to families of nondelinquents (see Alexander & Parsons, 1982). Improving these communication and support functions is a goal of treatment.

Characteristics of treatment. FFT requires that the family see the clinical problem from the relational function it serves within the family. The therapist points out interdependencies and contingencies between family members in their day-to-day functioning and with specific reference to the problem that has served as the basis for seeking treatment. Once the family sees alternative ways of viewing the problem, the incentive for interacting more constructively is increased.

The main goals of treatment are to increase reciprocity and positive reinforcement among family members, to establish clear communication, to help specify behaviors that family members desire from each other, to negotiate constructively and to help identify solutions to interpersonal problems. In therapy, family members identify behaviors they would like others to perform. Responses are incorporated into a reinforcement system in the home to promote adaptive behavior in exchange for privileges. However, the primary focus is within the treatment sessions, where family communication patterns are altered directly. During the sessions, the therapist provides social reinforcement (verbal and nonverbal praise) for communications that suggest solutions to problems, clarify problems or offer feedback.

Overview of the evidence. Relatively few outcome studies have evaluated FFT (see Alexander et al., 1994). However, the available studies have focused on difficult to treat populations (e.g. adjudicated delinquent adolescents, multiple offender delinquents) and have produced relatively clear effects. In controlled studies, FFT has led to greater change than other treatment techniques (e.g. client-centered family groups, psychodynamically oriented family therapy) and various control conditions (e.g. group discussion and expression of feeling, no-treatment control groups). Treatment outcome is reflected in improved family communication and interactions and lower rates of referral to and contact of youth with the courts. Moreover, gains have been evident in separate studies up to $2\frac{1}{2}$ years after treatment.

Research has examined processes in therapy to identify in-session behaviors of the therapist and how these influence responsiveness among family members (Alexander, Barton, Schiavo & Parsons, 1976; Newberry, Alexander & Turner, 1991). For example, providing support and structure and reframing (recasting the attributions and bases of a problem) can influence family member responsiveness and blaming of others. The relations among such variables are complex insofar as the impact of various type of statements (e.g. supportive) can vary as a function of gender of the therapist and family member. Evidence of change in processes proposed to be critical to FFT (e.g. improved communication in treatment, more spontaneous discussion) supports the conceptual view of treatment.

Overall evaluation. Several noteworthy points can be made about FFT. First, the outcome studies indicate that FFT can alter conduct problems among delinquent youth. Several studies have produced consistent effects. Second, the evaluation of processes that contribute to family member responsiveness within the sessions as well as to outcome represents a line of work rarely seen among treatment techniques for children and adolescents. Some of this process work has extended to laboratory (analog) studies to examine more precisely how specific types of therapist statements (e.g. reframing) can reduce blaming among group members (e.g. Morris, Alexander & Turner, 1991). Third, a treatment manual has been provided (Alexander & Parsons, 1982) to facilitate further evaluation and extension of treatment. Further work extending FFT to children and to clinic populations would be of interest in addition to the current work with delinquent adolescents. Also, further work on child, parent and family characteristics that moderate outcome would be a next logical step in the existing research program.

Multisystemic Therapy

Background and underlying rationale. Multisystemic therapy (MST) is a family-systems based approach to treatment (Henggeler & Borduin, 1990). Family approaches maintain that clinical problems of the child emerge within the context of the family and focus on treatment at that level. MST expands on that view by considering the family as one, albeit a very important, system. The child is embedded in a number of systems including the family (immediate and extended family members), peers, schools, neighborhood and so on. For example, within the context of the family, some tacit alliance between one parent and the child may contribute to disagreement and conflict over discipline in relation to the child. Treatment may be required to address the alliance and sources of conflict in an effort to alter child behavior. Also, child functioning at school may involve limited and poor peer relations; treatment may address these areas as well. Finally, the systems approach entails a focus on the individual's own behavior insofar as it affects others. Individual treatment of the child or parents may be included in treatment.

Because multiple influences are entailed by the focus of the treatment, many different treatment techniques are used. Thus, MST can be viewed as a package of interventions that are deployed with children and their families. Treatment procedures are used on an "as needed" basis directed toward addressing individual, family and system issues that may contribute to problem behavior. The conceptual view, focusing on multiple systems and their impact on the individual, serves as a basis for selecting multiple and quite different treatment procedures.

Characteristics of treatment. Central to MST is a family-based treatment approach. Several family therapy techniques (e.g. joining, reframing, enactment, paradox and assigning specific tasks) are used to identify problems, increase communication, build cohesion, and alter how family members interact. The goals of treatment are to help the parents develop behaviors of the adolescent, to overcome marital difficulties that impede the parents' ability to function as parents, to eliminate negative interactions between parent and adolescent and to develop or build cohesion and emotional warmth among family members.

MST draws on many other techniques as needed to address problems at the level of individual, family and extrafamily. As prominent examples, PSST, PMT, and marital therapy are used in treatment to alter the response repertoire of the adolescent, parent–child interactions at home and marital communication, respectively. In some cases, treatment consists of helping the parents address a significant domain through practical advice and guidance (e.g. involving the adolescent in prosocial peer activities at school, restricting specific activities with a deviant peer group). Although MST includes distinct techniques of other approaches, it is not a mere amalgamation of them. The focus of treatment is on interrelated systems and how they affect each other. Domains may be addressed in treatment (e.g. parent unemployment) because they raise issues for one or more systems (e.g. parent stress, increase in alcohol consumption) and affect how the child is functioning (e.g. marital conflict, child discipline practices).

Overview of the evidence. Several outcome studies have evaluated MST, primarily with delinquent youths with arrest and incarceration histories including violent crime (e.g. manslaughter, aggravated assault with intent to kill). Thus, this is a group of extremely antisocial and aggressive youth. Results have shown MST to be superior in reducing delinquency, emotional and behavioral problems and in improving family functioning in comparison to other procedures including "usual services" provided to such youths (e.g. probation, court-ordered activities that are monitored such as school attendance), individual counseling and community-based eclectic treatment (e.g. Borduin et al., 1995; Henggeler et al., 1986; Henggeler, Melton, & Smith, 1992). Follow-up studies up to 2, 4 and 5 years later with separate samples have shown that MST youths have lower arrest rates than youths who receive other services (see Henggeler, 1994).

Research has also shown that treatment affects critical processes proposed to contribute to deviant behavior (Mann, Borduin, Henggeler, & Blaske, 1990). Specifically, parents and teenage youths show a reduction in coalitions (e.g. less verbal activity, conflict and hostility) and increases in support, and the parents show increases in verbal communication and decreases in conflict. Moreover, decreases in adolescent symptoms are positively correlated with increases in supportiveness and decreases in conflict between the mother and father. This work provides an important link between theoretical underpinnings of treatment and outcome effects.

Overall evaluation. Several outcome studies are available for MST and they are consistent in showing that treatment leads to change in adolescents and that the changes are sustained. A strength of the studies is that many of the youths who are treated are severely impaired (delinquent adolescents with a history of arrest). Another strength is the conceptualization of conduct problems at multiple levels, namely, as dysfunction in relation to the individual, family and extrafamilial systems and the transactions among these. In fact, youths with conduct disorder experience dysfunction at multiple levels including individual repertoires, family interactions and extrafamilial systems (e.g. peers, schools, employment among later adolescents). MST begins with the view that may different domains are likely to be relevant; they need to be evaluated and then addressed as needed in treatment.

A challenge of the approach is deciding what treatments to use in a given case, among the many interventions encompassed by MST. Guidelines are available to direct the therapist, although they are somewhat general (e.g. focus on developing positive sequences of behaviors between systems such as parent and adolescent, evaluate the interventions during treatment so that changes can be made; see Henggeler, 1994). Providing interventions as needed is very difficult without a consistent way to assess what is needed, given inherent limits of decision making and perception, even among trained professionals. Related to this, the administration of MST is demanding in light of the need to provide several different interventions in a high-quality fashion. Individual treatments (e.g. PSST, PMT) alone are difficult to provide; multiple combinations invite problems related to providing treatments of high quality, strength and integrity. Yet there have been replications of MST beyond the original research program, indicating that treatment can be extended across therapists and settings (Henggeler, Schoenwald & Pickrel, 1995).

On balance, MST is quite promising given the quality of evidence and consistency in the effects that have been produced. The promise stems from a conceptual approach that examines multiple domains (systems) and their contribution to dysfunction, evidence on processes in therapy and their relation to outcome and the outcome studies themselves. The outcome studies have extended to youths with different types of problems (e.g. sexual offenses, drug use) and to parents who engage in physical abuse or neglect (e.g. Borduin, Henggeler, Blaske & Stein, 1990; Brunk, Henggeler & Whelan, 1987). Thus, the model of providing treatment may have broad applicability across problem domains among seriously disturbed children. In passing, it may be worth noting that other literatures are relevant to MST. Some of the techniques included in treatment are variations of PSST and PMT, already discussed, and hence have evidence on their own behalf as effective interventions.

Limitations of Promising Treatments

Each of the treatments just discussed has randomized, controlled trials on its behalf, includes replications of treatment effects in multiple studies, focuses on youths whose aggressive and antisocial behavior have led to impairment and referral to social services (e.g. clinics, hospitals, courts) and has assessed outcome over the course of follow-up, at least up to a year, but often longer. Even though these treatments have made remarkable gains, they also bear limitations worth highlighting.

Magnitude of therapeutic change. Promising treatments have achieved change, but is the change enough to make a difference in the lives of the youths who are treated? *Clinical significance* refers to the practical value or importance of the effect of an intervention, that is, whether it makes any "real" difference to the patients or to others with whom they interact (see Kazdin, 1992). Clinical significance is important because it is quite possible for treatment effects to be statistically significant, but not to have impact on most or any of the cases in a way that improves their functioning or adjustment in daily life.

There are several ways to evaluate clinical significance. As an example, one way is to consider the extent to which youths function at normative levels at the end of treatment (i.e. compared to same age and sex peers who are functioning well). This is particularly useful as a criterion in relation to children and adolescents because base rates of emotional and behavioral problems can vary greatly as a function of age. Promising treatments occasionally have shown that treatment returns individuals to normative levels in relation to behavioral problems and prosocial functioning at home and at school (see Kazdin, 1995b). Yet, the majority of studies, whether of promising or less well-evaluated treatments, have not examined whether youths have changed in ways that place them within normative range of functioning or have made gains that would reflect clinically significant changes (Kazdin, Bass, Ayers & Rodgers, 1990a).

Although the goal of treatment is to effect clinically significant change, other less dramatic goals are not trivial. For many conduct-disordered youths, symptoms may escalate, comorbid diagnoses (e.g. substance abuse, depression) may emerge and family dysfunction may increase. Also, such youths are at risk for teen marriage, dropping out of school and running away. If treatment were to achieve stability in symptoms and family life and prevent or delimit future dysfunction, that would be a significant achievement. The reason evaluation is so critical to the therapeutic enterprise is to identify whether treatment makes a difference because "making a difference" can have many meanings that are important in the treatment of conduct disorder.

Maintenance of change. Promising treatments have included follow-up assessment, usually up to a year after treatment. Yet, conduct disorder has a poor long-term prognosis, so it is especially important to identify whether treatment has enduring effects. Also, in evaluating the relative merit of different treatments, follow-up data play a critical role. When two (or more) treatments are compared, the treatment that is more (or most) effective immediately after treatment is not always the one that proves to be the most effective treatment in the long run (Kazdin, 1988). Consequently, the conclusions about treatment may be very different depending on the timing of outcome assessment. Apart from conclusions about treatment, follow-up may provide important information that permits differentiation among youths. Over time, youths who maintain the benefits of treatment may differ in important ways from those who do not. Understanding who responds and who responds more or less well to a particular treatment can be very helpful in understanding, treating and preventing conduct disorder.

The study of long-term effects of treatment is difficult in general, but the usual problems are exacerbated by focusing on conduct disorder. Among clinic samples, families of conduct-disordered youths have high rates of dropping out during treatment and during the follow-up assessment period, due in part to the many parent and family factors (e.g. socioeconomic disadvantage, stress) often associated with the problem (Kazdin, 1996b). As the sample size decreases over time, conclusions about the impact of treatment become increasingly difficult to draw. Nevertheless, evaluation of the long-term effects of treatment remains a high priority for research.

Limited assessment of outcome domains. In the majority of child therapy studies, child symptoms are the exclusive focus fo outcome assessment (Kazdin et al., 1990a). Other domains such as prosocial behavior and academic functioning are neglected, even though they relate to concurrent and long-term adjustment (e.g. Asher & Coie, 1990). Perhaps the greatest single deficit in the evaluation of treatment is absence of attention to impairment. Impairment reflects the extent to which the individual's functioning in everyday life is impeded. Impairment can be distinguished from symptoms insofar as individuals with similar levels of symptoms (e.g. scores), diagnoses and patterns of comorbidity are likely to be distinguishable based on their ability to function adaptively. School and academic functioning, peer relations, participation in activities and health are some of the areas included in impairment. In the context of treatment, an intervention may significantly reduce symptoms. Yet, is there any change or reduction in impairment? The impact of treatment on impairment is arguably as important as the impact on the conduct disorder symptoms.

Beyond child functioning, parent and family functioning may also be relevant. Parents and family members of conduct-disordered youths often experience dysfunction (e.g. psychiatric impairment, marital conflict). Also, the problem behaviors of the child are often part of complex, dynamic and reciprocal influences that affect all relations in the home. Consequently, parent and family functioning and the quality of life for family members are relevant outcomes and may be appropriate goals for treatment.

In general, there are many outcomes that are of interest in evaluating treatment. From existing research we already know that the conclusions reached about a given treatment can vary depending on the outcome criterion. Within a given study, one set of measures (e.g. child functioning) may show no differences between two treatments but another measure (e.g. family functioning) may show that one treatment is clearly better than the other (e.g. Kazdin, Bass, Siegel & Thomas, 1989; Kazdin, Siegel & Bass, 1992; Szapocznik et al., 1989). Thus, in examining different outcomes of interest, we must be prepared for different conclusions that these outcomes may yield.

General Comments

In light of these comments, clearly even the most promising treatments have several limitations. Yet it is critical to place these in perspective. The most commonly used treatments in clinical practice consist of "traditional" approaches including psychodynamic, relationship, play and family therapies (other than those mentioned earlier) (Kazdin, Siegel & Bass, 1990b). These treatments have rarely been tested in controlled outcome studies showing that they achieve therapeutic change in referred (or nonreferred) samples of youth with conduct problems. Many forms of behavior therapy have a rather extensive literature showing that various techniques (e.g. reinforcement programs, social skills training) can alter aggressive and other antisocial behaviors (Kazdin, 1985; McMahon & Wells, 1989). Yet the focus has tended to be on isolated behaviors, rather than a constellation of symptoms. Also, durable changes among clinical samples have rarely been shown.

Pharmacotherapy represents a line of work of some interest. For one reason, stimulant medication (e.g. methylphenidate), frequently used with children diagnosed with ADHD, has some impact on aggressive and other antisocial behaviors (see Hinshaw, 1994). This is interesting in part because such children often have a comorbid diagnosis of Conduct Disorder. Still no strong evidence exists that stimulant medication can alter the constellation of symptoms (e.g. fighting, stealing) associated with conduct disorder. A review of various medications for aggression in children and adolescents has raised possible leads, but the bulk of research consists of uncontrolled studies (see Campbell & Cueva, 1995; Stewart, Myers, Burket & Lyles, 1990). Controlled studies (e.g. random assignment, placebo-controls) have shown antiaggressive effects with some medications (e.g. lithium; Campbell et al., 1995) but not others (e.g. carbamazepine; Cueva et al., 1996). Reliable psychopharmacological treatments for aggression, leaving aside the constellation of conduct disorder (e.g. firesetting, stealing, and so on), remain to be developed.

There is a genre of interventions that are worth mentioning but are even less well evaluated than many of the psychotherapies and pharmacotherapies. Occasionally, interventions are advocated and implemented, such as sending conduct-disordered youths to a camp in the country where they learn how to "rough it," or how to take care of horses or to experience military (e.g. basic training) regimens. The conceptual bases of such treatments, research identifying processes involved in the onset of conduct disorders and related criteria (noted earlier in the paper) are rarely even approximated with this genre of interventions. Typically, such programs are not evaluated empirically. On the one hand, developing treatments that emerge outside of the mainstream of the mental health professions is to be encouraged precisely because traditional treatments have not resolved the problem. On the other hand, this genre of intervention tends to avoid evaluation. Evaluation is the key because well-intentioned and costly interventions can have little or no effect on the youths they treat (Weisz, Walter, Weiss, Fernandez & Mikow, 1990) and may actually increase antisocial behavior (e.g. see Lundman, 1984).

SALIENT CLINICAL ISSUES IN TREATMENT

There are a number of issues that emerge in treatment of conduct-disordered youths and decision-making about what interventions to provide to whom. These issues reflect obstacles in delivering treatment, lacunae in our knowledge base and limitations in the models of providing care.

Retaining Cases in Treatment

Dropping out from treatment is a significant problem in the treatment of children and adolescents.[3] Among families that begin treatment, 40–60% terminate prematurely (Armbruster & Kazdin, 1994; Wierzbicki & Pekarik, 1993). Youths with aggressive and antisocial behavior are particularly likely to drop out early (e.g. Capaldi & Patterson, 1987; Kaminer, Tarter, Bukstein & Kabene, 1992).

Many of the parent and family factors often associated with conduct disorder are likely to place families at risk for terminating treatment prematurely. These include: socioeconomic disadvantage, facets of the family constellation (younger mothers, single-parent families), high parent stress, adverse child-rearing practices (e.g. harsh punishment, poor monitoring and supervision of the child) and parent history of antisocial behavior (e.g. Kazdin, 1990; Kazdin, Mazurick & Bass, 1993; McMahon, Forehand, Griest & Wells, 1981). Child characteristics that predict early termination from treatment include comorbidity (multiple diagnoses and symptoms across a range of disorders), severity of delinquent and antisocial behavior and poor academic functioning. The accumulation of these factors places families at increased risk for dropping out of treatment within the first few sessions. Interestingly, many of the child, parent and family factors that predict premature termination from treatment are the same factors that portend a poor response to treatment and poor long-term prognosis (Dadds & McHugh, 1992; Dumas & Wahler, 1983; Kazdin, 1995a; Webster-Stratton, 1985).

The cases who terminate early are those who evince the greatest impairment in parent, family and child characteristics. In clinical work, the usual impression is that individuals

[3]Dropping out of treatment usually refers to prematurely terminating from ongoing therapy at a point where the patient ceases to come for treatment and when the therapist believes that this decision is ill-advised. In research, early termination usually refers to dropping out within the first few sessions of treatment, although the patient may leave the system at many different points (e.g. after being referred to the clinic, contacting the clinc by phone, scheduling an initial appointment, attending that appointment, beginning intake assessment).

who drop out of treatment are much worse off than those who have remained in treatment. Our own work suggests that this is true, but due primarily to the fact that those who drop out are more severely impaired to begin with (Kazdin, Mazurick & Siegel, 1994). Even so, evidence points to benefits of remaining in treatment. Those cases who remain in treatment but are equally impaired as those who have dropped out tend to fare better. Consequently, it is important to retain cases in treatment.

Even though treatment is designed to help families, several aspects of coming to treatment increase stress and demands on the family. Many of the burdens are associated with coming to the sessions and include procuring transportation, cajoling the identified patient (child) to agree to come to the session that day, arranging babysitting for other children and so on. In fact, parents will often cancel a session or not show up because of the difficulties of bringing the child and the child's siblings to the clinic. Financial costs associated with coming to treatment (e.g. babysitting, transportation, costs of treatment) also may be a significant burden in light of the disproportionate distribution of poverty among families of youths referred to treatment for conduct disorder.

There are a few leads for retaining cases better in treatment, although the empirical evidence in relation to child and adolescent treatment is sparse. Providing special sessions for the parents to address sources of stress and concern (e.g. job stress, personal worries, family disputes), when added to treatment of the child, reduces attrition (Prinz & Miller, 1994). Also, providing children with a special preparatory interview to convey why people go to therapy reduces the rate of dropping out (Holmes & Urie, 1975). Developing an alliance with all immediate family members (e.g. by extensive phone contacts) early in treatment, conveying the benefits that can accrue to each member as the child improves and making an effort to engage the family members in treatment as obstacles emerge have reduced attrition and improved treatment outcome (Santisteban et al., 1996; Szapocznik et al., 1988).

Clinically, adding interventions just to retain cases in treatment can place a burden on the therapy. Yet cases at high risk for dropping out can be identified, based on factors mentioned previously. In these cases, it may be feasible for the clinician to attack both fronts, namely, improvement of the conduct-disordered child and reduction of parental stress and the burden of treatment. It is unlikely that improvements in child functioning alone will help retain cases in treatment, given what we know about the factors that predict treatment termination. In fact, in our own clinical work, early improvement in treatment seems to increase the likelihood of attrition. Some parents perceive early changes as sufficient, even though many areas may require further attention.

What Treatments Do Not Work

With a few hundred or so treatments available for children, it would be quite helpful to know which among these do not work or do not work very well. Addressing the matter directly is not possible in light of the fact, noted previously, that the vast majority of treatment approaches have not been evaluated empirically. Thus, there is no accumulated body of evidence in which treatments have consistently emerged as weak or ineffective. Moreover, the nature of the dominant scientific research paradigm (inability to prove the null hypothesis) precludes firm demonstration of no effects of treatment. Most of the treatments currently used in clinical work (Kazdin et al., 1990b), including psychodynamic therapy, relationship-based treatment and play therapy, have not been evaluated empirically (Kazdin et al., 1990a). Occasionally, variations of these treatments have been used as comparative conditions and have been shown to be less effective than one of the promising treatments noted previously (e.g. Borduin et al., 1995; Kazdin, Esveldt-Dawson, French & Unis, 1987a, b). From this limited research, it is premature to conclude that these latter treatments are ineffective. Yet at best their benefits have still to be demonstrated and more promising treatments with firmer empirical bases are currently the treatments of choice.

The absence of empirical evidence is only one criterion, albeit an obviously important one. In advance of, and eventually along with, the evidence, scrutiny of the conceptual underpinnings of treatment and the treatment focus is important in relation to what we know about conduct disorder. We know, for example, that conduct-disordered youths usually show problems in multiple domains, including overt behavior, social relations (e.g. peers, teachers, family members) and academic performance. For a treatment to be effective, it is likely that several domains have to be addressed explicitly within the sessions or a conceptual model (with supporting evidence) is needed to convey why a narrow or delimited focus (e.g. on psychic conflicts or a small set of overt behaviors) is likely to have broad effects on domains not explicitly addressed in treatment. Although one cannot say for certain what techniques will not work, it is much safer to say that treatments that neglect multiple domains are likely to have limited effects.

Second, some evidence has emerged that is useful for selecting what treatments to avoid or to use with great caution. Often conduct-disordered youths are treated in group therapy, yet placing youths together could impede improvement. For example, Feldman, Caplinger and Wodarski (1983) randomly assigned youths (ages 8–17) to variations of group therapy. In one type of group, all members were referred for conduct disorder; in another type of group, conduct-disordered youths were placed with nonantisocial youths (without clinical problems). Those placed in a group of their deviant peers did not improve; those placed with nondeviant peers did improve. Interpretation of this is based on the likelihood that peer bonding to others can improve one's behavior, if those peers engage in more normative behavior; bonding to a deviant group can sustain deviant behavior.

Similarly, Dishion and Andrews (1995) evaluated several interventions for nonreferred youths (ages 10–14) with conduct problems. One of the treatment conditions included youths meeting in a group with a focus on self-regulation, monitoring and developing behavior-change programs. This condition, whether alone or in combination with parent training, was associated with increases in behavioral problems and substance use (cigarette smoking). Again, it appeared that placing conduct-problem teens in a group situation can exacerbate their problems. Other research has shown that individuals may become worse (e.g. increase in arrest rates) through association with deviant peers as part of treatment (O'Donnell, 1992).

Treatments for conduct-disordered youths in settings such as hospitals, schools and correctional facilities are often conducted in a group therapy format in which several conduct-problem youths are together to talk about or work on their problems or go to the country for some fresh air experience to get better. There may be conditions under which this arrangement is beneficial. However, current research suggests that placing several such youths together can impede therapeutic change and have deleterious effects.

Who Responds Well to Treatment

We have known for many years that the critical question of psychotherapy is not what technique is effective, but rather what technique works for whom, under what conditions, as administered by what type of therapists, and so on (Kiesler, 1971). The adult psychotherapy literature has focused on a range of questions to identify factors (e.g. patient, therapist, treatment process) that contribute to outcome. The child and adolescent therapy research has been devoted almost exclusively to questions about treatment technique, with scant attention to the role of child, parent, family and therapist factors that may moderate outcome (Kazdin et al., 1990a).

In the case of conduct disorder, a few studies have looked at who responds to treatment, mostly in the context of parent management training and problem-solving skills training. Current evidence suggests that risk factors for onset of conduct disorder and poor long-term prognosis also predict response to treatment (Dumas & Wahler, 1983; Kazdin, 1995a, Kazdin & Crowley, in press; Webster-Stratton, 1985). Multiple child, parent, family and contextual factors, including early onset and more severe child antisocial behavior, comorbid diagnoses, child academic impairment, socio-economic disadvantage, single-parent families, parental stress (perceived) and life events, and parent history of antisocial behavior in childhood are likely to influence responsiveness to treatment. These factors accumulate and increase risk for poor outcome in treatment. Our own work has shown that even those youths with multiple risk factors still improve with treatment, but the changes are not as great as those achieved for cases with fewer risk factors. The characteristics that have been studied in relation to treatment outcome (e.g. comorbidity) have not been examined across different treatments. Consequently, we do not know whether these factors affect responsiveness to any treatment or to particular forms of treatment.

In current subtyping of conduct-disordered youths, early (childhood) and later (adolescent) onset conduct disorder are distinguished (Hinshaw et al., 1993; Moffitt, 1993). Early-onset conduct-disordered youths are characterized by aggressive behavior, neuropsychological dysfunction (in "executive" functions), a much higher ratio of boys to girls and a poor long-term prognosis. Later-onset youths (onset at about age 15) are characterized more by delinquent activity (theft, vandalism), a more even distribution of boys and girls and a more favorable prognosis. The subtype and associated characteristics are by no means firmly established, but reflect current conceptual and empirical work in the area (e.g. Moffitt, 1993; Patterson, DeBaryshe & Ramsey, 1989). We can expect from this that youths with an early onset are more likely to be recalcitrant to treatment. At present, and in the absence of very much treatment research on the matter, a useful guideline to predict responsiveness to treatment is to consider loading of the child, parent and family on risk factors that portend a poor long-term prognosis (see Kazdin, 1995b; Robins, 1991).

In clinical work, there is frequent discussion about the importance of individualizing treatment to the needs of the child and family. At this point, the research is of little help in addressing the level of specificity in crafting treatment regiments to the individual. A possible exception is one of the treatments mentioned previously (multisystemic therapy), in which several different treatments, some with firm evidence on their behalf, are integrated as a treatment package. At present, perhaps the best strategy is to select the treatment that appears to be promising based on the evidence and applying that as the initial treatment of choice. Attempting to make decisions about what can be applied effectively among promising or unpromising techniques is difficult to do in an informed way in light of the current knowledge base and could very well lead to less effective clinical care for the individual child and family.

Addressing Comorbidity

An issue that has received attention in discussions of clinical dysfunction and treatment is the issue of comorbidity. As noted previously, conduct disorder is often comorbid with other diagnoses, most notably ADHD and ODD, but others as well. It is likely that comorbidity is the rule rather than the exception among cases referred for treatment. In our own clinic, for example, approximately 70% of the cases meet DSM criteria for two or more disorders (Kazdin, 1996b).

Comorbidity has been conceived of rather narrowly, namely, the presence of two or more disorders. In relation to treatment research and practice, there may be value in extending the notion more broadly. It is likely that children have many symptoms from many different disorders, even though they might not meet the criteria for each of the disorders. Indeed, in our research we have found the total number of symptoms across the range of disorders to be a more sensitive predictor of treatment outcome than merely counting the number of diagnoses (Kazdin & Crowley, in press). Although the number of disorders may be important, impairment across the full range of symptoms is noteworthy as well.

It may be useful to expand the notion of comorbidity well beyond symptoms and diagnoses. A central issue for treating conduct-disordered youth is the domains of impairment they experience. These domains can include other disorders (e.g. depression, substance abuse), learning difficulties (specific reading disorders, language delays, learning disability), dysfunctional peer relations (rejection, absence of prosocial friends) and perhaps deficits in prosocial activities (participation in school, athletic and extracurricular events). Problems or dysfunctions in each of these domains, apart from conduct-disorder symptoms themselves, can influence the effects of treatment and long-term prognosis.

At present, research has not provided guidelines for how to address comorbid conditions. Indeed, much of the treatment research has eschewed diagnosis, so the number or proportions of youth who meet criteria for any disorder is usually unclear (Kazdin et al., 1990a). We can say very little at this point about whether comorbid conditions invariably influence outcome, whether the influence and direction of that influence vary by the specific comorbid condition, or how to alter treatment in light of these conditions. This area of work represents a major deficiency in the knowledge base among even the most promising treatments for conduct disorder.

Combining Treatments

There is keen interest, both in clinical work and in research, in using combinations of treatment, i.e. multiple psychosocial and/or pharmacological interventions (see Kazdin,

1996a). In the case of conduct disorder, impetus stems from the scope of impairment evident in children (e.g. comorbidity, academic dysfunction) and families (e.g. stress, conflict) as well as limited effects of most treatments. The benefits of combined treatments can be identified in selected areas. For example, in the treatment of adult schizophrenia, combinations of treatment (e.g. medication and family counseling/therapy) surpasses the effects of the constituent components alone (e.g. Falloon, 1988).

In the case of child and adolescent therapy, combined treatments have not been well studied. I have argued elsewhere that there are many reasons to expect combined treatments not to surpass the effects of any promising single treatment (Kazdin, 1996a). Among the reasons, we know very little about the parameters of a given treatment that influence its effectiveness and the cases to whom the treatment is most suitably applied. Combining techniques of which we know relatively little, particularly in time-limited treatment, is not a firm base to build more effective treatments. Also, there are many obstacles in combining treatment that materially affect their likely outcome, such as decision rules regarding what treatments to combine, how to combine them (e.g. when, in what order), how to evaluate their impact and others.

An important assumption for combined treatments is that individual treatments are weak and, if combined, they would produce additive or synergistic effects. This is a reasonable, even if poorly tested, assumption. An alternative assumption is that the way in which treatment is usually administered, whether a single or a combined treatment, inherently limits the likelihood of positive outcome effects, a point discussed further later. As a general point, combining treatments itself is not likely to be an answer to developing effective treatment without more thought and evidence about the nature of these combinations.

Some of the promising treatments reviewed previously (MST, FFT) are combined treatments. For example, multisystemic therapy provides many different treatments for antisocial youths. Two points are worth noting. First, the constituent treatments that form a major part of treatment are those that have evidence on their behalf (e.g. PSST, PMT), so that not any combination is used. Second, we do not yet know that multisystemic therapy, as a combined treatment package, is more effective than the most effective constituent component administered for the same duration. The comparisons of multisystemic therapy have mostly included ordinary individual psychotherapy and counseling, important comparison groups to be sure. Although treatment has surpassed traditional therapy practices, this is not the same as showing that combinations of treatment per se are necessary to achieve therapeutic changes.

Combined treatments may be very useful and should be pursued. At the same time, a rash move to combine treatments is unwarranted. The effects of combined treatment obviously depend very much on the individual treatments that are included in the combination. For example, mentioned already was a study in which parent training and a teen-focused group were evaluated alone and in combination (Dishion & Andrews, 1995). Conditions that received the teen-group component, whether alone or in combination with parent training, became worse. Obviously, one cannot assume that combined treatments will automatically be neutral or better than their constituent treatments. There is another more subtle and perhaps worrisome facet of combined treatments. A danger in promoting treatment combinations is to continue to use techniques with little evidence on their behalf as an ingredient in a larger set of techniques. Old wine in new bottles is not bad if the original wine has merit.

However, without knowing if there is merit, the tendency to view the wine as new and improved would be unfortunate. With promising treatments available, we have a comparative base to evaluate novel treatments, treatment combinations, and unevaluated treatments in current use. If a promising treatment is not used in clinical work, we would want evidence that it has clearly failed, that other promising treatments for whatever reason cannot be used and that the treatment that is to be applied has a reasonable basis for addressing the scope of dysfunctions.

Models of Delivering Treatment

The model of treatment delivery in current research is to provide a relatively brief and time-limited intervention. For several clinical dysfunctions or for a number of children with a particular dysfunction such as conduct disorder, the course of maladjustment may be long-term. In such cases, the notion of providing a brief, time-limited treatment may very much limit outcome effects. Even if a great combination of various psychotherapies were constructed, administration in the time-limited fashion might have the usual, checkered yield. More extended and enduring treatment in some form may be needed to achieve clinically important effects with the greatest number of youths. Two ways of delivering extended treatment illustrate the point.

The first variation might be referred to as a *continued-care model*. The model of treatment delivery that may be needed can be likened to the model used in the treatment of diabetes mellitus. With diabetes, ongoing treatment (insulin) is needed to ensure that the benefits of treatment are sustained. The benefits of treatment would end with discontinuation of treatment. Analogously, in the context of conduct disorder, a variation of ongoing treatment may be needed. Perhaps after the child is referred, treatment is provided to address the current crises and to have impact on functioning at home, at school and in the community. After improvement is achieved, treatment is modified rather than terminated. At that point, the child could enter into maintenance therapy, i.e. continued treatment perhaps in varying schedules ("doses"). Treatment would continue but perhaps on a more intermittent basis. Continued treatment in this fashion has been effective as a model for treating recurrent depression in adults (see Kupfer et al., 1992).

The second variation might be referred to as a *dentalcare model* to convey a different way of extending treatment. After initial treatment and demonstrated improvement in functioning in everyday life, treatment is suspended. At this point, the child's functioning begins to be monitored regularly (e.g. every 3 months) and systematically (with standardized measures). Treatment could be provided *pro re nata* (PRN) based on the assessment data or emergent issues raised by the family, teachers or others. The approach might be likened to the more familiar model of dental care in the United States in which "check-ups" are recommended every 6 months; an intervention is provided if and as needed, based on these periodic checks.

Obviously, the use of ongoing treatment is not advocated in cases where there is evidence that short-term treatment is effective. A difficulty with most of the research on treatment of conduct disorder, whether promising, poorly investigated or combined treatments, is that the conventional treatment model of brief, time-limited therapy has been adopted. Without considering alternative models of delivery, current treatments may be quite limited in the effects they can produce. Although more effective treatments are sorely needed, the way of delivering currently available treatments ought to be reconsidered.

CONCLUSIONS

Many different types of treatment have been applied to conduct-disordered youths. Unfortunately, little outcome evidence exists for most of the techniques. Four treatments with the most promising evidence to date were highlighted: problem-solving skills training, parent management training, functional family therapy, and multisystemic therapy. Cognitive problem-solving skills training focuses on cognitive processes that underlie social behavior. Parent management training is directed at altering parent-child interactions in the home, particularly those interactions related to child-rearing practices and coercive interchanges. Functional family therapy utilizes principles of systems theory and behavior modification as the basis for altering interactions, communication and problem solving among family members. Multisystemic therapy focus on the individual, family and extrafamilial systems and their interrelations as a way to reduce symptoms and to promote prosocial behavior. Evidence on behalf of these interventions was reviewed; each has multiple controlled studies on its behalf and some of the techniques (e.g. PMT) have been extraordinarily well evaluated.

Significant issues remain to be addressed to accelerate advances in the area of treatment. The magnitude of change and durability of treatment effects raise multiple issues about how to evaluate treatment and the conclusions reached about any particular intervention. We cannot yet say that one intervention can ameliorate conduct disorder and overcome the poor long-term prognosis. On the other hand, much can be said. Much of what is practised in clinical settings is based on psychodynamically oriented treatment, general relationship counseling, family therapy and group therapy (with antisocial youths as members). These and other procedures, alone and in various combinations in which they are often used, have not been evaluated carefully in controlled trials. Of course, absence of evidence is not tantamount to ineffectiveness. At the same time, promising treatments have advanced considerably and a very special argument might be needed to administer treatments that have neither basic research on their conceptual underpinnings in relation to conduct disorder nor outcome evidence from controlled clinical trials on their behalf. Promising treatments, at best, leave important questions unanswered. Further development of treatments is clearly needed. Apart from treatment studies, further progress in understanding the nature of conduct disorder is likely to have very important implications for improving treatment outcome. Improved triage of patients to treatments that are likely to work will require understanding of characteristics of children, parents and families that will make them more or less amenable to current treatments.

REFERENCES

Alexander, J. F., Barton, C., Schiavo, R. S. & Parsons, B. V. (1976). Systems-behavioral intervention with families of delinquents: Therapist characteristics, family behavior, and outcome. *Journal of Consulting and Clinical Psychology*, *44*, 656–664.

Alexander, J. F., Holtzworth-Munroe, A. & Jameson, P. B. (1994). The process and outcome of marital and family therapy research: Review and evaluation. In A. E. Bergin & S. L. Garfield (Eds.), *Handbook of psychotherapy and behavior change* (4th edn.), (pp. 595–630). New York: John Wiley & Sons.

Alexander, J. F. & Parsons, B. V. (1982). *Functional family therapy*. Monterey, CA: Brooks/Cole.

American Psychiatric Association (1994). *Diagnostic and statistical manual of mental disorders* (4th edn.). Washington, DC: APA.

Armbruster, P., & Kazdin, A. E. (1994). Attrition in child psychotherapy. In T. H. Ollendick & R. J. Prinz (Eds.), *Advances in clinical child psychology, Vol. 16* (pp. 81–108). New York: Plenum.

Asher, S. R. & Coie, J. D. (Eds.) (1990). *Peer rejection in childhood*. New York: Cambridge University Press.

Baer, R. A. & Nietzel, M. T. (1991). Cognitive and behavioral treatment of impulsivity in children: A meta-analytic review of the outcome literature. *Journal of Clinical Child Psychology, 20*, 400–412.

Bank, L., Marlowe, J. H., Reid, J. B., Patterson, G. R. & Weinrott, M. R. (1991). A comparative evaluation of parent-training interventions for families of chronic delinquents. *Journal of Abnormal Child Psychology, 19*, 15–33.

Bell, R. Q. & Harper, L. (1977). *Child effects on adults*. New York: John Wiley & Sons.

Borduin, C. M., Henggeler, S. W., Blaske, D. M. & Stein, R. (1990). Multisystemic treatment of adolescent sexual offenders. *International Journal of Offender Therapy and Comparative Criminology, 34*, 105–113.

Borduin, C. M., Mann, B. J., Cone, L. T., Henggeler, S. W., Fucci, B. R., Blaske, D. M. & Williams, R. A. (1995). Multisystemic treatment of serious juvenile offenders: Long-term prevention of criminality and violence. *Journal of Consulting and Clinical Psychology, 63*, 569–578.

Brandt, D. E. & Zlotnick, S. J. (1988). *The psychology and treatment of the youthful offender*. Springfield, IL: Charles C Thomas.

Brunk, M., Henggeler, S. W. & Whelan, J. P. (1987). A comparison of multisystemic therapy and parent training in the brief treatment of child abuse and neglect. *Journal of Consulting and Clinical Psychology, 55*, 311–318.

Campbell, M., Adams, P. B., Small, A. M., Kafantaris, V., Silva, R. R., Shell, J., Perry, R. & Overall, J. E. (1995). Lithium in hospitalized aggressive children with conduct disorder: A double-blind and placebo-controlled study. *Journal of the American Academy of Child and Adolescent Psychiatry, 34*, 445–453.

Campbell, M. & Cueva, J. E. (1995). Psychopharmacology in child and adolescent psychiatry: A review of the past seven years. Part II. *Journal of the American Academy of Child and Adolescent Psychiatry, 34*, 1262–1272.

Capaldi, D. & Patterson, G. R. (1987). An approach to the problem of recruitment and retention rates for longitudinal research. *Behavioral Assessment, 9*, 169–187.

Cooper, J. O., Heron, T. E. & Heward, W. L. (1987). *Applied behavior analysis*. Columbus, OH: Merrill.

Crick, N. R. & Dodge, K. A. (1994). A review and reformulation of social information processing mechanisms in children's social adjustment. *Psychological Bulletin, 115*, 74–101.

Cueva, J. E., Overall, J. E., Small, A. M., Armenteros, J. L., Perry, R. & Campbell, M. (1996). Carbamazepine in aggressive children with conduct disorder: A double-blind and placebo controlled study. *Journal of the American Academy of Child and Adolescent Psychiatry, 35*, 480–490.

Cunningham, C. E., Bremner, R. & Boyle, M. (1995). Large group community-based parenting programs for families of preschoolers at risk for disruptive behavior disorders: Utilization, cost effectiveness, and outcome. *Journal of Child Psychology and Psychiatry, 36*, 1141–1159.

Dadds, M. R. & McHugh, T. A. (1992). Social support and treatment outcome in behavioral family therapy for child conduct problems. *Journal of Consulting and Clinical Psychology, 60*, 252–259.

Dadds, M. R., Schwartz, S. & Sanders, M. R. (1987). Marital discord and treatment outcome in behavioral treatment of child conduct disorders. *Journal of Consulting and Clinical Psychology, 55*, 396–403.

Dishion, T. J. & Andrews, D. W. (1995). Preventing escalation in problem behaviors with high-risk young adolescents: Immediate and 1-year outcomes. *Journal of Consulting and Clinical Psychology, 63*, 538–548.

Dishion, T. J. & Patterson, G. R. (1992). Age effects in parent training outcomes. *Behavior Therapy, 23*, 719–729.

Dishion, T. J., Patterson, G. R. & Kavanagh, K. A. (1992). An experimental test of the coercion model: Linking theory, measurement, and intervention. In J. McCord & R. E. Tremblay (Eds.), *Preventing antisocial behavior* (pp. 253–282). New York: Guilford.

Dumas, J. E. (1989). Treating antisocial behavior in children: Child and family approaches. *Clinical Psychology Review, 9*, 197–222.

Dumas, J. E. & Wahler, R. G. (1983). Predictors of treatment outcome in parent training: Mother insularity and socio-economic disadvantage. *Behavioral Assessment, 5*, 301–313.

Durlak, J. A., Fuhrman, T. & Lampman, C. (1991). Effectiveness of cognitive-behavioral therapy for maladapting children: A meta-analysis. *Psychological Bulletin, 110*, 204–214.

Falloon, I. R. (1988). Expressed emotion: Current status. *Psychological Medicine, 18*, 269–274.

Feindler, E. L. & Ecton, R. B. (1986). *Adolescent anger control: Cognitive-behavioral techniques*. Elmsford, NY: Pergamon.

Feldman, R. A., Caplinger, T. E. & Wodarski, J. S. (1983). *The St. Louis conundrum: The effective treatment of antisocial youths*. Englewood Cliffs, NJ: Prentice-Hall.

Fergusson, D. M., Horwood, L. J. & Lloyd, M. (1991). Confirmatory factor models of attention deficit and conduct disorder. *Journal of Child Psychology and Psychiatry, 32*, 257–274.

Finch, A. J., Jr., Nelson, W. M. & Ott, E. S. (1983). *Cognitive-behavioral procedures with children and adolescents: A practical guide*. Needham Heights, MA: Allyn & Bacon.

Forehand, R. & Long, N. (1988). Outpatient treatment of the acting out child: Procedures, long-term follow-up data, and clinical problems. *Advances in Behaviour Research and Therapy, 10*, 129–177.

Forehand, R. & McMahon, R. J. (1981). *Helping the non-compliant child: A clinician's guide to parent training*. New York: Guilford.

Griest, D. L., Forehand, R., Rogers, T., Breiner, J., Furey, W. & Williams, C. A. (1982). Effects of parent enhancement therapy on the treatment outcome and generalization of a parent training program. *Behaviour Research and Therapy, 20*, 429–436.

Henggeler, S. W. (1994). *Treatment manual for family preservation using multisystemic therapy*. Charleston, SC: Medical University of South Carolina, South Carolina Health and Human Services Finance Commission.

Henggeler, S. W. & Borduin, C. M. (1990). *Family therapy and beyond: A multisystemic approach to teaching the behavior problems of children and adolescents*. Pacific Grove, CA: Brooks/Cole.

Henggeler, S. W., Melton, G. B. & Smith, L. A. (1992). Family preservation using multisystemic therapy: An effective alternative to incarcerating serious juvenile offenders. *Journal of Consulting and Clinical Psychology*, *60*, 953–961.

Henggeler, S. W., Rodick, J. D., Borduin, C. M., Hanson, C. L., Watson, S. M. & Urey, J. R. (1986). Multisystemic treatment of juvenile offenders: Effects on adolescent behavior and family interaction. *Developmental Psychology*, *22*, 132–141.

Henggeler, S. W., Schoenwald, S. K. & Pickrel, S. A. G. (1995). Multisystemic therapy: Bridging the gap between university- and community-based treatment. *Journal of Consulting and Clinical Psychology*, *63*, 709–717.

Hinshaw, S. P. (1994). *Attention deficits and hyperactivity in children*. Thousand Oaks, CA: Sage.

Hinshaw, S. P., Lahey, B. B. & Hart, E. L. (1993). Issues of taxonomy and comorbidity in the development of conduct disorder. *Development and Psychopathology*, *5*, 31–49.

Holmes, D. S. & Urie, R. G. (1975). Effects of preparing children for psychotherapy. *Journal of Consulting and Clinical Psychology*, *43*, 311–318.

Kaminer, Y., Tarter, R. E., Bukstein, O. G. & Kabene, M. (1992). Comparison between treatment completers and non-completers among dually diagnosed substance-abusing adolescents. *Journal of the American Academy of Child and Adolescent Psychiatry*, *31*, 1046–1049.

Kazdin, A. E. (1985). *Treatment of antisocial behavior in children and adolescents*. Homewood, IL: Dorsey Press.

Kazdin, A. E. (1988). *Child psychotherapy: Developing and identifying effective treatments*. Needham Heights, MA: Allyn & Bacon.

Kazdin, A. E. (1990). Premature termination from treatment among children referred for antisocial behavior. *Journal of Child Psychology and Psychiatry*, *3*, 415–425.

Kazdin, A. E. (1992). *Research design in clinical psychology* (2nd edn.). Needham Heights, MA: Allyn & Bacon.

Kazdin, A. E. (1993). Treatment of conduct disorder: Progress and directions in psychotherapy research. *Development and Psychopathology*, *5*, 277–310.

Kazdin, A. E. (1994a). *Behavior modification in applied settings* (5th edn.). Pacific Grove, CA: Brooks/Cole.

Kazdin, A. E. (1994b). Psychotherapy for children and adolescents. In A. E. Bergin & S. L. Garfield (Eds.), *Handbook of psychotherapy and behavior change* (4th edn.) (pp. 543–594). New York: Wiley & Sons.

Kazdin, A. E. (1995a). Child, parent, and family dysfunction as predictors of outcome in cognitive-behavioral treatment of antisocial children. *Behaviour Research and Therapy*, *33*, 271–281.

Kazdin, A. E. (1995b). *Conduct disorder in childhood and adolescence* (2nd edn). Thousand Oaks, CA: Sage.

Kazdin, A. E. (1996a). Combined and multimodal treatments in child and adolescent psychotherapy: Issues, challenges, and research directions. *Clinical Psychology: Science and Practice*, *3*, 69–100.

Kazdin, A. E. (1996b). Dropping out of child psychotherapy: Issues for research and implications for practice. *Clinical Child Psychology and Psychiatry*, *1*, 133–156.

Kazdin, A. E., Bass, D., Ayers, W. A. & Rodgers, A. (1990a). Empirical and clinical focus of child and adolescent psychotherapy research. *Journal of Consulting and Clinical Psychology*, *58*, 729–740.

Kazdin, A. E., Bass, D., Siegel, T. & Thomas, C. (1989). Cognitive-behavioral treatment and relationship therapy in the treatment of children referred for antisocial behavior. *Journal of Consulting and Clinical Psychology, 57*, 522–535.

Kazdin, A. E. & Crowley, M. (in press). Moderators of treatment outcome in cognitively based treatment of antisocial children. *Cognitive Therapy and Research.*

Kazdin, A. E., Esveldt-Dawson, K., French, N. H. & Unis, A. S. (1987a). Problem-solving skills training and relationship therapy in the treatment of antisocial child behavior. *Journal of Consulting and Clinical Psychology, 55*, 76–85.

Kazdin, A. E., Esveldt-Dawson, K., French, N. H. & Unis, A. S. (1987b). The effects of parent management training and problem-solving skills training combined in the treatment of antisocial child behavior. *Journal of the American Academy of Child and Adolescent Psychiatry, 26*, 416–424.

Kazdin, A. E., Mazurick, J. L. & Bass, D. (1993). Risk for attrition in treatment of antisocial children and families. *Journal of Clinical Child Psychology, 22*, 2–16.

Kazdin, A. E., Mazurick, J. L. & Siegel, T. C. (1994). Treatment outcome among children with externalizing disorder who terminate prematurely versus those who complete psychotherapy. *Journal of the American Academy of Child and Adolescent Psychiatry, 33*, 549–557.

Kazdin, A. E., Siegel, T. C. & Bass, D. (1990b). Drawing upon clinical practice to inform research on child and adolescent psychotherapy: A survey of practitioners. *Professional Psychology: Research and Practice, 21*, 189–198.

Kazdin, A. E., Siegel, T. & Bass, D. (1992). Cognitive problem-solving skills training and parent management training in the treatment of antisocial behavior in children. *Journal of Consulting and Clinical Psychology, 60*, 733–747.

Kendall, P. C. (Ed.) (1991). *Child and adolescent therapy: Cognitive-behavioral procedures.* New York: Guilford.

Kiesler, D. J. (1971). Experimental designs in psychotherapy research. In A. E. Bergin & S. L. Garfield (Eds.), *Handbook of psychotherapy and behavior change: An empirical analysis* (pp. 36–74). New York: Wiley.

Kupfer, D. J., Frank, E., Perel, J. M., Cornes, C., Mallinger, A. G., Thase, M. E., McEachran, A. B. & Grochocinski, V. J. (1992). Five-year outcome for maintenance therapies in recurrent depression. *Archives of General Psychiatry, 49*, 769–773.

Lochman, J. E. & Dodge, K. A. (1994). Social-cognitive processes of severely violent, moderately aggressive, and non-aggressive boys. *Journal of Consulting and Clinical Psychology, 62*, 366–374.

Long, P., Forehand, R., Wierson, M. & Morgan, A. (1994). Does parent training with young noncompliant children have long-term effects? *Behaviour Research and Therapy, 32*, 101–107.

Lundman, R. J. (1984). *Prevention and control of juvenile delinquency.* New York: Oxford University Press.

Lytton, H. (1990). Child and parent effects in boys' conduct disorder: A reinterpretation. *Developmental Psychology, 26*, 683–697.

Mann, B. J., Borduin, C. M., Henggeler, S. W. & Blaske, D. M. (1990). An investigation of systemic conceptualizations of parent-child coalitions and symptom change. *Journal of Consulting and Clinical Psychology, 58*, 336–344.

McMahon, R. J., Forehand, R., Griest, D. L. & Wells, K. C. (1981). Who drops out of treatment during parent behavioral training? *Behavioral Counseling Quarterly, 1*, 79–85.

McMahon, R. J. & Wells, K. C. (1989). Conduct disorders. In E. J. Mash & R. A. Barkley (Eds.), *Treatment of childhood disorders* (pp. 73–132). New York: Guilford Press.

Miller, G. E. & Prinz, R. J. (1990). Enhancement of social learning family interventions for child conduct disorder. *Psychological Bulletin*, *108*, 291–307.

Moffitt, T. E. (1993). The neuropsychology of conduct problems. *Development and Psychopathology*, *5*, 135–151.

Morris, S. M., Alexander, J. F. & Turner, C. W. (1991). Do reattributions reduce blame? *Journal of Family Psychology*, *5*, 192–203.

Newberry, A. M., Alexander, J. F. & Turner, C. W. (1991). Gender as a process variable in family therapy. *Journal of Family Psychology*, *5*, 158–175.

O'Donnell, C. R. (1992). The interplay of theory and practice in delinquency prevention: From behavior modification to activity settings. In J. McCord & R. E. Tremblay (Eds.), *Preventing antisocial behavior* (pp. 209–232). New York: Guilford.

Offord, D. R., Boyle, M. H. & Racine, Y. A. (1991). The epidemiology of antisocial behavior. In D. J. Pepler & K. H. Rubin (Eds.), *The development and treatment of childhood aggression* (pp. 31–54). Hillsdale, NJ: Erlbaum.

Patterson, G. R. (1982). *Coercive family process*. Eugene, OR: Castalia.

Patterson, G. R., Capaldi, D. & Bank, L. (1991). An early starter model for predicting delinquency. In D. J. Pepler & K. H. Rubin (Eds.). *The development and treatment of childhood aggression* (pp. 139–168). Hillsdale, NJ: Erlbaum.

Patterson, G. R. & Chamberlain, P. (1994). A functional analysis of resistance during parent training therapy. *Clinical Psychology: Science and Practice*, *1*, 53–70.

Patterson, G. R., DeBaryshe, B. D. & Ramsey, E. (1989). A developmental perspective on antisocial behavior. *American Psychologist*, *44*, 329–335.

Patterson, G. R., Dishion, T. J. & Chamberlain, P. (1993). Outcomes and methodological issues relating to treatment of antisocial children. In T. R. Giles (Ed.), *Handbook of effective psychotherapy* (pp. 43–87). New York: Plenum.

Patterson, G. R., Reid, J. B. & Dishion, T. J. (1992). *Antisocial boys*. Eugene, OR: Castalia.

Pepler, D. J. & Rubin, K. H. (Eds.) (1991). *The development and treatment of childhood aggression*. Hillsdale, NJ: Erlbaum.

Prinz, R. J. & Miller, G. E. (1994). Family-based treatment for childhood antisocial behavior: Experimental influences on dropout and engagement. *Journal of Consulting and Clinical Psychology*, *62*, 645–650.

Robins, L. N. (1981). Epidemiological approaches to natural history research: Antisocial disorders in children. *Journal of the American Academy of Child Psychiatry*, *20*, 566–680.

Robins, L. N. (1991). Conduct disorder. *Journal of Child Psychology and Psychiatry, 32*, 193–212.

Rubin, K. H., Bream, L. A. & Rose-Krasnor, L. (1991). Social problem solving and aggression in childhood. In D. J. Pepler & K. H. Rubin (Eds.), *The development and treatment of childhood aggression* (pp. 219–248). Hillsdale, NJ: Erlbaum.

Rutter, M. & Giller, H. (1983). *Juvenile delinquency: Trends and perspectives*. New York: Penguin Books.

Sanders, M. R. & Dadds, M. R. (1993). *Behavioral family intervention*. Needham Heights, MA: Allyn & Bacon.

Santisteban, D. A. Szapocznik, J., Perez-Vidal, A., Kurtines, W. H., Murray, E. J. & LaPerriere, A. (1996). Efficacy of intervention for engaging youth and families into treatment and some variables that may contribute to differential effectiveness. *Journal of Family Psychology, 10,* 35–44.

Shirk, S. R. (Ed.) (1988). *Cognitive development and child psychotherapy.* New York: Plenum.

Shure, M. B. (1992). *I can problem solve (ICPS): An interpersonal cognitive problem solving program.* Champaign, IL: Research Press.

Spivack, G. & Shure, M. B. (1982). The cognition of social adjustment: Interpersonal cognitive problem solving thinking. In B. B. Lahey & A. E. Kazdin (Eds.), *Advances in clinical child psychology, Vol. 5* (pp. 323–372). New York: Plenum.

Stewart, J. T., Myers, W. C., Burket, R. C. & Lyles, W. B. (1990). A review of the psychopharmacology of aggression in children and adolescents. *Journal of the American Academy of Child and Adolescent Psychiatry, 29,* 269–277.

Szapocznik, J., Perez-Vidal, A., Brickman, A., Foote, F. H., Santisteban, D., Hervis, O. & Kurtines, W. H. (1988). Engaging adolescent drug abusers and their families into treatment: A strategic structural systems approach. *Journal of Consulting and Clinical Psychology, 56,* 552–557.

Szapocznik, J., Rio, A., Murray, E., Cohen, R., Scopetta, M., Rivas-Vasquez, A., Hervis, O., Posada, V. & Kurtines, W. (1989). Structural family versus psychodynamic child therapy for problematic Hispanic boys. *Journal of Consulting and Clinical Psychology, 57,* 571–578.

United States Congress, Office of Technology Assessment. (1991). *Adolescent health.* (OTA-H-468). Washington, DC: U.S. Government Printing Office.

Wahler, R. G. & Dumas, J. E. (1986). Maintenance factors in coercive mother-child interactions: The compliance and predictability hypotheses. *Journal of Applied Behavior Analysis, 19,* 13–22.

Walker, J. L., Lahey, B. B., Russo, M. F., Christ, M. A. G., McBurnett, K., Loeber, R., Stouthamer-Loeber, M. & Green, S. M. (1991). Anxiety, inhibition, and conduct disorder in children: I. Relation to social impairment. *Journal of the American Academy of Child and Adolescent Psychiatry, 30,* 187–191.

Webster-Stratton, C. (1985). Predictors of treatment outcome in parent training for conduct disordered children. *Behavior Therapy, 16,* 223–243.

Webster-Stratton, C. (1994). Advancing videotape parent training: A comparison study. *Journal of Consulting and Clinical Psychology, 62,* 583–593.

Webster-Stratton, C., Hollinsworth, T. & Kolpacoff, M. (1989). The long-term effectiveness and clinical significance of three cost-effective training programs for families with conduct-problem children. *Journal of Consulting and Clinical Psychology, 57,* 550–553.

Wierzbicki, M. & Pekarik, G. (1993). A meta-analysis of psychotherapy dropout. *Professional Psychology: Research and Practice, 24,* 190–195.

Weisz, J. R., Walter, B. R., Weiss, B., Fernandez, G. A. & Mikow, V. A. (1990). Arrests among emotionally disturbed violent and assaultive individuals following minimal versus lengthy intervention through North Carolina's Willie M. Program. *Journal of Consulting and Clinical Psychology, 58,* 720–728.

Part IV

PSYCHOSOCIAL ISSUES

The first paper in Part IV is a review of the cognitive and behavioral deficits associated with parental alcohol use. Weinberg reviews the literature from two areas, children of alcoholics, usually fathers, and prenatally exposed children of alcoholic women. She notes that alcoholic women tend to marry alcoholic men, such that these groups are often overlapping. Nonetheless, most researchers have treated these as distinct samples. She briefly covers epidemiological and societal cost data. The paper reviews the numerous ways in which alcohol exposure can lead to cognitive or behavioral deficits. These include fetal brain development, genetic factors, and a postnatal environment of inconsistent parenting and exposure to toxins. The deficits Weinberg covers in this paper include those associated with fetal alcohol syndrome, such as mental retardation, language disorder, learning disabilities, and behavioral difficulties associated with frontal lobe damage. Children of alcoholic parents have also been found to have learning disabilities, language disorders, and attention deficit and conduct disorder. Weinberg concludes her review by noting that there are few systematic interventions for children of alcoholic parents. In sum, this is an important topic with vast societal implications.

The next paper could have been included in Part I, Developmental Issues, with the meta-analysis of attachment and maternal sensitivity. However, we chose to include it in this section because of the broader societal questions it raises. The large, multisite collaborative study addresses whether child care experience is associated with attachment security and whether strange situation attachment classifications are valid for infants with extensive child care experience.

Participants were selected from among 31 hospitals at 10 sites around the country. Sampling was done to ensure demographic diversity. Over 1,300 families enrolled in the study. Beginning 1 month after the infant was born, researchers conducted home visits, telephone interviews, and visits to child care settings. The strange situation was conducted in a laboratory when the infants were 15 months old. Measures included beliefs about maternal employment, mother's psychological adjustment, maternal sensitivity, and difficult temperament. Numerous child care variables were collected, including age of entry, stability of care, type of care, and amount of care. The study was extremely well designed. For example, the attachment and play tapes were rated in a central location by experienced coders who were blind to child care status.

Results indicated that the strange situation was equally valid for children with and without extensive child care experience. There were no main effects of child care frequency or quality on attachment security. In other words, child care in the first year of life had no specific effect on infants' attachment security. There were significant interaction effects, such that low maternal sensitivity in conjunction with poor quality child care, multiple arrangements, or both was associated with insecure attachments. This important investigation into the effects of child care is continuing. Future developmental assessments are eagerly awaited.

The next paper by Olds and colleagues addresses a societal intervention to prevent developmental problems in economically disadvantaged children. Should home visitation services be provided to low-income, unmarried women before and after to the birth of a child? Is there a cost–benefit analysis to indicate that this type of program deserves to be funded? This paper presents 15-year longitudinal data of a home-visitation program. From the original sample of 400 first-time mothers, 80% ($n = 324$), were available for 15-year follow-up. There was probably less movement in this rural area than there would have been in an urban sample. There were four randomized comparison groups: (a) sensory and developmental screening at 12 and 24 months with referrals when needed, (b) screening plus transportation for well child visits, (c) the above plus a visiting nurse during the pregnancy, and (d) all of the above plus a visiting nurse for 2 years after the child's birth.

The home-visitation program provided to the fourth group was designed to promote three areas of maternal functioning: a healthy pregnancy, improved parenting, and maternal life-course development. Nurses made on average 9 visits during the pregnancy and 23 visits between birth and 24 months (approximately 1 visit per month). The follow-up study relied mostly on parental report but did have archived data for child abuse reports. When the fourth group was compared with the other groups, there were fewer subsequent pregnancies, a reduced use of welfare, a reduced incidence of child abuse and neglect, and reduced criminal behavior among the low-income, unmarried mothers 15 years after the child's birth.

Olds et al. note that many home-visitation programs have not had successful outcomes. Focusing on both the mother's life course and her parenting skills seems essential to creating positive outcomes, and replication studies are underway. This is an important paper that shows how a relatively brief intervention (the first 2 years of the child's life) can have a major impact on real-life indicators. This type of intervention represents a significant cost savings to society with respect to dollars saved on welfare as well as the savings in life potential.

The paper by Morrison, Griffith, and Alberts is intriguing because it addresses the frequently debated topic of school readiness and entrance age. Across North America, kindergarten entrance age varies from about 4 years, 6 months, to 5 years, 6 months. Educators are divided as to whether children are ready to learn to read at the younger ages. In addition, many parents choose to retain children who are close to the age cutoffs for entering school.

Morrison et al. posed the question: Do younger first-grade children make as much progress in reading and math as older first-grade children? This is a pre–post longitudinal design rather than a cross-sectional one. The sample consisted of 539 children attending public school in a Canadian city that has an extremely young school entry age (4.5 years for kindergarten). The authors studied older first graders, younger first graders, kindergarten children who just missed the first-grade cutoff, children who were voluntarily held out (a year prior to entering kindergarten), and children who were retained (repeated kindergarten for a second year). Kindergarten provided informal instruction in letter recognition and sounding out, and first grade provided a formal phonics-based curriculum. Morrison et al. used a standard reading decoding measure and multiple-choice math test to assess achievement levels in the early fall and late spring. Background variables did not significantly differentiate the groups. Children who were retained were less likely to have superior

IQ scores compared with children who were young first graders or who were voluntarily held out. Although older first-grade children finished the year with reading scores several months ahead of those of the younger first graders, the progress both groups made from pre- to posttesting was not significantly different. In sum, achievement testing revealed that when children were taught, they learned.

This study has some shortcomings. There were no achievement measures for the held-out and retained groups. It would be nice if there were follow-up data to determine if the achievement differences between older and younger children disappear. One study found that at the end of first grade, children who were 6 before first grade started were 9 percentile points ahead of children who were 5 at the beginning of the year. Although these findings are dismissed as statistically but not clinically significant, most parents would find them meaningful. After a few years of academic exposure, the age range should presumably be less important than other factors. Morrison et al. note that holding out intelligent children actually increases the range of variability in first-grade classrooms, thus making the legitimately younger children appear more immature.

The final paper in Part IV addresses an oft-neglected topic, the education of intellectually gifted children. There has been much attention and financial resources devoted to educating children with developmental and learning disabilities. Public laws require schools to provide "appropriate" education to children with special needs. Yet, little is known about the best ways to educate children with superior intellect. The educational system in the United States largely ignores those who stand to contribute the most to society.

Winner reviews the existing research on the types of educational programs currently available, including education in the regular classroom, pull-out programs, tracking, and specialized schools. She discusses definitions of giftedness and differentiates the moderately gifted (IQ between 130 and 150) and the profoundly gifted (IQ above 180). Some of the important issues in giftedness are whether the difference is qualitative or quantitative. Profoundly gifted students appear to have qualitatively different ways of problem solving and organizing complex material. Winner also describes indications of giftedness in infancy as well as the life course of giftedness. She delineates types of intellectual giftedness, including linguistic, mathematical, and intellectual unevenness (i.e., the gifted, learning-disabled student). Educational options for gifted students include acceleration (entering school early, skipping grades), ability grouping, and special schools, either private or public, with selective admissions policies. There is an interesting discussion of the virtues and criticisms of ability grouping. The paper highlights how little training teachers receive to provide an enriched environment for profoundly gifted children. One wonders about the ability of the average teacher to teach profoundly gifted children, children whose thinking is qualitatively different. In sum, this is an interesting paper that addresses an important but neglected topic. One wonders how many potential contributions are lost because children's intellectual talents are inadequately educated.

PART IV: PSYCHOSOCIAL ISSUES

16

Cognitive and Behavioral Deficits Associated With Parental Alcohol Use

Naimah Z. Weinberg

National Institute on Drug Abuse, Rockville, Maryland

Objective: *To review and synthesize the scientific literature on cognitive and behavioral deficits associated with parental alcohol use and to highlight areas for future attention.* **Method:** *Studies of children of alcoholic parents (generally fathers) and of children prenatally exposed to alcohol were reviewed, focusing on cognitive and behavioral findings. Relevant animal studies were also reviewed.* **Results:** *Large numbers of children may be affected by parental alcohol use. Prenatal alcohol exposure is frequently associated with specific cognitive and behavioral deficits. Children of alcoholic fathers also can present with difficulties in learning, language, and temperament. Similarities in the deficits of these two groups were noted.* **Conclusions:** *The problems associated with parental alcohol use merit much more clinical and research attention. Current clinical approaches often fail to recognize the diagnostic and therapeutic significance of this history, and subgroups of alcohol-affected children may confound research studies of other problems. Subtle deficits in learning, language, and self-regulation may be the most developmentally devastating and the least likely to be identified and addressed effectively. This is an important area in which to combine behavior genetic and environmental approaches to understanding development.*

The adverse effects that parental alcohol use may have on children are numerous, pervasive, costly, and often enduring. This review brings together information on developmental findings associated with alcohol use by either parent. It draws on two generally separate bodies of scientific literature, that on "children of alcoholics," usually of alcoholic fathers, and that on prenatally exposed children of alcoholic women. Both are clinically significant populations whose family history is frequently unrecognized. Critical reviews of the literature on

---

Reprinted with permission from the *Journal of the American Academy of Child and Adolescent Psychiatry*, 1997, Vol. 36(9), 1177–1186.

The author thanks the staff and patients of the Center for Learning and Its Disorders of the Kennedy Krieger Institute for their contributions to the development of this paper.

children of alcoholics from the early 1990s can be found in Galanter (1991), Sher (1991), and Windle and Searles (1990); recent publications on the effects of prenatal alcohol exposure include the report by the Institute of Medicine (IOM, 1996) and Spohr and Steinhausen (1996).

Epidemiology, Magnitude, and Costs

Estimates of the number of children affected by parental alcohol use, and of the societal costs, are difficult to obtain. The number of children under age 18 who have an alcoholic parent has been estimated at 6.6 million (Russell et al., 1985); together with approximately 22 million adult children of alcoholics, it is estimated that one in eight Americans is the child of an alcoholic parent. These children are overrepresented in mental health and general medical systems (Children of Alcoholics Foundation, 1990); studies have found children of alcoholics to have higher rates of injury, poisoning, admissions for mental disorders and substance abuse, and general hospital admissions; longer lengths of stay; and higher total health care costs (Children of Alcoholics Foundation, 1990).

Studies estimating the incidence of children affected by prenatal exposure to alcohol have resulted in widely varying figures, from 0.5 to 3 births per 1,000, and higher in some populations (IOM, 1996), which translates to 2,000 to 12,000 fetal alcohol syndrome births per year in the United States. The difficulties in diagnosing the condition, and the pitfalls of various surveillance methods, complicate this important public health issue. Cost estimates vary considerably as well, ranging up to nearly 10 billion dollars per year (IOM, 1996). All researchers agree, however, that the costs to society of this preventable disabling condition are quite high. These costs do not include the expense of foster care, which many of these children require because of parental neglect and/or death.

Definitions

Defining alcohol-related problems in adults is a complicated and at times controversial undertaking (Babor et al., 1992), beyond the scope of this review. Diagnostic labels such as "alcohol abuse" and "alcohol dependence" obscure the heterogeneity (presence of meaningful subtypes) of problematic drinking. Furthermore, much of the field of alcohol study has concentrated on men, who drink more predominantly; definitions, epidemiology, consequences, patterns, and treatment issues differ for women and have received less attention. In fact, some drinking patterns (for example, binge drinking early in pregnancy) may not merit a *DSM-IV* (American Psychiatric Association, 1994) diagnosis of alcohol abuse or dependence but may damage a developing fetus. The studies cited below vary widely in their definition of alcoholism and in their methods of measurement.

This review will use the terms "children of alcoholics" (COAs) and "prenatally exposed (children)" (PNE), recognizing that each of these groups is somewhat heterogeneous. In studies of COAs, it is most often the father who has been identified as having alcohol-related problems; prenatal alcohol use is usually not determined or reported in these studies. In studies of PNE children, there is evidence on physical examination or by history of significant alcohol use by the mother during pregnancy, usually without reference to paternal alcohol use patterns; it includes fetal alcohol syndrome and related conditions.

Although the following discussion focuses on deficits in COAs and PNE children, such individuals should not be automatically regarded as impaired, given the lack of epidemiological data. Some researchers have concluded that "most [COAs] emerge. . .relatively intact psychologically and emotionally" (Searles and Windle, 1990, p. 3) and that "only a relatively small proportion [of PNE infants]. . .are born with [fetal alcohol syndrome]" (Abel and Hannigan, 1996, p. 70).

Methodological Issues

A daunting assortment of factors complicates the study of parental alcohol use and its potential impact on children's development (Russell, 1990). These include definitions of problematic alcohol use, choice of instruments, recall and reporting biases, sampling, psychiatric comorbidity, choice of control groups, exposure to other teratogens, and socioeconomic and other conditions. Lumping together heterogeneous groups of alcohol-using adults further obscures useful findings; for example, several studies suggest that alcoholics with antisocial tendencies differ significantly from those without. Changing patterns of alcohol use in the general population over time also alter the generalizability of findings. The issue of assortative mating merits particular attention, as it potentially complicates this field greatly yet is rarely recognized (Abel, 1992; Russell, 1990); this is the tendency of alcoholic women to marry alcoholic men, which is not taken into account in most studies of COAs or PNE children.

SOURCES OF DEFICIT

Prenatal Alcohol Exposure

Both animal and human studies have established that prenatal alcohol exposure can adversely affect many aspects of fetal brain development. Timing of alcohol exposure, maternal drinking patterns, and blood alcohol levels are all factors affecting fetal outcome. Maternal alcohol ingestion can alter several important chemical, endocrine, and immunological functions of the fetal brain (U.S. Department of Health and Human Services, 1993). Although several of these biochemical systems underlie behavior regulation (e.g., dopamine and serotonin systems), their role in mediating the damaging effects of maternal alcohol use has not been firmly established (Abel, 1990).

Anatomical changes that have been confirmed include adverse fetal nerve development (U.S. Department of Health and Human Services, 1993) and neuropathological anomalies including incomplete cortical development, enlarged lateral ventricles, absent or underdeveloped corpus callosum, and rudimentary cerebellum (Abel, 1990). Of particular interest are changes in the hippocampus, given its role in learning, memory, and inhibitory behavior control.

Alcohol is considered directly fetotoxic; the major metabolite acetaldehyde may also be damaging. Three possible mechanisms of action have been proposed (Schencker et al., 1990; U.S. Department of Health and Human Services, 1993): hypoxia, disturbances in prostaglandin physiology, and direct alcohol effects on cells.

Other Prenatal Conditions

Several conditions commonly associated with maternal alcohol ingestion can potentiate the harmful effects of alcohol exposure or may be harmful in their own right. These include tobacco use (Abel and Hannigan, 1996; Milberger et al., 1996), caffeine use (Schencker et al., 1990), use of illegal drugs (Chiriboga, 1993; Kilbey and Asghar, 1992; Robins and Mills, 1993; Sonderegger, 1992; Wetherington et al., 1996), maternal malnutrition (Abel and Hannigan, 1996; Schencker et al., 1990), and lack of prenatal care (Day et al., 1993). Maternal parity affects outcome in PNE children, as the severity of defects generally increases with each subsequent alcohol-exposed pregnancy in affected families (Abel, 1984; IOM, 1996), even if maternal drinking levels remain constant. There may be some racial and sex differences in susceptibility to fetal alcohol exposure (Abel and Hannigan, 1996; Weinberg et al., 1992).

The above factors can be significant confounding variables in studies of offspring of alcoholic parents, and they need to be taken into account in studies of these children.

Genetic Factors

Genetics can play several roles in the development of PNE and COA children. First, genetic factors inherited from either parent can contribute to fetal susceptibility to alcohol damage in utero; this may help explain the diversity and unpredictability of fetal outcomes after alcohol exposure. Second, parental alcohol use may alter the genetic material passed on to offspring (Abel, 1992; Durcan and Goldman, 1993). In fact, some of the effects that have been attributed to maternal alcohol use may in fact be due to *paternal* drinking prior to conception (Abel, 1992). Third, reviews of the literature on COAs point to familial, and likely genetic, susceptibilities to alcoholism and other neuropsychological characteristics (Cadoret, 1990; Searles, 1990; Tarter, 1991).

Postnatal Environment

Unfortunately, exposure to adverse developmental circumstances generally does not stop with the end of pregnancy. Families affected by parental alcohol use are more likely to suffer myriad psychosocial stressors, including economic instability and disruption (West and Prinz, 1987). Children then lack consistent caretaking, healthy and secure attachments, and environmental stability (O'Connor et al., 1993; Sher, 1991). Many are physically and emotionally neglected. Children in alcoholic families may be exposed at greater rates to family violence and abuse (Kumpfer and Bays, 1995). COAs also have been found to suffer greater rates of injury, poisonings, and medical hospitalizations (Bijur et al., 1992; Children of Alcoholics Foundation, 1990). Tarter et al. (1984) found significantly higher rates of traumatic head injury in sons of alcoholics, which may constitute another source of impairment. Even substance exposure may not end with birth; children may be deliberately intoxicated for sedation or amusement (Bays, 1990) or accidentally dosed with alcohol when intoxicated parents leave unattended toddlers exposed to alcoholic beverages (Chiriboga, 1993). Other toxic exposures such as lead poisoning and second-hand tobacco smoke may also be associated with heavy parental alcohol use. All of these factors have profound implications for the biological, psychological, and social development of children in alcoholic families.

Furthering our understanding of the sources of deficit in children of alcoholic parents requires a comprehensive developmental psychopathological approach which integrates the complex biological, psychological, and social factors involved. The growing field of behavior genetics offers an approach to understanding such complex problems. As noted by Kendler (1995), "untangling of the common complex psychiatric conditions. . .will require an integration of genetic and epidemiologic strategies" (p. 899). Studying biological factors does not obviate the need to work on environmental influences; on the contrary, Pike and Plomin (1996) note that "genetic research provides the best evidence for the importance of environmental influences" (p. 568) (see also Searles, 1990). Our increasingly sophisticated understanding of environmental risk factors, e.g., nonshared environment (Pike and Plomin, 1996), quantitative (Rutter, 1979), and qualitative (Jensen et al., 1990) approaches, should also be applied to the study of these high-risk children.

DEFICITS

Multisystem

The effects of prenatal alcohol exposure on children's development are increasingly recognized. The term "fetal alcohol syndrome" (FAS) refers to a specific constellation of findings; however, it is sometimes used loosely and imprecisely. Other terms, particularly "fetal alcohol effects" and "alcohol-related birth defects," have been used commonly to signify those offspring with some but not all of the features of FAS. Inconsistency and controversy around these terms have contributed to poor communication and confusion for clinicians and researchers.

Three criteria are necessary for a strict diagnosis of FAS: (1) growth retardation; (2) CNS involvement, including neurological abnormalities, developmental delays, behavioral or intellectual impairments; and (3) characteristic facies, including short palpebral fissures, thin upper lip, and elongated, flattened midface and philtrum. Many other physical anomalies have been described, but are neither necessary nor sufficient for the diagnosis; these include cardiac anomalies, urogenital defects, skeletal malformations, visual and auditory deficits, and altered immunological function.

The features of FAS show great variability among the individuals affected. The findings can also change over time for a particular individual; the facial features are difficult to recognize at birth and may be less obvious after onset of puberty. Thus, along with the emergence of behavioral and cognitive difficulties, the full syndrome is most often recognized (if at all) between ages 2 and 11 years (Aase, 1994). The deficits endure, however, and despite the variability in presentation and impairment, there is no cure or "outgrowing" the syndrome.

Many individuals show some of the features of FAS without the full syndrome. Aase et al. (1995) have proposed eliminating the term "fetal alcohol effects" and simply recording the information that is verifiable in such cases, such as "prenatal alcohol exposure" and whatever deficits have been found. The Institute of Medicine report (IOM, 1996) discusses in detail the controversy, efforts, and needs for consistent terminology. They propose adoption of five diagnostic categories: (1) "FAS" (to which they would add a fourth criterion requiring a history of prenatal alcohol exposure); (2) "FAS without confirmed maternal alcohol exposure"; (3) "partial FAS," when there is a history of alcohol exposure and findings of at least one of the three FAS criteria; (4) "alcohol-related birth defects (ARBD)," designating a history of exposure and the presence of consistent physical anomalies; and (5) "alcohol-related neurodevelopmental disorder (ARND)," designating those with a history of exposure and neurodevelopmental abnormalities and/or behavioral or cognitive deficits. As in the *DSM*, more than one diagnosis can be made if criteria are met.

Cognitive

The following discussion of cognitive findings in children affected by parental alcohol use addresses separately the studies of PNE children and COAs. These two groups of children may overlap, a fact not always recognized by the study design; similarities between the two groups, however, may not all be attributable to assortative mating.

IQ and mental retardation. Prenatal alcohol exposure is generally cited as the most common nongenetic cause of mental retardation. (That it is completely preventable but receives little attention is also noted in the literature.) However, it must be kept in mind that retardation is *not* a criterion for the diagnosis of FAS. Studies of children with FAS have found IQ scores generally in the mild mentally retarded (60s) range (IOM, 1996). A wide variation, however, is noted. For "partial FAS," IQ is frequently in the borderline (70 to 85) range. As will be discussed below, behavior problems and deficits in judgment are frequently more problematic and adaptively impairing than the IQ would suggest. Where the prenatal alcohol exposure in a middle-class white population followed longitudinally was moderate to heavy, Streissguth's group has found lower IQ with specific weaknesses, but nonetheless average scores overall (Streissguth et al., 1990). Coles' group, working with African-Americans of lower socioeconomic status, found similar results (Coles et al., 1991). Streissguth et al. (1991) reported stability of IQ over extended periods of time and development, leading them to conclude that clinicians need to be realistic in planning for long-term behavioral and educational service needs; often what are described as the young child's bright appearance and good family resources lead to an unrealistic prognosis.

The literature on cognitive findings in COAs is characterized by Tarter et al. (1990) as "confusing and conflicting," reflecting all the difficulties of research in this area. No single conclusion can be drawn regarding overall IQ findings in COAs; specific areas of deficit that have been found are discussed below.

Learning disabilities. As reviewed by Driscoll et al. (1990), findings on learning deficits in PNE children derive from studies in animals as well as humans. In various studies, animals exposed to alcohol in utero demonstrated feeding difficulties, altered reflex development and motor functioning, hyperactivity and attention deficits, and impaired learning, including poorer associative and passive avoidance learning. Problems with spatial deficits were persistent. The findings were thought to be fairly congruent with those in PNE humans, who as infants take longer to extinguish on an operant task. Longitudinal studies of PNE children show some consistency in patterns of impairment, with those children exposed to lesser amounts of alcohol showing deficits similar to, but less severe than, those seen in

FAS children. Streissguth et al. (1990), in a longitudinal study of PNE middle-class white children, found significant weaknesses on arithmetic skills on the Wide Range Achievement Test among 7-year-olds. Neuropsychological tests showed impaired spatial memory and integration, impaired verbal memory, reduced flexible problem-solving skills, and poor attention. Teachers described these children as less cooperative, more impulsive, and with poor grammar, information retention, and comprehension. Data further suggested that binge-drinking patterns in pregnancy were associated with poorer reading and math skills, and risk for learning disabilities, in 7-year-olds; there were suggestions of a dose-response relationship. A pattern of nonverbal learning disabilities, with poor spatial organization and math skills, memory, and problem-solving, was also described. Deficits persisted into adolescence (Streissguth et al., 1994). Coles et al. (1991), working with an African-American population of low socioeconomic status, found that maternal alcohol use, regardless of the timing of the drinking, was associated with poor sequential processing, early math, and pre-reading skills. The pattern of learning problems, as well as behavioral problems discussed below, is noted to resemble those resulting from frontal lobe damage (IOM, 1996). Of note, a case-control study by Marino et al. (1987) found that children identified as learning-disabled were more than seven times as likely to show the physical stigmata of prenatal alcohol exposure when specifically examined for it; this suggests that indeed special education settings serve a large number of PNE children, despite the failures to recognize them as such.

There is also a body of literature, albeit limited, on learning and behavior in animals whose *fathers* were exposed to alcohol prior to conception. Too few studies are available to generalize; however, the findings are tantalizing, holding the potential for changes in our thinking about the mechanisms and source of deficits in offspring of alcohol-using parents (Abel, 1992). For example, Abel (1993) found that rats sired by alcohol-treated males demonstrated increased activity levels, and a differential response to amphetamine, in comparison with the offspring of ad libitum and pair-fed controls.

Efforts to study patterns of learning difficulties in COAs (children of alcoholic men) have been complicated by numerous factors. Nonetheless, the available studies suggest some consistent patterns of weakness and a surprising degree of overlap with the studies of PNE children. Studies by Tarter and colleagues (Tarter et al., 1984, 1990) found weaknesses in verbal ability and abstraction/conceptual reasoning in the presence of normal range IQ. In reviewing this area, Tarter et al. (1990) state that COAs appear to experience cognitive impairments, although the etiology, pattern, and substrate cannot currently be defined. They cite Danish adoption studies as supporting the presence of deficits in academic achievement, verbal information processing, and planning and abstraction abilities even when the COA child is raised in a nonalcoholic environment. Reich et al. (1993) were surprised to find only a weakness in reading on achievement testing in children with one alcoholic parent. Schandler et al. (1993) studied adolescent children of alcoholic fathers, who demonstrated poorer visuospatial learning, deficits which resembled those in detoxified alcoholics they studied. Garland et al. (1993) reported that adult male COAs showed poorer visual-spatial learning. In a review of studies on sons of male alcoholics, Pihl et al. (1990) found frequent reports of reduced performance on tests involving abstraction or problem-solving; studies have also found deficits in Performance IQ, visual-spatial skills, perceptual-motor skills, and auditory-visual attention span. Both Pihl et al. (1990) and Tarter et al. (1990) note how the constellation of impairments resembles that in prefrontal cortical trauma. Thus, the literature reviewed suggests some congruency in findings between PNE children and COAs.

Language disorder. Those studies that have examined language functioning in PNE children suggest that there are patterns of deficit; however, as noted in reviews by Abkarian (1992) and the Institute of Medicine (1996), there is a paucity of studies in this very important area. Some have found deficits in semantics, syntax, and pragmatics of speech. The clinical description is of good superficial speech and sociability that belie later deficits in both language and peer relationships. Given the significance that language skills have for ego development and self-regulation, further studies are clearly indicated, with attention given to the possible role of language disorder in the behavioral and social problems of these children.

With regard to COAs, Pihl et al. (1990) note numerous studies characterizing sons of male alcoholics as performing poorly on tests of linguistic ability. Both this group (Peterson et al., 1992) and Tarter's group (Tarter et al., 1990) relate these weaknesses to those of abstraction, problem-solving, and self-regulation, again pointing to possible deficits in the prefrontal cortex and to similarities to the PNE children.

Behavioral

Adaptive functioning. Studies on PNE children and on COAs note patterns of difficulties resembling deficits which accompany frontal lobe damage. Clinical reports repeatedly describe PNE children and adolescents as showing impaired judgment and poor adaptive behavior. Failure to learn from experience, affecting social, moral, and academic functioning, is often noted (IOM, 1996; LaDue et al., 1992), a very painful, frustrating, and vexing developmental impairment poignantly described by Dorris (1989). Such difficulties have no clear label and are not themselves the target of interventions, yet "maladaptive behaviors" are noted by Streissguth et al. (1991) to persist and to present the *greatest* difficulty in management of the PNE individual.

Several prominent researchers studying the neurological characteristics of COAs have noted a pattern of behavior problems corresponding to prefrontal cortical trauma (Pihl et al., 1990; Tarter et al., 1990). Impulsivity, impairments in regulation of social behavior, and poor emotional modulation are noted (Pihl et al., 1990); deficits in language and other executive functions may play a role in these failures of self-regulation (Tarter et al., 1990).

Attention-deficit hyperactivity disorder. Clinical and anecdotal reports frequently note symptoms of impulsivity, poor attention, and restlessness in both PNE children and COAs. However, rigorous studies have *not* confirmed a link between parental alcohol use and attention-deficit hyperactivity disorder (ADHD) in offspring. Several factors cloud this area of research, including the shifts in diagnostic criteria, environmental contributions, and mislabeling of conduct, oppositionality, and anxiety problems as ADHD.

In PNE children, controlled tests on vigilance tasks have yielded contradictory results among various study groups (IOM, 1996). Several have found no impairments relative to control children, despite clinical descriptions and teacher ratings suggesting otherwise.

Streissguth et al. (1995a), however, found that a measure of individual variation in reaction time on vigilance testing was enduring from ages 4 to 14 years, related to prenatal alcohol exposure, and predictive of later behavior ratings. Some clinicians who focus on children with PNE believe that these children may constitute an important subgroup among children with ADHD, differentially responsive to traditional treatments (O'Malley, 1994). Clarren (1995) characterizes children with FAS as having an "atypical attention deficit disorder" that shows no response or an idiosyncratic response to methylphenidate; it is reported that about half the children will respond to an alternative medication.

Many studies have looked at symptoms of ADHD in COAs (see reviews by Russell et al., 1985; Sher, 1991; West and Prinz, 1987; Windle, 1990). Methodology has varied greatly, as have study populations, resulting in some confusion. Studies on sons of male alcoholics have repeatedly described hyperactivity, impulsivity, hypersensitivity to stimuli, difficultics with self-regulation, impaired concentration, and poor self-control (Pihl et al., 1990). Genetic links have been considered (Cantwell, 1976; West and Prinz, 1987). In a comprehensive study of psychopathology in COAs, using standardized diagnostic interview techniques, Reich et al. (1993) did not find a clear association between ADHD and parental alcoholism; these authors suggest that some features of COA children (oppositionality, conduct disorder, anxiety) may be misdiagnosed as ADHD in other studies. This issue merits further elucidation.

Conduct disorder. Despite the descriptions of poor judgment, impulsivity, and early alcohol use, clear studies on conduct disorder in PNE offspring are lacking. In contrast, many studies have looked at conduct disturbances in COAs (see reviews by Pihl et al., 1990; Sher, 1991; West and Prinz, 1987). Reich et al. (1993) found a "very strong connection between parental alcoholism and. . .conduct disorder in children" (p. 998). Environmental factors account for much of the association; however, genetic links are still considered possible (Russell et al., 1985; Sher, 1991; West and Prinz, 1987). The shifting definitions of conduct disorder and an emerging understanding of behavioral genetics make this a challenging area of study.

Temperament. The literature on PNE children describes irritability in babies and gregariousness in pre-school children, but few studies have examined issues of personality and temperament (see O'Connor et al., 1993). Among COA researchers, however, much interest has focused on features of personality and temperament that may predict problematic alcohol use (Sher, 1991; Windle, 1990). Tarter (1991) describes the largely heritable temperament characteristics that predispose to alcoholism and how they interact with the environment. Recent genetic studies of traits such as novelty seeking may have significance for understanding the development of alcohol and drug abuse (Cloninger et al., 1996).

Risk for alcohol/substance use. Children of parents with alcohol-related difficulties face an increased risk of alcohol problems themselves. Studies have focused on risks and early alcohol use in COAs; among PNE adolescents, the combination of genetic predisposition and poor judgment is likely dangerous (Dorris, 1989; IOM, 1996) but has not been systematically studied (Streissguth et al., 1995b). Streissguth and her colleagues warn that the failures to recognize the multiple handicaps in PNE patients presenting for alcoholism treatment and to provide appropriate treatment accommodations are very costly for society (Streissguth et al., 1995b).

COAs are at risk for earlier onset of alcohol use, problematic drinking at younger ages, and heavier alcohol use than peers (Russell, 1990). Among adolescents, the disinhibition and impaired judgment associated with alcohol intoxication contribute to suicide, accidents (automobile and diving), unintended pregnancies, and exposure to human immunodeficiency virus, as well as social and school failure. COAs are also at greater risk for other substance abuse (Hawkins et al., 1992) and associated problems.

Not all COAs develop alcohol problems, however. While COAs should be aware of their increased risk, the wide array of environmental and genetic factors should be kept in mind when assessing an individual. Areas of resilience should be noted and nurtured as well (Kumpfer, in press; Weinberg, 1997).

Other psychiatric conditions. Several studies have looked at disorders of mood and anxiety and other features of COAs; a few have studied these problems in PNE children. These findings, and the associated methodological problems, are beyond the scope of this review; the interested reader is referred to Hill and Muka (1996), O'Connor et al. (1993), Reich et al. (1993), Sher (1991), Spohr and Steinhausen (1996), and Weinberg (1997).

INTERVENTIONS

Few scientific studies exist to guide treatment interventions with PNE children or children of alcoholic parents, despite the prevalence of these conditions. Lack of clinical recognition (diagnosis) is the first barrier to evaluating and designing appropriate interventions. The subtle and variable nature and the daunting psychosocial complications also inhibit enthusiasm for rigorous research on these populations. Thus, it is not currently known what benefits may derive from appropriate interventions with these vulnerable populations.

The treatment needs and related research needs of PNE children are outlined in the Institute of Medicine report (1996) and by Smith and Coles (1991). The available information points to the need for (1) early identification, for purposes of early intervention; (2) provision of special education services for the learning and language disabilities and other appropriate services such as supervised work and living situations, through and beyond adolescence, if necessary, to address the maladaptive behavior problems; (3) parent work and coordination with social and mental health services (Kumpfer et al., 1996; Smith and Coles, 1991); and (4) alternative medication trials. PNE children may constitute an unrecognized *subgroup* of ADHD, one that does *not* respond well to methylphenidate (Clarren, 1995; IOM, 1996). Until systematic research takes place, clinicians need to consider switching to other classes of medication that may prove more effective (Clarren, 1995).

There is virtually no *scientific* literature to guide treatment of young COAs. Appropriate interventions depend on the specific problems and deficits found; awareness of the family history can enhance treatment, even if it is not clear whether children improve when parents stop drinking (Russell et al., 1985; Williams, 1990). General treatment principles for working with COAs, which do not address specific cognitive or behavioral deficits, can be found in Rivinus (1991), Weinberg (1997), and Williams (1990); these are based on inference from the research base on characteristics of COAs and on clinical observation, and they need to be tested empirically. They include (1) education of COAs regarding their alcoholism risk; (2) work on problem-solving and coping skills; (3) referral to appropriate community resources, including Alateen, school-based student assistance programs, and parent or family skills training (Kumpfer et al., 1996; Weinberg, 1997); and (4) viewing the child as an individual with potential and supporting his or her resilience.

CONCLUSIONS

1. More children may be affected by parental alcohol use than are recognized by clinical, educational, and social institutions. They may, in fact, represent significant subgroups of children with ADHD, learning disabilities, language disorders, and other psychiatric conditions, for whom conventional treatments may be ineffective and may need to be altered.

2. The subtle deficits, particularly in adaptive functioning, in some PNE children and COAs, often represent the *greatest* risks to development. More attention is needed to identify and intervene with these risks.

3. A surprising degree of congruence appears to exist between some areas of cognitive and behavioral deficits in PNE children and in children of alcoholic fathers. It is not clear whether these two groups represent the same children (because of assortative mating) or whether there are biological and/or environmental factors affecting each group independently, leading to similar deficits. It appears likely that genetic or other biological factors underlie many of the common deficits, particularly those problem areas related to executive (frontal lobe) functioning, such as aggression, poor judgment, and impaired language skills. Teasing out the sources of these deficits holds potential for developing appropriate preventive interventions.

FUTURE NEEDS RELEVANT TO CHILD PSYCHIATRY

1. Further research is needed on the treatment of PNE children and COAs. The presence of possible subgroups in clinical studies merits particular attention. Development of effective interventions for the deficits in adaptive skills and judgment is particularly needed.

2. Studies of high-risk children need to take family alcohol history into account.

3. More epidemiological data are needed on the prevalence, characteristics, and severity of deficits associated with parental alcohol use. The inclusion of appropriate measures in population-based, clinically based, and services research studies can contribute toward a needed base of knowledge.

4. Professionals from the many disciplines who deal with these children need to communicate and coordinate to a greater extent, for both service and research purposes. Child psychiatrists in particular should join the research efforts on young PNE and COA populations.

5. The problems of children affected by parental alcohol use merit greater recognition in clinical training, practice, and continuing medical education (see Streissguth et al., 1992).

6. Clinician involvement is needed in prevention efforts, by (a) recognizing PNE characteristics in children whose mothers are still of childbearing age, to refer the mother for treatment and try to prevent increased damage in future children, and (b) counseling young COAs about their risk for later alcohol problems.

7. These children should also be studied for their sources of resilience and strength; those who have overcome their deficits and adverse backgrounds can shed light on the factors needed to enhance competence and success.

REFERENCES

Aase JM (1994), Clinical recognition of FAS: difficulties of detection and diagnosis. *Alcohol Health Res World* 18:5–9

Aase JM, Jones KL, Clarren SK (1995), Do we need the term "FAE"? *Pediatrics* 95:428–430

Abel EL (1984), *Fetal Alcohol Syndrome and Fetal Alcohol Effects*. New York: Plenum

Abel EL (1990), *Fetal Alcohol Syndrome*. Oradell, NJ: Medical Economics Company

Abel EL (1992), Paternal exposure to alcohol. In: *Perinatal Substance Abuse: Research Findings and Clinical Implications*, Sonderegger TB, ed. Baltimore: Johns Hopkins University Press, pp 132–160

Abel EL (1993), Paternal alcohol exposure and hyperactivity in rat offspring: effects of amphetamine. *Neurotoxicol Teratol* 15:445–449

Abel EL, Hannigan JH (1996), Risk factors and pathogenesis. In: *Alcohol, Pregnancy and the Developing Child*, Spohr HL, Steinhausen HC, eds. Cambridge, England: Cambridge University Press, pp 63–96

Abkarian GG (1992), Communication effects of prenatal alcohol exposure. *J Commun Disord* 25:221–240

American Psychiatric Association (1994), *Diagnostic and Statistical Manual of Mental Disorders, 4th edition (DSM-IV)*. Washington, DC: American Psychiatric Association

Babor TF, Hofmann M, DelBoca FK et al. (1992), Types of alcoholics, I: evidence for an empirically derived typology based on indicators of vulnerability and severity. *Arch Gen Psychiatry* 49:599–608

Bays J (1990), Substance abuse and child abuse: impact of addiction on the child. *Pediatr Clin North Am* 37:881–904

Bijur PE, Kurzon M, Overpeck MD, Scheidt PC (1992), Parental alcohol use, problem drinking, and children's injuries. *JAMA* 267:3166–3171

Cadoret RJ (1990), Genetics of alcoholism. In: *Alcohol and the Family: Research and Clinical Perspectives*, Collins RL, Leonard KE, Searles JS, eds. New York: Guilford, pp 39–78

Cantwell DP (1976), Genetic factors in the hyperactive syndrome. *J Am Acad Child Psychiatry* 15:214–223

Children of Alcoholics Foundation (1990), *Children of Alcoholics in the Medical System: Hidden Problems, Hidden Costs*. New York: Children of Alcoholics Foundation

Chiriboga CA (1993), Fetal effects. *Neurol Clin* 11:707–728

Clarren SK (1995), Fetal alcohol syndrome. Invited presentation at the conference on the Spectrum of Developmental Disabilities XVII: Behavior Belongs in the Brain—Neurobehavioral Syndromes. Baltimore: Johns Hopkins Medical Institutions

Cloninger CR, Adolfsson R, Svrakic NM (1996), Mapping genes for human personality. *Nat Genet* 12:3–4

Coles CD, Brown RT, Smith IE, Platzman KA, Erickson S, Falek A (1991), Effects of prenatal alcohol exposure at school age, I: physical and cognitive development. *Neurotoxicol Teratol* 13:357–367

Day NL, Cottreau CM, Richardson GA (1993), The epidemiology of alcohol, marijuana, and cocaine use among women of childbearing age and pregnant women. *Clin Obstet Gynecol* 36:232–245

Dorris M (1989), *The Broken Cord*. New York: Harper & Row

Driscoll CD, Streissguth AP, Riley EP (1990), Prenatal alcohol exposure: comparability of effects in humans and animal models. *Neurotoxicol Teratol* 12:231–237

Durcan MJ, Goldman D (1993), Genomic imprinting: implications for behavioral genetics. *Behav Genet* 23:137–143

Galanter M, ed (1991), *Recent Developments in Alcoholism*, Vol 9: *Children of Alcoholics*. New York: Plenum

Garland JA, Parsons OA, Nixon SJ (1993), Visual-spatial learning in nonalcoholic young adults with and those without a family history of alcoholism. *J Stud Alcohol* 54:219–224

Hawkins JD, Catalano RF, Miller JY (1992), Risk and protective factors for alcohol and other drug abuse in adolescence and early adulthood: implications for substance abuse prevention. *Psychol Bull* 112:64–105

Hill SY, Muka D (1996), Childhood psychopathology in children from families of alcoholic female probands. *J Am Acad Child Adolesc Psychiatry* 35:725–733

Institute of Medicine, Committee to Study Fetal Alcohol Syndrome (1996), *Fetal Alcohol Syndrome: Diagnosis, Epidemiology, Prevention, and Treatment*, Stratton K, Howe C, Battaglia F, eds. Washington, DC: National Academy Press

Jensen PS, Bloedau L, Degroot J, Ussery T, Davis H (1990), Children at risk, I: risk factors and child symptomatology. *J Am Acad Child Adolesc Psychiatry* 29:51–59

Kendler KS (1995), Genetic epidemiology in psychiatry (commentary). *Arch Gen Psychiatry* 52:895–899

Kilbey MM, Asghar K, eds (1992), *Methodological Issues in Epidemiological, Prevention, and Treatment Research on Drug-Exposed Women and Their Children*. Rockville, MD: US Department of Health and Human Services

Kumpfer KL (in press), Factors and processes contributing to resilience: the resilience framework. In: *Resilience and Development: Positive Life Adaptations*, Glantz M, Johnson J, Huffman L, eds. New York: Plenum

Kumpfer KL, Bays J (1995), Child abuse and tobacco, alcohol and other drug abuse: causality, coincidence or controversy? In: *The Encyclopedia of Drugs and Alcohol*, Jaffe JH, ed. New York: MacMillan, pp 217–222

Kumpfer KL, Molgaard V, Spoth R (1996), Strengthening Families Program for the prevention of delinquency and drug use. In: *Preventing Childhood Disorders, Substance Abuse, and Delinquency*, Peters RD, McMahon RJ, eds. Thousand Oaks, CA: Sage

LaDue RA, Streissguth AP, Randels SP (1992), Clinical considerations pertaining to fetal alcohol syndrome. In: *Perinatal Substance Abuse: Research Findings and Clinical Implications*, Sonderegger TB, ed. Baltimore: Johns Hopkins University Press, pp 104–131

Marino RV, Scholl TO, Karp RJ, Yanoff JM (1987), Minor physical anomalies and learning disability: what is the prenatal component? *J Natl Med Assoc* 79:37–39

Milberger S, Biederman J, Faraone SV, Chen L, Jones J (1996), Is maternal smoking during pregnancy a risk factor for attention deficit hyperactivity disorder in children? *Am J Psychiatry* 153:1138–1142

O'Connor MJ, Sigman M, Kasari C (1993), Interactional model for the association among maternal alcohol use, mother–infant interaction, and infant cognitive development. *Infant Behav Dev* 16:177–192

O'Malley KD (1994), Fetal alcohol effect and ADHD (letter). *J Am Acad Child Adolesc Psychiatry* 33:1059–1060

Peterson JB, Finn PR, Pihl RO (1992), Cognitive dysfunction and the inherited predisposition to alcoholism. *J Stud Alcohol* 53:154–160

Pihl RO, Peterson J, Finn P (1990), Inherited predisposition to alcoholism: characteristics of sons of male alcoholics. *J Abnorm Psychol* 99:291–301

Pike A, Plomin R (1996), Importance of nonshared environmental factors for childhood and adolescent psychopathology. *J Am Acad Child Adolesc Psychiatry* 35:560–570

Reich W, Earles F, Frankel O, Shayka JJ (1993), Psychopathology in children of alcoholics. *J Am Acad Child Adolesc Psychiatry* 32:995–1002

Rivinus TM, ed (1991), *Children of Chemically Dependent Parents: Multiperspectives From the Cutting Edge*. New York: Brunner/Mazel

Robins LN, Mills JL, eds (1993), Effects of in utero exposure to street drugs. *Am J Public Health* 3(suppl)

Russell M (1990), Prevalence of alcoholism among children of alcoholics. In: *Children of Alcoholics: Critical Perspectives*, Windle M, Searles JS, eds. New York: Guilford, pp 9–38

Russell M, Henderson C, Blume SB (1985), *Children of Alcoholics: A Review of the Literature*. New York: Children of Alcoholics Foundation

Rutter M (1979), Protective factors in children's response to stress and disadvantage. In: *Social Competence in Children*, Kent MW, Rolf JE, eds. Hanover, NH: University Press of New England

Schandler SL, Brannock JC, Cohen MJ, Mendez J (1993), Spatial learning deficits in adolescent children of alcoholics. *Exp Clin Psychopharmacol* 1:207–214

Schencker S, Becker HC, Randall CL, Phillips DK, Baskin GS, Henderson GI (1990), Fetal alcohol syndrome: current status of pathogenesis. *Alcohol Clin Exp Res* 14:635–647

Searles JS (1990), Behavior genetics research and risk for alcoholism among children of alcoholics. In: *Children of Alcoholics: Critical Perspectives*, Windle M, Searles JS, eds. New York: Guilford, pp 99–128

Searles JS, Windle M (1990), Introduction and overview: salient issues in the children of alcoholics literature. In: *Children of Alcoholics: Critical Perspectives*, Windle M, Searles JS, eds. New York: Guilford, pp 1–8

Sher KJ (1991), *Children of Alcoholics: The Critical Appraisal of Theory and Research*. Chicago: University of Chicago Press

Smith IE, Coles CD (1991), Multilevel intervention for prevention of fetal alcohol syndrome and effects of prenatal alcohol exposure. In: *Children of Alcoholics*, Galanter M, ed. New York: Plenum, pp 165–180

Sonderegger TB, ed (1992), *Perinatal Substance Abuse: Research Findings and Clinical Implications*. Baltimore: Johns Hopkins University Press

Spohr H, Steinhausen H, eds (1996), *Alcohol, Pregnancy, and the Developing Child*. New York: Cambridge University Press

Streissguth AP, Aase JM, Clarren SK, Randels SP, LaDue RA, Smith DF (1991), Fetal Alcohol syndrome in adolescents and adults. *JAMA* 265:1961–1967

Streissguth AP, Barr HM, Olson HC, Sampson PD, Bookstein FL, Burgess DM (1994), Drinking during pregnancy decreases word attack and arithmetic scores on standardized test: adolescent data from a population-based prospective study. *Alcohol Clin Exp Res* 18:248–254

Streissguth AP, Barr HM, Sampson PD (1990), Moderate prenatal alcohol exposure: effects on child IQ and learning problems at age 71/2 years. *Alcohol Clin Exp Res* 14:662–669

Streissguth AP, Bookstein FL, Sampson PD, Barr HM (1995a), Attention: prenatal alcohol and continuities of vigilance and attentional problems from 4 through 14 years. *Dev Psychopathol* 7:419–446

Streissguth AP, Moon-Jordan A, Clarren SK (1995b), Alcoholism in four patients with fetal alcohol syndrome: recommendations for treatment. *Alcohol Treat Q* 13:89–102

Streissguth AP, Randels SP, Smith DF (1992), "Fetal alcohol syndrome": reply. *J Am Acad Child Adolesc Psychiatry* 31:563–564

Tarter RE (1991), Developmental behavior-genetic perspective of alcoholism etiology. In: *Children of Alcoholics*, Galanter M, ed. New York: Plenum, pp 53–67

Tarter RE, Hegedus AM, Goldstein G, Shelly D, Alterman AI (1984), Adolescent sons of alcoholics: neuropsychological and personality characteristics. *Alcohol Clin Exp Res* 8:216–221

Tarter RE, Laird SB, Moss HB (1990), Neuropsychological and neurophysiological characteristics of children of alcoholics. In: *Children of Alcoholics: Critical Perspectives*, Windle M, Searles JS, eds. New York: Guilford, pp 79–106

US Department of Health and Human Services (1993), *Eighth Special Report to the US Congress on Alcohol and Health.* Rockville, MD: US Department of Health and Human Services

Weinberg J, Zimmerberg B, Sonderegger TB (1992), Gender-specific effects of perinatal exposure to alcohol and other drugs. In: *Perinatal Substance Abuse: Research Findings and Clinical Implications*, Sonderegger, TB, ed. Baltimore: Johns Hopkins University Press, pp 51–89

Weinberg NZ (1997), Developmental effects of parental alcohol use. In: *Handbook of Child and Adolescent Psychiatry*, Noshpitz JD, editor in chief, Vol 4: *Varieties of Development*, Alessi N, ed. New York: Wiley, pp 171–187

West MO, Prinz RJ (1987), Parental alcoholism and childhood psychopathology. *Psychol Bull* 102:204–218

Wetherington CL, Smeriglio VL, Finnegan LP, eds (1996), *Behavioral Studies of Drug-Exposed Offspring: Methodological Issues in Human and Animal Research.* Rockville, MD: US Department of Health and Human Services

Williams CN (1990), Prevention and treatment approaches for children of alcoholics. In: *Children of Alcoholics: Critical Perspectives*, Windle M, Searles JS, eds. New York: Guilford, pp 187–216

Windle M (1990), Temperament and personality attributes of children of alcoholics. In: *Children of Alcoholics: Critical Perspectives*, Windle M, Searles JS, eds. New York: Guilford, pp 129–167

Windle M, Searles JS (1990), Summary, integration, and future directions: toward a life-span perspective. In: *Children of Alcoholics: Critical Perspectives*, Windle M, Searles JS, eds. New York: Guilford, pp 217–238

17

The Effects of Infant Child Care on Infant-Mother Attachment Security: Results of the NICHD Study of Early Child Care

NICHD Early Child Care Research Network
Bethesda, Maryland

The aims of this investigation were to determine whether Strange Situation attachment classifications were equally valid for infants with and without extensive child-care experience in the first year of life and whether early child-care experience, alone or in combination with mother/child factors, was associated with attachment security, and specifically with insecure-avoidant attachment. Participants were 1,153 infants and their mothers at the 10 sites of the NICHD Study of Early Child Care. Mothers were interviewed, given questionnaires, and observed in play and in the home when their infants were from 1 to 15 months of age; infants were observed in child care at 6 and 15 months and in the Strange Situation at 15 months. Infants with extensive child-care experience did not differ from infants without child care in the distress they exhibited during separations from mother in the Strange Situation or in the confidence with which trained coders assigned them attachment classifications. There were no

Reprinted with permission from *Child Development*, 1997, Vol. 68(5), 860–879.

This study is directed by a steering committee and supported by NICHD through a cooperative agreement (U10), which calls for scientific collaboration between the grantees and the NICHD staff. The participating investigators are listed in alphabetical order with their institutional affiliations designated by number: Mark Appelbaum (14), Dee Ann Batten (14), Jay Belsky (2), Cathryn Booth (12), Robert Bradley (4), Celia Brownell (9), Bettye Caldwell (4), Susan Campbell (9), Alison Clarke-Stewart (5), Jeffrey Cohn (9), Martha Cox (8), Kaye Fendt (1), Sarah Friedman (1), Kathryn Hirsh-Pasek (3), Aletha Huston (6), Bonnie Knoke (1), Nancy Marshall (15), Kathleen McCartney (7), Marion O'Brien (6), Margaret Tresch Owen (10), Deborah Phillips (11), Henry Ricciuti (1), Susan Spieker (12), Deborah Lowe Vandell (13), Marsha Weinraub (3). The institutional affiliations, in alphabetical order, are the National Institute of Child Health and Human Development (1), Pennsylvania State University (2), Temple University (3), University of Arkansas at Little Rock (4), University of California, Irvine (5), University of Kansas (6), University of New Hampshire (7), University of North Carolina—Chapel Hill (8), University of Pittsburgh (9), University of Texas—Dallas (10), University of Virginia (11), University of Washington (12), University of Wisconsin—Madison (13), Vanderbilt University (14), Wellesley College (15). We wish to express our appreciation to the study coordinators at each site who supervised the data collection, to the research assistants who collected the data, and especially to the families and child-care providers who welcomed us into their homes and workplaces with good grace, and cooperated willingly with our repeated requests for information.

significant main effects of child-care experience (quality, amount, age of entry, stability, or type of care) on attachment security or avoidance. There were, however, significant main effects of maternal sensitivity and responsiveness. Significant interaction effects revealed that infants were less likely to be secure when low maternal sensitivity/responsiveness was combined with poor quality child care, more than minimal amounts of child care, or more than one care arrangement. In addition, boys experiencing many hours in care and girls in minimal amounts of care were somewhat less likely to be securely attached.

INTRODUCTION

The prospect that routine nonmaternal care in the first year of life might adversely affect the security of the infant's attachment to mother has been a subject of much discussion and debate (Belsky & Steinberg, 1978; Fox & Fein, 1990; Karen, 1994; Rutter, 1981). Evidence linking institutional rearing in the early years of life with affective and cognitive deficits led to early concerns that the experience of maternal deprivation posed hazards for the emotional well-being of young children (Bowlby, 1973). Later, these same concerns were voiced about day-care. Indeed, Barglow, Vaughn, and Molitor (1987) interpreted findings linking child care with elevated rates of insecure attachment, especially insecure-avoidant relationships, as evidence that babies experience daily separations as maternal rejection. Others drew attention to the possibility that nonmaternal care might affect proximal processes of mother-infant interaction and thus interfere with the infant-mother attachment relationship (Jaeger & Weinraub, 1990; Owen & Cox, 1988). Time away from baby, Brazelton argued (1985), might undermine a mother's ability to respond sensitively to the child, which would itself reduce the probability that a secure relationship would develop, and Sroufe (1988, p. 286) suggested that daily separations might both cause the infant to lose confidence in the availability and responsiveness of the parent and reduce the opportunities for "ongoing tuning of the emerging infant-caregiver interactive system."

Irrespective of the mechanisms responsible, it is notable that several multistudy analyses have documented statistically significant associations between routine nonmaternal care in the first year and elevated rates of insecure attachment as measured in the Strange Situation (Ainsworth & Wittig, 1969). In one of the first multistudy analyses of published research linking infant child care and attachment classifications, Belsky and Rovine (1988) evaluated child-care effects in five homogeneous samples of maritally intact, middle- and working-class families ($N = 491$). They found that infants who experienced 20 or more hours per week of routine child care in the first year were significantly more likely to be classified as insecurely attached to their mothers between 12 and 18 months of age than were infants with more limited child-care experience. The difference was particularly marked for insecure avoidance. In a subsequent analysis of 1,247 infants from a more heterogeneous set of studies, some of them unpublished, Clarke-Stewart (1989) documented a similar significant association. This pattern was confirmed by Lamb and Sternberg (1990), who included 790 cases from a subset of the studies compiled by Clarke-Stewart. Quite consistent across these multistudy investigations was the extent to which early and extensive child care, defined as 20 or more hours per week of routine child care in the first year, increased the risk of insecure infant-mother attachment. In Belsky and Rovine's (1988) analysis, 43% of the infants in early and extensive care were classified as insecurely attached; in the Clarke-Stewart (1989) analysis, the comparable figure was 36%; and in the data compiled by Lamb and Sternberg (1990), it was 40%. For infants with more limited child-care experience, the percentages of insecure attachment were 26%, 29%, and 27%, respectively, in the three investigations.

Despite the relative consistency of findings across these three compilations of multiple data sets, a more recent investigation of 105 infants revealed no significant relation between child-care experience and attachment security (Roggman, Langlois, Hubbs-Tait, & Rieser-Danner, 1994). One interpretation of Roggman et al.'s failure to replicate is that the studies in the compilations of Belsky, Clarke-Stewart, and Lamb were all published in the 1980s, when it was less common for mothers of infants to work full time than it is today. Perhaps now that a majority of mothers in the United States are employed outside the home in the infant's first year, there is no longer a difference in the likelihood of attachment insecurity. This could certainly be the case if mothers employed today represent a population that is demographically different (e.g., older) or more inclusive than those similarly employed a decade or more ago. A second possibility is that mothers placing their infants in child care in the 1990s are better informed about child-care issues and controversies. These mothers may attempt to compensate for potential deleterious effects of child care discussed at length in scholarly journals and the popular media over the past decade by being (on average) more sensitive, responsive, and involved with their infants when they are not at work, which could increase the probability of secure attachment in this group. Also worth considering are the possibilities that child-care providers have been affected by the ongoing discussion about the effects of infant care and of the importance of high-quality care, that employed mothers receive more social support today than they did in the past, and that families now have more work options and child-care choices.

The NICHD Study of Early Child Care, which was conducted in the 1990s, can shed light on this cohort issue. The study is nearly as large in terms of sample size ($N = 1,153$) as the largest of the multistudy analyses. It has the additional advantage of being a prospective, longitudinal investigation, in which infants were identified at birth and followed through their first 3 years—thus reducing selection biases. The kinds and amount of child care the children experienced were determined solely by their parents and tracked and observed by the researchers over this time period. The design of the NICHD Study was also unique in the opportunity it provided to examine the effects of child care "in context."

Examining child care in context is important because even multistudy analyses documenting elevated rates of insecurity among groups of infants with early and extensive child-care experience do not suggest that insecurity is inevitable. Although infants with early and extensive child care were more likely to be insecure than other infants, the majority—about 60%—of the infants with early and extensive childcare experience developed secure attachments to their mothers. Whether infant child-care experience is associated with increased rates of insecurity (or security) may depend on the nature of the care received and the ecological context—broadly conceived—in which it is embedded. More specifically, characteristics of child care (type, quality, amount, age of entry, and stability), as well as characteristics of the child (especially sex and temperament) and characteristics of the family (including social, psychological and economic resources), may interact with one another when it comes to shaping developmental outcomes, including attachment security.

Two types of hypotheses were advanced in this investigation regarding how this myriad of potentially influential factors might operate. Main effects hypotheses stipulated that features of child care in and of themselves would affect attachment security. More specifically, main effects hypotheses predicted that children in (1) early, (2) extensive, (3) unstable, or (4) poor quality care would have an increased likelihood of insecure attachment independent of conditions at home or in the child. Interactive effect hypotheses stipulated that child-care features would exert their influence on attachment security principally in interaction with aspects of the family and/or the child. One set of interaction effect hypotheses predicted that large amounts of child care, poor quality of child care, or frequent changes in care arrangements over time would promote insecure infant-mother attachment relationships principally when the child was otherwise at risk—by having a difficult temperament, being a male (Zaslow & Hayes, 1986), or residing in a home in which the mother had poor psychological adjustment or provided less sensitive and responsive care to the infant. Another set of interaction effect hypotheses predicted that when family or child risks were high (e.g., a poorly adjusted mother, a difficult infant, unresponsive caregiving), child care would serve a compensatory function in fostering the formation of a more secure infant-mother attachment bond, particularly when child care began early in life, and was stable, extensive, and of high quality.

To test these hypotheses and examine relations between the complex ecology of infant child care and infant-mother attachment security, the NICHD Study of Early Child Care analyzed measures of multiple features of the family, the child, and the child-care experience. Main effects and interaction effects involving child-care variables were tested over and above main effects of mother and child variables. Our goal was to determine the conditions (in the mother and the child) under which routine child-care experience in the first 15 months of life could lead to increased or decreased rates of infant-mother attachment insecurity, as well as avoidant insecurity in particular.

The data from previous studies of infant child-care experience and infant-mother attachment security have been subject to varied interpretations. One interpretation is that early and extensive child care as routinely experienced in the United States is a risk factor for the development of insecure infant-mother attachment relationships (e.g., Belsky, 1990). An alternative interpretation is that the results might be an artifact of the measurement strategy used for assessing attachment security (e.g., Clarke-Stewart, 1989). The latter interpretation suggests that the apparent elevated rates of insecurity, and especially of avoidant insecurity, might be a result of the fact that children who have experienced the multiple separations associated with child care are not especially stressed by the Strange Situation episodes designed to elicit attachment behavior. Thus, the Strange Situation may not be a valid measure of attachment for these children.

A meta-analysis and a review of attachment studies revealed no significant differences in distress or exploration for children with and without child-care experience (Clarke-Stewart & Fein, 1983; McCartney & Phillips, 1988), and two more recent attempts to investigate this issue did not find that avoidant behavior in the Strange Situation was an artifact of past experience with separations and reunions. Belsky and Braungart (1991) found that the infants with extensive child-care experience who were classified as insecure-avoidant were no less distressed or more exploratory in the reunion episodes than similarly classified infants with limited child-care experience, and Berger, Levy, and Compaan (1995) found that classifications of children's attachment security in a standard pediatric check-up were highly concordant with Strange Situation classifications whether the infants had extensive child-care experience in the first year or not. However, these studies were based on small samples, and the issue merits further investigation.

One purpose of the current inquiry was to explore further the validity of the Strange Situation for assessing the attachment security of infants with extensive experience in child care. A subsample of infants who experienced more than 30 hr per week of child care from 4 months to 15 months was compared with a sample of infants who had fewer than 10 hr per week of child care during this period, in terms of (1) their distress during separations in the Strange Situation, and (2) the confidence with which coders assigned them secure or insecure classifications.

In brief, then, the aims of this investigation were fourfold: (1) to determine if attachment classifications made on the basis of Strange Situation behavior were equally valid for infants with and without extensive child-care experience in the first year of life; (2) to identify differences in the probability of attachment security in infants with varying child-care experience (in terms of quality, amount, age of entry, stability, and type of care); (3) to identify the combination of factors (mother/child and child-care) under which child-care experience was associated with increased or decreased rates of attachment security; and (4) to determine whether early child-care experience was associated specifically with insecure-avoidant attachment.

METHOD

Participants

Participants in the NICHD Study of Early Child Care were recruited throughout 1991 from 31 hospitals near the following sites: Little Rock, AR; Orange County, CA; Lawrence and Topeka, KS; Boston, MA; Philadelphia, PA; Pittsburgh, PA; Charlottesville, VA; Morganton and Hickory, NC; Seattle, WA; and Madison, WI. Potential participants were selected from among 8,986 mothers giving birth during selected 24 hr sampling periods. Participants were selected in accordance with a conditionally random sampling plan that was designed to ensure that the recruited families reflected the demographic diversity (economic, educational, and ethnic) of the catchment area at each site. The recruited families included 24% ethnic-minority children, 10% low-education mothers, and 14% single mothers (note that these percentages are not mutually exclusive), and did not differ significantly from the families in the catchment areas on these variables. Participants were excluded from the sample if (1) the mother was under 18; (2) the mother did not speak English; (3) the family planned to move; (4) the child was hospitalized for more than 7 days following birth or had obvious disabilities; or (5) the mother had a known or acknowledged substance abuse problem. A total of 1,364 families with healthy newborns were enrolled; 58% of the families

TABLE 1
Sample Characteristics for Families Included in Attachment Analyses

Characteristics	%
Child ethnicity:	
European American, non-Hispanic	81.5
African American, non-Hispanic	11.9
Hispanic	5.7
Other	.9
Child sex:	
Girls	49.4
Boys	50.6
Maternal education:	
<12 years	8.4
High school or GED	20.2
Some college	34.2
B.A.	21.9
Postgraduate	15.3
Husband/partner in the home	86.9
Child-care plans at birth:	
Full-time	53
Part-time	23
None	24

who were asked agreed to participate in the study. Of the mothers recruited, 53% planned to work full time, 23% part time, and 24% did not intend to be employed during the child's first year.

Strange Situation data for 1,153 infants (84.5% of those recruited) are included in the major analyses in this report. (The Strange Situation was administered to 1,201 dyads; six were uncodable due to technical errors; 42 cases were eventually excluded because they received an Unclassifiable "U" code.) Characteristics of these families are presented in Table 1. (Note that analyses specifically pertaining to the effects of child care on the attachment security of ethnic-minority children will be included in a forthcoming paper addressing a broader set of outcomes for these children.) The 211 mother-infant dyads who did not contribute Strange Situation data were compared with the rest of the sample on seven variables measured when the infants were 1 month old. There were no differences between the two groups on income-to-needs ratio, maternal depression, and mother's or child's race (European American versus non-European American). However, those who did not contribute Strange Situation data, compared with those who did, were more likely to have boys (61.7% versus 50.6%, likelihood chi-square ratio $= 5.74$, $p < .02$), to be single mothers (22.9% versus 12.9%, likelihood chi-square $= 14.45$, $p < .001$), and to have more positive attitudes about the benefits of maternal employment for children (20.0% versus 19.1%), $F(1, 1279) = 10.19$, $p < .002$. (See below for description of these measures.)

Overview of Data Collection

Visits to the families occurred when the infants were 1, 6, and 15 months old. Observations in child-care arrangements were conducted when the infants were 6 and 15 months old. The Strange Situation assessment of infant attachment security (Ainsworth, Blehar, Waters, & Wall, 1978) was conducted in a laboratory playroom visit when the infants were 15 months old (± 1 month). Telephone interviews to update maternal employment and child-care information were conducted when the infants were 3, 9, and 12 months old, and phone calls to update information on child care and to schedule the 6 and 15 month observations occurred when the infants were 5 and 14 months old.

At all home visits, mothers reported on a variety of factors, including household composition and family income. In addition, at the 1 month visit, mothers completed a modified Attitude toward Maternal Employment Questionnaire (Greenberger, Goldberg, Crawford, & Granger, 1988). At 6 months, they completed a modified Infant Temperament Questionnaire (ITQ; Carey & McDevitt, 1978), and selected scales of the NEO Personality Inventory (Costa & McCrae, 1985), and at 1, 6, and 15 months, the Center for Epidemiologic Studies Depression Scale (CES-D; Radloff, 1977). At the 6 and 15 month home visits, mothers and infants were videotaped in a 15 min semistructured play interaction adapted from a procedure used by Vandell (1979), and the home visitor completed the Infant/Toddler HOME Scale (HOME; Caldwell & Bradley, 1984).

Infants in child care at 6 and 15 months were observed for 2 half-days in the child-care arrangement in which they spent the most time, using the Observational Record of the Caregiving, Environment (ORCE) developed for this project (see NICHD Early Child Care Research Network, 1996).

Overview of Measures

The presentation of measures is conceptually organized to reflect how variables functioned in the analyses. We first present measures used as control variables in the substantive analyses of the effects of child care, followed by mother and child measures that are employed as ecological parameters likely to interact with child-care variables, then child-care variables themselves, and, finally, the dependent construct of the study, attachment security.

Control variables. To reduce the risk of generating spurious findings, a number of possible control variables tapping family and mother characteristics were used in correlational analyses with the child-care parameters under study and with attachment security. These included family income and structure, and maternal child-rearing beliefs, locus of control, feelings about the pregnancy, separation anxiety, parenting stress, education, race, and beliefs about the benefits of maternal employment.[1] Two variables met our criteria for control variables in that they were related to both attachment security and child-care parameters: an income-to-needs ratio and a measure of the mother's beliefs about the benefits of maternal employment.

The income-to-needs ratio is an index of family economic resources, with higher scores indicating greater financial resources per person in the household. It was computed from

[1]These measures are described in NICHD Early Child Care Research Network (1997).

maternal interview items collected at each home visit. Family income (exclusive of welfare payments) was divided by the poverty threshold, which was based on total family size. This variable was averaged across the three assessments at 1, 6, and 15 months to create an overall *average income-to-needs* ratio. Higher average income-to-needs ratios significantly predicted younger age of entry into care, $r(1,149) = -.16$, $p < .001$. They also predicted higher-quality care, $r(690) = .18$, $p < .001$, for positive caregiving frequency, and $r(688) = .16$, $p < .001$, for positive caregiving ratings, the two measures of child-care quality described below; more hours of care, $r(1,149) = .17$, $p < .001$; and more starts of different care arrangements, $r(1,149) = .07$, $p < .05$. Families of secure infants had higher average income-to-needs ratios than did families of insecure infants, $t(1,149) = 2.24$, $p < .05$.

The *beliefs about benefits of maternal employment* measure was created by summing five 6 point items from the Attitude toward Maternal Employment Questionnaire administered at the 1 month visit (Greenberger et al., 1988). Cronbach's alpha was .80. Higher scores reflected the belief that maternal employment was beneficial for children (e.g., "Children whose mothers work are more independent and able to do things for themselves"). Stronger beliefs in the benefits of maternal employment for children's development were associated with earlier entry into child care, $r(1,151) = -.26$, $p < .001$; more hours of care, $r(1,151) = .38$, $p < .001$; more care starts, $r(1,151) = .18$, $p < .001$; and lower-quality care, $r(691) = -.12$, $p = .001$, for positive caregiving frequency and $r(689) = -.19$, $p < .001$ for positive caregiving ratings. Mothers of secure infants had weaker beliefs about the benefits of maternal employment for child development than did mothers of insecure infants, $t(1,151) = 2.68$, $p < .01$.

Child and family measures. To reduce the number of variables analyzed, increase measurement reliability, and increase sample size by including participants with some missing values, five composite variables were created from the mother and child measures.

A composite measure of the mother's *psychological adjustment* was created by summing the average of the three CES-D depression scores (reverse-scored) from the three ages plus scores on three scales of the NEO Personality Inventory: neuroticism, the extent to which the mother indicated she is anxious, hostile, and depressed (reverse-scored); extraversion, the extent to which she is sociable, fun-loving, and optimistic; and agreeableness, the extent to which she is trusting, helpful, and forgiving. Cronbach's alpha was .80.

Mothers' sensitivity is a central construct for the study of attachment. For this reason, two measures of sensitivity were included. The first was derived from observations of mother-child interaction in a play task, in which tapes were rated for qualities such as positive regard and intrusiveness. The second measure was derived from a home observation using the HOME. These approaches to the study of sensitivity are very different, and the correlation between the two sensitivity indexes (described below) was only moderate, $r(1,148) = .41$. To determine whether effects replicated across these measures, it was important to keep them separate.

One of the composite measures of the mothers' sensitivity and responsiveness was constructed on the basis of ratings of videotaped episodes of mother-child play. Tapes from all sites were shipped to a central location for coding. Mother's sensitivity to distress and nondistress, intrusiveness, detachment/disengagement, stimulation of cognitive development, positive and negative regard for the child, and flatness of affect were rated by a single team of coders using 4 point scales. A composite variable was created by summing the individual scales for sensitivity to nondistress, positive regard, and intrusiveness (reverse-scored). Sensitivity to distress, negative regard, and detachment/disengagement were not considered for this composite due to kurtosis problems. Intercoder reliability on the composite was .87 at 6 months and .83 at 15 months, based on 17% and 16% of the cases, respectively. Cronbach's alphas were .75 and .70 for the 6 and 15 month composites, respectively. These two scores were averaged to create the overall *sensitivity in play* composite used in these analyses.

The second composite measure representing the mothers' sensitivity and responsiveness was constructed on the basis of data obtained from the Infant/Toddler HOME. The HOME is a semistructured interview/observational procedure in which a home visitor answers a set of binary questions based on maternal response to specific queries and makes observations of materials in the home and the mother's behavior toward the child. This instrument was used by research assistants who had passed two certification procedures: (1) agreement with the scoring of a "gold-standard" videotape of a HOME administration on 41 of 45 items prior to the onset of data collection, and (2) agreement with a certified HOME trainer on 41 of 45 items for three videotaped home visits during the course of data collection. In addition, research assistants submitted a tape and score sheet from a HOME administration for evaluation every 4 months. A composite score was computed by summing the positive involvement factor score (Cronbach's alpha = .52 at 6 months and .56 at 15 months; e.g., "Parent's voice conveys positive feelings toward child," "Parent caresses or kisses child at least once," "Parent responds to child's vocalizations") and the lack of negativity factor score (Cronbach's alpha = .50 at 6 months and .54 at 15 months; e.g., "Parent does not shout at child," "Parent is not hostile"). The 6 and 15 month scores were averaged to create the *sensitivity in the HOME* score used in these analyses (Cronbach's alpha = .60 and .64).

A measure of infant temperament was based on 55 6-point items from the Infant Temperament Questionnaire, administered at 6 months. The items represented the following subscales: approach, activity, intensity, mood, and adaptability. The composite measure, *difficult temperament*, was created by calculating the mean of the nonmissing items with appropriate reflection of items, so that numerically large scores consistently reflected a more "difficult" temperament (e.g., "My baby is fussy or cries during the physical examination by the doctor"). Cronbach's alpha was .81.

Child-care variables. At 5 and 14 months, mothers were telephoned and asked about their current child-care arrangements, if any, and if changes were anticipated. If no changes were anticipated, information about the child-care setting was obtained. This information was used to classify the *type of care* of the arrangement observed at 6 and 15 months: mother (i.e., those children not in any regular child care), father, other relative, in-home nonrelative, child-care home, and child-care center. Information provided in the telephone calls and interviews was used to calculate the monthly average for number of hours in care per week. A composite measure of *amount of care* was created by computing the mean hours per week from the monthly care average from 4 through 15 months.[2] Children who

[2]The decision to begin counting hours of care at 4 months rather than 1 month was made because this was the age by which the majority of infants who were in care during the first year had started care, and we did not want to deflate our estimate of hours of care by the "zeros" infants received in months 1–3.

received no regular nonmaternal care through 15 months received scores of "0." On the basis of maternal reports, two additional measures were generated. One was *age of entry* into routine child care (1 = entered care at 0–3 months, 2 = entered care at 4–6 months, 3 = entered care at 7–15 months, 4 = children who had not entered care by 15 months when the Strage Situation procedure was conducted). The second one was *frequency of care starts*, a measure of stability of care, which reflected the number of different arrangements the child experienced through 15 months.

Observations of the child-care settings were conducted on 2 half-days that were scheduled within a 2 week interval. During these sessions, observers scored child-care quality using the Observational Record of the Caregiving Environment (ORCE; see NICHD Early Child Care Research Network, 1996). Because the ORCE is used to assess the quality of caregiving for an individual child rather than what happens at the level of caregivers or classrooms, it is an instrument that can be used in home and center settings alike.

Data collection using the ORCE consisted of four 44 min cycles spread over 2 days. Each 44 min cycle was broken into four 10 min observation periods, plus a 4 min period for rating global quality. Observers recorded the occurrence of specific behaviors directed by the caregiver to the study infant for each minute during the first three 10 min cycles. These behaviors focused on positive caregiving and included the following: positive affect, positive physical contact, response to distress, response to vocalization, positive talk, asking questions, other talk, stimulation of cognitive or social development, facilitation of the infant's behavior. At each age a composite variable was created by summing standardized scores for these behavior scales. This composite was based on an a priori conceptualization of positive caregiving and was supported by the results of factor analysis. It had good internal consistency (alphas = .87 at 6 months and .79 at 15 months).

At the end of the fourth cycle, observers made qualitative ratings of the observed caregiving. A second composite was based on 4 point qualitative ratings of the same dimensions of caregiving behavior that were rated for the mothers in the structured play task with their infants. This qualitative rating composite was created by summing ratings for sensitivity to nondistress, stimulation of cognitive development, positive regard, and the reflection of detachment and flatness of affect. This composite also had good internal consistency (alphas = .89 at 6 months and .88 at 15 months).

Both positive frequency scores and qualitative ratings had adequate interobserver reliability with "gold standard" videotapes and with live reliability partners at 6 and 15 months (.86 to .98). At 6 and 15 months, each observer participated in three rounds of gold standard reliability tests, consisting of six tapes each, at regular intervals throughout the year of data collection. In addition, live reliability was conducted on 17% of the cases at 6 months and 11% of the cases at 15 months. Two overall composite measures of the quality of child care were created by computing the mean of the behavior composites at 6 and 15 months (*positive caregiving frequency*) and the mean of the qualitative composites at 6 and 15 months (*positive caregiving ratings*). Although these two composites were highly correlated, $r(689) = .73$, they were designed to tap somewhat different aspects of the caregiving environment, namely, the frequency of caregiving behaviors viewed as positive (e.g., response to vocalization, positive physical contact) and ratings of the quality of caregiving behavior. The decision to retain the separate composites reflects the design of the ORCE, as well as a concern that measures of amount and quality would be differentially related to attachment security.

Attachment security. The Strange Situation is a 25 min procedure containing brief episodes of increasing stress for the infant, including two mother-infant separations and reunions. It is designed to elicit and measure infants' attachment behavior. Attachment behaviors may be categorized as secure (B) or insecure (A, C, D, or U; Main & Solomon, 1990). When stressed, secure (B) infants seek comfort from their mothers, which is effective and permits the infant to return to play. Avoidant (A) infants tend to show little overt distress and turn away from or ignore the mother on reunion. Resistant (C) infants are distressed and angry, but ambivalent about contact, which does not effectively comfort and allow the children to return to play. Examples of disorganized/disoriented (D) behaviors are prolonged stilling, rapid vacillation between approach and avoidance, sudden unexplained changes in affect, severe distress followed by avoidance, and expressions of fear or disorientation at the entrance of the mother. A case that cannot be assigned an A, B, C, or D classification is given the unclassifiable (U) code. The U classifications (3.5% of the sample) have been eliminated from the major analyses in this report.

The Strange Situation was administered according to standard procedures (Ainsworth et al., 1978) by research assistants who had been trained and certified according to a priori criteria to assure that the assessments were of very high quality. These research assistants were trained so that the child's child-care status was not discussed during the Strange Situation (so as not to bias coders). Videotapes of the Strange Situation episodes from all sites were shipped to a central location (different from the one responsible for coding mother-child interaction) and rated by a team of three coders who were blind to child-care status, although not to the fact that this was a study of the effects of child care. The three workers, all with a minimum of 4 years previous experience coding Strange Situations from a variety of low- and high-risk samples, received additional training using master-coded tapes (including tapes coded by Mary Main), and intensive supervision continued during formal scoring to maintain expertise. Before beginning formal scoring, coders also passed the University of Minnesota Attachment Test Tapes for ABC classifications.

Coders rated their *confidence* in each classification on a 5 point scale. A score of 5 reflected the view that the child was a "classic" exemplar of a particular subcategory (e.g., B3, A2). A rating of 1 reflected the view that the child's behavior was ambiguous or that the assessment was difficult to code for technical reasons. Distress during the three mother-absent episodes was rated with a 5 point scale for each episode. A rating of 1 reflected no overt distress and no attenuation of the child's exploration. A rating of 5 reflected immediate, high distress resulting in termination of the separation. These ratings were summed across episodes to create a total Distress score, which could range from 3 to 15. Cronbach's alpha was .84.

The three coders double-coded 1,201 Strange Situation assessments. Disagreements were viewed by the group and discussed until a code was assigned by consensus. Across all coder pairs, before conferencing, agreement for the five-category classification system (ABCDU) was 83% (kappa = .69) and agreement for the two-category classification system (secure/insecure) was 86% (kappa = .70). Distress was coded by a single worker based on the written notes by all coders. A second worker coded 47 cases from the notes for reliability. Pearson correlations between the two ratings ranged from .93 for Episode 6 to .96 for Episode 7.

The 5 point confidence rating was related to interrater agreement in expectable ways. When both coders' confidence ratings were 3 or higher, agreement on ABCDU was very good (94%, kappa = .86). When both coders had confidence ratings below 3 (13% of the cases), agreement was low (53%, kappa = .35). Overall, the correlation between the confidence ratings across coders was .53.

RESULTS

Two sets of analyses were performed. The first set was designed to assess the internal validity of the Strange Situation, and the second set tested the effects of child care on attachment security.

Assessing the Validity of the Strange Situation

The issue of the internal validity of the Strange Situation was addressed for children with routine separation experience by investigating the infant's distress during mother-absent episodes of the Strange Situation, and the confidence of coders assigning attachment classifications. Two extreme groups of children were selected for these analyses: those with less than 10 hr of child care per week every month from 0 to 15 months ("low-intensity" child-care group, $n = 251$) and those with 30 or more hr per week in every month from 3 to 15 months ("high-intensity" child-care group, $n = 263$). In these validity analyses, the five-category attachment classification (ABCDU) was used.

One theoretical challenge to the validity of the Strange Situation for children with extensive child care is that these children are not as distressed by their mother's absence as are children without routine, daily separation experience, and therefore the Strange Situation, designed as a mild stressor for children in maternal care, is not sufficiently stressful to activate the attachment system and tap secure-base behavior for these children. This hypothesis would be supported if it were found that children with extensive child care showed less distress in the mother-absent episodes of the Strange Situation than the children with no child care, or if, among children classified as avoidant (A), those with extensive child care showed less distress in the mother-absent episodes, compared with children with no child care.

Results of a 2 (high/low child-care intensity) × 5 (attachment classification) ANOVA for the distress rating provided no support for the hypothesis that the Strange Situation was a less valid measure of attachment for children with extensive child-care experience. As expected, children classified as Cs showed the most distress (13.6) and As the least (6.3), $F(4, 492) = 37.34$, $p < .001$. However, there was no significant main effect for child-care experience. The mean distress level of children in high-intensity child care was 6.5, and in low-intensity child care was 6.0. (See Appendix for cell means.)

The validity of the Strange Situation as a measure of attachment for children with extensive child-care experience would also be called into question if coders were less confident about the classification given these children. This was not the case. A 2 × 5 ANOVA for the confidence rating revealed that Bs were rated with higher confidence (3.9) than any other classification (3.1 to 3.3), $F(4, 510) = 18.64$, $p < .001$, but there was no significant main effect for child-care experience on rater confidence. Moreover, D and U infants in the high-intensity child-care group were coded with higher confidence (3.9, 3.3) than were D and U infants in the low-intensity child-care group (2.8, 2.6) rather than the reverse, $F(4, 510) = 2.94$, $p < .02$. Thus, there was no evidence in these analyses that the Strange Situation was less valid for children with extensive child-care experience than for those without.

Effects of Child Care on Attachment Security

Analysis plan. A number of approaches to analyzing the effects of child care on Strange Situation classifications were considered. A primary issue was the selection/construction of dependent variables from the attachment classification categories that would provide the most direct test of our major hypotheses as well as address the results of previous studies. Two parameterizations of attachment categories were selected: secure (B) versus insecure (A, C, and D), and secure (B) versus insecure-avoidant (A). The secure/insecure dependent variable afforded the testing of child-care effects at the most global level of adaptive versus maladaptive child outcomes. The secure/avoidant dependent variable provided a means for testing the proposition that infant child-care experiences were specifically related to the incidence of insecure-avoidant attachment.

A second issue concerned the type of analyses to be performed. Due to the categorical, binary nature of the dependent variables, logistic regression analyses were employed (with secure = 1 and insecure = 0, or avoidant = 0). In a series of analyses, the dependent variable (secure/insecure or secure/avoidant) was predicted from (1) one of five characteristics of the mother (psychological adjustment, sensitivity in play, sensitivity in the HOME) or the child (difficult temperament, sex), (2) one of five characteristics of child care (positive caregiving frequency, positive caregiving ratings, amount of care, age of entry, and frequency of care starts), and (3) the interaction between the two selected (mother/child and child care) variables.

This analysis plan was preferred to a single analysis that included all five mother/child variables, all five child-care variables, and all possible interactions among these variables because of multicollinearity among the measures. In addition, it was impossible to include all participants in a single analysis because some of the child-care variables (age of entry, amount of care, stability of care) involved the total sample, whereas others (positive caregiving frequency, positive caregiving ratings) were available only for those infants in child care. Alpha was set at .05 for all analyses, rather than adjusting alpha for the number of analyses, because of a concern regarding Type II errors.

In performing the logistic regression analyses, the order of entry of predictor variables was guided by our theoretical rationale and our major hypotheses. In each analysis, control variables reflective of selection effects (income-to-needs ratio, beliefs about the benefits of maternal employment) were entered into the regression equation first, and then the main effect of a mother or child characteristic was tested. The main effect of a child-care variable was tested next, and then the interaction between (i.e., the product of) the mother/child variable and the child-care variable. When these two-way interactions proved significant, subsequent analyses were undertaken to determine whether they could be clarified by considering selected additional child-care predictors within the context of the two-way interaction.

After analyses of continuous child-care variables were completed, attention was turned to the categorical variable of type of child care. Chi-square analyses were performed to determine whether attachment security was related to type of care at 5 and at 14 months, and additional logistic regression analyses were used to evaluate the effects of child-care variables on attachment outcomes within types of care.

Descriptive statistics. Descriptive statistics and intercorrelations among control and predictor variables appear in Table 2. Table 3 presents unadjusted descriptive statistics for predictor variables by attachment classification (ABCD).

Secure/insecure analyses. Results of the secure/insecure analyses are presented in Tables 4 and 5. These tables show the association of attachment security with each mother and child predictor (top panel of Table 4), each child-care predictor (bottom panel of Table 4), and each interaction term (Table 5). The Wald chi-square for each variable indicates the effect of adding that variable following entry of prior variables; the odds ratio is the ratio of the probability that an event will occur to the probability that it will not (i.e., the closer to 1.00, the smaller the effect).

Among the five mother/child variables, two were significant predictors of attachment security: psychological adjustment and sensitivity in the HOME. As expected, mothers who exhibited greater sensitivity and responsiveness toward their infants and mothers who had better psychological adjustment were more likely to have securely attached infants. Child temperament, sex, and sensitivity in play were not significantly related to attachment security in these analyses.

None of the five child-care variables, entered after the mother/child variables, significantly predicted attachment security. That is, variations in the observed quality of care, the amount of care, the age of entry, and the frequency of care starts did not increase or decrease a child's chances of being securely attached to mother.[3] Thus, the "main effects" hypotheses for child care received no support.[4]

Of the 25 interaction terms included in the logistic regression analyses (Table 5), six were significant predictors of attachment security: (1) maternal sensitivity in play × positive caregiving ratings, (2) maternal sensitivity in the HOME × positive caregiving ratings, (3) maternal sensitivity in play × positive caregiving frequency, (4) maternal sensitivity in the HOME × amount of care, (5) maternal sensitivity in play × care starts, and (6) child sex × amount of care. Although significant (see Wald chi-squares), these interaction effects were relatively small (see odds ratios).

To explore the nature of the significant interactions in as simple a way as possible, categorical groupings were formed from the variables involved. It should be understood,

---

[3]The same results were obtained when child-care variables were entered prior to mother/child variables or prior to control variables, and when the two measures of child-care quality were aggregated.

[4]In a logistic regression predicting attachment security from income-to-needs ratio, beliefs about the benefits of maternal employment, sensitivity—HOME, and cumulative child-care risk (low quality, high amount, and frequent starts), the Wald chi-square for the cumulative child-care risk variable was .49 (*ns*).

TABLE 2

Intercorrelations among Control and Predictor Variables, and Descriptive Statistics

	Intercorrelations											
	Inc.	Work	Psych. Adj.	Sens. Play	Sens. HOME	Temp.	Sex	PCF	PCR	Amt.	Age	Starts
Controls:												
Income-to-needs												
Benefits of work	.01											
Mother/child predictors:												
Psychological adjustment	.30***	−.01										
Sensitivity—Play	.37***	−.09**	.28***									
Sensitivity—HOME	.31***	−.06*	.25***	.41***								
Temperament	−.16***	−.04	−.27***	−.14***	−.13***							
Sex[a]	.02	−.01	−.01	.04	.06*	.04						
Child-care predictors:												
Positive caregiving frequency (PCF)	.18***	−.12***	.05	.10**	.10**	.01	.07					
Positive caregiving ratings (PCR)	.16***	−.19***	.05	.13***	.12***	.02	.09*	.73***				
Amount of care	.17***	.38***	.08**	.02	.05	−.09**	.02	−.14***	−.19***			
Age of entry[b]	−.16***	−.26***	−.11***	−.06*	−.03	.08**	.01	.04	.05	−.67***		
Frequency of care starts	.07*	.18***	.09**	.03	−.01	−.01	−.01	.01	−.02	.44***	−.57***	
	Descriptive Statistics											
n	1,151	1,153	1,131	1,151	1,150	1,138	1,153	693	691	1,153	1,153	1,153
M	3.28	19.06	−.02	.01	.00	3.17	50.60[c]	.07	14.76	23.13	1.84[b]	2.54
SD	2.80	3.13	2.85	.82	.63	.40	. . .	2.59	2.67	18.19	1.13	2.00

[a] 1 = boys, 2 = girls.

[b] 1 = 0–3 months, 2 = 4–6 months, 3 = 7–15 months, 4 = not entered by 15 months.

[c] % boys.

$^{*}p < .05$; $^{**}p < .01$; $^{***}p < .001$.

TABLE 3
Descriptive Statistics for Mother, Child, and Child-Care Variables, by ABCD Classification

	Classification											
	A			B			C			D		
Predictors	*n*	*M* or %	(*SD*)	*n*	*M* or %	(*SD*)	*n*	*M* or %	(*SD*)	*n*	*M* or %	(*SD*)
Mother variables:												
Psychological adjustment	156	−.44	(3.05)	700	.14	(2.76)	101	−.10	(3.05)	174	−.28	(2.86)
Sensitivity—Play	161	−.25	(.56)	711	.06	(.79)	102	.21	(.78)	177	−.08	(.88)
Sensitivity—HOME	161	−.22	(.87)	710	.05	(.58)	102	.03	(.56)	177	−.02	(.58)
Child variables:												
Temperament	157	3.16	(.44)	705	3.18	(.40)	101	3.16	(.38)	175	3.19	(.37)
Sex (%):												
Boys	94	16.12		352	60.38		58	9.95		79	13.55	
Girls	68	11.93		360	63.16		44	7.72		98	17.19	
Child-care variables:												
Positive caregiving frequency	111	−.20	(2.70)	422	−.01	(2.58)	53	.78	(2.43)	107	.30	(2.52)
Positive caregiving ratings	111	14.36	(2.84)	420	14.74	(2.59)	53	15.66	(2.70)	107	14.79	(2.67)
Amount of care (hr/week)	162	25.42	(18.06)	712	22.97	(18.33)	102	19.42	(17.27)	177	23.80	(18.02)
Age of entry[a]	162	1.84	(1.11)	712	1.85	(1.14)	102	1.80	(1.13)	177	1.83	(1.12)
Frequency of care starts	162	2.37	(1.91)	712	2.56	(2.01)	102	2.25	(1.82)	177	2.76	(2.13)
Type of care—5 months (%):												
Mother	47	11.24		259	61.96		40	9.57		72	17.22	
Father	20	15.04		79	59.40		17	12.78		17	12.78	
Other relative	38	21.23		106	59.22		11	6.15		24	13.41	
In-home nonrelative	9	10.00		56	62.22		8	8.89		17	18.89	
Child-care home	31	14.69		137	64.93		15	7.11		28	13.27	
Child-care center	11	10.78		67	65.69		9	8.82		15	14.71	
Type of care—14 months (%):												
Mother	44	13.10		204	60.71		36	10.71		52	15.48	
Father	27	16.17		103	61.68		10	5.99		27	16.17	
Other relative	28	17.61		89	55.97		14	8.81		28	17.61	
In-home nonrelative	14	13.86		60	59.41		12	11.88		15	14.85	
Child-care home	34	14.47		147	62.55		18	7.66		36	15.32	
Child-care center	11	7.97		97	70.29		11	7.97		19	13.77	

[a] 1 = 0–3 months, 2 = 4–6 months, 3 = 7–15 months, 4 = not entered in care by 15 months.

TABLE 4
Mother/Child and Child-Care Predictors (Main Effects) of Secure (B) versus Insecure (A, C, D) Attachment

Predictors	n	Wald χ^2	Odds Ratio
Mother/child variables:			
Psychological adjustment	1,129	3.90*	1.05
Sensitivity—Play	1,149	2.82	1.14
Sensitivity—HOME	1,148	7.25**	1.32
Temperament	1,136	.26	1.08
Sex	1,151	.77	1.11
Child-care variables:			
Positive caregiving frequency	692	2.24	.96
Positive caregiving ratings	690	.64	.98
Amount of care	1,151	.06	1.00
Age of entry	1,151	.01	.99
Frequency of care starts	1,151	.82	1.03

Note: In all analyses, income-to-needs ratio and work beliefs were entered first as control variables. For ease of presentation, reported Wald chi-square values for child-care predictors reflect the main effect of each variable on attachment security, following entry of control variables. In fact, child-care variables were entered following control variables and mother/child variables, yielding nonsignificant results similar to those reported above.
$^*p < .05$; $^{**}p < .01$.

however, that the particular groupings are solely for the purpose of illuminating the nature of the already established interactions, and should not be reified. For maternal sensitivity and quality-of-care variables, the continuous variables were transformed into categories reflecting low, moderate, and high sensitivity or quality. Participants who were in the highest quartile on any variable were in the "high" group, and participants in the lowest quartile were in the "low" group. The "moderate" group comprised participants in the middle 50% of the distribution. For amount of care, three categories were formed: full-time care (>30 hr/week), part-time care (10–30 hr/week), and minimal or no care (<10 hr/week). For care starts, the categories were 0, 1, and more than 1 start.

The results of these categorical breakdowns are presented in Table 6*a*–*f*. The tabled entries are mean security proportions (adjusted for the effects of the control variables), standard errors, and the *n* in each cell. The three sections of the table displaying the significant maternal sensitivity × child-care quality interactions (6*a*–*c*) indicate a consistent pattern related to low maternal sensitivity and low-quality child care. In each section, the lowest proportion of secure attachment was obtained when both maternal sensitivity and child-care quality were low (top left cell in each section). For these three interactions, the proportions of secure children among those receiving low scores on both maternal sensitivity and positive caregiving were .44, .45, and .51; the mean proportion of secure attachment for the rest of the children, collapsed across all the other cells, was .62 in each of the three sections.

TABLE 5

Child-Care × Mother/Child Interactions Predicting Secure (B) versus Insecure (A, C, D) Attachment

Predictors	n	Wald χ^2	Odds Ratio
Psychological adjustment × . . . :			
Positive caregiving frequency	683	1.10	1.01
Positive caregiving ratings	681	.05	1.00
Amount of care	1,129	.14	1.00
Age of entry	1,129	2.67	1.03
Frequency of care starts	1,129	.06	1.00
Sensitivity—play × . . . :			
Positive caregiving frequency	692	4.28*	.93
Positive caregiving ratings	690	3.92*	.93
Amount of care	1,149	.00	1.00
Age of entry	1,149	.05	.98
Frequency of care starts	1,149	3.88*	1.08
Sensitivity—HOME × . . . :			
Positive caregiving frequency	692	.84	.95
Positive caregiving ratings	690	4.09*	.89
Amount of care	1,148	4.52*	1.01
Age of entry	1,148	1.34	.91
Frequency of care starts	1,148	1.97	1.07
Temperament × . . . :			
Positive caregiving frequency	689	.12	1.03
Positive caregiving ratings	687	2.49	1.14
Amount of care	1,136	.36	1.00
Age of entry	1,136	.28	1.07
Frequency of care starts	1,136	.17	.97
Sex × . . . :			
Positive caregiving frequency	692	.20	1.03
Positive caregiving ratings	690	.01	1.00
Amount of care	1,151	4.19*	1.01
Age of entry	1,151	.07	.97
Frequency of care starts	1,151	.71	1.05

Note: In all analyses, income-to-needs ratio and benefits of work were entered first as control variables, followed by the mother/child variable, then the child-care variable, and then the interaction term. The main effects of the mother/child variables when all terms were included in the model were as follows: sensitivity—play, positive caregiving frequency analysis: Wald $\chi^2 = 2.97$, $p = .08$, odds ratio = 1.20; sensitivity—play, positive caregiving ratings analysis: Wald $\chi^2 = 5.12$, $p < .05$, odds ratio = 3.42; sensitivity—play, frequency of care starts analysis: Wald $\chi^2 = .24$, $p > .10$, odds ratio = .94; Sensitivity—HOME, positive caregiving ratings analysis: Wald $\chi^2 = 6.25$, $p = .01$, odds ratio = 7.67; Sensitivity—HOME, amount of care analysis: Wald $\chi^2 = .04$, $p > .10$, odds ratio = 1.03; sex, amount of care analysis: Wald $\chi^2 = 1.16$, $p > .10$, odds ratio = .81.

$^*p < .05$.

TABLE 6

Adjusted Proportion of Securely Attached Children by Group for Significant Secure/Insecure Interactions

a: Sensitivity—Play × Positive Caregiving Ratings

	Positive Caregiving Ratings								
	Low			Mod.			High		
	p	*SE*	*n*	*p*	*SE*	*n*	*p*	*SE*	*n*
Sensitivity—play:									
Low	**.44**	.07	(48)	**.62**	.06	(80)	**.53**	.09	(30)
Mod.	**.65**	.06	(76)	**.65**	.04	(192)	**.59**	.06	(77)
High	**.73**	.08	(37)	**.54**	.05	(86)	**.61**	.06	(64)

b: Sensitivity—HOME × Positive Caregiving Ratings

	Positive Caregiving Ratings								
	Low			Mod.			High		
	p	*SE*	*n*	*p*	*SE*	*n*	*p*	*SE*	*n*
Sensitivity—HOME:									
Low	**.45**	.07	(44)	**.57**	.06	(78)	**.63**	.08	(35)
Mod.	**.64**	.05	(80)	**.60**	.03	(202)	**.55**	.05	(85)
High	**.72**	.08	(37)	**.70**	.06	(78)	**.62**	.07	(51)

c: Sensitivity—Play × Positive Caregiving Frequency

	Positive Caregiving Frequency								
	Low			Mod.			High		
	p	*SE*	*n*	*p*	*SE*	*n*	*p*	*SE*	*n*
Sensitivity—Play:									
Low	**.51**	.07	(49)	**.56**	.06	(75)	**.58**	.08	(35)
Mod.	**.73**	.05	(83)	**.62**	.04	(184)	**.58**	.05	(79)
High	**.69**	.08	(36)	**.61**	.05	(89)	**.53**	.06	(62)

d: Sensitivity—HOME × Amount of Care

	Amount of Care (hr)								
	>30			10–30			<10		
	p	*SE*	*n*	*p*	*SE*	*n*	*p*	*SE*	*n*
Sensitivity—HOME:									
Low	**.54**	.05	(94)	**.52**	.05	(83)	**.62**	.05	(105)
Mod.	**.63**	.03	(264)	**.64**	.04	(141)	**.59**	.04	(198)
High	**.66**	.05	(113)	**.73**	.06	(63)	**.66**	.05	(87)

(*Continued*)

TABLE 6 (*Continued*)

e: Sensitivity—Play × Frequency of Care Starts

	Frequency of Care Starts								
	>1			1			0		
	p	*SE*	*n*	*p*	*SE*	*n*	*p*	*SE*	*n*
Sensitivity—Play:									
Low	**.56**	.04	(182)	**.60**	.07	(53)	**.60**	.07	(44)
Mod.	**.66**	.02	(366)	**.59**	.04	(124)	**.64**	.05	(91)
High	**.64**	.04	(198)	**.54**	.07	(54)	**.62**	.08	(37)

f: Sex × Amount of Care

	Amount of Care (hr)								
	>30			10–30			<10		
	p	*SE*	*n*	*p*	*SE*	*n*	*p*	*SE*	*n*
Sex:									
Boys	**.58**	.03	(233)	**.60**	.04	(150)	**.65**	.04	(198)
Girls	**.66**	.03	(238)	**.65**	.04	(137)	**.58**	.04	(195)

For purposes of this article, this and similar patterns will be referred to as "dual-risk" effects, in the sense that they involve both child-care and maternal conditions that might be expected to have a negative effect on the development of secure attachment.

In Table 6*d*–*e*, the dual-risk pattern was evident but less pronounced for the interactions between the mother's sensitivity in the HOME and the amount of care, and for the mother's sensitivity in play and the number of care starts. In these analyses, the rates of security in the dual-risk cells, when low maternal sensitivity was coupled with more than 10 hr/week of care or more than one care arrangement, were among the lowest in the table (.54/.52 in the dual-risk cells versus .62 for the rest of the cells in section 6*d*, and .56 in the dual-risk cell versus .63 for the rest of the cells in section 6*e*).

A different pattern was evident in section 6*f*, which shows the sex × amount of care interaction. This section reveals that the proportion of security was lowest among boys in more than 30 hr of care per week and girls in less than 10 hr of care per week.[5]

Inspection of Table 6*a*–*c* also reveals some evidence of a compensatory interaction pattern in relation to high-quality child care. The proportions of secure attachment in the top rows of the three sections show that for children with less sensitive and responsive mothers, security proportions were higher if the children were in high-quality child care (.53, .63, .58) than if they were in low-quality child care (.44, .45, and .51), and a linear

[5] In a separate analysis, we tested whether children in dual-risk groups for one analysis were also members of the dual-risk groups in other analyses. The majority of these children (65%, or 289) were in only one of the six dual-risk groups, 19% (83) were in two, and 16% (73) were in three or more.

increase in security as child-care quality increased was observed in two of the three analyses. However, a compensatory effect was not found for amount of child care. Section 6*d* shows that the less time children of less sensitive and responsive mothers spent in child care, the more likely they were to be securely attached. If amount of child care were compensating for low maternal sensitivity, we would expect security to be less probable in this group.

A final pattern, one that was unanticipated but was indicated in the three sections pertaining to maternal sensitivity and child-care quality (6$a-c$), is that the influence of the mother appears to vary as a function of quality of child care. Specifically, the proportions of secure attachment in the left columns of the three sections show that, for children in low-quality child care, security proportions were higher if the mother was highly sensitive (.73, .72, .69 in sections 6*a*, 6*b*, and 6*c*, respectively) than if she was insensitive (.44, .45, .51), whereas for children in high-quality child care, maternal sensitivity did not appear to be related to attachment security (proportions ranged from .53 to .63 regardless of maternal sensitivity). (To be noted, however, is the finding that maternal sensitivity remained a significant predictor of security even after accounting for the interaction term.)

Secure/insecure—follow-up analyses. For the secure/insecure analyses yielding significant two-way interactions, we sought to determine whether consideration of additional child-care conditions would further illuminate the dual-risk pattern of results. For example, among children experiencing low maternal sensitivity and responsiveness and low-quality child care, could the increased risk of insecurity be explained by the number of hours in child care? For the subsample of participants experiencing a dual risk in any given analysis, attachment security was crossed with an additional child-care variable (quality, amount of care, age of entry, care starts, type of care at 5 months, type of care at 14 months) grouped into the discrete categories described above. For example, security (secure, insecure) was crossed with amount of care (<10 hr, 10–30 hr, >30 hr) within the group of children at dual risk due to low maternal sensitivity and poor-quality child care. Chi-square analyses provided no evidence that low quality of care at home and in child care was associated with increased rates of insecurity only, or principally, when children were in care for longer hours, were in less stable care, or were in a particular type of care. There was no evidence that boys with more hours in care were more likely to be insecure than boys with fewer hours of care because they received poorer quality or less stable care. There was no evidence that children who received extensive child care and insensitive maternal care were more likely to be insecure because the child care they received was of poorer quality, less stable, or of a certain type. In sum, although significant two-way interactions were obtained, we did not find evidence that these interactions were moderated by additional features of child care.

Secure/avoidant analyses. The set of logistic regression analyses used to predict secure/insecure attachment was repeated for secure/avoidant attachment. Two of the five mother/child predictors were significant: sensitivity in play, Wald $\chi^2(1, N = 871) = 7.16$, $p < .01$, odds ratio = 1.36, and sensitivity in the HOME, Wald $\chi^2(1, N = 870) = 10.54$, $p < .01$, odds ratio = 1.51. Infants whose mothers were more sensitive and responsive toward them were more likely to be securely attached than insecure-avoidant. The main effects of psychological adjustment, temperament, and sex were not significant. Paralleling the results of the secure/insecure analyses, none of the five child-care variables was significant as a main-effect predictor of secure/avoidant attachment.[6] Only one of the 25 interaction terms was significant—sensitivity in play × care starts, Wald $\chi^2(1, N = 871) = 6.24$, $p < .05$, odds ratio = 1.17. Examination of the data indicated that the group with low maternal sensitivity and more than one care start (i.e., the dual-risk condition) had one of the lowest proportions of secure attachment (.76 versus .83).

Type-of-care analyses. Chi-square analyses were performed on attachment security × type of care at 5 months and at 14 months of age. The types of care used were mother, father, other relative, in-home nonrelative, child-care home, and child-care center. The results indicated that type of care was not significantly related to secure/insecure or secure/avoidant attachment at either age. Similar analyses grouping type of care into mother versus all other types, and relative versus nonrelative care, yielded nonsignificant results. The proportion of secure attachment for children in mother care was identical to the proportion secure for the rest of the sample (.62).

Additional analyses were performed to determine whether various aspects of child care—quality, amount, age of entry, and care starts—were related to attachment security within types of care. Because of sample size limitations, only two types of care were used in these analyses—relative care (mother, father, other relative) and nonrelative care (in-home nonrelative, child-care home, and child-care center). These analyses were designed to determine whether child-care parameters would have different effects on attachment security depending on the caregiver's relationship with the child. A logistic regression procedure was employed in which each child-care variable was used to predict attachment security separately within the two types of care. None of the analyses yielded significant results.

DISCUSSION

The NICHD Study of Early Child Care was undertaken to study associations between infant child care and developmental outcomes in a comprehensive and detailed way (see NICHD Early Child Care Network, 1994). One of its main goals was to illuminate the conditions under which infant child care increases or decreases rates of security of infant-mother attachment. Notable and unique design features of the study include its large sample size, the diversity of its participants (varying in SES, race, and family structure, and living in nine different states), the breadth of naturally occurring child-care types included (fathers, other relatives, in-home caregivers, child-care homes, and centers), the variety of child-care settings observed (from a single child with a formally trained nanny to a center with 30 children in the class), the extensiveness of the observational procedures used to assess both child-care contexts and maternal behavior, the prospective and longitudinal design, and the multivariate statistical analyses that allowed us to explore interactions between mother/child and child-care factors as well as main effects. At the same time, it is important to note that one limitation of the present study is that the sample was not designed to be nationally representative. Nor did it include mothers under 18, infants with perinatal

[6]The same results were obtained when child-care variables were entered prior to mother/child variables or prior to control variables.

problems requiring extensive hospitalization, or mothers who declined to participate (42% of those invited). Of those in the study, 15.5% did not contribute Strange Situation data to this report (12% dropped out or did not have a 15 month laboratory assessment; 3% had "U" Strange Situation classifications; the remainder had assessments that were not coded due to technical problems). Families who did not contribute Strange Situation data were more likely to have boys, to have single mothers, and to have more positive attitudes about the benefits of maternal employment for children. All of these variables are related to either attachment security or child-care parameters in this study. Taken together, the factors described above may limit the generalizability of the results.

Validity of the Strange Situation

The first purpose of the present study was to evaluate the internal validity of the Strange Situation assessment procedure. This was necessary because concerns have been raised about the appropriateness of using the separation-based Strange Situation to assess the attachment of infants in child care, who presumably have had more experience with absences from their mothers. It was predicted that if the Strange Situation was invalid for children with routine separation experiences, these children would exhibit less distress during the mother's absence or be more difficult to classify than children without regular absences from mother. No significant differences in ratings of infants' distress during mothers' absence in the Strange Situation or in coders' ratings of their own confidence in assigning attachment classifications were observed between children with less than 10 hr of care per week versus children with more than 30 hr of care over the first year of life. Thus, these tests did not reveal any differential internal validity for the Strange Situation as a function of child-care experience.

Another issue pertaining to the validity of the Strange Situation in the present study is the extent to which the distribution of attachment classifications parallels distributions reported in previous research. However, a comparison of absolute levels of particular categories is problematic, because in earlier studies the A, B, C classification system was used rather than the A, B, C, D classifications used in the present study. When the four-category system is used, children who are given a D classification are recruited from any one of the other classifications—A, B, or C. The result is that the proportions of A, B, and C in the present study (14, 62, 9) are all lower than those reported for normative populations (21, 65, 14) (van IJzendoorn & Kroonenberg, 1988).

Selection Effects

Before we could examine differences in the rates of attachment security and insecurity for infants with varying child-care experiences, it was necessary to control for selection effects—because child-care experience is not randomly assigned, and family factors affect whether children receive child care, when such care begins, the type of care, and its quality (Clarke-Stewart, Gruber, & Fitzgerald, 1994; Howes, 1990; McCartney, 1984; Melhuish, Moss, Mooney, & Martin, 1991; NICHD Early Child Care Research Network, 1997; Owen & Henderson, 1989). In examining these factors, we found that children reared in economically disadvantaged homes were more likely to be insecurely attached to their mothers. This finding is consistent with evidence indicating that poorer children are more likely to be classified as insecurely attached in the Strange Situation (Spieker & Booth, 1988), as well as with data showing that economic stress undermines the quality of care that parents provide their offspring (for review, see McLoyd, 1990).

We also discovered that when mothers more strongly endorsed statements supporting the possible benefits of maternal employment for children's development, their infants were more likely to be insecurely attached. These mothers were also observed to be less sensitive and responsive and to have their children in poorer quality care, at earlier ages, for more hours per week (see Table 2). One might speculate that maternal concern about the effects of child care fosters the mother's sensitive attentiveness to the infant at home and leads her to a more careful and cautious selection of care, thereby increasing the likelihood that the infant will experience security-promoting interactions and develop a secure attachment.

Main Effects of Mother and Child Characteristics

Results of the study indicated that children's attachment security was related to the mother's sensitivity and responsiveness, especially observed in the natural setting of the home, and to her overall positive psychological adjustment. These findings are consistent with a substantial theoretical and empirical literature linking infants' attachment security to their mothers' psychological adjustment (e.g., Spieker & Booth, 1988; for a review see Belsky, Rosenberger, & Crnic, 1995) and sensitive and responsive caregiving (e.g., Ainsworth et al., 1978; for reviews, see Belsky & Cassidy, 1994; Clarke-Stewart, 1988). Also, security of attachment was not related to the child's sex or to the mother-rated index of difficult temperament, results which are consistent with theorizing about the relation between temperament and attachment (e.g., Sroufe, 1985).

Main Effects of Infant Child Care

After selection effects were taken into account, along with child effects (i.e., temperament, sex) and mother effects (i.e., psychological adjustment, sensitivity), results pertaining to main effects of child care were clear and consistent: There were no significant differences in attachment security related to child-care participation. Even in extensive, early, unstable, or poor-quality care, the likelihood of infants' insecure attachment to mother did not increase, nor did stable or high-quality care increase the likelihood of developing a secure attachment to mother.

It is unclear why the results of this inquiry are different from those of past studies, especially the multistudy analyses of Belsky and Rovine (1988) and Clarke-Stewart (1989) in which the Strange Situation classifications of hundreds of infants were examined. Perhaps as Roggman et al. (1994) suggested, null findings that would have reduced the multistudy analyses to nonsignificance were relegated to the "file drawer" (i.e., not published). However, Clarke-Stewart's analysis did include available unpublished data. Alternatively, as mentioned in the Introduction, it may be that the population of families using infant child care today is different from those families of a decade or more ago, on whom the multistudy analyses were based. It may also be the case that the past decade's scholarly debate about adverse effects of child care, which has been discussed widely in the popular media, has sensitized parents using infant care. That is, these parents may make special efforts to provide "quality interaction" when they are with their infants, thereby increasing the likelihood that their infants will develop secure attachments. Another possible explanation is that in the present study, extensive statistical controls were employed to eliminate spurious effects. However, no main effects of child care emerged even without such controls.

Comparison of our results with those of earlier studies must give substantial weight to the present findings because of the advantages of this study—its methodological strengths, its control for family selection effects, its recency, and its "quality control" (in which, for example, Strange Situation coders were highly trained, reliable, and blind to the child's care arrangement). Nevertheless, it should be noted that the present study shares a limitation with previous studies, namely, that it was not possible to conduct observations in all eligible child-care arrangements. Approximately 16% of the care providers contacted at 6 and 15 months were unwilling, unable, or unavailable to be observed. These unobserved care arrangements may have been of lower quality than observed arrangements. In the unobserved settings, the average child-adult ratio—a predictor of higher levels of positive caregiving (see NICHD Early Child Care Research Network, 1996)—was 3.1 children per adult, compared with 2.5 for the observed arrangements. It is possible that with a wider range of care arrangements, an effect of child care on attachment security might have been obtained. Nevertheless, this seems quite unlikely, given the complete lack of association between attachment security and quality of care in this study. In the 1990s, it appears, child care in the first year of life does not have a direct, main effect on infants' attachment security.

Interaction Effects with Child and Mother Characteristics

Although analyses revealed no significant main effects of child care, it was not the case that child care was totally unrelated to attachment security. Consistent with Bronfenbrenner's (1979, p. 38) assertion that "in the ecology of human development the principal main effects are likely to be interactions," results revealed that six of the 25 two-way interactions tested (five child-care measures × five mother/child measures) achieved conventional levels of statistical significance, and yielded small but consistent effects.

A consistent pattern observed across five of the six significant interactions supported the proposition that children's attachment is affected by a combination of maternal and child-care factors. Children with the highest rates of insecurity with their mothers experienced conditions that could be considered to constitute a dual risk. This was most clearly demonstrated by children whose mothers and caregivers were least sensitive and responsive to their needs and behavior. Children who received less sensitive and responsive caregiving in child care (as measured by ratings and by frequencies of caregivers' positive behaviors) as well as less sensitive and responsive care from their mothers (as measured by less frequent and responsive positive behavior in a semistructured play session and at home) had the highest rates of insecurity (ranging from .49 to .56, depending on the analysis). Children in less risky conditions (better child care or better maternal care) had a rate of insecurity that averaged only .38. Parallel but less pronounced effects were observed for children who experienced the dual risks of less sensitive and responsive mothering combined with more time spent in child care (rate of insecurity of .47 compared with .38 in the other cells) or more care arrangements over time (rate of insecurity of .44, compared with .37). These results support a dual risk model of development (see Belsky & Rovine, 1988; Werner & Smith, 1992).

Beyond the dual-risk effects, other significant interactions were observed. One is that children in low-quality child care were more strongly affected by their mothers' behavior than were children in high-quality care. For children in low-quality child care, the probability of a secure attachment was low (.44–.51) if the mother was less sensitive and responsive and high (.69–.73) if she was highly sensitive and responsive. For children in high-quality care, the security proportions were moderate (.53–.63) regardless of the mothers' behavior. This pattern, suggesting that child care had a moderating effect on the link between maternal sensitivity and attachment security, was not predicted a priori. A tentative explanation might be that the mother's behavior is more salient and significant in the lives of children in low-quality child care, who would be less likely to form secure attachments to their alternative caregivers (Howes & Hamilton, 1992).

A second pattern pertains to the interaction between maternal sensitivity and amount of child care. Children whose mothers exhibited less sensitive and responsive behavior toward them in the HOME observation and interview were more likely to be securely attached if they spent more time with mother (and less time in child care). This finding may, at first, appear to be counterintuitive. Why should spending more time with a relatively insensitive and unresponsive mother increase the probability of establishing a secure relationship with her? Our tentative explanation is that there may be a "dosage effect" for maternal sensitivity and involvement: Children with less involved mothers may need more time with them in order to develop the internalized sense that the mother is responsive and available, whereas children with more sensitive and responsive mothers may require less time to develop confidence in the mother's availability.

A third interaction pattern suggested different developmental processes for boys and girls. Whereas more time in child care was associated with a somewhat higher rate of insecurity for boys, less time in care was associated with a somewhat higher rate of insecurity for girls. These data bring to mind two sets of findings in the developmental literature. Relevant to the elevated rate of insecurity for boys in child care is evidence that boys tend to be more vulnerable than girls to psychosocial stress generally (Zaslow & Hayes, 1986). Perhaps, for the boys in this study, the experience of spending a lot of time in child care was stressful enough to tip the balance toward a lower likelihood of secure attachment. Consistent with the elevated rate of insecurity for girls not in child care is evidence that girls lacking child-care experience in infancy score lower on later intelligence tests (Desai, Chase-Lansdale, & Michael, 1989; Mott, 1991). The reasons why girls in child care would benefit in terms of their attachment security remain unclear. Further analyses of child outcome measures in the NICHD Study will shed light on these possible developmental differences.

The interaction analyses provided evidence that high-quality child care served a compensatory function for children whose maternal care was lacking: The proportion of attachment security among children with the least sensitive and responsive mothers was higher in high-quality child care than in low-quality care. However, there was no evidence that amount of time in child care compensated for the mother's lack of sensitivity and involvement, because the proportion of secure attachment among the children with the least sensitive and responsive mothers was higher in minimal hours of child care than in many hours of care.

Effect of Child Care on Avoidance

Previous studies (compiled by Belsky & Rovine, 1988, and Clarke-Stewart, 1989) suggested that effects of child care were most likely to increase the rate of one particular form of insecurity—insecure avoidance. Indeed, Barglow et al. (1987) contended that this was the case because infants interpreted the routine separations associated with child care as maternal rejection, which is theorized to foster insecure-avoidant attachment. Analyses of secure versus insecure-avoidant children in the present study revealed no main effects of child care, and only one of the 25 interactions tested was significant. Thus, in contrast to the results of earlier research, there was no evidence that child-care experience is associated with avoidance per se.

Conclusion

The results of this study clearly indicate that child care by itself constitutes neither a risk nor a benefit for the development of the infant-mother attachment relationship as measured in the Strange Situation. However, poor quality, unstable, or more than minimal amounts of child care apparently added to the risks already inherent in poor mothering, so that the combined effects were worse than those of low maternal sensitivity and responsiveness alone. Such results suggest that the effects of child care on attachment, as well as the nature of the attachment relationship itself, depend primarily on the nature of ongoing interactions between mother and child (Ainsworth, 1973; Sroufe, 1988). Another finding of the study was that the influence of amount of care on attachment security varied as a function of the child's sex.

Our continuing, longitudinal investigation of children's development in the NICHD Study of Early Child Care will determine the ultimate importance of these findings for developmentalists, policy-makers, and parents, as we consider the effects of early child care on longer-term outcomes and on the broader variety of social-emotional, cognitive, and health outcomes the study was designed to assess. To the extent that evidence emerges in future analyses that early child care is associated with problem behavior or developmental deficits at older ages, these infant-mother attachment findings will take on greater importance. To the extent, however, that evaluations of child-care effects in the longitudinal follow-up to this investigation provide no evidence of developmental disadvantages associated with early care, then even concerns raised in this inquiry about dual risks with respect to attachment security would be mitigated. In sum, the full meaning of the child-care findings reported here will not become clear until more is known about the development of the children participating in the NICHD Study of Early Child Care.

APPENDIX

Mean Distress Ratings for Low- and High-Child-Care Intensity Groups by Five-Category Attachment Classification

	A		B		C		D		U		Total	
	n	*M*	*n*	*M*	*n*	*M*	*n*	*M*	*n*	*M*	*n*	*M*
Low intensity	26	6.0	164	10.5	27	13.4	33	9.3	13	9.4	263	9.7
High intensity	42	6.5	153	10.4	15	13.7	38	11.8	9	8.8	257	10.3
Total	68	6.3	317	10.5	42	13.6	71	10.6	22	9.1	520	...

Note: The results for the two main effects tests and the interaction were as follows: intensity child-care group $F(1, 492) = .04$, $p > .1$; attachment group $F(4, 492) = 37.34$, $p < .001$; intensity child-care group × attachment group $F(4, 492) = 2.50$, $p < .05$. There was no main effect of intensity and no difference between the low-intensity and high-intensity As, the group for which a difference could theoretically be predicted. The interaction between intensity and attachment classification appeared to involve the D group: Low-intensity Ds showed less separation distress than high-intensity Ds. Because this difference was not theoretically predicted, we concluded that the Strange Situation was equally valid for children with and without early child-care experience.

REFERENCES

Ainsworth, M. D. S. (1973). The development of infant-mother attachment. In B. Caldwell & H. Ricciuti (Eds.), *Review of child development research* (Vol. *3*, pp. 1–94). Chicago: University of Chicago Press.

Ainsworth, M. D., Blehar, M., Waters, E., & Wall, S. (1978). *Patterns of attachment: A psychological study of the Strange Situation.* Hillsdale, NJ: Erlbaum.

Ainsworth, M. D. S., & Wittig, B. (1969). Attachment and exploratory behavior of one-year-olds in a strange situation. In B. M. Foss (Ed.), *Determinants of infant behavior* (Vol. *4*, pp. 129–173). London: Methuen.

Barglow, P., Vaughn, B., & Molitor, N. (1987). Effects of maternal absence due to employment on the quality of infant-mother attachment in a low-risk sample. *Child Development, 58,* 945–954.

Belsky, J. (1990). Developmental risks associated with infant day-care: Attachment insecurity, non-compliance, and aggression? In S. Chehrazi (Ed.), *Psychosocial issues in day-care* (pp. 37–68). New York: American Psychiatric Press.

Belsky, J., & Braungart, J. (1991). Are insecure-avoidant infants with extensive day-care experience less stressed by and more independent in the Strange Situation? *Child Development, 62,* 567–571.

Belsky, J., & Cassidy, J. (1994). Attachment: Theory and evidence. In M. Rutter, D. Hay, & S. Baron-Cohen (Eds.), *Developmental principles and clinical issues in psychology and psychiatry* (pp. 373–402). London: Blackwell.

Belsky, J., Rosenberger, K., & Crnic, K. (1995). The origins of attachment security: Classical and contextual determinants. In S. Goldberg, R. Muir, & J. Kerr (Eds.), *Attachment theory: Social developmental and clinical perspectives* (pp. 153–184). Hillsdale, NJ: Analytic Press.

Belsky, J., & Rovine, M. (1988). Nonmaternal care in the first year of life and the security of infant-parent attachment. *Child Development, 59,* 157–167.

Belsky, J., & Steinberg, L. (1978). The effects of day-care: A critical review. *Child Development, 49,* 929–949.

Benn, R. K. (1986). Factors promoting secure attachment relationships between employed mothers and their sons. *Child Development, 57,* 1224–1231.

Berger, S., Levy, A., & Compaan, K. (1995, March). *Infant attachment outside the laboratory: New evidence in support of the Strange Situation.* Paper presented at the biennial meetings of the Society for Research in Child Development, Indianapolis, IN.

Bowlby, J. (1973). *Attachment and loss: Vol. 3. Separation: Anxiety and anger.* New York: Basic.

Brazelton, T. B. (1985). *Working and caring.* New York: Basic.

Bronfenbrenner, U. (1979). *The ecology of human development.* Cambridge, MA: Harvard University Press.

Caldwell, B. M., & Bradley, R. H. (1984). *Home Observation for Measurement of the Environment.* Little Rock: University of Arkansas.

Carey, W., & McDevitt, S. (1978). Revision of the Infant Temperament Questionnaire. *Pediatrics, 61,* 735–739.

Clarke-Stewart, K. A. (1988). Parents' effects on children's development: A decade of progress? *Journal of Applied Developmental Psychology, 9,* 41–84.

Clarke-Stewart, K. A. (1989). Infant day-care: Maligned or malignant? *American Psychologist, 44,* 266–273.

Clarke-Stewart, K. A., & Fein, G. G. (1983). Early childhood programs. In M. Haith & J. Campos (Eds.), P. H. Mussen (Series Ed.), *Handbook of child psychology: Vol. 2. Infancy and developmental psychobiology* (pp. 917–1000). New York: Wiley.

Clarke-Stewart, K. A., Gruber, C. P., & Fitzgerald, L. M. (1994). *Children at home and in day-care.* Hillsdale, NJ: Erlbaum.

Costa, P. T., & McCrae, R. R. (1985). *The NEO Personality Inventory manual.* Odessa, FL: Psychological Assessment Resources.

Desai, S., Chase-Lansdale, P. L., & Michael, R. (1989). Mother or market? Effects of maternal employment on the intellectual ability of four-year-old children. *Demography, 26,* 545–561.

Fox, N., & Fein, G. (1990). *Infant day-care: The current debate.* Norwood, NJ: Ablex.

Greenberger, E., Goldberg, W., Crawford, T. J., & Granger, J. (1988). Beliefs about the consequences of maternal employment for children. *Psychology of Women Quarterly, 12,* 35–59.

Howes, C. (1990). Current research on early day-care. In S. S. Chehrazi (Ed.), *Psychosocial issues in day-care* (pp. 21–53). Washington, DC: American Psychiatric Press.

Howes, C., & Hamilton, C. E. (1992). Children's relationships with caregivers: Mothers and child-care teachers. *Child Development, 63,* 859–866.

Jaeger, E., & Weinraub, M. (1990). Early maternal care and infant attachment: In search of process. In K. McCartney (Ed.), *Child care and maternal employment: A social ecology approach* (pp. 71–90). San Francisco: Jossey-Bass.

Karen, R. (1994). *Becoming attached.* New York: Warner.

Lamb, M., & Sternberg, K. (1990). Do we really know how day-care affects children? *Journal of Applied Developmental Psychology, 11,* 351–379.

Main, M., & Solomon, J. (1990). Procedures for identifying disorganized/disoriented infants in the Ainsworth Strange Situation. In M. Greenberg, D. Cicchetti, & M. Cummings (Eds.), *Attachment in the preschool years: Theory, research, and intervention* (pp. 121–160). Chicago: University of Chicago Press.

McCartney, K. (1984). The effect of quality of day-care environment upon children's language development. *Developmental Psychology, 20,* 244–260.

McCartney, K., & Phillips, D. (1988). Motherhood and child care. In B. Birns & D. Hay (Eds.), *The different faces of motherhood* (pp. 157–183). New York: Plenum.

McLoyd, V. C. (1990). The impact of economic hardship on black families and children: Psychological distress, parenting, and socioemotional development. *Child Development, 61,* 311–436.

Melhuish, E. C., Moss, P., Mooney, A., & Martin, S. (1991). How similar are day-care groups before the start of day-care? *Journal of Applied Developmental Psychology, 12,* 331–335.

Mott, F. L. (1991). Developmental effects of infant care: The mediating role of gender and health. *Journal of Social Issues, 47,* 139–158.

NICHD Early Child Care Network. (1994). Child care and Child Development: The NICHD Study of Early Child Care. In S. Friedman & H. C. Haywood (Eds.), *Developmental follow-up: Concepts, domains, and methods* (pp. 377–396). New York: Academic Press.

NICHD Early Child Care Research Network. (1996). Characteristics of infant child care: Factors contributing to positive caregiving. *Early Childhood Research Quarterly, 11,* 269–306.

NICHD Early Child Care Research Network. (1997). Familial factors associated with the characteristics of nonmaternal care for infants. *Journal of Marriage and Family, 59,* 389–408.

Owen, M. T., & Cox, M. J. (1988). Maternal employment and the transition to parenthood: Family functioning and child development. In A. E. Gottfried & A. W. Gottfried (Eds.), *Maternal employment and children's development: Longitudinal research* (pp. 85–119). New York: Plenum.

Owen, M. R., & Henderson, B. K. (1989, April). *Relations between child care qualities and child behavior at age 4: Do parent-child interactions play a role*? Paper presented at the biennial meetings of the Society for Research in Child Development, Kansas City, MO.

Radloff, L. (1977). The CES-D Scale: A self-report depression scale for research in the general population. *Applied Psychological Measurement, 1,* 385–410.

Roggman, L., Langlois, J., Hubbs-Tait, L., & Rieser-Danner, L. (1994). Infant day-care, attachment, and the "file drawer problem." *Child Development, 65,* 1429–1443.

Rutter, M. (1981). Socioemotional consequences of day-care for preschool children. *American Journal of Orthopsychiatry, 51,* 4–28.

Spieker, S. J., & Booth, C. L. (1988). Maternal antecedents of attachment quality. In J. Belsky & T. Nezworski (Eds.), *Clinical implications of attachment* (pp. 95–135). Hillsdale, NJ: Erlbaum.

Sroufe, L. A. (1985). Attachment classification from the perspective of infant-caregiver relationships and infant temperament. *Child Development, 56,* 1–14.

Sroufe, L. A. (1988). A developmental perspective on day-care. *Early Childhood Research Quarterly, 3,* 283–291.

Vandell, D. L. (1979). The effects of playgroup experiences on mother-son and father-son interactions. *Developmental Psychology, 15,* 379–385.

van IJzendoorn, M. H., & Kroonenberg, P. M. (1988). Cross-cultural patterns of attachment: A meta-analysis of the Strange Situation. *Child Development, 59,* 147–156.

Werner, E. E., & Smith, R. S. (1992). *Overcoming the odds*. Ithaca, NY: Cornell University Press.

Zaslow, M. S., & Hayes, C. D. (1986). Sex differences in children's responses to psychosocial stress: Toward a cross-context analysis. In M. Lamb & B. Rogoff (Eds.), *Advances in developmental psychology* (Vol. 4, pp. 289–337). Hillsdale, NJ: Erlbaum.

18

Long-Term Effects of Home Visitation on Maternal Life Course and Child Abuse and Neglect: Fifteen-Year Follow-Up of a Randomized Trial

David L. Olds
University of Colorado Health Sciences Center, Denver, Colorado
John Eckenrode and Charles R. Henderson
Cornell University, New York, New York
Harriet Kitzman
University of Rochester, Rochester, New York
Jane Powers
Cornell University, New York, New York
Robert Cole and Kimberly Sidora
University of Rochester, Rochester, New York

Reprinted with permission from *Journal of the American Medical Association*, 1997, Vol. 278, 637–643.

This research was supported by a Senior Research Scientist Award (1-K05-MH01382-01) (Dr Olds) and grants from the Prevention Research and Behavioral Medicine Branch of the National Institute of Mental Health, Rockville, Md (R01-MH49381), and the Assistant Secretary for Planning and Evaluation, US Department of Health and Human Services, Washington, DC (grant 96ASPE278A).

The following federal agencies and private foundations contributed to earlier phases of this research: the Bureau of Community Health Services, Maternal and Child Health Research Division, Rockville, Md; the Carnegie Corporation, New York, NY; The Commonwealth Fund, New York; the Ford Foundation, New York; The Pew Charitable Trusts, Philadelphia, Pa; The Robert Wood Johnson Foundation, Princeton, NJ; and the William T. Grant Foundation, New York.

We thank John Shannon, PhD, for his support of the program and data gathering; Alise Mahr, Darlene Batroney, RN, Karen Hughes, Barbara Lee, Sherry Mandel, and Barbara Ganzel for tracing and interviewing the families; Kathleen Buckwell, Sondra Thomas, and Sharon Holmberg, RN, PhD, for coding the data; Robert Chamberlin, MD, and Robert Tatelbaum, MD, for their contributions to the earlier phases of this research; the New York Department of Social Services, in particular Renee Hallock for assistance with the coding of CPS records; Anthony Stack, Jim Blake, David J. van Alstyne, and the NYS Division of Criminal Justice Services for their assistance with extraction and coding of the criminal justice data; Del Elliott, PhD, Zorika Henderson, Dave Huizinga, PhD, and Richard Jessor, PhD, for their comments on the manuscript; Jackie Roberts, RN, Liz Chilson, RN, Lyn Scazafabo, RN, Georgie McGrady, RN, and Diane Farr, RN, for their home-visitation work with the families; and the families who participated in the research.

Pamela Morris

Cornell University, New York, New York

Lisa M. Pettitt

University of Denver, Denver, Colorado

Dennis Luckey

University of Colorado Health Sciences Center, Denver, Colorado

Context: *Home-visitation services have been promoted as a means of improving maternal and child health and functioning. However, long-term effects have not been examined.* **Objective:** *To examine the long-term effects of a program of prenatal and early childhood home visitation by nurses on women's life course and child abuse and neglect.* **Design:** *Randomized trial.* **Setting:** *Semirural community in New York.* **Participants:** *Of 400 consecutive pregnant women with no previous live births enrolled, 324 participated in a follow-up study when their children were 15 years old.* **Intervention:** *Families received a mean of 9 home visits during pregnancy and 23 home visits from the child's birth through the second birthday.* **Data Sources and Measures:** *Women's use of welfare and number of subsequent children were based on self-report; their arrests and convictions were based on self-report and archived data from New York State. Verified reports of child abuse and neglect were abstracted from state records.* **Main Results:** *During the 15-year period after the birth of their first child, in contrast to women in the comparison group, women who were visited by nurses during pregnancy and infancy were identified as perpetrators of child abuse and neglect in 0.29 vs 0.54 verified reports ($P < .001$). Among women who were unmarried and from households of low socioeconomic status at initial enrollment, in contrast to those in the comparison group, nurse-visited women had 1.3 vs 1.6 subsequent births ($P = .02$), 65 vs 37 months between the birth of the first and a second child ($P = .001$), 60 vs 90 months' receiving Aid to Families With Dependent Children ($P = .005$), 0.41 vs 0.73 behavioral impairments due to use of alcohol and other drugs ($P = .03$), 0.18 vs 0.58 arrests by self-report ($P < .001$), and 0.16 vs 0.90 arrests disclosed by New York State records ($P < .001$).* **Conclusions:** *This program of prenatal and early childhood home visitation by nurses can reduce the number of subsequent pregnancies, the use of welfare, child abuse and neglect, and criminal behavior on the part of low-income, unmarried mothers for up to 15 years after the birth of the first child.*

In recent years, home-visitation services have been promoted widely as a means of preventing a range of health and developmental problems in children from vulnerable families. The US Advisory Board on Child Abuse and Neglect, for example, has recommended that home-visitation services be made available to all parents of newborns as a means of preventing child abuse and neglect.[1]

Many of these recommendations have been based on the results of a randomized trial of a comprehensive program of prenatal and early childhood home visitation by nurses that was conducted in Elmira, NY.[2-11] Findings from this trial indicated that the program reduced the rates of subsequent pregnancy, increased labor force participation, and reduced government spending for low-income unmarried women from the birth of the first child through the child's fourth birthday, ie, through 2 years after the program ended.[8,9] Although the rates of state-verified cases of child maltreatment among high-risk families were reduced while the program was in operation (through age 2 years),[5] the effects were attenuated during a 2-year period after the program ended,[6] most likely because of increased surveillance for child abuse and neglect set in motion among the nurse-visited families.[7] Children's health care encounters in which injuries were detected also were reduced from ages 1 through 4 years.[5,6]

Although this program produced positive effects on maternal and child health from pregnancy through the child's fourth year of life,[4-11] its long-term effects remain unexamined. The present study was conducted to determine the extent to which the beneficial effects of the program instituted early in the life cycle altered the life-course trajectories of the mothers through the child's 15th birthday. We examined the long-term effects of the program on 2 domains of maternal functioning: (1) maternal life course (subsequent number of children, use of Aid to Families With Dependent Children [AFDC], employment, substance abuse, and encounters with the criminal justice system) and (2) perpetration of child abuse and neglect. We hypothesized that the program effects, as in earlier phases of the study, would be greater for families in which the mothers experienced a larger number of chronic stressors and had fewer resources to manage the challenges of living in poverty and being a parent.

DESIGN AND METHODS

Setting

The study was originally conducted in and around Elmira, NY, a small city with a population of 40 000 in a semirural area of central New York State (NYS). Patients were recruited from a clinic offering free antepartum services sponsored by the county health department and the offices of private obstetricians.

Participants

From April 1978 through September 1980, 500 consecutive eligible women were invited to participate. Pregnant women were actively recruited for the study if they had no previous live births, could register in the study prior to the 25th week of gestation, and had at least one of the following sociodemographic risk characteristics: young age (<19 years at registration), unmarried, or low socioeconomic status (SES) (Medicaid status or no private insurance). To avoid creating a program stigmatized as being exclusively for the poor, any woman who asked to participate and had no previous live birth was accepted into the study. Approximately 10% of the target population (low income, unmarried, or teenaged) was not recruited because of late registration for prenatal care, and another 10% was not recruited because they were not referred from the offices of private obstetricians.

Four hundred of the 500 women enrolled in the study. All enrollees completed approved informed consent procedures. There were no differences in the age, education, or marital status of women who chose to enroll and those who declined; there was a difference by race, with 80% of white women vs 96% of the African-American women agreeing to participate.

Eighty-five percent of the sample originally recruited had at least 1 of the 3 risk characteristics used for recruitment. Fortyeight percent were younger than 19 years, 62% were unmarried, and 59% were from households classified as low SES[12] at registration during pregnancy. Eleven percent of the sample was African American.

Treatment Conditions

The research design included 4 treatment conditions. Families randomized to treatment 1 (n = 94) were provided sensory and developmental screening for the children at 12 and 24 months of age. Based on these screenings, the children were referred for further clinical evaluation and treatment when needed. Families randomized to treatment 2 (n = 90) were provided the screening services offered those in treatment 1, plus free transportation (using a taxicab voucher system) for prenatal and well-child care through the child's second birthday. There were no differences between participants in treatments 1 and 2 in their use of prenatal and well-child care (both groups had high rates of completed appointments). Therefore, these 2 groups were combined to form a single comparison group as in earlier reports. Families randomized to treatment 3 (n = 100) were provided the screening and transportation services offered those in treatment 2 in addition to being provided a nurse who visited them at home during pregnancy. Families randomized to treatment 4 (n = 116) were provided the same services as those in treatment 3, except that the nurse continued to visit through the child's second birthday.

Randomization

Women were stratified by marital status, race, and 7 geographic regions within the county (based on census tract boundaries). At the end of the intake interview, women drew their treatment assignments from a deck of cards and placed them in a sealed envelope. The cards were transferred to a research associate who managed the randomization. The stratification was executed by using separate decks of cards for the groups defined by the women's race, marital status at intake, and, for white women, the geographic region in which they resided. To ensure reasonably balanced subclasses, the decks were reconstituted periodically to overrepresent those treatment groups with smaller numbers of subjects, a procedure similar to the Efron biased coin designs.[13] Women in treatments 3 and 4 subsequently were assigned on a rotating basis, within their stratification blocks, to 1 of 5 nurse home visitors.

There were 2 deviations from this randomization procedure. First, 6 women who were enrolled were living in the same household as were other women who were already participating in the study. To avoid potential horizontal diffusion of the treatment in case of different assignments within households, the 6 new enrollees were assigned to the same treatment as their housemates. Second, during the last 6 months of the 30-month enrollment period, the number of cards representing treatment 4 was increased in each of the decks to enlarge the size of that group and to enhance the statistical power of the design to compare the infancy home-visitation program with treatments 1 and 2 on infant health and developmental outcomes. A thorough analysis conducted at earlier phases of the trial indicated that this slight confounding of treatments with time did not affect the treatment effects.

Program Plan and Implementation

The experimental home-visitation program was administered by Comprehensive Interdisciplinary Developmental Services, Inc, of Elmira. In the home visits, the nurses promoted 3 aspects of maternal functioning: (1) health-related behaviors during pregnancy and the early years of the child's life; (2) the care parents provided to their children; and (3) maternal personal life-course development (family planning, educational achievement, and participation in the workforce). In the service of these 3 goals, the nurses linked families with needed health and human services and attempted to involve other family members and friends in the pregnancy, birth, and early care of the child. The program was based on theories of self-efficacy, human ecology, and human attachment.[14] The nurses used detailed assessments, record-keeping forms, and protocols to guide their work with families, but adapted the content of their home visits to the individual needs of each family. They provided a comprehensive educational program designed to promote parents' and other family members' effective physical and emotional care of their children. The nurses also helped women clarify their goals and develop problem-solving skills to enable them to cope with the challenges of completing their education, finding work, and planning future pregnancies. Developing a close working relationship with the mother and her family, the nurses helped mothers identify small achievable objectives that could be accomplished between visits that, if met, would build mothers' confidence and motivation to manage the demands of caregiving and become economically self-sufficient. The nurses completed an average of 9 (range, 0-16) visits during the pregnancy and 23 (range, 0-59) visits from the child's birth to second birthday. Details of the program can be found elsewhere.[14,15]

Overview of Follow-up Study

The present phase of the study consists of a longitudinal follow-up of those 400 families who were randomized to treatment and comparison conditions and in which the mother and child were still alive and the family had not refused participation in earlier phases. The flow of patients from recruitment through the 15-year follow-up is presented in Table 1. As this table indicates, we completed assessments at 15 years on 81% of participants originally randomized and on 90% of women for whom there was no miscarriage, stillbirth, death (infant, child, or maternal), or child adoption. There were no treatment differences in the rates of completed assessments at the 15-year follow-up. Table 1 also shows that reviews of children's Child Protective Service (CPS) records were completed for an average of 13.4

TABLE 1
Profile of the Trial: Flow of Patients From Recruitment During Pregnancy Until 15 Years After Birth of First Child*

	Treatments 1 and 2 (n = 184)	Treatment 3 (n = 100)	Treatment 4 (n = 116)
Program implementation			
Completed prenatal home visits, mean (range)	. . .	8.6 (0–16)	8.6 (0–16)
Completed postnatal home visits, mean (range)	. . .	. . .	22.8 (0–59)
Intervening years			
Fetal, infant, or child death	10	7	9
Child adopted†	7	6	2
Maternal death‡	1	1	0
15-y follow-up study			
Missing (mothers)	12	1	4
Refused to participate§			
Mothers	6	5	4
Adolescents	10	8	7
Completed assessments			
Mothers	148	79	97
Adolescents	144	77	94
Cases with CPS data‖	142	77	95
Years of complete CPS data, mean (SD) [range]	13.4 (3.2) [2.6–15.0]	13.3 (3.1) [2.9–15.0]	13.4 (3.1) [0.7–15.0]

*Of 500 eligible patients, 100 refused participation. The 400 participants were randomized to treatment conditions: treatments 1 and 2 were combined to form a comparison group; treatment 3, nurse visitation during pregnancy; and treatment 4, nurse visitation during pregnancy and infancy. Data are given as number, unless otherwise indicated.
†There were 2 adoptions in which interviews were conducted with the child but not the mother. They are not shown in this table.
‡For both cases in which the mother died, the adolescents were interviewed.
§Refusals include 8 mothers who refused to participate during earlier phases and were not approached for the 15-year follow-up.
‖Child Protective Service (CPS) data were used to determine the number of state-verified reports of child abuse and neglect.

years for those cases on which 15-year interviews were conducted with the mother. There were no treatment differences in the number of years for which we had CPS data.

Statistical Power

Sample size and power were determined by the original design and subsequent attrition of subjects. Power calculations are given here for 3 key outcomes (number of months receiving AFDC, subsequent births, and verified reports of child abuse or neglect) with the assumption of $\alpha = .05$ and $\beta = .20$ (2-tailed tests); sample sizes as realized in the present study; and means and SDs obtained from the comparison subjects in the present study. The calculations were performed for the contrast of women in the comparison condition (treatment 1 + treatment 2) vs those in the nurse-visited-during-pregnancy-and-infancy condition (treatment 4)—for both the total sample and for the unmarried, low-SES subsample.

For the number of months receiving AFDC, a normal variable, we can detect a mean difference of 19 months in the total sample and 30 months in the higher-risk sample. For the number of subsequent births, also a normal variable, we can detect differences of 0.36 and 0.57 in the total and high-risk samples, respectively.

For the count of number of verified reports of abuse and neglect, the smallest detectable differences are 0.21 and 0.33, respectively. The actual analyses in this report use more fully specified models than those used for the power calculations, and thus have greater power.

Masking

The mothers were informed that they were being interviewed as part of a follow-up to their participation in a study in which they originally enrolled when they were pregnant with their first child. All data were gathered by staff members who had no access to the families' treatment assignments, except in a few cases in which the mothers in-advertently revealed that they were visited by a nurse. Staff members who gathered data were told that the 15-year follow-up study was designed to assess the long-range effects of prenatal and early childhood services, including home visitation by nurses. The principal investigators and statisticians had access to the families' treatment assignments, although the operationalization of variables was made explicitly without reference to this information.

Assessments and Definitions of Variables

Assessments conducted at earlier phases are specified in previous publications.[5,6,8] Intake interviews, which were conducted with women before randomization, included assessments of women's sociodemographic and personality characteristics (including a short-form measure of the locus of control scale of Rotter[16]), health-related behaviors, and health conditions. Women's household SES was estimated by using the Hollingshead 4-factor method[12]; families were classified into low SES (III and IV) and higher SES (I and II) levels.

At the 15th-year interview, mothers completed a life-history calendar that was designed to help them recall major life events (such as births of additional children, marriages, employment, household moves, and housing arrangements). Women were asked to estimate the number of months that they used AFDC, Medicaid, and food stamps, as well as the number of times that they were arrested or convicted from the time of the birth of their first child to the child's 15th birthday.

Women also were asked a series of questions adapted from the National Comorbidity Survey[17] regarding the impact of alcohol and other drug use on major aspects of their lives since the birth of their child. A variable was constructed that summarized a count of 6 domains of women's lives that were affected by their use of alcohol (missing work, experiencing trouble at work, having a motor vehicle crash or traffic violation, having compromised care of their children, having received treatment). The same set of questions were repeated for their use of illegal and prescription drugs. The counts of domains affected by their use of alcohol and other drugs were summarized to create a "substance use behavioral impairment" scale with values ranging from 0 to 12.

Mothers provided consent for the research staff to review CPS records from states in which they resided during thc interval from the birth of their first child (focal child) to that child's 15th birthday. All reports involving either the mother or the focal child were recorded.

Substantiated reports were abstracted to ascertain key features of the maltreatment incident. All NYS records were searched, as well as those of most othe states in which families resided during the 15-year period. In some states, data were not available for the entire 15-year period because these states expunge their records on a periodic basis. A few other states prohibit the release of case-level information. Six cases had fewer than 4 years of CPS data, and although none was indicated for abuse or neglect, they are retained as valid cases for this analysis. As shown in Table 1, our search covered an average of more than 13 years of the 15-year period in each treatment group, and there were no treatment differences in the amount of time searched, either for the sample as a whole or for the low-SES, unmarried subgroups. The primary outcome variable reported herein is the total number of substantiated reports during the entire 15-year period involving the mother as perpetrator.

Mothers' records of arrests and criminal convictions were abstracted from the NYS Division of Criminal Justice Services, after the principal investigator (D.O.) signed a nondisclosure agreement. Cases were matched based on the women's names, birth dates, ethnicity, and Social Security numbers. Data on the number of arrests and convictions and types of offenses were abstracted from this data-base. Arrests were separated by whether they occurred before randomization or between the child's birth and 15th birthday. (No arrests occurred between randomization and the child's birth.)

Statistical Models and Methods

The study was conducted with an intent-to-treat approach. After examination of a large number of classification factors and covariates, a core statistical model was derived that was consistent with the one used in the earlier phases of this research. It consisted of a $3 \times 2 \times 2$ factorial structure and 6 covariates. The classification factors were treatments (1 and 2 vs 3 vs 4), maternal marital status (married vs unmarried, at registration), and social class (Hollingshead I and II vs III and IV, at registration). All interactions among these factors were included. The basic conclusions reported herein were not modified by or limited to one race, and race was not included in final models.

The 6 covariates included in the final model were maternal age, education, locus of control, husband or boyfriend support, mother's employment status, and father's public-assistance status, all measured at registration. These covariates had consistently significant relationships with many of the outcomes examined in this report. All covariates were tested for homogeneity of regressions for the hypothesized contrasts.[18]

Dependent variables for which a normal distribution was assumed were analyzed in the general linear model and low-frequency count data (eg, number of substantiated reports of child maltreatment) in the log-linear model (assuming a Poisson distribution). In the log-linear model, the analysis was performed and estimates obtained in terms of the logs of the incidence. We use the term *incidence* in referring to the actual count or mean of counts over specific periods of measurement.

The distributions of each of the dependent variables were carefully examined, and cases with outlying values (above 20) were truncated to 20 to reduce the likelihood that the differences observed were the result of a few extreme values. This was done for 1 outcome variable, number of days jailed.

All treatment contrasts focused on the comparison of the combination of treatments 1 and 2 (the comparison group) with treatment 4 (the pregnancy and infancy nurse-visited group), because we hypothesized that the greatest treatment effect would be exerted by the combination of prenatal and postnatal home visitation, as found in earlier evaluations.[8,9] We also show treatment effects for the group defined by women's being unmarried and from low-SES households at registration during pregnancy; this constitutes our operationalization of women's experiencing higher levels of chronic stress (being from a low-SES household) and having few personal resources to manage stress (being unmarried).

RESULTS

We conducted detailed examinations of 17 background variables to determine the extent to which the treatment groups were equivalent for families on which 15-year assessments were completed. As indicated in Table 2, the treatment groups were equivalent both for the sample as a whole and for women who were unmarried and form low-SES households at registration.

Rates of Subsequent Births and Use of Welfare

As indicated in Table 3, in contrast to their counterparts in the comparison group, nurse-visited unmarried women from low-SES households had fewer subsequent pregnancies ($P = .03$) and live births ($P = .02$) and greater spacing between first and second births ($P = .001$). In addition, they reported using AFDC and food stamps fewer months than did unmarried, low-SES women in the comparison group ($P = .005$ and $P = .001$, respectively).

Substance Abuse, Criminal Justice Encounters, and Child Abuse and Neglect

Table 4 shows that nurse-visited, low-SES, unmarried women reported being impaired in fewer domains by alcohol or other drug use, having been arrested fewer times, having been convicted fewer times, and having spent fewer days in jail ($P = .005$, $P < .001$, $P = .008$, and $P < .001$, respectively) since the birth of their first child than did low-SES unmarried women in the comparison group. Data from NYS showed that nurse-visited, low-SES, unmarried women had fewer actual arrests ($P < .001$) and fewer convictions ($P < .001$).

New York State arrests were classified into 3 categories: property crimes (eg, theft), person crimes (assault, robbery), and other (eg, vice, major traffic offenses). Overall, 67%

TABLE 2

Equivalence of Treatment Conditions on Background Characteristics Measured at Registration for Women Assessed at 15-Year Follow-up*

Dependent Variables	Whole Sample			Low-SES Unmarried Sample		
	Treatments 1 and 2 (n = 148)	Treatment 3 (n = 79)	Treatment 4 (n = 97)	Treatments 1 and 2 (n = 62)	Treatment 3 (n = 30)	Treatment 4 (n = 38)
Unmarried, %	62	59	64	...	...	...
Low-SES household, %	64	70	61	...	...	...
White, %	90	91	86	87	87	77
Smoker (>4 cigarettes/d), %	47	46	58	51	60	59
Male child, %	55	44	55	44	53	49
Mother working, %	39	36	31	24	20	20
Mother receiving public assistance, %	9	10	13	23	29	20
Father working, %	70	70	67	42	50	52
Father receiving public assistance, %	4	3	3	10	6	2
Husband or boyfriend in house, %	58	76	60	21	47	22
Maternal age, mean (SD), y	19.3 (2.9)	19.5 (3.1)	19.4 (3.7)	18.6 (2.5)	19.0 (2.8)	18.2 (3.3)
Maternal education, mean (SD), y	11.2 (1.5)	11.6 (1.5)	11.1 (1.6)	10.7 (1.4)	10.9 (1.4)	10.3 (1.5)
Husband or boyfriend education, mean (SD), y	11.4 (1.4)	11.7 (1.7)	11.5 (1.6)	11.1 (1.4)	11.0 (1.8)	10.8 (1.5)
Grandmother support†‡	100.4 (10.1)	97.7 (9.2)	101.3 (10.3)	101.6 (10.9)	98.1 (10.3)	104.1 (11.2)
Husband or boyfriend support†‡	99.6 (10.5)	102.0 (9.0)	99.0 (9.9)	94.2 (10.6)	98.6 (9.4)	96.8 (9.3)
Locus of control†	99.3 (10.1)	100.6 (9.5)	100.6 (10.2)	97.5 (10.2)	99.2 (10.3)	99.1 (9.9)
Incidence of maternal arrests in New York State prior to randomization§	0.09 (−2.50)	0.13 (−5.41)	0.06 (−8.98)	0.13 (−2.03)	0.13 (−2.02)	0.18 (−1.71)

*See first footnote to Table 1 for explanation of treatment groups. SES indicates socioeconomic status.

†Standardized to mean = 100 and (SD) = 10.

‡Locally developed scale that assesses degree to which individual provides emotional and material support to mother.

§Incidence (log incidence) represents the mean number of infrequently occurring events within stated period. Individual cases may have values greater than 1, although the range is small.

TABLE 3

Adjusted Maternal Life-Course Outcomes From Birth of First Child to 15 Years*

Dependent Variables	Whole Sample				Low-SES Unmarried Sample			
	Mean No.				Mean No.			
	Treatments 1 and 2	Treatment 3	Treatment 4	Estimate† (95% CI), vs Treatment 4	Treatments 1 and 2	Treatment 3	Treatment 4	Estimate† (95% CI), Treatments 1 and 2 vs Treatment 4
Subsequent pregnancies	2.1	1.9	1.7	0.4 (−0.1 to 0.8)	2.2	2.0	1.5	0.7‡ (0.1 to 1.3)
Subsequent births	1.6	1.4	1.3	0.3 (−0.0 to 0.6)	1.6	1.4	1.1	0.5‡ (0.1 to 1.0)
Months between birth of first and second child	37.3	39.8	41.7	−4.4 (−14.9 to 6.1)	37.3	46.6	64.8	−27.5§ (−44.1 to −10.9)
Months receiving AFDC	65.9	70.2	52.8	13.1 (−0.9 to 27.0)	90.3	81.8	60.4	29.9§ (9.0 to 50.7)
Months employed	89.7	87.5	96.4	−6.7 (−20.4 to 7.0)	80.0	74.9	95.9	−15.9 (−36.6 to 4.6)
Months receiving food stamps	56.4	62.0	47.9	8.5 (−6.3 to 23.3)	83.5	84.0	46.7	36.8§ (14.6 to 59.0)
Months receiving Medicaid	70.0	71.1	61.8	8.2 (−7.6 to 24.0)	95.4	92.4	72.3	23.1 (−0.6 to 46.8)

*Adjusted for socioeconomic status (SES), marital status, maternal age, education, locus of control, support from husband or boyfriend, working status, and husband or boyfriend use of public assistance at registration. See first footnote to Table 1 for explanation of treatment groups. AFDC indicates Aid to Families With Dependent Children; CI, confidence interval.

†Estimate = (treatments 1 and 2 mean) − (treatment 4 mean).

‡$P < .05$.

§$P < .01$.

TABLE 4

Adjusted Rates of Maternal Substance Abuse, Arrests, Convictions, and Child Abuse and Neglect Reports From Birth of First Child to 15 Years*

Dependent Variables	Whole Sample				Low-SES Unmarried Sample			
	Incidence (Log Incidence)†			Estimate‡ (95% CI), Treatments 1 and 2 vs Treatment 4	Incidence (Log Incidence)†			Estimate‡ (95% CI), Treatments 1 and 2 vs Treatment 4
	Treatments 1 and 2	Treatment 3	Treatment 4		Treatments 1 and 2	Treatment 3	Treatment 4	
Substance use impairments§	0.43 (−1.09)	0.45 (−0.82)	0.34 (−1.33)	0.24 (−0.39 to 0.87)	0.73 (−0.31)	0.61 (−0.49)	0.41 (−0.89)	0.58‖ (0.04 to 1.11)
Arrests	0.22 (−2.02)	0.16 (−2.17)	0.09 (−5.21)	3.19 (−99.66 to 106.04)	0.58 (−0.55)	0.36 (−1.01)	0.18 (−1.74)	1.19‖ (0.49 to 1.89)
Convictions	0.13 (−2.29)	0.05 (−9.48)	0.03 (−9.62)	7.33 (−408.24 to 422.91)	0.28 (−1.28)	0.11 (−2.22)	0.06 (−2.74)	1.46‖ (0.38 to 2.54)
Days in jail	0.65 (−4.36)	0.13 (−9.20)	0.01 (−13.36)	9.00 (−481.52 to 499.53)	1.11 (0.10)	0.47 (−0.76)	0.04 (−3.22)	3.32‖ (2.16 to 4.48)
NYS arrests	0.38 (−1.57)	0.34 (−1.12)	0.12 (−5.03)	3.46 (−105.59 to 112.50)	0.90 (−0.11)	0.39 (−0.95)	0.16 (−1.85)	1.74‖ (0.94 to 2.54)
NYS convictions	0.27 (−4.92)	0.28 (−1.32)	0.12 (−5.30)	0.38 (−226.81 to 227.57)	0.69 (−0.37)	0.29 (−1.25)	0.13 (−2.02)	1.65‖ (0.79 to 2.52)
Substantiated reports of child abuse and neglect	0.54 (−0.63)	0.35 (−1.26)	0.29 (−1.40)	0.77‖ (0.34 to 1.19)	0.53 (−0.64)	0.63 (−0.47)	0.11 (−2.25)	1.61‖ (0.87 to 2.35)

*Adjusted for socioeconomic status (SES), marital status, maternal age, education, locus of control, support from husband or boyfriend, working status, and husband or boyfriend use of public assistance at registration. See first footnote to Table 1 for explanation of treatment groups. NYS indicates New York State; CI, confidence interval.

†Incidence represents the mean number of Infrequently occurring events within stated period. Individual cases may have values greater than 1, although the range is small.

‡Estimate = (treatments 1 and 2 log incidence) − (treatment 4 log incidence).

§Scale summarizes the counts of behavioral impairments (eg, missing work, motor vehicle crash) reported by women resulting from their use of alcohol and illegal drugs.

‖$P < .01$.

of the crimes were for property offenses, 14% were for person crimes, and 19% were for other offenses. The treatment differences for low-SES, unmarried women were present for arrests for property offenses (0.12 vs 0.60; $P < .001$), but not at conventional levels of statistical significance for person offenses (0.02 vs 0.13; $P = .10$), and other offenses (0.02 vs 0.17; $P = .12$) (data not shown).

Table 4 also shows that in contrast to women in the comparison group, those visited during pregnancy and the first 2 years of the child's life were identified as perpetrators of child abuse and neglect in fewer verified reports during the 15-year interval ($P < .001$). This effect was greater for women who were unmarried and from low-SES households at registration ($P < .001$). The effect of the program on number of verified reports was especially strong for the 4- to 15-year period after the birth of the child—ie, the period not assessed in previous reports (data not shown).

COMMENT

In contrast to women in the comparison group, those visited by nurses during pregnancy and the first 2 years after the birth of their first child were identified as perpetrators of child abuse and neglect in fewer verified reports. Among women who were unmarried and from low-SES households at registration, those who were visited by nurses during pregnancy and infancy had fewer subsequent children, months receiving AFDC and food stamps, behavioral impairments from use of alcohol and other drugs, arrests, convictions, and number of days jailed during the 15-year period after birth of their first child. For most outcomes, the group that was visited only during pregnancy exhibited levels of functioning that fell in between the comparison group and the group that was visited during pregnancy and infancy, indicating a dose-response relationship for level of home visitation.

These findings have some limitations. First, most of the positive results were concentrated among mothers who were unmarried and from low-SES households at registration during pregnancy. While we hypothesized originally that the effects would be greater for women who experienced higher levels of stress and who had fewer personal resources, we did not fully operationalize the stress and resource variables prior to the beginning of the trial. We chose to employ characteristics used for sample recruitment as indicators of chronic stress (coming from a low-SES household) and having few personal resources (being unmarried). The marital status and poverty variables chosen to reflect the personal resource and stress constructs, however, are both well-established risk factors for several adverse outcomes. The concentration of program effects in women who are unmarried and of lower SES suggests that they need these services and benefit from them to a greater extent than do those who are married and of higher SES. Consequently, such services should be made available to communities with high concentrations of low-income, unmarried women.

The second limitation is that several of the outcomes were based on self-report, which may be subject to treatment-related reporting bias. The data on maternal use of AFDC and food stamps, for example, were based on self-reports and covered up to 15-year time periods. We attempted to validate maternal report of welfare use by reviewing state and county records but found that they often were incomplete. Fortunately, we were able to obtain archived data from independent sources on other critical outcomes.

The child abuse and neglect findings, for example, were based on state archived data, which makes them less susceptible to reporting bias. Although we were unable to achieve complete reviews of these archived records for all families, they are substantially complete, and there is no indication that missing data resulted in any bias in favor of the nurse-visited groups. It should be noted, moreover, that the effects of the program overrode a tendency for nurse-visited families to be identified for maltreatment at lower thresholds of caregiving dysfunction than were families in the comparison group during the first 4 years of the child's life—a form of detection bias that worked against the hypothesis of program efficacy.[7]

Although it would have been preferable to have criminal records to corroborate the mothers' reports of all arrests and convictions, the analysis of their arrests and convictions archived in NYS produced a pattern of treatment effects that was even stronger than was found with maternal report. Thus, in spite of the knowledge nurse-visited women had of the purpose of this study, they were at least as accurate in reporting this undesirable behavior as were women in the comparison group.

Finally, one may reasonably question the extent to which the findings of this study may be generalized to a wider range of low-SES, unmarried women today. This question led to a recently completed replication of this trial in Memphis, Tenn, with a sample of predominantly low-income, unmarried African-American mothers and their families.[19] The findings of the replications are congruent with the Elmira trial for the 2-year period after birth of the first child and indicate that the benefits of the program, at least through the first child's second birthday, are not limited by time, geography, or the sociodemographic characteristics of the families served. We believe that the results of these 2 trials now provide sufficient evidence to form a rationale for preliminary stages of program dissemination.

One of the most fundamental considerations in planning program dissemination is cost. As indicated in a forthcoming report, the reduction in family size, use of welfare, incidence of child abuse and neglect, and maternal criminality 15 years after the birth of the first child found for this program will lead to substantial savings to government in several domains of spending.[20] In considering the cost of the program (estimated to be $3300 in 1980 dollars and $6700 in 1997 dollars for $2\frac{1}{2}$ years of service), it is important to note that the investment in the service, from the standpoint of government spending, was recovered for low-SES families before the child reached 4 years of age.[9] It would take longer for the investment to be recovered today because costs for such a program have increased more rapidly than costs of welfare benefits.

It is also important to note that the effects reported herein were produced in the context of a controlled experiment, in which the program was conducted with high levels of fidelity to the underlying theoretical and clinical model.[14] The next challenge is to determine the extent to which this progam can be replicated.[21] A modest dissemination effort is currently being conducted under the auspices of the US Departments of Justice and Health and Human Services that will shed light on community and organizational factors that contribute to or undermine fidelity of program implementation in new program sites.

Finally, it should be emphasized that although many different kinds of home-visitation programs have been promoted, it is incorrect to assume that our results can be applied to home-visitation programs that are not based on this model. While some other types of home-visitation programs have shown some promise,[22,23] most have failed.[3] At least 2 well-designed trials of other home-visitation programs are under way that should give us a better understanding of the range of program characteristics that can affect important aspects of maternal, child, and family functioning.[24,25] In the meantime, as health and social welfare policy is redesigned in the near future, we believe that it makes sense to being with programs that have been tested, replicated, and found to work.

REFERENCES

1. US Advisory Board on Child Abuse and Neglect. *Creating Caring Communities: Blueprint for an Effective Federal Policy on Child Abuse and Neglect*. Washington, DC: US Dept of Health and Human Services, Administration for Children and Families; 1991.
2. Olds D, Kitzman H. Can home-visitation improve the health of women and children at environmental risk? *Pediatrics*. 1990;86:108-116.
3. Olds D, Kitzman H. Review of research on home visiting for pregnant women and parents of young children. *Future Child*. 1993;3:53-92.
4. Olds D, Henderson C, Tatelbaum R, Chamberlin R. Improving the delivery of prenatal care and outcomes of pregnancy: a randomized trial of nurse home visitation. *Pediatrics*. 1986;77:16-28.
5. Olds D, Henderson C, Chamberlin R, et al. Preventing child abuse and neglect: a randomized trial of nurse home visitation. *Pediatrics*. 1986;78:65-78.
6. Olds D, Henderson C, Kitzman H. Does prenatal and infancy nurse home visitation have enduring effets on qualities of parental caregiving and child health at 25 to 50 months of life? *Pediatrics*. 1994;93:89-98.
7. Olds D, Henderson C, Kitzman H, et al. Effects of prenatal and infancy nurse home visitation on surveillance of child maltreatment. *Pediatrics*. 1995;95:365-372.
8. Olds D, Henderson C, Tatelbaum R, et al. Improving the life-course development of socially disadvantaged mothers: a randomized trial of nurse home visitation *Am J Public Health*, 1988;78:1436-1445.
9. Olds D, Henderson C, Phelps C, et al. Effects of prenatal and infancy nurse home visitation on government spending. *Med Care*. 1993;31:155-174.
10. Olds D, Henderson C, Tatelbaum R. Intellectual impairment in children of women who smoke cigarettes during pregnancy. *Pediatrics*. 1994;93:221-227.
11. Olds D, Henderson C, Tatelbaum R. Prevention of intellectual impairment in children of women who smoke cigarettes during pregnancy. *Pediatrics*. 1994;93:228-233.
12. Hollingshead A. *Four Factor Index of Social Status*. New Haven, Conn: Yale University Social Sciences Library; 1976. Manuscript.
13. Efron B. Forcing a sequential experiment to be balanced. *Biometrika*. 1971;58:403-417.
14. Olds D, Kitzman H, Cole R, et al. Theoretical and empirical foundations of a program of home visitation for pregnant women and parents of young children. *J Community Psychol*. 1997;25:9-25.
15. Olds D. The Prenatal/Early Infancy Project. In: Price R, Cowen E, Lorion R, Ramos-McKay J, eds. *Fourteen Ounces of Prevention: A Case Book of Practitioners*. Washington, DC: American Psychological Association; 1988.

16. Rotter JB. Generalized expectancies for internal versus external control of reinforcement. *Psychol Monogr Gen Appl.* 1966;80:1.
17. Kessler R. The National Comorbidity Survey: preliminary results and future directions. *Int Rev Psychiatry.* 1994;6:365-376.
18. Henderson C. Analysis of covariance in the mixed model: higher level, nonhomogeneous, and random regressions. *Biometrics.* 1982;38:623-640.
19. Kitzman H, Olds DL, Henderson CR Jr, et al. Effect of prenatal and infancy home visitation by nurses on pregnancy outcomes, childhood injuries, and repeated childbearing: a randomized controlled trial. *JAMA.* 1997;278:644-652.
20. Karoly LA, Everingham SS, Hoube J, et al. *Benefits and Costs of Early-Childhood Interventions: A Documented Briefing.* Santa Monica, Calif: RAND; 1997.
21. Olds D, O'Brien R, Racine D, et al. Increasing the policy and program relevance of results from randomized trials of home visitation. *J Community Psychol.* In press.
22. Gutelius MF, Kirsch AD, MacDonald S, et al. Controlled study of child health supervision: behavioral results. *Pediatrics.* 1977;60:294-304.
23. Black MM, Nair P, Kight C, Wachtel R, Roby P, Schuler M. Parenting and early development among children of drug-abusing women: effects of home intervention. *Pediatrics.* 1994; 94(4, pt1):440-448.
24. Landsverk J, Carrilio T. *San Diego Healthy Families America Clinical Trial.* San Diego, Calif: Children's Hospital and Health Center; 1995.
25. Duggan AK, Buchbinder SB, Fuddy L, Young E, Sia C. Hawaii's Healthy Start Home Visiting Program: engagement of at-risk families. Presented at the annual meetings of the Ambulatory Pediatric Association; May 7, 1996; Washington, DC.

19

Nature–Nurture in the Classroom: Entrance Age, School Readiness, and Learning in Children

Frederick J. Morrison
Loyola University, Chicago, Illinois
Elizabeth M. Griffith
University of Denver, Colorado
Denise M. Alberts
McGill University, Montreal, Quebec

The impact of entrance age on reading and mathematics achievement in 1st grade was examined. Methodological problems with past research were identified, including small size of achievement differences, failure to take background variables into account, and confusion of achievement levels with degree of learning. Using a pre–post design, growth of reading and mathematics was examined in younger 1st graders, older 1st graders, and older kindergarteners. Comparisons of background information on these groups with children who were either held out prior to or retained an extra year in kindergarten, produced minimal background differences. Results revealed that younger 1st graders made as much progress over the school year as did older 1st graders and made far more progress than older kindergarteners. Overall, findings demonstrated that, in itself, entrance age was not a good predictor of learning or academic risk.

The role of genetic or maturational versus experiential influences on psychological development surfaces regularly in efforts to explain important psychological phenomena. In recent years, the intensity of the "nature–nurture" debate has heated up in both academic and applied settings. Findings from work in quantitative behavior genetics (Plomin, 1995; Rowe, 1994) have revealed substantial genetic influences across a range of intellectual and

---

Reprinted with permission from *Developmental Psychology*, 1997, Vol. 33(2), 254–262.

Support for this research was provided by grants from the National Sciences and Engineering Research Council of Canada and Grant HD 27176 from the National Institute of Child Health and Human Development. We would like to thank Ghislaine Boucher and Kate Murie for assistance in data collection.

personality dimensions, including IQ, introversion–extraversion, depression, and aggression (Plomin, 1990; Scarr, 1992). Moreover, the unique impact of environmental influences has also been highlighted recently, including schooling effects on memory and language skills (Ferreira & Morrison, 1994; Morrison, Smith, & Dow-Ehrensberger, 1995) as well as on selected narrative and quantitative problem-solving skills (Bisanz, Morrison, & Dunn, 1995; Varnhagen, Morrison, & Everall, 1994). As a consequence of these advances, debate has been reawakened among basic developmental scientists on the unique and interactive effects of genetic and environmental influences (Wahlsten, 1996) as well as on the most fruitful theoretical conceptualization of their impact on psychological development (Bronfenbrenner, Ceci, & Lenzenweger, in press).

In reality, the nature–nurture debate is by no means limited to academic circles. Important social problems have also generated controversy over the roles of genetic versus environmental factors. Recent examples include the debates over the success or failure of compensatory education (Jensen, 1969), over genetic versus social factors underlying criminal behavior (Wilson & Herrnstein, 1985), and over the bases for cross-cultural differences in academic achievement (Stevenson & Lee, 1990). This classic dichotomy has surfaced again in recent years in educational circles, surrounding the question of school readiness and entrance age. Specifically, concerns have been expressed in the scientific and popular literature that children who are young when they enter Grade 1 (effectively, 5 years old) may be at risk for academic underachievement, lowered self-esteem, and later adaptation problems. Yet, research findings in this area have not uniformly supported this claim, leading to a confusing and contradictory picture.

On one side, a number of reports have claimed that the youngest children in a class are more likely to perform less well academically (Breznitz & Teltsch, 1989; Davis, Trimble, & Vincent, 1980), to repeat a grade (Langer, Kalk, & Searls, 1984), to be referred to special education (Di Pasquale, Moule, & Flewelling, 1980; Maddux, 1980), and to be labeled as learning disabled (Maddux, 1980). The maturationalist theme underlying such claims is that young children entering Grade 1 are not developmentally ready to benefit from formal schooling (Gesell, 1940). Consequently, researchers have argued that these children progress little academically, their poorer performance compared with older classmates results in feelings of anxiety and lowered self-esteem, and subsequent emotional and motivational difficulties produce a spiralling circle of increasing academic and social failure throughout elementary and junior high school.

On the other side, careful review reveals a number of logical and methodological problems with these studies (Shepard & Smith, 1986, 1988). In addition, not all studies found age to be a major, independent predictor of early school success (Alexander & Entwistle, 1988; Gredler, 1980; Jones & Mandeville, 1990; Shepard & Smith, 1986). Still, in other studies with cross-sectional designs, researchers have noted that age differences in achievement in the early grades diminish or disappear in later grades (Langer, Kalk, & Searls, 1984; Miller & Norris, 1967; Shepard & Smith, 1986; but see Breznitz & Teltsch, 1989).

Examination of the rather extensive and contradictory literature on this question reveals at least three major problems with existing research that could contribute to the currently confused picture.

MAGNITUDE OF AGE DIFFERENCES

First, the size of the achievement differences found in many studies comparing younger with older first graders, although statistically significant, is seldom very large and, hence, of dubious educational significance (Shepard & Smith, 1986). For example, using sample sizes of over 8,000 children per grade, Davis et al. (1980) found that, at the end of first grade, children who were fully 6 years old at the beginning of the year were only 9 percentile points ahead of children who were 5 years old at the beginning of the year. Similarly, Shepard and Smith (1985), examining data from 700 first graders in 10 separate schools, found an average of only a 9 and a 6 percentile point difference in reading and math, respectively, between youngest and oldest first graders. In a recent investigation of factors contributing to the risk of reading failure in elementary school children, Jones and Mandeville (1990) found that the proportion of total risk attributed to socioeconomic and racial factors was 13 times larger than that contributed by chronological age. These findings reinforce the view that achievement differences between younger and older children are small in absolute magnitude and in educational relevance compared with other factors.

ASSESSMENT OF BACKGROUND CHARACTERISTICS

Second, few studies have attempted to systematically control for potentially biasing background variables (e.g., IQ, day-care experience, and parental education and occupation). There are several potentially important problems in this area. Differential rates of participation in research studies as a function of socioeconomic, racial, or other factors may yield group differences in background characteristics for younger versus older entrants, which could in turn influence the direction and magnitude of the achievement differences observed. Depending on the nature and sources of the bias, real group differences may be eliminated, or nonexistent group differences may be artifactually created.

In addition, differential rates of holding out and retaining younger rather than older students could produce different background characteristics in the two samples that might yield a biased picture. Younger children are held out for a year prior to kindergarten and retained an extra year in kindergarten to a greater degree than are older children (Shephard & Smith, 1985). Consequently, depending on the policies of local school boards and the existing stereotypes in communities about the importance of entrance age on development, background characteristics of younger versus older children entering school may differ substantially sometimes in counterintuitive ways. Certainly, in some cases, children deemed to be cognitively, academically, or socially at risk may be held out or retained. Such practices could yield residual samples of younger school entrants with more favorable background characteristics on average (like IQ or socioeconomic status [SES]) than older entrants (Cahan & Cohen, 1989), thereby reducing the magnitude of the age effect. In some communities, however, substantial numbers of relatively affluent, educated parents of comparatively bright, mature children opt to hold them out prior to kindergarten or have them repeat kindergarten simply to avoid any possible disadvantage to their child. This removal of young, high SES children serves to lower the background characteristics of the residual group of younger age entrants as compared with older children, thereby magnifying the size of the age differences.

Finally, although some studies claimed that achievement differences diminished in later grades (Langer, Kalk, & Searls, 1984), higher retention rates over the elementary school years for younger versus older entrants could systematically eliminate the poorest performing younger entrants from the later comparisons, thereby minimizing the true size of the age effect on growth of academic achievement. Overall, without gathering systematic information on younger versus older entrants, one cannot be certain to what degree and in what direction potential group differences in background characteristics might be produced nor can their subsequent impact on academic achievement be predicted beforehand.

MEASURING DEGREE OF PROGRESS

Third, by focusing attention on age differences in absolute levels of academic achievement, most research has systematically overlooked the more central question, namely, are relatively young children learning? It is entirely possible that younger entrants, being in some cases almost a full year younger than older entrants, start out first grade slightly behind their older classmates but make as much (or more) progress during the course of the school year, concluding first grade only a few percentile points lower. Without some way to assess degree of progress in children (e.g., with a pre–post design), one cannot draw valid conclusions about whether younger children are learning as well as older children.

Taking into account these methodological issues, in this study, we attempted to reexamine the influence of entrance age on academic achievement. To compare degree of learning, three groups of children were chosen for study: younger Grade 1 children (those with birthdates within 2 months prior to the official cutoff date for school entry); older Grade 1 children (those with birthdates falling 2 months after the official cutoff date for school entry); and older kindergarten children (those with birthdates falling 2 months after the official cutoff date for entry into kindergarten). This latter group comprise children who just missed the cutoff for Grade 1 but were very close in age to the younger Grade 1 children (in this study, they averaged 58 days apart in age). Children were tested in reading and mathematics performance in the early fall and late spring of the school year.

This pre–post design with three groups of children permitted two fundamental questions to be asked. First, do younger Grade 1 children make as much progress in reading and math as do older Grade 1 children? Second, do younger first graders make any more progress in reading and math than a closely age-matched group of kindergarten children who just missed the cutoff for Grade 1? Put another way, the latter question asks whether younger Grade 1 children make any more progress than they would have if they had been in kindergarten. On the surface, the comparison between younger first graders and older kindergarteners may seem unfair, because kindergarteners really do not receive the same degree of formal schooling in reading and math as do first graders. Yet the strong form of the claim that younger first graders are not ready for formal schooling would necessarily predict that the degree of learning exhibited by younger first graders should be no greater than that exhibited by an age-matched group of children not exposed to the formal schooling experience (i.e., older kindergarteners who just missed the cutoff date).

In one final question addressed in this study, we examined the magnitude of predicted schooling effects in reading versus mathematics. Accumulating evidence (Stevenson & Lee, 1990) suggests that American schools and families place more emphasis and spend more instructional time on reading and related activities than on mathematics in the elementary grades. Consequently, we anticipated that schooling effects for reading achievement would be more pronounced than on mathematics achievement.

To assess potential differences in background characteristics, we gathered data on children's IQ, amount of day-care experience, and parental occupation and education. These data were crucial for examining whether differential rates of holding out or retaining younger age entrants might produce group differences in important background characteristics that could influence academic performance.

Because of the potential importance of these types of subject selection biases with the present research design (Bentin, Hammer, & Cahan, 1991; Cahan & Cohen, 1989), we directly compared the background characteristics of the group of younger first graders with two other groups of children. The first was a *held-out* group, composed of children identical in age to younger first graders and therefore eligible for school entry but who had been held out for a year prior to entry into kindergarten. The second was a *retained* group, composed of children identical in age to younger first graders but who had spent an additional year in kindergarten. Unfortunately, limitations on the number of testers available did not permit collection of comparable achievement data on the samples of held-out and retained groups in this study.

It is worth noting that the first graders in this study represent the youngest group of children in North America receiving formal Grade 1 schooling (as far as we can ascertain). The cutoff date for school entry in the locale under study is March 1 (i.e., they must have turned 5 years of age by this date to be allowed entry to kindergarten the previous September). Therefore, young school entrants could have started kindergarten as young as 4 years 6 months of age. Hence, to the degree that being relatively young is a major hindrance, this group of younger first graders should be more at risk than any other children on the continent receiving Grade 1 instruction.

METHOD

Participants

A total of 539 children participated in the study: 152 young Grade 1 children (87 girls and 65 boys), 114 old Grade 1 children (66 girls and 48 boys), 126 old kindergarten children (60 girls and 66 boys), 103 held-out children (40 girls and 63 boys), and 44 retained children (17 girls and 27 boys). Children were recruited into the study over a 3-year period from 26 public elementary schools in a moderately large city in western Canada. Participating schools represented a broad spectrum of socioeconomic levels and geographic areas within the city. All participating children spoke fluent English and were judged by teachers to be free of serious medical, neurological, behavioral, and emotional problems.

Young first-grade children were defined as those whose birthdates fell within 2 months prior to the official March 1 cutoff date for school entry. Old kindergarten children's birthdates fell within 2 months following the official cutoff date. Old first-grade children were identical to old kindergarten children, but were a year older. Held-out children included those with birthdates 2 months prior to the official cutoff (and hence eligible the year before for school entry) but who had been held out of kindergarten for a year. Retained children were those with birthdates 2 months prior to the official cutoff date, who had entered kindergarten at the appropriate time but had been retained an extra year in kindergarten. The latter two groups, then, were identical in age to the young first-grade group but had not proceeded to first grade according to an age-appropriate schedule.

Educational Setting

Examination of the curriculum guidelines and discussions with teachers and administration officials revealed that the instructional environment in kindergarten was grounded in a philosophy featuring *learning through play* activities, in which teachers emphasized developmentally appropriate practices to promote children's learning and development. Although the definition of *developmentally appropriate* was not entirely clear or consistent across teachers, in practice, instruction in kindergarten emphasized informal student arrangements coupled with individual choice by students of the activity on which they would focus. Teachers attempted to facilitate children's learning within the context of these child-initiated activitives. As a consequence, relatively little time was spent in kindergarten on formal drills in component reading and mathematics skills (such as sound blending, initial consonant stripping, and adding and subtracting). Informal instruction in kindergarten provided experiences in alphabet recognition, sounding out letters, narrative skills, number recognition, and counting.

In contrast, more formal instruction was reserved for first grade. Here, seating arrangements at tables were more permanent and periods of whole-group instruction were scheduled daily, along with more child-initiated sessions. Curricular guidelines emphasized direct instruction in alphabet recognition, letter–sound associations, initial consonant stripping, sound blending, and addition and subtraction. Overall, more instructional time was spent in first grade on reading and related skills than in mathematical skills, consistent with findings in other North American school districts (Stevenson, Lee, & Stigler, 1986; Stevenson & Lee, 1990).

In general, while kindergarten emphasized learning through child-initiated playlike activities facilitated by the teacher, first grade introduced more formal instruction in early reading and mathematics skills. As a result, although some measurable influence of schooling was predicted following kindergarten, more substantial changes were anticipated following first grade. Further, we expected schooling effects to be relatively greater in reading compared with mathematics, given the relatively greater instructional time spent in reading and related activities.

Materials and Procedure

As part of a larger battery, three tests were administered to the kindergarten, young first-grade and old first-grade children. In the early fall and late spring of the school year, the Reading subtest of the Wide Range Achievement Test—Revised (WRAT–R; Jastak,

1978) and the Mathematics subtest of the Peabody Individual Achievement Test—Revised (PIAT–R; Markwardt, 1989) were given to each child individually. Order of test administration was counterbalanced within groups. The WRAT–R measures children's skills in letter knowledge and elementary word decoding. The PIAT–R measures a range of mathematical knowledge and skills in kindergarten and first grade, including number recognition, counting, cardinality and ordinality, and addition and subtraction. We chose these tests for their strong psychometric validity and reliability and because the focus of inquiry of this study was on general academic achievement and not on more specific components of reading and mathematical skills. During the middle of the year, each child received the six-subtest short form of the Stanford–Binet Intelligence Scale—4th edition (Thorndike, Hagen, & Sattler, 1986). Reliability indices for this version range from .95 to .97 for children in this age span. All tests were administered by research assistants trained by a licensed, clinical psychologist. Also, parents were asked to complete a questionnaire, developed by the experimenters, which yielded information on parental occupation derived from Pineo–Porter–McRoberts 16-point scale (Pineo, Porter, & McRoberts, 1977) on parental education and on each child's preschool experience.

RESULTS

Background Variables for Old Kindergarten, Young First-Grade, and Old First-Grade Groups

The old kindergarten, young first-grade, and old first-grade groups were compared on several background factors that could potentially differentiate the groups and contribute significantly to academic achievement. Specifically, child IQ, day-care experience, paternal and maternal occupation, and paternal and maternal education were compared in a series of one-way analyses of variance (ANOVAs). Because of the number of pairwise comparisons conducted on each measure (three), a Bonferroni correction was applied to hold the overall probability of a Type I error at $p < .05$. Across all comparisons, only mother's occupational status yielded a reliable effect, $F(2, 207) = 3.365$, $p < .03$. Follow-up comparisons revealed that the occupational status of mothers of young first graders was relatively higher than that of older first graders, $t(207) = 2.53$, $p < .01$ (see Table 1; note that lower scores mean higher occupational status). With that exception, examination of these samples of children and families failed to reveal major systematic differences in important background characteristics that could influence academic achievement results. Similar comparisons on a number of other background variables (e.g., maternal employment status, number of siblings, single-parent homes) yielded no evidence of any differences among the old kindergarten, young first-grade and old first-grade groups of children.

Comparisons of Background Variables for Young First-Grade, Held-Out, and Retained Groups

Like the previous analyses, results of a series of one-way ANOVAs revealed only one statistically reliable difference among the young first-grade, held-out, and retained groups. Paternal occupational status of young first graders was reliably higher than that of retained

TABLE 1
Background Characteristics of the Five Groups of Children in the Study

Variable	Old K ($n = 126$)	Young G1 ($n = 152$)	Old G1 ($n = 114$)	Held-out ($n = 103$)	Retained ($n = 44$)
Entrance age[a]					
M	65.0	67.0	77.0	67.0	67.0
SD	0.7	0.7	0.7	0.7	0.7
IQ					
M	105.0	109.0	107.0	109.0	105.0
SD	11.6	10.6	11.4	9.3	8.6
Paternal occupational status[b]					
M	8.8	9.5	9.4	9.1	7.3
SD	4.4	4.1	4.4	4.1	3.9
Maternal occupational status[b]					
M	9.4	8.3	10.1	9.2	9.9
SD	4.1	4.1	4.1	4.1	4.1
Paternal education[c]					
M	14.0	13.6	13.9	13.4	12.6
SD	2.5	2.9	2.6	2.8	2.6
Maternal education[c]					
M	13.2	12.8	13.4	13.2	12.7
SD	2.5	2.2	2.3	2.2	2.0
Day-care experience[d]					
M	9.4	9.6	6.7	11.9	10.2
SD	15.4	16.3	13.6	18.8	17.8

Note: K = kindergarten; G1 = Grade 1.
[a]Age of child (in months) at beginning of the school year. [b]Derived from Pineo-Porter-McRoberts (1977) 16-point scale (1981). [c]Number of years of formal schooling. [d]Number of months of day-care experience.

children, $t(212) = 2.67$, $p < .05$. Overall, minimal differences emerged in this study in the background characteristics of groups of identically aged children either promoted according to the appropriate age schedule, held out for 1 year prior to kindergarten entry, or retained an extra year in kindergarten.

Because relying exclusively on examination of mean differences can sometimes obscure group differences in the range or distribution of scores, frequency histograms of the scores for each major background variable were examined for young first-grade, held-out, and retained groups. In each case, there were no obvious differences across groups in overall distribution of scores. For example, Figure 1 depicts the frequency distribution of IQ scores for the young first-grade, held-out, and retained groups. As is readily discernible, the overall shape of the distributions is quite similar across groups, approximating a normal curve. The only possible difference among groups was a slight tendency for fewer, very high IQ scores in the group of retained children. Nevertheless, substantial numbers of children with normal

```
                YOUNG FIRST GRADE       HELDOUT               RETAINED
MIDPOINTS...............................+.....................+...............

   142.5
   140.0
   137.5                                *
   135.0
   132.5
   130.0                                **
   127.5  ***                           *
   125.0  *******                       ***                   *
   122.5  *********                     **
   120.0  ***********                   *****
   117.5  ***************               ***                   *
   115.0  **************                **************        ********
   112.5  ******                        **                    **
   110.0  ********************          ***********           ******
   107.5  *************                 ******************    ****
   105.0  ***********                   ***************       *******
   102.5  *****                         *******               **
   100.0  ************                  *******               **
    97.5  ***                           **                    *
    95.0  ***********                   ****                  ****
    92.5  ****                          **                    ***
    90.0  *                             **                    **
    87.5  ***                           *                     *
    85.0  **                            *
    82.5  *
    80.0  *
```

Figure 1. Distribution of IQ scores for young first-grade, held-out, and retained groups. Each asterisk represents one child.

and above average IQ scores were in the retained and, especially, the held-out group. One held-out child had an IQ of 138!

Overall, our examination of background variables gleaned little evidence that major differences existed among the groups of promoted, held-out, and retained children, which was consistent with the failure to find differences among the three study groups—old kindergarten, young first grade, and old first grade.

Academic Achievement in the Old Kindergarten, Young First-Grade, and Old First-Grade Groups

We conducted a three-way mixed ANOVA on mean raw scores for reading and mathematics achievement, with group (old kindergarten, young first grade, old first grade) and gender as between-subject variables and test phase (pretest, posttest) as the within-subject variable. As in previous analyses, given the number of pairwise comparisons conducted on each measure (nine), a Bonferroni correction was applied within each area (i.e., reading and math) to hold the overall probability of a Type I error to $p < .05$. Gender did not yield any significant main effects or interactions on reading achievement scores. A reliable main effect of gender, $F(1, 386) = 10.020$, $p < .002$, and a significant Gender × Group interaction, $F(2, 386) = 3.280$, $p < .04$, on mathematics achievement scores revealed that, for old first-grade students only, boys outperformed girls, $t(386) = 3.29$, $p < .05$, whereas no gender differences were found for the other two groups.

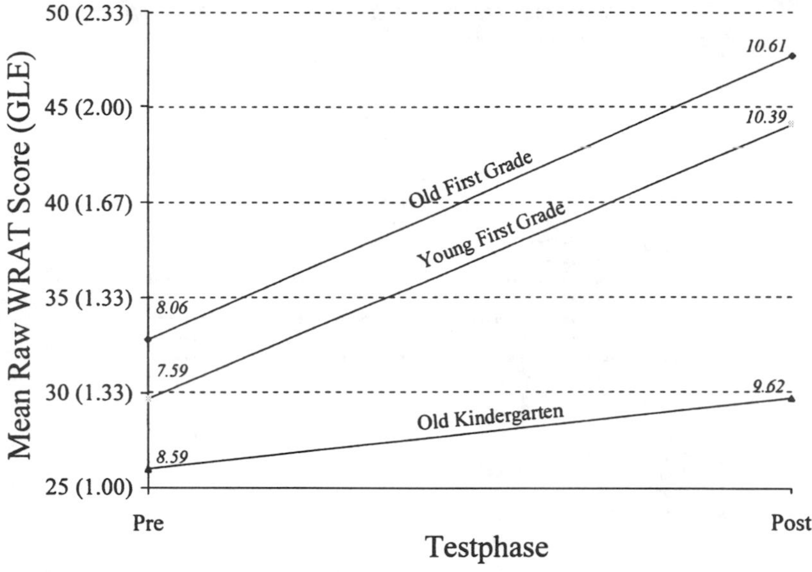

Figure 2. Mean levels of achievement in reading on the Wide Range Achievement Test (WRAT; raw scores and grade-level equivalents [GLE]) attained by the old kindergarten, young first-grade, and old first-grade groups at pretest (fall) and posttest (spring). Standard deviations are in italics.

Reading. Results for reading scores yielded significant group, $F(2, 386) = 70.860$, $p < .0001$, and test phase, $F(1, 386) = 899.920$, $p < .0001$, effects, both qualified by a significant Group × Test Phase interaction, $F(2, 386) = 98.280$, $p < .0001$. As depicted in Figure 2, small but statistically reliable group differences in reading were observed at pretest. Old first-grade children outperformed young first-grade children, $t(389) = 3.11$, $p < .05$, who exceeded performance of old kindergarten children, $t(389) = 3.88$, $p < .01$. Although raw reading scores for the old first-grade and young first-grade groups differed significantly, for both groups, grade-level equivalent scores were 1.33, whereas the old kindergarten children performed at Grade 1.00. At posttest, again old first-grade children displayed a small but significant superiority in reading over young first-grade children, $t(389) = 2.88$, $p < .05$. Both young first-grade and old first-grade groups showed marked superiority over old kindergarten children at posttest, $t(389) = 11.65$ and 13.62, for comparisons of old kindergarten with young first-grade and old first-grade groups, $p < .01$. In grade-level equivalents, old kindergarten children ended their year reading at Grade 1.33, whereas young first-grade and old first-grade children were reading at Grades 2.00 and 2.33, respectively. Most important, a separate ANOVA performed on the change scores from pretest to posttest revealed that the degree of improvement exhibited by young first-grade and old first-grade children in reading achievement was not reliably different. In contrast, the degree of improvement of both young first-grade and old first-grade groups was reliably greater than that exhibited by the old kindergarten group, $t(389) = 12.35$ and 12.10, $p < .01$, respectively, for comparison of the old kindergarten group with young first-grade and old first-grade groups.

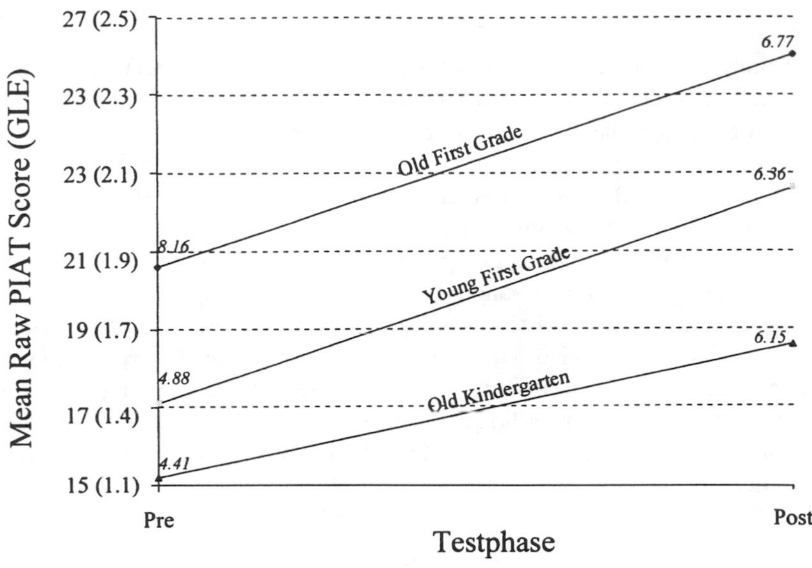

Figure 3. Mean levels of achievement in mathematics on the Peabody Individual Achievement Test (PIAT; raw scores and grade-level equivalents [GLE]) attained by the old kindergarten, young first-grade, and old first-grade groups at pretest (fall) and posttest (spring). Standard deviations are in italics.

Mathematics. Separate examination of achievement in mathematics yielded significant group, $F(2, 386) = 50.570$, $p < .00001$, and test phase, $F(1, 386) = 312.560$, $p < .00001$, effects and a significant interaction, $F(2, 386) = 6.700$, $p < .002$. As depicted in Figure 3, at pretest, old first-grade children showed modest but significant superiority over young first-grade children, $t(389) = 5.50$, $p < .01$, who outperformed old kindergarten children, $t(389) = 3.05$, $p < .05$. In grade-level terms, old kindergarten, young first-grade, and old first-grade children at pretest were performing at about Grades 1.1, 1.4, and 1.9, respectively. At posttest, old first-grade children showed a similar trend with modest, but significant, superiority over young first-grade children, $t(389) = 4.25$, $p < .01$, with grade levels of 2.4 and 2.1, respectively. In contrast, the posttest scores of both young first-grade and old first-grade children exceeded those of old kindergarten children, who had attained a grade level of 1.7, $t(389) = 5.17$ and 8.89, $p < .01$, respectively, for comparisons of old kindergarten group with young first-grade and old first-grade children. Finally, separate analyses on the change scores from pretest to posttest confirmed that the degree of improvement in mathematics performance during Grade 1 was not reliably different in young first-grade versus old first-grade children. In contrast, the degree of improvement made by both young first-grade and old first-grade groups was reliably greater than that manifested by the old kindergarten group, $t(389) = 3.31$ and 2.89, respectively, for comparisons of old kindergarten children with young first-grade and old first-grade children, $p < .01$ and $p < .05$.

DISCUSSION

In this study, we sought to examine whether children who were relatively young when they entered first grade made as much progress as older children and whether they made any more progress than they would have if they had been in kindergarten. Findings from comparisons of growth of reading and mathematics skills for young first-grade children versus old first-grade and old kindergarten groups yielded strongly affirmative answers to these two questions. Further, in this research, we attempted to ascertain whether evidence demonstrating progress in younger first graders might be compromised by serious selection biases resulting from more younger first graders being held out from or retained an extra year in kindergarten. Comparisons of background variables for young first-grade, old kindergarten, old first-grade, held-out, and retained children failed to reveal any evidence of serious participant selection biases in the present samples. Overall, findings from this study demonstrated clearly that younger first graders, as a group, made normal progress over the course of first grade. Entrance age, in and of itself, did not appear to constitute a major risk factor in school readiness.

Growth of Academic Skills

Results from the reading and mathematics tests confirmed earlier findings (Davis et al., 1980; Shepard & Smith, 1985) that, at the end of first grade, achievement levels of younger first graders were slightly below those of older first graders. Yet, this study clearly demonstrated that virtually the same degree of difference existed between younger and older first graders at the beginning of first grade. Further, the degree of progress made by the younger first graders, given their starting point, was identical to that made by older students. In grade-level terms, the younger school entrants made a good year's worth of progress in reading and close to a year's worth of progress in math. Perhaps more revealing, the degree of progress exhibited by the younger first graders surpassed that shown by the older kindergarten group. As stated earlier, if relatively young children (around 5 years of age) were not ready to benefit from formal Grade 1 schooling in reading and math, they should have demonstrated no more progress over the course of their year in Grade 1 than an almost identical age-matched group of children who had just missed the cutoff and had gone to kindergarten. Clearly, findings from this study strongly disconfirmed that notion. The progress of younger first graders as a group clearly surpassed that of their kindergarten counterparts.

Finding group differences between old kindergarten and young first-grade children at pretest demonstrated that instructional experiences in kindergarten also served to enhance growth of elementary reading and mathematics skills, although to a lesser degree. Interpretation of the pretest differences between young first-grade and old first-grade children is more difficult. It is possible that the old first-grade group benefited more from the kindergarten experience the year before. It is equally likely that the old first-grade group, being approximately 10 months older than the young first-grade group, started out the kindergarten year slightly ahead of the young first-grade group and remained so when they entered this study at the beginning of first grade. A clear answer to that question would require conducting a study similar to this one but starting with assessments at the beginning of kindergarten.

The relative magnitude of the schooling influence on reading versus mathematics performance deserves comment. In particular, instruction in first grade appeared to produce greater progress in reading than in mathematics. This difference is consistent with recent evidence from Stevenson, Lee, and Stigler (1986) demonstrating that teachers in early elementary classrooms in American schools spent much more instructional time in reading and language arts than in mathematics. Differential emphasis on reading versus mathematics may help explain the poorer performance of American elementary students compared with Asian students in mathematics as well as the smaller influence of schooling on progress in mathematics observed in this study.

In a related vein, the exact pattern of schooling effects observed in this study may have been largely due to the educational practices and emphases operating at the time the children were tested. For example, minimal formal instruction in either reading or mathematics occurred in kindergarten, consistent with the emphasis in the district on "developmentally appropriate" practices for this age group. A different pattern of results may have emerged for children in more traditional, "academic" kindergartens. Yet, depending on one's philosophy of early education, either larger or smaller effects of traditional kindergarten schooling could be predicted. On the one hand, larger influences of traditional kindergarten might be predicted because earlier formal instruction in elementary decoding skills is introduced. On the other hand, to the extent that formal instruction is not appropriate for children at this age, smaller influences in kindergarten might be expected. A third alternative is also possible, namely that different educational philosophies and practices will influence cognitive and academic skills in different ways and at different times. For example, traditional practices may produce schooling effects on elementary letter and word decoding skills (including spelling), whereas they may have little or no effect on higher order narrative comprehension or storytelling skills. In contrast, a "whole language" approach may produce more substantial schooling influences on narrative skills, with relatively little effect on more elementary decoding or spelling skills.

One concern in this study is the possibility that differences in levels of performance between younger first-grade and older kindergarten children might be due to differential familiarity with formal testing procedures like those used in school settings. Such practices are not common in preschool settings and only become an integral part of most school practices around first grade. Although plausible, recent evidence from other studies with the same methodology casts doubt on this simple interpretation. Using the method of comparing old kindergarten with young first-grade children in a pre–post design (the so-called cutoff methodology), researchers in a series of studies have examined growth of a variety of cognitive and language skills with formal testing procedures similar to those used in the present study: free recall of pictures (Morrison, Smith, & Dow-Ehrensberger, 1995), conservation of number and number addition (Bisanz, Morrison, & Dunn, 1995), story recall and production (Varnhagen, Morrison, & Everall, 1994), and syntactic processing (Ferreira & Morrison, 1994). The pattern of findings across studies clearly refuted the notion that old kindergarten children uniformly performed more poorly than young first-grade children. In each case, patterns of performance were consistent with theoretical predictions about the relative influence of schooling-related or age-related factors contributing to development of the cognitive or linguistic skills under investigation. Hence, group differences between old kindergarten and young first-grade children in this study were most likely due to real differences in the acquisition of reading and math skills in the two groups. Regardless of how one interprets the performance differences between the old kindergarten and young first-grade groups, the separate finding of identical progress for young first-grade and old first-grade groups constitutes additional direct evidence that younger first graders were benefiting substantially from formal schooling in first grade.

Question of Background Variables

A separate attempt was made to examine whether group differences in background variables contributed to achievement outcomes. Using two separate assessments, in this research, we found almost no evidence that background variables contaminated the results or conclusions. Younger first graders were slightly higher than older first graders on maternal occupational status but did not differ at all from older first graders or older kindergartners on measures of general cognitive ability, parental educational levels, paternal occupational status, or amount of day-care experience. Other comparisons revealed that, with the exception of paternal occupational status, the group of younger first graders did not differ significantly on the same set of background characteristics from identically age-matched groups of children held out from or retained an extra year in kindergarten. On the surface, the latter findings are surprising, given the reasonable assumption that parents and teachers must be holding out or retaining these children for some reason. Notwithstanding the fact that some younger students eligible for school entry are thought by parents and teachers to be relatively cognitively or socially immature and, hence, would benefit from being held out or repeating a year, significant numbers of parents of bright, mature, younger children have elected in recent years to postpone school entry or have their child repeat a year in kindergarten for reasons other than fears about their child's readiness to learn in school. Full consideration of the nature and consequences of current practices of retaining and holding out children is beyond the scope of this article (for analysis and review of this complex issue, see Shepard & Smith, 1988). For present purposes, it is sufficient to note that substantial numbers of bright, mature children from economically and educationally advantaged families were not entering school at the age-appropriate time. Given this fact, it is not surprising that the background characteristics of groups of promoted, retained, and held-out children would not differ substantially.

Implications

Findings from this study have implications for future research as well as for selected social policy questions in early education.

Research. Although these findings document clearly that younger first graders as a group were progressing academically as well as their older peers, the results raise additional important questions for future consideration. First, although entrance age failed to produce a main effect on academic achievement, might not entrance age interact with other variables (e.g., child IQ, gender, and social maturity) to yield smaller subgroups of children at risk for poor academic progress? Many teachers and parents commonly assume that younger boys are more at risk than younger girls and that socially immature, younger boys are the most vulnerable of all younger entrants. Shepard and Smith (1985) found that differences in reading and math performance between older and younger age entrants were pronounced only for students in the lowest 25th percentile of performance. The authors concluded that the purported disadvantage exhibited by younger school entrants may be produced by younger children of lower intellectual ability. An important direction for future studies will be closer examination of the interactive role of entrance age with other psychological variables.

Second, findings from the present study are limited to performance in kindergarten and first grade, leaving open the possibility that entrance-age problems may not surface until later in elementary school or even in the transition to high school. Academic demands of the first two school years are relatively light, hence younger age entrants may be able to hold their own during this period. As school becomes more difficult, younger entrants may possibly begin to experience more academic problems. Longitudinal data comparing younger with older entrants over the course of early elementary school are needed to address this question.

Third, despite the successful levels of learning and achievement of younger age entrants in this study, we did not examine learning and achievement in the held-out and retained groups. It is possible that these two groups might have benefited from the extra year before entering first grade and, as a consequence, might have outperformed their promoted peers. Nevertheless, it should be noted that recent reviews of the effects of nonpromotion on children (Gredler, 1984; Shepard & Smith, 1986, 1988) have uniformly failed to find either academic or social–emotional benefits of retaining immature children.

Finally, in the present study, we used relatively global measures of achievement. Hence, it is possible that age differences might have emerged for selected components of reading and mathematics. For example, Morrison, Smith, and Dow-Ehrensberger (1995) found age-related differences in phonemic awareness in spring of the kindergarten year. Yet, in that study, age differences disappeared by the end of first grade. On balance, the present findings leave open the possibility of age-related effects on selected reading and mathematics skills.

Educational policy. In conjunction with other findings (Alexander & Entwistle, 1988; Jones & Mandeville, 1990; Shepard & Smith, 1985), the present results raise doubts about the validity of recent claims that entrance age may contribute substantially to the academic and literacy problems of American children (Davis et al., 1980). Moreover, the findings caution against facile solutions like raising the entrance age, holding out or retaining young entrants, or adding "transition" years for "young fives." As several authors have repeatedly made clear (May, Kundert, & Brent, 1995; Meisels, 1992), such policies may actually be counterproductive. For example, the present findings revealed that substantial numbers of bright children from relatively affluent homes were being held out or retained prior to first grade. As Shepard and Smith (1988) have pointed out, such practices actually increase the range of variation among children in kindergarten and first-grade classrooms, thereby significantly exacerbating the relative immaturity and perceived unreadiness of the youngest children in the class. Clearly, wholesale retention of sizable numbers of younger school entrants is not warranted by existing data and is of dubious educational benefit.

REFERENCES

Alexander, K. L., & Entwistle, D. R. (1988). Achievement in the first two years of school: Patterns and processes. *Monographs of the Society for Research in Child Development, 53,* (2, Serial No. 217).

Bentin, S., Hammer, R., & Cahan, S. (1991). The effects of aging and first grade schooling on the development of phonological awareness. *Psychological Science, 2,* 271–274.

Bisanz, J., Morrison, F. J., & Dunn, M. (1995). The effects of age and schooling on the acquisition of elementary quantitative skills. *Developmental Psychology, 31,* 221–236.

Breznitz, Z., & Teltsch, T. (1989). The effect of school entrance age on academic achievement and social–emotional adjustment of children: Follow-up study of fourth graders. *Psychology in the Schools, 26,* 62–68.

Bronfenbrenner, U., Ceci, S. J., & Lenzenweger, M. F. (in press). Nature–nurture reconceptualized in developmental perspective: Toward a new theoretical and operational model. *Psychological Review.*

Cahan, S., & Cohen, N. (1989). Age versus schooling effects on intelligence development. *Child Development, 60,* 1239–1249.

Davis, B. G., Trimble, C. S., & Vincent, D. R. (1980). Does age of entrance affect school achievement? *The Elementary School Journal, 80,* 133–143.

Di Pasquale, G. W., Moule, A. D., & Flewelling, R. W. (1980). The birthdate effect. *Journal of Learning Disabilities, 13,* 234–238.

Dunn, L. M., & Markwardt, F. (1970). *Peabody Individual Achievement Test.* Circle Pines, MN: American Guidance Service.

Ferreira, F., & Morrison, F. J. (1994). Children's knowledge of syntactic constituents: Effects of age and schooling. *Developmental Psychology, 30,* 663–678.

Gesell, A. (1940). *The first five years of life* (9th ed.). New York: Harper & Row.

Gredler, G. R. (1980). The birthdate effect: Fact or artifact? *Journal of Learning Disabilities, 13,* 239–242.

Gredler, G. R. (1984). Transition classes: A viable alternative for the at-risk child? *Psychology in the Schools, 21,* 463–470.

Jastak, S. (1978). *Wide Range Achievement Test—Revised.* Wilmington, DE: Jastak Associates.

Jensen, A. R. (1969). How much can we boost I.Q. and scholastic achievement? *Harvard Educational Review, 39,* 1–123.

Jones, M. M., & Mandeville, G. K. (1990). The effect of age at school entry on reading achievement scores among South Carolina students. *Remedial and Special Education, 11,* 56–62.

Langer, P., Kalk, J. M., & Searls, D. T. (1984). Age of admission and trends in achievement: A comparison of Blacks and Caucasians. *American Educational Research Journal, 21,* 61–78.

Maddux, C. D. (1980). First-grade entry age in a sample of children labeled learning disabled. *Learning Disability Quarterly, 3,* 79–83.

Markwardt, F. C. (1989). *Peabody Individual Achievement Test—Revised.* Circle Pines, MN: American Guidance Service.

May, D. C., Kundert, D. K., & Brent, D. (1995). Does delayed school entry reduce later grade retentions and use of special education services? *Remedial and Special Education, 16,* 288–294.

Meisels, S. J. (1992). Doing harm by doing good: Iatrogenic effects on early childhood enrollment and promotion policies [Special issue: Research on kindergarten]. *Early Childhood Research Quarterly, 7,* 155–174.

Miller, D. W., & Norris, R. (1967). Entrance age and school success. *Journal of School Psychology, 6,* 47–60.

Morrison, F. J., Smith, L., & Dow-Ehrensberger, M. (1995). Education and cognitive development: A natural experiment. *Developmental Psychology, 31,* 789–799.

Pineo, P. C., Porter, J., & McRoberts, H. A. (1977). The 1971 census and the socioeconomic classification of occupation. *Canadian Review of Sociology and Anthropology, 14,* 91–102.

Plomin, R. (1990). *Nature and nurture: An introduction to human behavioral genetics.* Pacific Groves, CA: Brooks/Cole.

Plomin, R. (1995). Molecular genetics and psychology. *Psychological Science, 4,* 114–117.

Rowe, D. C. (1994). *The limits of family influence.* New York: Guilford Press.

Scarr, S. (1992). Developmental theories for the 1990's: Developmental and individual differences. *Child Development, 63,* 1–19.

Shepard, L. A., & Smith, M. L. (1985, March). *Boulder valley kindergarten study: Retention practices and retention effects.* Boulder, CO: Boulder Valley Public Schools.

Shepard, L. A., & Smith, M. L. (1986). Synthesis of research on school readiness and kindergarten retention. *Educational Leadership, 44,* 78–86.

Shepard, L. A., & Smith, M. L. (1988). Escalating academic demand in kindergarten: Counterproductive policies. *The Elementary School Journal, 89,* 135–145.

Stevenson, H. W., & Lee, S. Y. (1990). Contexts of achievement. *Monographs of the Society for Research in Child Development, 55*(1–2, Serial No. 221).

Stevenson, H. W., Lee, S. Y., & Stigler, J. W. (1986, February). Mathematics achievement of Chinese, Japanese and American children. *Science, 231,* 693–699.

Thorndike, R. L., Hagen, E. P., & Sattler, J. M. (1986). *Stanford-Binet Intelligence Scale—4th edition.* Chicago: Riverside.

Varnhagen, C., Morrison, F. J., & Everall, R. (1994). Age and schooling effects in story recall and production. *Developmental Psychology, 30,* 969–979.

Wahlsten, D. (1996). Evaluating genetic models of cognitive evolution and behavior. *Behavioral Process, 35,* 183–194.

Wilson, J. Q., & Herrnstein, R. J. (1985). *Crime and human nature.* New York: Touchstone.

20

Exceptionally High Intelligence and Schooling

Ellen Winner
Boston College, Chestnut Hill, Massachusetts

Exceptionally intelligent children differ qualitatively from their peers and often are socially isolated and underchallenged in the classroom. Research on educational options for these children shows existing programs to be effective. Little money is spent in the United States on education for gifted children, and distribution of special programs varies widely, with nonurban areas and disadvantaged children being the least likely to receive special services and with the most common option being the weakest one—the pullout program. There is a growing movement to disband existing programs. Instead of calling for more of the existing programs, it is argued that first, standards should be elevated for all children. Those children who still remain underchallenged should then receive advanced classes in their domain of ability. Thus, fewer children would be identified as being in need of special services, and those identified would be the more profoundly gifted children who would receive the strongest kind of intervention.

Stories about Jonathan Estrada have appeared off and on in the national news, describing a young child with extraordinary abilities. Jonathan began to talk at nine months; by two-and-a-half years of age, he was reading at the second-grade level and speaking with an eight-year-old's vocabulary. At age seven, he had an intense intellectual curiosity and a passion for geography (Nieves, 1996).

When Jonathan was five years old, his parents tried to get him admitted into the gifted-and-talented program in their local school district. Jonathan refused to complete the necessary IQ test because he was upset that he was asked to do "easy" things with blocks. When his mother tried to explain to the school officials that he found the test too easy, they told her that there was nothing wrong with the test and that she probably had an inflated view of her child's intelligence. Had Jonathan been accepted into the program, he would have had two hours a week of "enrichment" activities outside of the regular classroom, activities designed for gifted children. Instead, his parents enrolled him in a school for gifted children, where he would get a challenging curriculum full time rather than once or twice a week.

Reprinted with permission from *American Psychologist*, 1997, Vol. 52(10), 1070–1081.

When children like Jonathan reach school age, their parents face a crisis. It is difficult for schools to meet the needs of children who are so out of step with their age-mates in their abilities and interests. What educational choice is most likely to ensure that Jonathan will fulfill his intellectual potential? Should he be placed in a regular classroom so that he is with his age-mates? Would a two-hour enrichment program be an adequate way to deal with his special needs? Should he skip grades so that he is with his mental-age peers, even if that means he is many years younger than his classmates? Should schools have special classes for such children?

The difficulty Jonathan's parents faced in finding an appropriate school did not evoke sympathy in others. Most people thought the parents were bragging and suspected that Jonathan's prodigious abilities had been artificially created by pushy parents. This kind of reaction reflects people's deep-seated ambivalence about intellectual giftedness, arising perhaps from an anti-intellectual strain in American culture (de Tocqueville, 1945) as well as from America's democratic antielitist tradition, which leads to fear of hierarchies as a threat to the egalitarian American dream (Hofstadter, 1963). Although the belief that all people should be treated the same way is one way of interpreting the democratic ideal, another interpretation is that each person should be helped to fulfill his or her individual potential. These two interpretations of democracy lead to clashing visions of how exceptionally intelligent students should be educated.

GIFTED CHILDREN IN REGULAR CLASSROOMS

Exceptionally intelligent students (hereafter referred to as gifted students) face a variety of problems in ordinary classrooms. They often are ostracized as being different and weird and are labeled as *nerds* and *geeks* (Silverman, 1993a, 1993b). In addition, they face the problem of boredom due to lack of an appropriate level of challenge (Csikszentmihalyi, Rathunde, & Whalen, 1993; Gross, 1993). Teachers often make little accommodation to the needs of these children, and many teachers have little or no special training in how to teach such exceptional children (Westberg, Archambault, Dobyns, & Salvin, 1993). A gifted child in the regular classroom may be the only such child in the room; hence, he or she will not have the opportunity to learn with others of like ability. When such classrooms have been observed, the gifted students generally have been bored and inattentive (Westberg et al., 1993). Meta-analyses have shown only modest benefits for this kind of instruction (Bangert, Kulik, & Kulik, 1983).

Many eminent adults report that school was a negative experience for them; they were bored and often knew more than their teachers (Bloom, 1985; Cox, Daniel, & Boston, 1985; Goertzel & Goertzel, 1962). Of course, the lack of appropriate control groups makes it impossible to know whether such negative reconstructions of school are typical of all children or are particularly typical of gifted children. Nonetheless, although one might expect children who lack intellectual interests to find school boring, it is particularly disturbing that the most able students often dislike school and feel they get little out of it. The lack of appropriate instruction for high-ability students is especially problematic for economically disadvantaged children whose families do not have the resources for extracurricular lessons, concerts, museum visits, and so forth.

The findings about gifted children and schooling, discussed below, are almost always based on research with scholastically gifted children and with those who are moderately gifted. Moderately gifted children are very different from profoundly gifted children, like Jonathan Estrada. Moderately gifted children perform one or two years above the level of their age-mates; in IQ terms, which is often how such children are classified, a moderately gifted child has an IQ between about 130 and 150, whereas a profoundly gifted child has an IQ of about 180 or above. Recommendations derived from research with moderately gifted children cannot be assumed to apply to profoundly gifted children because these two kinds of children are as different from one another as are moderately gifted from average children.

THE NATURE OF GIFTEDNESS

Researchers and educators differ in how they define *giftedness*. Traditionally, researchers have defined giftedness as high general intelligence as measured by a high global IQ score (Hollingworth, 1942; Terman, 1925). Since then, arguments have been advanced for expanding and differentiating conceptions of giftedness. For instance, Sternberg's (1981, 1985, 1991) triarchic theory of intelligence allows for three very different kinds of gifts: analytic, synthetic, and practical. Davidson and Sternberg's (1984) theory makes insight central to scholastic giftedness: Gifted children excel at solving insight problems because they are skilled at selectively encoding information (sifting out what is relevant to solve a problem) and selectively combining and comparing information. Renzulli's (1978) theory defines giftedness not only in terms of high ability but also by task commitment and creativity; Getzels and Jackson's (1962) theory makes creativity a part of giftedness. And Gardner's (1983, in press) theory of intelligence, which consists of eight independent abilities (linguistic, logical–mathematical, spatial, interpersonal, intrapersonal, musical, bodily kinesthetic, and naturalist), suggests that giftedness can occur separately in any one of these domains; this modular view of intelligence is inconsistent with a definition of giftedness in terms of general intelligence.

Because my concern here is with the problem of how gifted children should be schooled, I focus only on scholastic, or intellectual, forms of giftedness—that is, on giftedness in language, abstract logical thinking, and mathematics (in Gardner's [1983] terms, these would be gifts in the first two intelligences listed above; in other terms, these would be high-IQ children). Although children with artistic, musical, or athletic gifts also have special educational needs, America's schools do not even try to address these needs. Such children usually seek extra training outside of school (in the case of music and art) or in after-school, extracurricular programs (in the case of athletics).

Theorists of intellectual giftedness differ not only in how they define giftedness but also in terms of whether they view gifted children as differing qualitatively or just quantitatively from average children. In a review of studies investigating the quantitative versus the qualitative question, Rogers (1986) identified the following areas in which gifted children (identified by high IQ) excel: (a) higher order thinking processes, such as recognizing problems and generating and monitoring solutions; (b) encoding, mapping, inference, and justification on analogical-thinking tasks; and (c) transferring skills to new problems and solving insight problems (Davidson & Sternberg, 1984; Sternberg, 1981). In addition, Rogers found that gifted children differ from average children in cognitive style: They are more likely to think independently, to take an active approach toward problem solving, and to persist at tasks; furthermore, they have less need than do average children for structure and adult scaffolding, and they score higher on self-efficacy and internal locus of control.

One could argue that the aforementioned differences between gifted and average children are simply quantitative. Jackson and Butterfield (1986) have argued that there is no evidence for qualitative differences: For example, gifted children use the same memory strategies as do average children, but gifted children simply use these strategies more efficiently. However, many of the studies showing no qualitative differences have been based on artificial tasks such as memory for letters in series (Jackson & Butterfield, 1986), and, for the most part, the gifted children in these studies have been moderately rather than profoundly gifted (as defined by IQ). Moreover, when differences are large, they may lead to qualitative differences in thinking. It seems quite reasonable to assume that although moderately gifted children may not think in a qualitatively different way than ordinary children, profoundly gifted children like Jonathan Estrada may well do so. There have been reports that profoundly gifted children as young as three or four years of age have induced rules of algebra on their own (Winner, 1996), have memorized almost instantly entire musical scores (Feldman & Goldsmith, 1991) and have figured out on their own how to identify all prime numbers (Winner, 1996). Feats such as these just do not feel like faster variants of normal processes; they seem qualitatively different.

I think it is useful to suggest two ways in which profoundly gifted children may think qualitatively differently than average children. One way in which they seem different is suggested by the aforementioned examples: their ability to intuit solutions to challenging problems without help and their striking memories for complex information in their domain. A second way in which they are different is in their passion, their "rage to master," and their intrinsic drive to immerse themselves in a domain (Winner, 1996). These children often cannot be torn away from work in their domain of ability, and they achieve flow by setting challenges for themselves (Kanevsky, 1992).

It should be noted that when educational interventions for scholastically gifted children are being considered, it is important to distinguish between moderately and profoundly gifted children; it also is important to distinguish among kinds of scholastically gifted children (e.g., those who excel in creativity and imagination and those who excel in analytic ability, speed of learning, and memory). Educational options that are ideal for one kind of scholastically gifted child may not work for children with other kinds of scholastic gifts.

INDICATIONS OF SCHOLASTIC (OR INTELLECTUAL) GIFTEDNESS

Moderately as well as profoundly gifted children show early signs of being exceptional. Some of the indications of intellectual giftedness in infancy include long attention spans, good recognition memory, preference for novelty, overreactivity to sensations, and early onset of language (Bornstein & Sigman, 1986; Fagan & McGrath, 1981; Lewis & Brooks-Gunn, 1981; Piechowski, 1995). Indications of the unusual learning styles of these children also emerge early: They show intense curiosity, persistence, drive, obsessive interests, and a metacognitive awareness of their problem-solving strategies, making it possible for them to transfer strategies to new and unfamiliar problems (Kanevsky, 1992; Rogers, 1986; Shore & Kanevsky, 1993). School-related abilities also emerge early: Many (although not all) read one or more years before entering kindergarten, demonstrate a fascination with numbers and numerical patterns, and excel at abstract logical thinking (Jackson, 1992; Krutetskii, 1976).

These children differ socially and affectively in three major respects from the norm. First, they are more likely to be solitary and introverted than are typical children. They like playing alone because they are stimulated by their own minds. When they do play with others, they prefer older children, for obvious reasons, but they have difficulty finding like-minded peers of any age with whom to play (Albert, 1978; Csikszentmihalyi et al., 1993; A. Gallagher, 1990; Janos & Robinson, 1985b; Silverman, 1993b; Storr, 1988). Perhaps because of their sense of isolation and sometimes because of their ostracism, children who are extremely gifted have a rate of social and emotional problems about twice as high as that of average children; more moderately gifted children with less extreme abilities seem to have a slightly lower than average rate of emotional difficulties (Janos & Robinson, 1985b). In one study comparing popular and unpopular gifted children, Cornell (1990) found that these two groups did not differ in academic achievement. However, he noted that the achievement tests used may not have been sensitive enough to pick out profoundly gifted children. In addition, he reported that several children in the unpopular group had IQs higher than 148. Thus, it does appear likely that with extreme levels of ability, social and emotional problems can develop (Hollingworth, 1931, 1942).

Second, these children are often fiercely independent and nonconforming (Janos & Robinson, 1985b; Silverman, 1993a, 1993c; Winner, 1996). And finally, these children are intrinsically motivated to achieve mastery, they derive pleasure from work, and they often have high self-esteem about their intellectual capacities (Bloom, 1985; Csikszentmihalyi et al., 1993; Gross, 1993; Janos & Robinson, 1985b). Those children whose families combine nurturance and stimulation appear to be most likely to remain motivated to achieve, and those who persist in their area of ability report being more engaged and satisfied in high school (Csikszentmihalyi et al., 1993). Some very highly gifted children underachieve, however, often because of lack of appropriate challenges in school. Underachievers are not motivated, and they develop low self-esteem about their intellectual capacities (Butler-Por, 1987).

This picture of giftedness does not, of course, fit all gifted children. To begin with, many eminent adults were late bloomers (Darwin is an oft-cited example) who did not show many of these signs in childhood (Simonton, 1994). As children, their gifts were hidden. In addition, many children present a more one-sided, uneven profile of giftedness. Although many gifted children are globally gifted in the academic realm and balanced in their intellectual skills, it appears that at least as many, if not more, gifted children have a domain-specific gift in either language or mathematics (Benbow & Minor, 1990; Detterman & Daniel, 1989; Mueller, Dash, Matheson, & Short, 1984; Silver & Clampit, 1990; Wilkinson, 1993). For instance, among a thousand intellectually gifted adolescents, more than 95% showed a sharp disparity between their mathematical and verbal abilities (Achter, Lubinski, & Benbow, 1996). And a study of intellectually gifted middle school students revealed three separate kinds of gifts: linguistic, logical–mathematical, and social (D. J. Matthews & Keating, 1995). The kinds of memories and information-processing skills possessed by mathematically gifted children are different than those possessed by verbally gifted children (Dark & Benbow, 1991). Thus, educational interventions need to be tailored to the kind of gift the child possesses. Mathematically gifted children should not be treated the same way as linguistically gifted children. In addition, gifted children who are highly creative and imaginative may benefit from certain kinds of educational interventions, whereas those who are highly analytic or who excel in memory and speed of learning may benefit from other kinds of educational interventions. In short, there are different kinds of intellectual gifts; hence, there must be different kinds of interventions.

Gifted children also may possess a combination of intellectual giftedness in one area and learning disability in another. A common combination is a gift in a spatial area as well as a language-based disability such as dyslexia (Feiring & Taft, 1985; Fox, 1983; Reis, Neu, & McGuire, 1995; Yewchuk, 1985). Students with a combination of gifts and disabilities face particular problems in school: They are excluded from gifted programs (their unevenness can lower overall IQ scores) but are considered too smart for remedial education (Reis et al., 1995). And because they excel in some areas, teachers sometimes write them off as simply being unmotivated.

THE LIFETIME COURSE OF GIFTEDNESS

It is tempting to argue that intellectually gifted children need special schooling so that they can become eminent and creative geniuses as adults. The development of any kind of gift is a long-term endeavor, fostered by early identification, supportive and encouraging parents, and teachers who are at first nurturant and later demanding and tough (Bloom, 1995). However, most gifted children do not grow into eminent adults and do not ever make major contributions to the way people think about a particular domain (Richert, 1997). The lack of correlation between childhood giftedness and adult eminence was first revealed in Terman's longitudinal study of high-IQ children (Terman & Oden, 1959). Most of the participants in this study grew up to be successful but not major creators. And those participants with IQs of 170 or above were no more likely to become eminent than were those with lower IQs (Feldman, 1984). Above the level of 120, IQ cannot predict adult eminence (Barron & Harrington, 1981; Guilford, 1967). And the correlation between school achievement and eminence is either zero or only weakly positive (Cohen, 1984; Hudson, 1958; McClelland, 1973).

There are many reasons why childhood giftedness does not typically grow into adult eminence. Eminence requires drive, and although gifted children are driven, not all of them persist in the kind of hard work that is one of the preconditions for achieving eminence (Ericsson, Krampe, & Tesch-Romer, 1993). Eminence requires creativity, dissatisfaction with the status quo, and a desire to shake things up, and these personality traits are not necessarily reflected in high academic achievement or high IQ (Gardner, 1993). Eminence also is associated with higher than average rates of psychopathology (Eysenck, 1995; Jamison, 1993; Ludwig, 1995; Simonton, 1994). Perhaps the high-IQ children in Terman and Oden's (1959) study did not achieve eminence because to be admitted into the study, they first had to be nominated by their teachers, a procedure that may have weeded out odd children with psychopathological tendencies (Simonton, 1997). Finally, extremely gifted children may have social and emotional difficulties, as mentioned above, and these difficulties can lead to maladaption and dropping out. Numerous individual case studies of maladjusted prodigies exist: One famous case is that of William James Sidis, a math prodigy who dropped out of math after graduating from Harvard University at age 15 (Montour, 1977).

THE CASE FOR SPECIAL EDUCATION FOR GIFTED CHILDREN

Although the most appropriate kind of schooling cannot ensure that intellectually gifted children become eminent adults, for some of the reasons just cited, it is certainly likely that inappropriate schooling, in which instruction is not matched to children's needs, will result in less than optimal intellectual development (as well as an unhappy school experience). The most gifted students in the United States perform far worse than high-ability students in other countries, and about half of the top U.S. students (in the top 5% of the IQ range) are underachieving (Reis, 1994; VanTassel-Baska, 1991). Although international comparisons suggest that most U.S. children are underachieving because at all ability levels they perform poorly as compared with the children in many European and East Asian nations (Stevenson, Chen, & Lee, 1993; Stevenson, Lee, & Stigler, 1986; Stevenson & Stigler, 1992), the gap between potential and performance is probably the greatest for the most gifted children (Ross, 1993). Thus, the most intellectually gifted students are the most underchallenged group, and cross-cultural comparisons suggest that these students could be performing at a far higher level.

If America's democratic ideals are interpreted to mean that each child should receive an education that matches his or her intellectual needs, then it is clear that children like Jonathan should not be placed in ordinary classrooms. Whether more moderately gifted children should be placed in ordinary classrooms is a matter for more debate and is a question I address later in this article.

EXISTING OPTIONS FOR GIFTED CHILDREN

Schools have considered and attempted a variety of options for educating children who are years ahead of their peers in abilities and interests. In the first half of the 20th century, a few special schools for gifted children existed, but it was far more common to accelerate gifted children than to group them together (Kulik & Kulik, 1997). The movement to establish formal "gifted programs" in which gifted children of the same age are grouped together began in reaction to Sputnik in 1957 (Tannenbaum, 1993).

Policies for educating gifted children are determined by states; thus, they vary considerably. During the past 25 years, the number of programs for gifted children offered by the public school system has grown considerably. According to a federal report in 1972, only 4% of gifted children were getting any kind of special service (Marland, 1972), and 20 years ago, only 7 states had legislation and funding for gifted education (Ross, 1993). However, by 1990, 38 states served more than two million gifted children in Grades kindergarten through 12; the other 12 states did not report figures, but every state offers some programs.

According to the 1988 National Education Longitudinal Study, 75% of 8th graders in public schools had some opportunities for gifted education, and almost 9% of 8th graders in public schools participated in some gifted-and-talented programs (Ross, 1993). However, selection for such programs was unevenly distributed across ethnic backgrounds (18% of Asians, 9% of Whites, 8% of African Americans, 7% of Hispanics, and 2% of Native Americans were selected) and income levels (only 9% of identified children came from the bottom quartile of family income in contrast to 47% from the top quartile). In addition, school districts in small towns and rural areas had the fewest such programs (Ross, 1993). The federal Jacob K. Javits Gifted and Talented Students Act of 1988 was passed to address this disparity: The act provides support for research on gifted education, with priority given to efforts to serve gifted children with economic disadvantages or with disabilities.

Although the number of gifted programs has grown dramatically since the 1970s, only 2 cents out of every 100 government dollars allocated for education are spent on gifted programs (Ross, 1993). The number of children participating in some kind of gifted school program is also only about half the number of children participating in some kind of special program for children with disabilities. According to a report by the U.S. Department of Education (1996), in the 1993–1994 school year, 6% of children in Grades kindergarten through 12 in public schools participated in some gifted program, as compared with 12% of children ages 0–21 years who were enrolled in federally supported programs for disabled persons (a category that includes, among other things, individuals with learning disabilities, mental retardation, and emotional disturbances).

Today, there is a growing movement to disband special programs for gifted children (Purcell, 1993; Renzulli & Reis, 1991). The arguments for and against gifted programs are polarized and bitter, and sharp clashes occur between those in favor of ability grouping and those who see it as racist and elitist and who argue for heterogeneous grouping with cooperative learning and between those in favor of grade skipping and those who insist that such acceleration stunts children's social development and robs them of a normal childhood. Even among those who favor special education for gifted children, disagreements form between advocates of enrichment and advocates of acceleration and between those who favor grade skipping, which means placing a gifted child with nongifted older children, and those who promote ability grouping, which means grouping together gifted children who are similar in age. There is no unified approach to gifted education in the United States, which is not surprising given that there also is no unified approach to education in general, no national standards, and no central educational philosophy. Various kinds of services for gifted children can be found in school districts, although many schools have no services at all and only some programs have been adequately evaluated. Next, I describe the major kinds of approaches and review the evidence for the effectiveness of each type.

It is useful first to distinguish between two broad classes of programs: (a) those that supplement education in the regular classroom and thereby help to improve a gifted child's educational experience and (b) those that make fundamental alterations. In the former category are pullout programs (the most common kind of elementary school gifted programs) and out-of-school summer (and sometimes weekend) programs for children selected by talent searches. In the latter category are full-time ability grouping—clustered within a regular classroom, in a special classroom, or in a special school—and acceleration in the form of early school entrance, grade skipping, and courses taken at an above grade level without grade skipping. With some exceptions, including the talent searches for out-of-school programs, gifted children are typically selected for special programs on the basis of global test scores (whether IQ or some other aptitude test).

PROGRAMS THAT SUPPLEMENT

Pullout Programs

Most children selected for gifted programs spend the bulk of their time in regular classrooms but are pulled out for up to several hours a week to participate in programs for gifted children. Seventy-two percent of elementary school districts have adopted this kind of solution for gifted children (Ross, 1993). These children are identified on the basis of global IQ scores (the cutoff may be 130 or somewhat lower) or by some other kind of aptitude or achievement test. Often, other measures such as teacher recommendations and checklists also are used. For the most part, participants are moderately, not profoundly, gifted.

Pullout programs, often called enrichment programs, come in a number of varieties. Schiever and Maker (1997) identified three kinds: (a) Process-oriented programs teach creative problem solving and critical thinking but often not in the context of any particular kind of subject matter, (b) content-oriented approaches offer minicourses or mentorships in a specific subject area, and (c) product-oriented approaches involve students in projects culminating in reports and presentations.

One of the most widely used approaches to pullout education is the schoolwide enrichment model (SEM) developed by Renzulli and Reis (1997). SEM has three phases: exposure, the development of critical and creative thinking skills, and the opportunity to pursue a self-selected area of study. Children are identified by multiple criteria (including creativity and commitment). Up to 20% of children in a school may be admitted to Phase 1, and these children have been shown to do as well in Phase 3 as the top 3%–5% identified by traditional IQ measures (Renzulli & Reis, 1997).

Pullout programs have been criticized for generally not leading to the development of a systematic knowledge base in the area in which a child is gifted because these programs are not grounded in a particular subject area. For the same reason, they have been criticized for not being tailored to the student's particular area of giftedness. Informal research on these programs suggests they are not highly effective: Children often show poor recall of what they did in these sessions (Fetterman, 1988), and schools with such programs often are dissatisfied with them, dismissing them as too superficial and unsystematic (Cox et al., 1985; J. J. Gallagher, Weiss, Oglesby, & Thomas, 1983). The main problem seems to be that even the most exciting curriculum cannot accomplish much if students are exposed to it for only several hours a week. Thus, such programs are weak solutions to large problems (Feldhusen, 1997; Gagné, 1995; Winner, 1996).

Yet, these programs do have some positive effects. Children in these programs show moderately higher achievement gains on standardized tests as compared with children with equal abilities who are not in such programs (Delcourt, Loyd, Cornell, & Goldberg, 1994; Treffinger, Callahan, & Baughn, 1991; Vaughn, Feldhusen, & Asher, 1991). In Vaughn et al.'s study, for example, students gained in achievement, critical thinking, and creativity, and achievement gains were greatest when the curriculum in the pullout program extended that in the regular classroom. Evaluations of SEM have shown that participation in this program improved attitudes toward learning and helped underachievers and that students who went through all three phases remained interested in the same subject areas in college (Renzulli & Reis, 1997). However, students in such studies were not always randomly assigned to an enrichment class; thus, some of the gains shown may have been due to preexisting ability. More important, it is probable that students of all ability levels would benefit from such programs. Thus far, there certainly is no evidence that they would not. Renzulli (1994) argued that the best features of enrichment programs should be taken (e.g., project-based learning) and infused into school for all children.

Talent Searches for Summer and Weekend Programs

A very different kind of selection for special programs was pioneered by Julian Stanley with the founding of the Study of Mathematically Precocious Youth (SMPY) at Johns Hopkins University. Students selected for this program were identified on the basis of a domain-specific achievement test rather than a high overall score on an IQ test or another aptitude test (which cannot predict the specific academic area or areas in which a student may excel). Middle school students were given an "out-of-level" test (the Scholastic Assessment Test [SAT] designed for college-bound seniors in high school) to qualify for fast-paced summer courses in which an entire year of a high school course is compacted into three weeks. There are now four regional centers that conduct talent searches based on out-of-level SATs: the Center for Talented Youth at Johns Hopkins University (now a part of the Institute for the Advancement of Academically Talented Youth), the Talent Identification Program at Duke University, the Center for Talent Development at North-western University, and the Rocky Mountain Talent Search at the University of Denver. Many other local talent-search programs can now be found in every state and even in some other countries, such as China. Middle school students are eligible to participate in talent searches if they score in the upper 3% on a standardized achievement test (elementary school students qualify in the upper 5%). They then take the SAT. Many of these students do extraordinarily well. Twenty percent of these seventh graders do as well or better than average collegebound seniors (Assouline & Lupkowski-Shoplik, 1997; Center for Talented Youth, 1995).

Originally, the courses offered were in mathematics, but now courses in all areas of the curriculum are offered. About 150,000 students per year participate in these programs, which are mostly residential summer programs but sometimes are offered on weekends during the school year. Students who participate find the experience to be very positive, particularly because of the opportunity to have social and intellectual contact with like-minded peers, which for many of them may be a first-time experience (Benbow & Lubinski, 1997; Enersen, 1993).

Currently, SMPY is conducting a longitudinal study of 5,000 students who enrolled in these fast-paced courses (Benbow & Lubinski, 1997; Lubinski & Benbow, 1994). Preliminary findings have shown that these students have maintained a positive self-concept about work and that 85% of the first cohort of SMPY graduated from college with excellent academic records. Thus, students as young as 13 can be identified as having high mathematical abilities and as being likely to go on to be high scholastic achievers. SMPY students also took advanced-placement exams earlier, were more likely to take college courses in high school, and attended more selective colleges than did students matched in gender and SAT scores who chose not to participate (Barnett & Durden, 1993). Thus, students who participate in these summer courses continue to be high achievers in high school and college. And the greatest benefit, in terms of a commitment to advanced courses, higher education, and a full-time career, has been for girls who took courses in math (Fox, Brody, & Tobin, 1985; Olszewski-Kubilius & Grant, 1994). One cannot conclude, however, that the high achievement of these students is causally related to SMPY participation, because those who chose not to participate in SMPY may have been less achievement oriented to begin with.

PROGRAMS THAT MAKE FUNDAMENTAL ALTERATIONS

Ability Grouping in the Classroom

Classroom ability grouping for gifted children can take a number of forms. It can mean placing children in self-contained classes for gifted children, grouping high-ability children together within a classroom (or even across grades) for specific subject matters (cluster grouping), or placing children in schools designed only for gifted children.

Ability grouping is often confused with tracking, a term that evokes strong controversy. *Tracking* usually refers to the practice of assigning high school students to a college preparatory, general, or vocational track on the basis of career goals (Kulik & Kulik, 1997). Although students often choose the track that they prefer (Jencks, 1972), once they are assigned, it is difficult to move into a different track. Critics of tracking, such as Oakes (1985), have argued that such practice leads to segregation by class and race and that the curriculum for the low-tracked students is boring and unchallenging and is taught by the poorest quality of teachers. However, although Oakes showed that low-tracked students learned little, she did not have a control group of similar ability students who were not tracked. Would these students have learned more if they had been in a mixed-ability classroom? It is possible that the lower level of challenge may have been appropriate for the lower ability levels of these students.

Ability grouping is more flexible than tracking, as students can be readily regrouped when appropriate. In addition, grouping may occur only for specific subject matters or for the entire curriculum, as in self-contained classrooms for gifted children. Although ability grouping is also often attacked as being elitist and robbing lower ability students of high-achieving role models (R. Good & Brophy, 1993), it is surprising how common ability grouping actually is. Some form of within-class ability grouping is used in about 90% of elementary schools (McPartland, Coldiron, & Braddock, 1987), and most teachers favor some kind of ability grouping (National Education Association, Research Division, 1968; Slavin, 1989/1990; Wilson & Schmits, 1978).

Meta-analyses of evaluations of self-contained classes for gifted children have shown that ability grouping per se, without appropriate curriculum modifications, leads either to very minimal gains (Kulik, 1992; Kulik & Kulik, 1982, 1991, 1992) or to no gains at all

(Slavin, 1987, 1990). But when curriculum is appropriately strengthened, the effects are quite positive. Kulik (1992) found that (a) the typical gain for gifted students in accelerated, ability-grouped classes was almost one year more on standardized tests than gains made by equivalent-ability students in heterogeneous classrooms and (b) the typical gain for gifted students in enriched, ability-grouped classes was about four to five months greater than gains by matched students in regular classrooms (see also Allan, 1991; Feldhusen, 1989; Fiedler, Lange, & Winebrenner, 1993; Rogers, 1991, 1993, for research showing positive gains made by ability-grouped students).

Meta-analyses of within-class and cross-grade groupings by subject matter again show benefits. More than 80% of studies analyzed by Kulik (1992) reported a positive gain, and the average gain was two to three months greater than that made by equivalent students who were not grouped. Slavin (1987) also reported positive effects of such subject-matter grouping. Even students in middle- and low-ability groups apparently benefit but to a lesser degree (Kulik & Kulik, 1997). The argument that nongifted children will do worse because they lack the role models of the high-achieving students is thus not supported. Perhaps this is because high-ability students cannot serve as effective role models for those who do not feel similar enough to these students to try to emulate them (Schunk, 1987).

Critics of ability grouping argue that cooperative learning in heterogeneous classrooms is a fairer solution (Slavin, 1989/1990). But research demonstrating positive effects of cooperative learning is typically based on a comparison between a cooperative-learning classroom and a traditional classroom with a basic-skills orientation (A. Robinson, 1990a, 1990b, 1991, 1997). Thus, these studies cannot indicate what the effects are of cooperative learning per se on gifted children. Cooperative learning can, of course, be used in a heterogeneous or an ability-grouped classroom, and it is not known whether cooperative learning among equally high-ability students is more or less beneficial than an individualistic approach. However, although most studies of cooperative learning have not looked separately at how this style affects gifted students, one study has shown that gifted high school students dislike cooperative learning, preferring both individualistic and competitive approaches (Li & Adamson, 1992). In addition, qualitative studies of gifted students in cooperative-learning groups report that these students are frustrated by having to explain concepts to uninterested students and feel that they do all of the work (Clinkenbeard, 1991; M. Matthews, 1992; Mulryan, 1992). Gifted students dominate in such groups, and lower ability students remain passive (T. L. Good, Reys, Grouws, & Mulryan, 1989–1990). Even some high-ability students become passive in such groups because they are bored or feel slowed by others (Mulryan, 1992).

Special Schools for Gifted Children

There always have been special schools for gifted children. Many private schools do not label themselves as such, but because they require achievement (or even IQ tests) for admission, they are, in effect, schools for high-ability students. Some private schools officially designate themselves as schools for gifted children and require IQ scores of at least 125 or 130 for admission. Public magnet schools for gifted children at the elementary and middle school level (such as Hunter College Elementary School in New York City) are rare, but state-supported high schools for gifted students are more common (e.g., Bronx High School of Science, Stuyvesant High School, Hunter College High School). In the 1970s, a number of state-supported residential high schools for juniors and seniors began to develop (see Cox et al., 1985; Eilber, 1987; Kolloff, 1997; Stanley, 1987). The North Carolina School of Science and Math, founded in 1980, has served as a model for such schools, and now a number of others have been founded (e.g., Texas Academy of Math and Science; Illinois Math and Science Academy; Louisana School for Math, Science, and the Arts). These high schools are for the most highly gifted students—those for whom advanced-placement and honors courses in regular high schools are insufficient. Teachers at these schools are specialists in their subject area (often they have PhDs); classes are often longer than in regular schools; and students engage in independent, in-depth research. These schools have high-achieving students and typically place a large number of students in the annual Science Talent Search sponsored by Westinghouse (Stanley, 1987). At the Illinois Math and Science Academy, 33% of the students recently were National Merit semifinalists (Kolloff, 1997).

The successful outcome of the graduates speaks well for these schools. But no research has compared students of equally high ability randomly assigned to such schools versus ordinary schools, and no such studies are likely. It seems unreasonable to suggest, however, that high-ability students would do just as well in less rigorous schools. Such a suggestion would mean that there are no benefits to being challenged by one's teachers and peers.

Acceleration

Acceleration can mean taking a fast-paced course (in a regular or special class), early entrance to school, or grade skipping. Although acceleration is often pitted against enrichment as an alternative approach to gifted education, this is not a necessary dichotomy—a class can be fast-paced and enriched (Davis & Rimm, 1994).

Grade skipping is one of the cheapest ways to accommodate gifted students, and evidence for the effects of modest acceleration is positive. Terman (1925) believed that gifted children should be allowed to skip several grades and enter college by age 16. He opposed more radical grade skipping for his high-IQ participants, fearing its negative social effects. Students in the Terman sample who skipped grades went on to achieve more in their careers (Terman & Oden, 1947). Of course, these are correlational data, and it is not known whether the grade skipping led to the achievement or whether the most able students chose to skip grades. But this comparison at least suggests that moderate acceleration is not harmful in the long run. As mentioned, Kulik (1992) showed in a meta-analysis that gifted students who were accelerated outperformed nonaccelerated students (matched in age and IQ) by one year on achievement tests. Many other studies have corroborated these conclusions (e.g., Brody & Stanley, 1991; Feldhusen, 1989; Janos & Robinson, 1985a; Rogers, 1991; Swiatek & Benbow, 1991).

But grade skipping has potential problems. The major concern is that it involves placing children with others who are more physically advanced and with others who are very different socially and emotionally. Schools often resist grade skipping for fear of causing social maladjustment (Gross, 1993; Southern, Jones, & Fiscus, 1989). Although some studies have reported no social or emotional problems for accelerated students (Brody & Benbow, 1987; N. M. Robinson & Janos, 1986), one study of girls in a residential early college entrance program reported an alarming amount of stress and depression (Cornell, Callahan, & Loyd, 1991). These findings do not show that acceleration causes problems, but they do suggest caution and the need to evaluate the individual child before deciding on whether he or she should be accelerated.

Acceleration also is based on the assumption that gifted children are not different but rather just faster than their peers, that is, just like older average children. Moreover, although many studies have shown positive effects of a 1- or 2-year grade skip, a profoundly gifted child like Jonathan, who was described earlier, would need a far more radical grade skip. This would mean placing him with children many years older (as in the muchpublicized case of Michael Kearney, who attended college between the ages of 6 and 10; Castro & Grant, 1994). In addition, if profoundly gifted children are more likely to think in qualitatively different ways than older average students, then placing a 6-year-old prodigy with a 12-year-old average child may not accomplish the intended goal of grouping the prodigy with others of like ability. Grade skipping, then, seems to be a riskier solution for children with extreme levels of intellectual ability who would require radical acceleration. In addition, a gifted child who is very creative and imaginative might have more difficulty with acceleration than a gifted child who is not particularly creative but who is a rapid learner with an excellent memory. Assouline, Colangelo, and Lupowski (1993) pointed out the importance of evaluating the child for acceleration not only in terms of academic ability but also in terms of the child's social and emotional maturity and the child's own attitude toward acceleration.

CONCLUSIONS

Special educational programs for scholastically gifted students have been shown to have positive effects, and a strong case can be made that intellectually gifted students need more than what most regular classrooms in the United States can offer today. One major problem that gifted students face is that American schools hold low expectations for students in general and make minimal demands, as compared with, say, schools in many Western European and East Asian countries. In my view, if America's schools were able to be modeled on the more regorous approaches in such countries, it seems likely that many of America's moderately gifted students, currently bored and languishing, would be appropriately challenged in regular classrooms. Perhaps it is for this reason that countries such as France and Japan, whose schools are more demanding than are U.S. schools, have far fewer gifted programs than the United States does. There is certainly evidence that when standards in classrooms are raised, many students, not just the brightest ones, rise to meet the challenge (Edmonds, 1982; Levin, 1987; Rutter, Maughan, Mortimore, & Ouston, 1979).

International comparisons also show that higher standards lead to higher achievement for all ability levels. If the standards were raised for all students, I believe the gap between high- and low-achieving students would be narrowed. In my view, gifted education requires a two-pronged approach. First, standards for all students need to be radically elevated. If this endeavor were successful, then the children who still remained bored and underchallenged could be identified, and they could be offered advanced classes. Instead of the term *gifted class*, the more precise and less precious term *advanced class* might be used. Students should be identified as needing advanced instruction in mathematics or reading, for instance, rather than be labeled as *gifted* in general.

Even with a more challenging curriculum, the research on ability grouping suggests that students at all levels would benefit from being so grouped. Ideally, students might be placed in flexible, non-age-graded ability groups for all subjects. Children in elementary school who need more advanced courses in a specific subject matter could take courses in middle school; those in high school could take college courses while still in high school. This recommendation for domain-specific, advanced classes also has been made by Stanley and Benbow (1986) and by Feldhusen (1993), who called for accelerated, enriched, challenging instruction in a child's particular talent area. Similarly, Renzulli (1994) argued for making the regular curriculum more challenging, forming enrichment clusters for children with similar interests, and also retaining special services for those at the highest level—services such as independent work and mentors. Furthermore, Ross (1993) recommended that all children be given more challenging material and be allowed to proceed at their own pace with flexible ability grouping.

In my view, young children do not need to be given an IQ test to determine what group they should be placed in. Instead, curriculum-based identification should be used. When children are given a challenging curriculum, high abilities make themselves visible (Ramos-Ford & Gardner, 1997). Teachers can look for signs of boredom, curiosity, drive, and a desire for more work. A 10-year-old boy whom I know, after quickly and effortlessly completing his homework one afternoon, turned to his mother and said, "I think I need more work!" I would take such a statement as a clear sign that this child needed a higher level of challenge. No IQ test would be called for. And groups can and should be flexible; children who are overwhelmed can be regrouped. The use of such curriculum-based identification seems more likely to lead to a fairer representation of minority and poor students in high-ability groups than there are now, given the problems that such students often have with paper-and-pencil tests (Richert, Alvino, & McDonnel, 1982).

But none of these alterations will help children like Jonathan Estrada. Profoundly gifted children are often underchallenged in gifted programs (including special schools for gifted children, which have many moderately gifted children) and do not find their appropriate level of stimulation until they reach college (Winner, 1996). Children like this will continue to need special classrooms or special schools.

When schools cannot or will not meet the needs of high-ability students, families can seek mentors for their children. Highly successful adults often report having had mentors who played a very important role in their intellectual development (Bloom, 1985; Gardner, 1993; Kaufman, 1981), and mentors have been shown to play a particularly important role for disadvantaged students and for girls who enter traditionally male fields (Clasen & Clasen, 1997; McIntosh & Greenlaw, 1990).

Most researchers in the area of gifted education recommend identifying more students as gifted and providing more special services. Because the most common kind of special service is a pullout program, this recommendation can be taken to mean more of the same. In conclusion, I offer a different recommendation, one that does not represent the mainstream of those in the field of gifted education. I suggest that the expectations for all students be considerably elevated and that children be flexibly grouped by subject matter within regular classrooms. Furthermore, special full-time classrooms or special schools should be provided for those children who continue to be underchallenged despite the greater rigor.

This would likely mean that fewer children would be identified as being in need of gifted programming, because many more of the moderately gifted children would be appropriately challenged in regular classrooms if the curriculum were genuinely altered in favor of higher standards. Those identified would then be the more highly gifted children. This solution also would mean that children like Jonathan would not be taught in the same way as moderately gifted children. The difference between children like Jonathan and moderately gifted children should be recognized to be as great or greater than the difference between an average and a moderately gifted child.

REFERENCES

Achter, J., Lubinski, D., & Benbow, C. P. (1996). Multipotentiality among the intellectually gifted: "It was never there and already it's vanishing." *Journal of Counseling Psychology, 43,* 65–76.

Albert, R. S. (1978). Observations and suggestions regarding giftedness, familial influence and the achievement of eminence. *Gifted Child Quarterly, 28,* 201–211.

Allan, S. (1991). Ability grouping research reviews: What do they say about grouping and the gifted? *Educational Leadership, 48*(6), 60–65.

Assouline, S. G., Colangelo, N., & Lupowski, A. E. (1993). *Iowa Acceleration Scale.* Iowa City: University of Iowa, Belin–Blank Center.

Assouline, S. G., & Lupkowski-Shoplik, A. (1997). Talent searches: A model for the discovery and development of academic talent. In N. Colangelo & G. A. Davis (Eds.), *Handbook of gifted education* (2nd ed., pp. 170–179). Boston: Allyn & Bacon.

Bangert, R., Kulik, J. A., & Kulik, C.-L. C. (1983). Individualized systems of instruction in secondary schools. *Review of Educational Research, 53,* 143–158.

Barnett, L. B., & Durden, W. G. (1993). Education patterns of academically talented youth. *Gifted Child Quarterly, 37,* 161–168.

Barron, F., & Harrington, D. M. (1981). Creativity, intelligence, and personality. *Annual Review of Psychology, 32,* 439–476.

Benbow, C. P., & Lubinski, D. (1997). Intellectually talented children: How can we best meet their needs? In N. Colangelo & G. A. Davis (Eds.), *Handbook of gifted education* (2nd ed., pp. 155–169). Boston: Allyn & Bacon.

Benbow, C. P., & Minor, L. L. (1990). Cognitive profiles of verbally and mathematically precocious students: Implications for identification of the gifted. *Gifted Child Quarterly, 34,* 21–26.

Bloom, B. (Ed.). (1985). *Developing talent in young people.* New York: Ballantine Books.

Bornstein, M., & Sigman, M. (1986). Continuity in mental development from infancy. *Child Development, 57,* 251–274.

Brody, L. E., & Benbow, C. P. (1987). Accelerative strategies: How effective are they for the gifted? *Gifted Child Quarterly, 31,* 105–110.

Brody, L. E., & Stanley, J. C. (1991). Young college students: Assessing factors that contribute to success. In W. T. Southern & E. D. Jones (Eds.), *Academic acceleration of gifted children* (pp. 102–132). Baltimore: Johns Hopkins University Press.

Butler-Por, N. (1987). *Underachievers in school: Issues and intervention*. Chichester, England: Wiley.

Castro, P., & Grant, M. (1994, October 24). Small wonder. *Psychology Today,* 99–100.

Center for Talented Youth. (1995). *1995 talent search report*. Baltimore: Johns Hopkins University Press.

Clasen, D. R., & Clasen, R. E. (1997). Mentoring: A time-honored option for education of the gifted and talented. In N. Colangelo & G. A. Davis (Eds.), *Handbook of gifted education* (2nd ed., pp. 218–229). Boston: Allyn & Bacon.

Clinkenbeard, P. R. (1991). Unfair expectations: A pilot study of middle school students' comparisons of gifted and regular classes. *Journal for the Education of the Gifted, 15,* 56–63.

Cohen, P. A. (1984). College grades and adult achievement: A research synthesis. *Research in Higher Education, 20,* 281–293.

Cornell, D. G. (1990). High ability students who are unpopular with their peers. *Gifted Child Quarterly, 34,* 155–160.

Cornell, D. G., Callahan, C. M., & Loyd, B. H. (1991). Socioemotional adjustment of adolescent girls enrolled in a residential acceleration program. *Gifted Child Quarterly, 35,* 58–66.

Cox, J., Daniel, N., & Boston, B. O. (1985). *Educating able learners: Programs and promising practices*. Austin: University of Texas Press.

Csikszentmihalyi, M., Rathunde, K., & Whalen, S. (1993). *Talented teenagers: The roots of success and failure*. New York: Cambridge University Press.

Dark, V. J., & Benbow, C. P. (1991). Differential enhancement of working memory with mathematical versus verbal precocity. *Journal of Educational Psychology, 83,* 48–60.

Davidson, J. E., & Sternberg, R. J. (1984). The role of insight in intellectual giftedness. *Gifted Child Quarterly, 28,* 58–64.

Davis, G. A., & Rimm, S. B. (1994). *Education of the gifted and talented*. Boston: Allyn & Bacon.

Delcourt, M. A. B., Loyd, B., Cornell, D. G., & Goldberg, M. L. (1994). Evaluation of the effects of programming arrangements on student learning outcomes. *Monograph of the National Research Center on the Gifted and Talented* (No. 94107). Storrs: University of Connecticut.

de Tocqueville, A. (1945). *Democracy in America*. New York: Knopf.

Detterman, D. F., & Daniel, M. (1989). Correlations of mental tests with each other and with cognitive variables are highest for low IQ groups. *Intelligence, 15,* 349–359.

Edmonds, R. (1982). Programs of school improvement: An overview. *Educational Leadership, 40,* 4–11.

Eilber, C. R. (1987). The North Carolina School of Science and Mathematics. *Phi Delta Kappan, 68,* 773–777.

Enersen, D. (1993). Summer residential programs: Academics and beyond. *Gifted Child Quarterly, 37,* 169–176.

Ericsson, K. A., Krampe, R. T., & Tesch-Romer, C. (1993). The role of deliberate practice in the acquisition of expert performance. *Psychological Review, 100,* 363–406.

Eysenck, H. J. (1995). *Genius: The natural history of creativity*. Cambridge, England: Cambridge University Press.

Fagan, J., & McGrath, S. (1981). Infant recognition and later intelligence. *Intelligence, 5,* 121–130.

Feiring, C., & Taft, L. (1985). The gifted learning disabled child: Not a paradox. *Pediatric Annals, 14,* 729–732.

Feldhusen, J. F. (1989). Synthesis of research on gifted youth. *Educational Leadership, 46*(6), 6–11.

Feldhusen, J. F. (1993). Talent Identification and Development in Education (TIDE). *Gifted Education International, 10*(1), 10–15.

Feldhusen, J. F. (1997). Secondary services, opportunities, and activities for talented youth. In N. Colangelo & G. A. Davis (Eds.), *Handbook of gifted education* (2nd ed., pp. 189–197). Boston: Allyn & Bacon.

Feldman, D. H. (1984). A follow-up study of subjects who scored above 180 IQ in Terman's "Genetic Studies of Genius." *Exceptional Children, 50,* 518–523.

Feldman, D. H. (with Goldsmith, L. T.). (1991). *Nature's gambit: Child prodigies and the development of human potential.* New York: Teachers College Press.

Fetterman, D. M. (1988). *Excellence and equality: A qualitatively different perspective on gifted and talented education.* Albany: State University of New York Press.

Fiedler, E., Lange, R., & Winebrenner, S. (1993). In search of reality: Unraveling the myths about tracking, ability grouping, and the gifted. *Roeper Review, 16,* 4–7.

Fox, L. H. (1983). Gifted students with reading problems: An empirical study. In L. H. Fox, L. Brody, & D. Tobin (Eds.), *Learning disabled/gifted children: Identification and programming* (pp. 117–140). Baltimore: University Park Press.

Fox, L. H., Brody, L., & Tobin, D. (1985). The impact of early intervention programs upon course-taking and attitudes in high school. In S. F. Chipman, L. R. Brush, & D. M. Wilson (Eds.), *Women and mathematics: Balancing the equation* (pp. 249–274). Hillsdale, NJ: Erlbaum.

Gagné, F. (1995). Hidden meaning of the "Talent Development" concept. *Educational Forum, 59,* 349–362.

Gallagher, A. (1990). Personality patterns of the gifted. *Understanding Our Gifted, 3*(1), 11–13.

Gallagher, J. J., Weiss, P., Oglesby, K., & Thomas, T. (1983). *The status of gifted/talented education: United States survey of needs, practices and policies.* Los Angeles: Leadership Training Institute.

Gardner, H. (1983). *Frames of mind: The theory of multiple intelligences.* New York: BasicBooks.

Gardner, H. (1993). *Creating minds: An anatomy of creativity seen through the lives of Freud, Einstein, Picasso, Stravinsky, Eliot, Graham, and Gandhi.* New York: BasicBooks.

Gardner, H. (in press). Are there additional intelligences? In J. Kane (Ed.), *Education, information, and transformation.* New York: Prentice Hall.

Getzels, J. W., & Jackson, P. W. (1962). *Creativity and intelligence: Explorations with gifted students.* New York: Wiley.

Goertzel, V., & Goertzel, M. G. (1962). *Cradles of eminence.* Boston: Little, Brown.

Good, R., & Brophy, J. (1993). *Looking in classrooms* (6th ed.). New York: HarperCollins College.

Good, T. L., Reys, B., Grouws, D. A., & Mulryan, C. M. (1989–1990). Using work groups in mathematics in an attempt to improve students' understanding and social skills. *Educational Leadership, 47*(4), 56–62.

Gross, M. U. M. (1993). *Exceptionally gifted children.* London: Routledge.

Guilford, J. P. (1967). *The nature of human intelligence.* New York: McGraw-Hill.

Hofstadter, R. (1963). *Anti-intellectualism in American life.* New York: Knopf.

Hollingworth, L. S. (1931). The child of very superior intelligence as a special problem in social adjustment. *Mental Hygiene, 29,* 3–16.

Hollingworth, L. S. (1942). *Children above 180 IQ, Stanford–Binet origin and development.* Yonkers, NY: World Book.

Hudson, L. (1958). Undergraduate academic record of fellows of the Royal Society. *Nature, 182,* 1326.

Jackson, N. E. (1992). Precocious reading of English: Origins, structure, and predictive significance. In P. S. Klein & A. J. Tannenbaum (Eds.), *To be young and gifted* (pp. 171–203). Norwood, NJ: Ablex.

Jackson, N., & Butterfield, E. (1986). A conception of giftedness designed to promote research. In R. J. Sternberg & J. E. Davidson (Eds.), *Conceptions of giftedness* (pp. 151–181). New York: Cambridge University Press.

Jamison, K. R. (1993). *Touched with fire: Manic-depressive illness and the artistic temperament.* New York: Free Press.

Janos, P. M., & Robinson, N. M. (1985a). The performance of students in a program of radical acceleration at the university level. *Gifted Child Quarterly, 29,* 175–179.

Janos, P. M., & Robinson, N. M. (1985b). Psychosocial development in intellectually gifted children. In F. D. Horowitz & M. O'Brien (Eds.), *The gifted and talented: Developmental perspectives* (pp. 149–195). Washington, DC: American Psychological Association.

Jencks, C. (1972). *Inequality.* New York: BasicBooks.

Kanevsky, L. (1992). The learning game. In P. S. Klein & A. J. Tannenbaum (Eds.), *To be young and gifted* (pp. 204–243). Norwood, NJ: Ablex.

Kaufman, F. (1981). The 1964–68 presidential scholars: A follow-up study. *Exceptional Children, 18,* 164–169.

Kolloff, P. B. (1997). Special residential high schools. In N. Colangelo & G. A. Davis (Eds.), *Handbook of gifted education* (2nd ed., pp. 198–206). Boston: Allyn & Bacon.

Krutetskii, V. (1976). *The psychology of mathematical abilities in school children.* Chicago: University of Chicago Press.

Kulik, J. A. (1992). An analysis of the research on ability grouping: Historical and contemporary perspectives. *Monograph of the National Research Center on the Gifted and Talented* (No. 9204). Storrs: University of Connecticut.

Kulik, J. A., & Kulik, C.-L. C. (1982). Effects of ability grouping on secondary school students: A meta-analysis of evaluation findings. *American Educational Research Journal, 19,* 415–428.

Kulik, J. A., & Kulik, C.-L. C. (1991). Ability grouping and gifted students. In N. Colangelo & G. A. Davis (Eds.), *Handbook of gifted education* (pp. 178–196). Boston, MA: Allyn & Bacon.

Kulik, J. A., & Kulik, C.-L. C. (1992). Meta-analytic findings on grouping programs. *Gifted Child Quarterly, 36,* 73–77.

Kulik, J. A., & Kulik, C.-L. C. (1997). Ability grouping. In N. Colangelo & G. A. Davis (Eds.), *Handbook of gifted education* (2nd ed., pp. 230–242). Boston: Allyn & Bacon.

Levin, H. (1987). Accelerating schools for disadvantaged students. *Educational Leadership, 44*(6), 19–21.

Lewis, M., & Brooks-Gunn, J. (1981). Attention and intelligence. *Intelligence, 5,* 231–238.

Li, A. K. F., & Adamson, G. (1992). Gifted secondary students' preferred learning style: Cooperative, competitive, or individualistic? *Journal for the Education of the Gifted, 16,* 46–54.

Lubinski, D., & Benbow, C. P. (1994). The Study of Mathematically Precocious Youth (SMPY): The first three decades of a planned fifty-year longitudinal study of intellectual talent. In R. Subotnik & K. Arnold (Eds.), *Beyond Terman: Longitudinal studies in contemporary gifted education* (pp. 255–281). Norwood, NJ: Ablex.

Ludwig, A. M. (1995). *The price of greatness: Resolving the creativity and madness controversy*. New York: Guilford Press.

Marland, S. P., Jr. (1972). *Education of the gifted and talented: Report to the Congress of the United States by the Commissioner of Education*. Washington, DC: U.S. Government Printing Office.

Matthews, D. J., & Keating, D. P. (1995). Domain specificity and habits of mind: An investigation of patterns of high-level development. *Journal of Early Adolescence, 15,* 319–343.

Matthews, M. (1992). Gifted students talk about cooperative learning. *Educational Leadership, 50*(2), 48–50.

McClelland, D. C. (1973). Testing for competence rather than for "intelligence." *American Psychologist, 28,* 1–14.

McIntosh, M., & Greenlaw, M. (1990). Fostering the post-secondary aspirations of gifted urban minority students. In S. Berger (Ed.), *ERIC flyer files*. Reston, VA: ERIC Clearinghouse on Handicapped and Gifted Children.

McPartland, J. M., Coldiron, J. R., & Braddock, J. H. (1987). *School structures and classroom practices in elementary, middle, and secondary schools* (ERIC Document Reproduction Service No. ED 291-703). Baltimore: Johns Hopkins University, Center for Research on Elementary and Middle Schools.

Montour, K. (1977). William J. Sidis, the broken twig. *American Psychologist, 32,* 265–279.

Mueller, H., Dash, U., Matheson, D., & Short, R. (1984). WISC–R subtest patterning of below average, average and above average IQ children: A meta-analysis. *Alberta Journal of Educational Research, 30,* 68–85.

Mulryan, C. M. (1992). Student passivity during cooperative small groups in mathematics. *Journal of Educational Research, 85,* 261–273.

National Education Association, Research Division. (1968). *Ability grouping (Research summary 1968–1973)*. Washington, DC: National Education Association.

Nieves, E. (1996, November 29). Being a 7-year-old genius can be tough and costly. *The New York Times,* p. B1.

Oakes, J. (1985). *Keeping track: How schools structure inequality*. New Haven, CT: Yale University Press.

Olszewski-Kubilius, P. M., & Grant, B. (1994). Academically talented females in mathematics: The role of special programs and support from others in acceleration, achievement and aspiration. In K. D. Noble & R. G. Subotnik (Eds.), *Remarkable women: Perspectives on female talent development*. Creskill, NJ: Hampton Press.

Piechowski, M. M. (1995). Emotional giftedness: The measure of intrapersonal intelligence. In N. Colangelo & G. A. Davis (Eds.), *Handbook of gifted education* (2nd ed., pp. 366–381). Boston: Allyn & Bacon.

Purcell, J. H. (1993). The effects of the elimination of gifted and talented programs on participating students and their parents. *Gifted Child Quarterly, 37,* 177–187.

Ramos-Ford, V., & Gardner, H. (1997). Giftedness from a multiple intelligences perspective. In N. Colangelo & G. A. Davis (Eds.), *Handbook of gifted education* (2nd ed., pp. 54–66). Boston: Allyn & Bacon.

Reis, S. M. (1994, April). How schools are shortchanging the gifted. *MIT Technology Review,* 39–45.

Reis, S. M., Neu, T., & McGuire, J. (1995). Talents in two places: Case studies of high ability students with learning disabilities who have achieved. *Monograph of the National Research Center on the Gifted and Talented* (No. 95113). Storrs: University of Connecticut.

Renzulli, J. S. (1978). What makes giftedness? Reexamining a definition. *Phi Delta Kappan, 60,* 180–184, 261.

Renzulli, J. S. (1994). *Schools for talent development: A practical plan for total school improvement.* Mansfield Center, CT: Creative Learning Press.

Renzulli, J. S., & Reis, S. M. (1991). The reform movement and the quiet crisis in gifted education. *Gifted Child Quarterly, 35,* 26–35.

Renzulli, J. S., & Reis, S. M. (1997). The schoolwide enrichment model: New directions for developing high-end learning. In N. Colangelo & G. A. Davis (Eds.), *Handbook of gifted education* (2nd ed., pp. 136–154). Boston: Allyn & Bacon.

Richert, E. S. (1997). Excellence with equity in identification and programming. In N. Colangelo & G. A. Davis (Eds.), *Handbook of gifted education* (2nd ed., pp. 75–88). Boston: Allyn & Bacon.

Richert, E. S., Alvino, J. J., & McDonnel, R. C. (1982). *The national report on identification: Assessment and recommendation for comprehensive identification of gifted and talented youth.* Sewell, NJ: Educational Information and Resource Center.

Robinson, A. (1990a). Cooperation or exploitation: The argument against cooperative learning for talented students. *Journal for the Education of the Gifted, 14,* 9–27.

Robinson, A. (1990b). Response to Slavin: Cooperation, consistency, and challenge for academically talented youth. *Journal for the Education of the Gifted, 14,* 31–36.

Robinson, A. (1991). Cooperative learning and the academically talented student. *Monograph of the National Research Center on the Gifted and Talented.* Storrs: University of Connecticut.

Robinson, A. (1997). Cooperative learning for talented students: Emergent issues and implications. In N. Colangelo & G. A. Davis (Eds.), *Handbook of gifted education* (2nd ed., pp. 243–252). Boston: Allyn & Bacon.

Robinson, N. M., & Janos, P. M. (1986). Psychological adjustment in a college level program of marked academic acceleration. *Journal of Youth and Adolescence, 15,* 51–60.

Rogers, K. B. (1986). Do the gifted think and learn differently? A review of recent research and its implications for instruction. *Journal for the Education of the Gifted, 10,* 17–39.

Rogers, K. B. (1991). *The relationship of grouping practices to the education of the gifted and talented learner.* Storrs: University of Connecticut, National Research Center on the Gifted and Talented.

Rogers, K. B. (1993). Grouping the gifted and talented. *Roeper Review, 16,* 8–12.

Ross, P. O. (1993). *National excellence: A case for developing America's talent.* Washington, DC: U.S. Department of Education, Office of Educational Research and Improvement.

Rutter, M., Maughan, B., Mortimore, P., & Ouston, J. (1979). *Fifteen thousand hours: Secondary schools and their effects on children.* Cambridge, MA: Harvard University Press.

Schiever, S. W., & Maker, C. J. (1997). Enrichment and acceleration: An overview and new directions. In N. Colangelo & G. A. Davis (Eds.), *Handbook of gifted education* (2nd ed., pp. 113–125). Boston: Allyn & Bacon.

Schunk, D. H. (1987). Peer models and children's behavioral change. *Review of Educational Research, 57,* 49–174.

Shore, B. M., & Kanevsky, L. (1993). Thinking processes: Being and becoming. In K. A. Heller, F. J. Monks, & A. H. Passow (Eds.), *International handbook of research and development of giftedness and talent* (pp. 133–147). Oxford, England: Pergamon Press.

Silver, S., & Clampit, M. (1990). WISC–R profiles of high ability children: Interpretation of verbal-performance discrepancies. *Gifted Child Quarterly, 34,* 76–79.

Silverman, L. K. (1993a). Counseling families. In L. K. Silverman (Ed.), *Counseling the gifted and talented* (pp. 43–89). Denver, CO: Love.

Silverman, L. K. (1993b). A developmental model for counseling the gifted. In L. K. Silverman (Ed.), *Counseling the gifted and talented* (pp. 51–78). Denver, CO: Love.

Silverman, L. K. (1993c). The gifted individual. In L. K. Silverman (Ed.), *Counseling the gifted and talented* (pp. 3–28). Denver, CO: Love.

Simonton, D. K. (1994). *Greatness: Who makes history and why.* New York: Guilford Press.

Simonton, D. K. (1997). When giftedness becomes eminence: How does talent achieve eminence? In N. Colangelo & G. A. Davis (Eds.), *Handbook of gifted education* (2nd ed., pp. 335–349). Boston: Allyn & Bacon.

Slavin, R. E. (1987). Ability grouping and student achievement in elementary schools: A best-evidence synthesis. *Review of Educational Research, 57,* 292–336.

Slavin, R. E. (1989/1990). Research on cooperative learning: Consensus and controversy. *Educational Leadership,* 52–54.

Slavin, R. E. (1990). Achievement effects of ability grouping in secondary schools: A best-evidence synthesis. *Review of Educational Research, 60,* 471–499.

Southern, W. T., Jones, E. D., & Fiscus, E. D. (1989). Practitioner objections to the academic acceleration of gifted children. *Gifted Child Quarterly, 33,* 29–35.

Stanley, J. C. (1987). State residential high schools for mathematically talented youth. *Phi Delta Kappan, 68,* 770–773.

Stanley, J. C., & Benbow, C. P. (1986). Youths who reason exceptionally well in mathematics. In R. J. Sternberg & J. E. Davidson (Eds.), *Conceptions of giftedness* (pp. 361–387). New York: Cambridge University Press.

Sternberg, R. J. (1981). A componential theory of intellectual giftedness. *Gifted Child Quarterly, 25,* 86–93.

Sternberg, R. J. (1985). *Beyond IQ: A triarchic theory of human intelligence.* New York: Cambridge University Press.

Sternberg, R. J. (1991). Giftedness according to the triarchic theory of human intelligence. In N. Colangelo & G. A. Davis (Eds.), *Handbook of gifted education* (2nd ed., pp. 45–54). Boston: Allyn & Bacon.

Stevenson, H., Chen, C., & Lee, S. (1993). Motivation and achievement of gifted children in East Asia and the United States. *Journal for the Education of the Gifted, 16,* 223–250.

Stevenson, H., Lee, S., & Stigler, J. (1986, February). Mathematics achievement of Chinese, Japanese, and American children. *Science, 231,* 693–699.

Stevenson, H., & Stigler, J. (1992). *The learning gap: Why our schools are failing and what we can learn from Japanese and Chinese education.* New York: Simon & Schuster.

Storr, A. (1988). *Solitude.* New York: Free Press.

Swiatek, M. A., & Benbow, C. P. (1991). Ten-year longitudinal follow-up of ability-matched accelerated and unaccelerated gifted students. *Journal of Educational Psychology, 83,* 528–538.

Tannenbaum, A. J. (1993). History of giftedness and "gifted education" in world perspective. In K. A. Heller, F. J. Monks, & A. H. Passow (Eds.), *International handbook of research and development of giftedness and talent* (pp. 3–27). Oxford, England: Pergamon Press.

Terman, L. (1925). *Genetic studies of genius: Vol. 1. Mental and physical traits of a thousand gifted children.* Stanford, CA: Stanford University Press.

Terman, L., & Oden, M. H. (1947). *Genetic studies of genius: Vol. 4. The gifted child grows up.* Stanford, CA: Stanford University Press.

Terman, L., & Oden, M. H. (1959). *Genetic studies of genius: Vol. 5. The gifted group at mid-life: Thirty-five years' follow-up of the superior child.* Stanford, CA: Stanford University Press.

Treffinger, D. J., Callahan, C. M., & Baughn, V. (1991). Research on enrichment efforts in gifted education. In M. Wang, M. Reynolds, & H. J. Walberg (Eds.), *Handbook of special education: Research and practice: Vol. 4. Emerging programs* (pp. 37–55). Oxford, England: Pergamon Press.

U.S. Department of Education. (1996). *National Center for Education Statistics: Schools and staffing in the United States: A statistical profile, 1993–94* (NCES 96-124). Washington, DC: Author.

VanTassel-Baska, J. (1991). Research on special populations of gifted learners. In M. Wang, M. Reynolds, & H. J. Walberg (Eds.), *Handbook of special education: Research and practice: Vol. 4. Emerging programs* (pp. 77–101). Oxford, England: Pergamon Press.

Vaughn, V., Feldhusen, J. F., & Asher, J. W. (1991). Meta-analysis and review of research on pull-out programs in gifted education. *Gifted Child Quarterly, 35,* 92–98.

Westberg, K. L., Archambault, F. X., Dobyns, S. M., & Salvin, T. (1993). The Classroom Practices Observational Study. *Journal for the Education of the Gifted, 16,* 120–146.

Wilkinson, S. (1993). WISC–R profiles of children with superior intellectual ability. *Gifted Child Quarterly, 37,* 84–91.

Wilson, B., & Schmits, D. (1978). What's new in ability grouping? *Phi Delta Kappan, 60,* 535–536.

Winner, E. (1996). *Gifted children: Myths and realities.* New York: BasicBooks.

Yewchuk, C. (1985). Gifted/learning disabled children: An overview. *Gifted Education International, 3*(2), 122–126.